STANDARD EDITION

2017 HCPCS Level II

Carol J. Buck
MS, CPC, CCS-P

Former Program Director
Medical Secretary Programs
Northwest Technical College
East Grand Forks, Minnesota

ELSEVIER

ELSEVIER

3251 Riverport Lane
St. Louis, Missouri 63043

2017 HCPCS LEVEL II, STANDARD EDITION ISBN: 978-0-323-43074-6

Notices

Knowledge and best practice in this field are constantly changing. As new research and experience broaden our understanding, changes in research methods, professional practices, or medical treatment may become necessary.

Practitioners and researchers must always rely on their own experience and knowledge in evaluating and using any information, methods, compounds, or experiments described herein. In using such information or methods they should be mindful of their own safety and the safety of others, including parties for whom they have a professional responsibility.

With respect to any drug or pharmaceutical products identified, readers are advised to check the most current information provided (i) on procedures featured or (ii) by the manufacturer of each product to be administered, to verify the recommended dose or formula, the method and duration of administration, and contraindications. It is the responsibility of practitioners, relying on their own experience and knowledge of their patients, to make diagnoses, to determine dosages and the best treatment for each individual patient, and to take all appropriate safety precautions.

To the fullest extent of the law, neither the Publisher nor the authors, contributors, or editors, assume any liability for any injury and/or damage to persons or property as a matter of products liability, negligence or otherwise, or from any use or operation of any methods, products, instructions, or ideas contained in the material herein.

International Standard Book Number: 978-0-323-43074-6

Director, Private Sector Education & Professional/Reference: Jeanne Olson
Content Development Manager: Luke Held
Associate Content Development Specialist: Anna Miller
Publishing Services Manager: Jeffrey Patterson
Project Manager: Lisa A. P. Bushey
Design Manager: Julia Dummitt

Printed in the United States of America

Last digit is the print number: 9 8 7 6 5 4 3 2 1

DEVELOPMENT OF THIS EDITION

Editorial Consultant

Jenna Price, BA, CPC-A
President
Price Editorial Services, LLC
St. Louis, Missouri

Technical Collaborators

Jackie L Grass, CPC
Coding and Reimbursement Specialist
Grand Forks, North Dakota

Nancy Maguire, ACS, CRT, PCS, FCS, HCS-D, APC, AFC
Physician Consultant for Auditing and Education
Palm Bay, Florida

Patricia Cordy Henricksen, MS, CHCA, CPC-I, CPC, CCP-P, ACS-PM
AAPC/AHIMA Approved ICD-10-CM Trainer
Auditing, Coding, and Education Specialist
Soterion Medical Services/Merrick Management
Lexington, Kentucky

DEDICATION

To all who require of themselves the highest level of accuracy, integrity, and professionalism. You enhance our profession and are a tremendous asset to health care. May this manual be of assistance to you.
With Greatest Admiration.

Carol J. Buck, MS, CPC, CCS-P

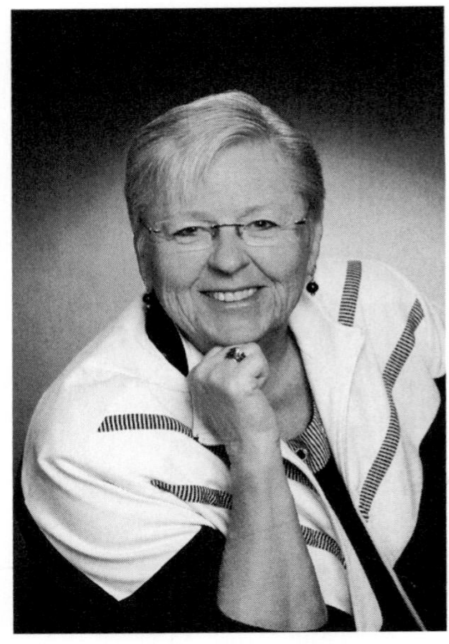

CONTENTS

Updates will be posted on codingupdates.com when available.

Check the Centers for Medicare and Medicaid Services (www.cms.gov/Manuals/IOM/list.asp) website and codingupdates.com for full and select IOMs.

HCPCS level II codes - HCPCS Workgroup maintains the permanent codes that are available for use by all government and private payers.

Temporary Codes can be added, changed or deleted on a quarterly basis. Ones that begin with C, G, H, K, Q, S & T are updated quarterly.

Each January HCPCS level II codes are updated, except temporary.

* HCPCS Level II - identifies products, services, & supplies not included in CPT

Medicare has 4 Regional Durable Medical Equip Regional Carriers or DMERCS - Durable Medical Equipment (DME)

Claims go to a regional DMEMAC

INTRODUCTION

2017 HCPCS quarterly updates available on the companion website at: www.codingupdates.com

The Centers for Medicare and Medicaid Services (CMS) (formerly Health Care Financing Administration [HCFA]) Healthcare Common Procedure Coding System (HCPCS) is a collection of codes and descriptors that represent procedures, supplies, products, and services that may be provided to Medicare beneficiaries and to individuals enrolled in private health insurance programs. The codes are divided as follows:

Level I: Codes and descriptors copyrighted by the American Medical Association's (AMA's) Current Procedural Terminology, ed. 4 (CPT-4). These are 5 position numeric codes representing physician and nonphysician services.

Level II: Includes codes and descriptors copyrighted by the American Dental Association's current dental terminology, seventh edition (CDT-7/8). These are 5 position alpha-numeric codes comprising the D series. All other Level II codes and descriptors are approved and maintained jointly by the alpha-numeric editorial panel (consisting of CMS, the Health Insurance Association of America, and the Blue Cross and Blue Shield Association). These are 5 position alpha-numeric codes representing primarily items and nonphysician services that are not represented in the Level I codes.

Level III: The CMS eliminated Level III local codes. See Program Memorandum AB-02-113.

Headings are provided as a means of grouping similar or closely related items. The placement of a code under a heading does not indicate additional means of classification, nor does it relate to any health insurance coverage categories.

HCPCS also contains modifiers, which are two-position codes and descriptors used to indicate that a service or procedure that has been performed has been altered by some specific circumstance but not changed in its definition or code. Modifiers are grouped by the levels. Level I modifiers and descriptors are copyrighted by the AMA. Level II modifiers are HCPCS modifiers. Modifiers in the D series are copyrighted by the ADA.

HCPCS is designed to promote uniform reporting and statistical data collection of medical procedures, supplies, products, and services.

HCPCS Disclaimer

Inclusion or exclusion of a procedure, supply, product, or service does not imply any health insurance coverage or reimbursement policy.

HCPCS makes as much use as possible of generic descriptions, but the inclusion of brand names to describe devices or drugs is intended only for indexing purposes; it is not meant to convey endorsement of any particular product or drug.

Updating HCPCS

The primary updates are made annually. Quarterly updates are also issued by CMS.

GUIDE TO USING THE 2017 HCPCS LEVEL II CODES

Medical coding has long been a part of the health care profession. Through the years medical coding systems have become more complex and extensive. Today, medical coding is an intricate and immense process that is present in every health care setting. The increased use of electronic submissions for health care services only increases the need for coders who understand the coding process.

2017 HCPCS Level II was developed to help meet the needs of today's coder.

All material adheres to the latest government versions available at the time of printing.

Annotated

Throughout this text, revisions and additions are indicated by the following symbols:

- ◀ **New:** Additions to the previous edition are indicated by the color triangle.
- ↩ **Revised:** Revisions within the line or code from the previous edition are indicated by the color arrow.
- ✔ **Reinstated** indicates a code that was previously deleted and has now been reactivated.
- ✖ ~~deleted~~ words have been removed from this year's edition.

HCPCS Symbols

- ⚙ **Special coverage instructions** apply to these codes. Usually these special coverage instructions are included in the Internet Only Manuals (IOM). References to the IOM locations are given in the form of Medicare Pub. 100 reference numbers listed below the code. IOM select references are located at codingupdates.com.
- ⊘ **Not covered or valid by Medicare** is indicated by the "No" symbol. Usually the reason for the exclusion is included in the Internet Only Manuals (IOM) select references at codingupdates.com.
- * **Carrier discretion** is an indication that you must contact the individual third-party payers to find out the coverage available for codes identified by this symbol.
- *NDC* Drugs approved for Medicare Part B are listed as NDC (National Drug Code). All other FDA-approved drugs are listed as Other.
- Ⓑ Bill local carrier.
- Ⓑ Bill DME MAC.

Color typeface terms within the Table of Drugs and tabular section are terms added by the publisher and do not appear in the official code set. Information supplementing the official HCPCS Index produced by CMS is *italicized*.

SYMBOLS AND CONVENTIONS

HCPCS Symbols

Special coverage instructions apply to these codes. Usually these instructions are included in the Internet Only Manuals (IOM). References to the IOM locations are given in the form of Medicare Pub. 100 reference numbers listed below the code. IOM select references are located at codingupdates.com.

L3540 Miscellaneous shoe additions, sole, full
IOM: 100-2, 15, 290

The Internet Only Manuals (IOM) give instructions regarding use of the code. IOM select references are located at codingupdates.com.

Not covered or valid by Medicare is indicated by the "No" symbol. Usually the reason for the exclusion is included in the IOM references located at codingupdates.com.

⃠ **A65331** Gradient compression stocking, thigh length, 18–30 mm Hg, each
IOM: 100-02, 15, 130; 100-03, 4, 280.1

Carrier discretion is an indication that you must contact the individual third-party payers for the coverage for these codes.

* **A6154** Wound pouch, each

A4650 Implantable radiation dosimeter; each

Bill local carrier.

A4606 Oxygen probe for use with oximeter device; replacement

Bill DME MAC.

Codes shown are for illustration purposes only and may not be current codes.

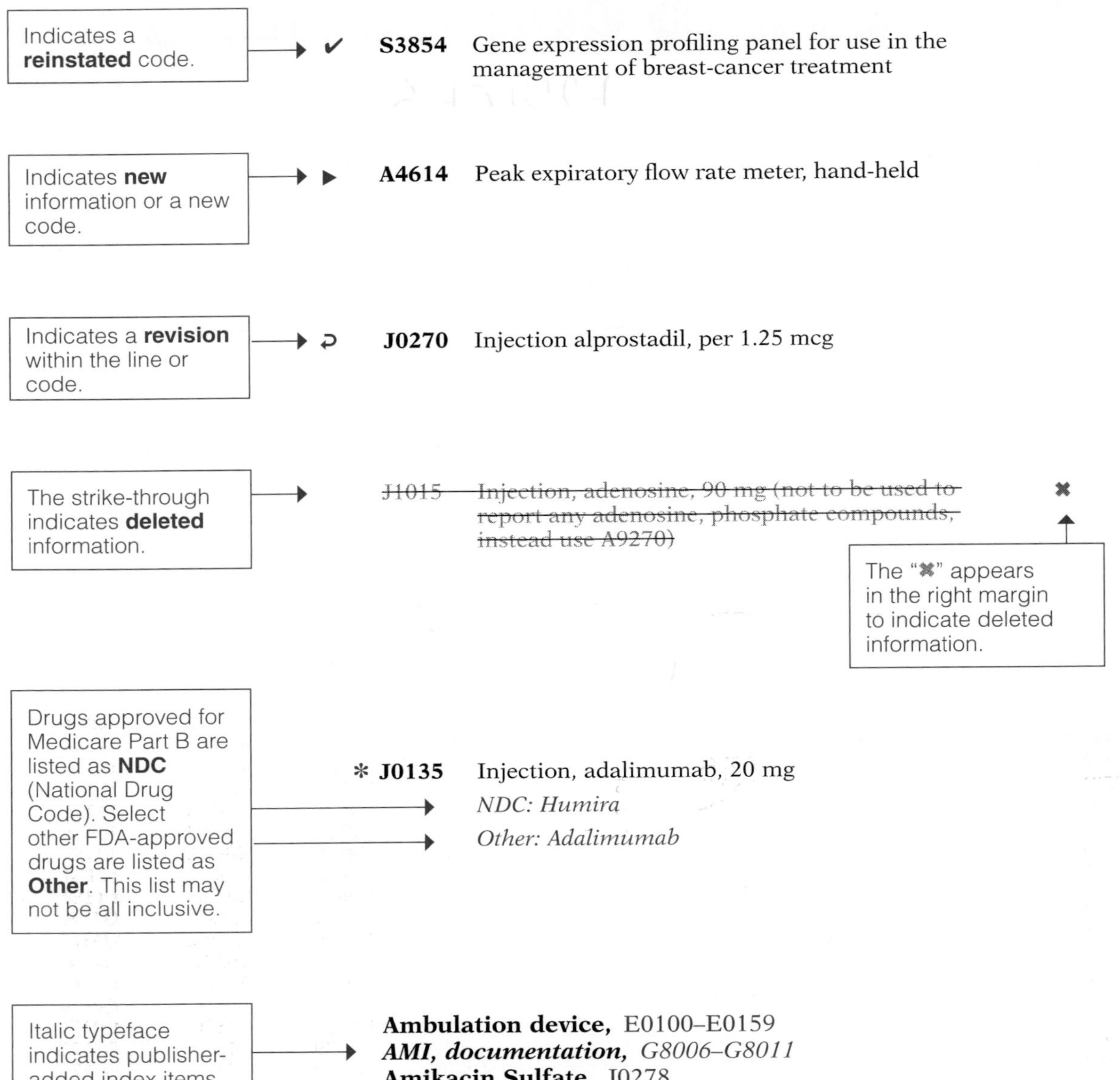

Indicates a **reinstated** code.
✔ S3854 Gene expression profiling panel for use in the management of breast-cancer treatment
Indicates **new** information or a new code.
▶ A4614 Peak expiratory flow rate meter, hand-held
Indicates a **revision** within the line or code.
J0270 Injection alprostadil, per 1.25 mcg
The strike-through indicates **deleted** information.
~~J1015 Injection, adenosine, 90 mg (not to be used to report any adenosine, phosphate compounds, instead use A9270)~~ ✖
The "✖" appears in the right margin to indicate deleted information.
Drugs approved for Medicare Part B are listed as **NDC** (National Drug Code). Select other FDA-approved drugs are listed as **Other**. This list may not be all inclusive.
✻ J0135 Injection, adalimumab, 20 mg
NDC: Humira
Other: Adalimumab
Italic typeface indicates publisher-added index items.
Ambulation device, E0100–E0159
AMI, documentation, *G8006–G8011*
Amikacin Sulfate, J0278

Codes shown are for illustration purposes only and may not be current codes.

2017 HCPCS UPDATES

2017 HCPCS New/Revised/Deleted Codes and Modifiers

HCPCS quarterly updates are posted on the companion website (www.codingupdates.com) when available.

NEW CODES/MODIFIERS

FX	G0496	G9684	G9712	G9740	G9768	G9796	G9824	G9852	J9034
PN	G0499	G9685	G9713	G9741	G9769	G9797	G9825	G9853	J9145
V1	G0500	G9686	G9714	G9742	G9770	G9798	G9826	G9854	J9176
V2	G0501	G9687	G9715	G9743	G9771	G9799	G9827	G9855	J9205
V3	G0502	G9688	G9716	G9744	G9772	G9800	G9828	G9856	J9295
ZB	G0503	G9689	G9717	G9745	G9773	G9801	G9829	G9857	J9325
A4224	G0504	G9690	G9718	G9746	G9774	G9802	G9830	G9858	J9352
A4225	G0505	G9691	G9719	G9747	G9775	G9803	G9831	G9859	L1851
A4467	G0506	G9692	G9720	G9748	G9776	G9804	G9832	G9860	L1852
A4553	G0507	G9693	G9721	G9749	G9777	G9805	G9833	G9861	Q4166
A9285	G0508	G9694	G9722	G9750	G9778	G9806	G9834	G9862	Q4167
A9286	G0509	G9695	G9723	G9751	G9779	G9807	G9835	J0570	Q4168
A9515	G9481	G9696	G9724	G9752	G9780	G9808	G9836	J0883	Q4169
A9587	G9482	G9697	G9725	G9753	G9781	G9809	G9837	J0884	Q4170
A9588	G9483	G9698	G9726	G9754	G9782	G9810	G9838	J1130	Q4171
A9597	G9484	G9699	G9727	G9755	G9783	G9811	G9839	J1942	Q4172
A9598	G9485	G9700	G9728	G9756	G9784	G9812	G9840	J2182	Q4173
C1889	G9486	G9701	G9729	G9757	G9785	G9813	G9841	J2786	Q4174
C9140	G9487	G9702	G9730	G9758	G9786	G9814	G9842	J2840	Q4175
C9482	G9488	G9703	G9731	G9759	G9787	G9815	G9843	J7175	Q5102
C9483	G9489	G9704	G9732	G9760	G9788	G9816	G9844	J7179	Q9982
C9744	G9490	G9705	G9733	G9761	G9789	G9817	G9845	J7202	Q9983
G0490	G9678	G9706	G9734	G9762	G9790	G9818	G9846	J7207	S0285
G0491	G9679	G9707	G9735	G9763	G9791	G9819	G9847	J7209	S0311
G0492	G9680	G9708	G9736	G9764	G9792	G9820	G9848	J7320	T1040
G0493	G9681	G9709	G9737	G9765	G9793	G9821	G9849	J7322	T1041
G0494	G9682	G9710	G9738	G9766	G9794	G9822	G9850	J7342	
G0495	G9683	G9711	G9739	G9767	G9795	G9823	G9851	J8670	

REVISED CODES/MODIFIERS

Change in Coverage and Long Description

PO

Change in Long Description

Q2
A4221
A9599
B9002
E0627
E0629
E0740
E0967
E0995
E2206
E2220
E2221
E2222
E2224
G0202
G0204
G0206
G8427
G8428
G8430
G8431
G8432
G8433
G8510
G8511
G8598
G8599
G8649
G8653
G8655
G8656
G8657
G8658
G8659
G8660
G8661
G8662
G8665
G8669
G8671
G8672
G8673
G8674
G8697
G8815
G8924
G8925
G8968
G9229
G9231
G9232
G9239
G9264
G9307
G9308
G9326
G9327
G9359
G9361
G9381
G9416
G9417
G9497
G9500
G9501
G9519
G9520
G9531
G9532
G9547
G9549
G9551
G9554
G9555
G9556
G9557
G9584
G9585
G9595
G9596
G9607
G9609
G9610
G9611
G9625
G9626
G9627
G9628
G9629
G9630
G9632
G9633
G9642
J0573
J1745
J3357
J7201
J7297
J7298
J7301
J7340
J9033
K0019
K0037
K0042
K0043
K0044
K0045
K0046
K0047
K0050
K0051
K0052
K0069
K0071
K0072
K0077
K0098
K0552
L1906
P9072
Q2039
Q4105
Q4131

Change in Coverage

UJ

Change in Payment

C9250
E0140
E0149
E0197
E0955
E0985
E1020
E1028
E2228
E2368
E2369
E2370
E2375
G0429
J0882
J1212
J1364
J1410
J1455
J1460
J1560
J1730
J1826
J2260
J2265
J2510
J2515
J2730
J3365
J7182
J7503
J7505
J8510
J9218
J9351
K0015
K0070
Q0139

Change in Short Description

E0292
E0293

Miscellaneous Change

J7325
J7326
J7328
J8501

REINSTATED CODES/MODIFIERS

S3854

DELETED CODES/MODIFIERS

L1
A4466
A9544
A9545
B9000
C9121
C9349
C9458
C9459
C9742
C9743
C9800
E0628
G0154
G0163
G0164
G0389
G0436
G0437
G3001
G8401
G8458
G8460
G8461
G8485
G8486
G8487
G8489
G8490
G8491
G8494
G8495
G8496
G8497
G8498
G8499
G8500
G8544
G8545
G8548
G8549
G8551
G8634
G8645
G8646
G8725
G8726
G8728
G8757
G8758
G8759
G8761
G8762
G8765
G8784
G8848
G8853
G8868
G8898
G8899
G8900
G8902
G8903
G8906
G8927
G8928
G8929
G8940
G8948
G8953
G8977
G9203
G9204
G9205
G9206
G9207
G9208
G9209
G9210
G9211
G9217
G9219
G9222
G9233
G9234
G9235
G9236
G9237
G9238
G9244
G9245
G9324
G9435
G9436
G9437
G9438
G9439
G9440
G9441
G9442
G9443
G9463
G9464
G9465
G9466
G9467
G9499
G9572
G9581
G9619
G9650
G9652
G9653
G9657
G9667
G9669
G9670
G9671
G9672
G9673
G9677
J0760
J1590
K0901
K0902
Q4119
Q4120
Q4129
Q9980
Q9981
S8032

ADDED AND DELETED DURING 2016

C9137
C9138
C9139
C9461
C9470
C9471
C9472
C9473
C9474
C9475
C9476
C9477
C9478
C9479
C9480
C9481
Q9981

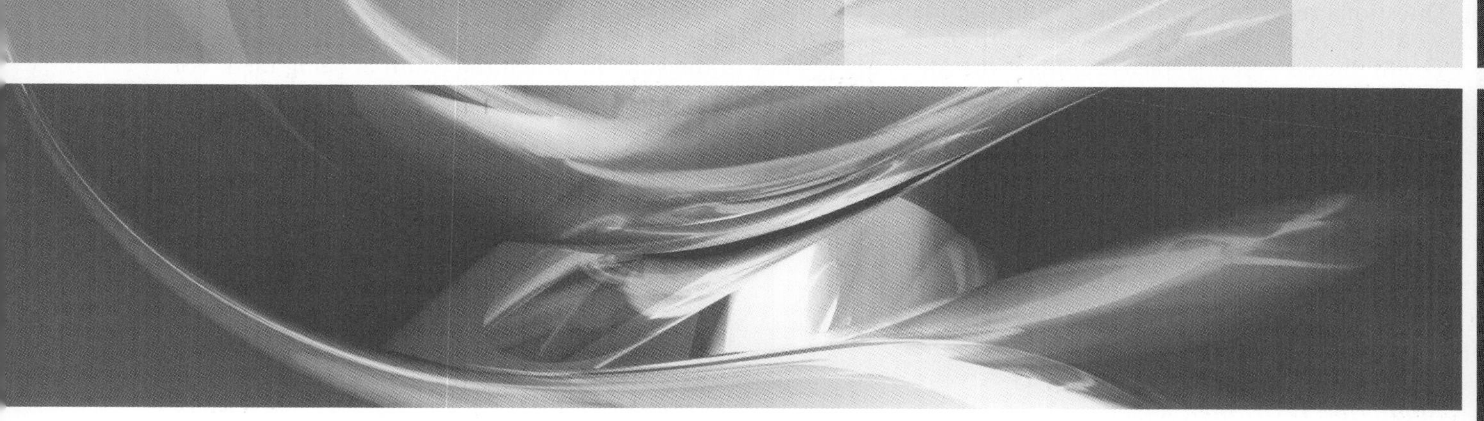

HCPCS 2017 INDEX

Questions regarding coding and billing guidance should be submitted to the insurer in whose jurisdiction a claim would be filed. For private sector health insurance systems, please contact the individual private insurance entity. For Medicaid systems, please contact the Medicaid Agency in the state in which the claim is being filed. For Medicare, contact the Medicare contractor.

A

Abatacept, J0129
Abciximab, J0130
Abdomen
dressing holder/binder, A4462
pad, low profile, L1270
Abduction control, each, L2624
Abduction restrainer, *A4566*
Abduction rotation bar, foot, L3140–L3170
adjustable shoe style positioning device, L3160
including shoes, L3140
plastic, heel-stabilizer, off-shelf, L3170
without shoes, L3150
AbobotulinumtoxintypeA, J0586
Absorption dressing, A6251–A6256
Access, site, occlusive, device, *G0269*
Access system, A4301
Accessories
ambulation devices, E0153–E0159
crutch attachment, walker, E0157
forearm crutch, platform attachment, E0153
leg extension, walker, E0158
replacement, brake attachment, walker, E0159
seat attachment, walker, E0156
walker, platform attachment, E0154
wheel attachment, walker, per pair, E0155
artificial kidney and machine (*see also* ESRD), E1510–E1699
adjustable chair, ESRD patients, E1570
automatic peritoneal dialysis system, intermittent, E1592
bath conductivity meter, hemodialysis, E1550
blood leak detector, hemodialysis, replacement, E1560
blood pump, hemodialysis, replacement, E1620
cycler dialysis machine, peritoneal, E1594
deionizer water system, hemodialysis, E1615
delivery/instillation charges, hemodialysis equipment, E1600
hemodialysis machine, E1590
hemostats, E1637
heparin infusion pump, hemodialysis, E1520
kidney machine, dialysate delivery system, E1510
peritoneal dialysis clamps, E1634
portable travel hemodialyzer, E1635
reciprocating peritoneal dialysis system, E1630
replacement, air bubble detector, hemodialysis, E1530
replacement, pressure alarm, hemodialysis, E1540
reverse osmosis water system, hemodialysis, E1610
scale, E1639
Accessories *(Continued)*
artificial kidney and machine *(Continued)*
sorbent cartridges, hemodialysis, E1636
transducer protectors, E1575
unipuncture control system, E1580
water softening system, hemodialysis, E1625
wearable artificial kidney, E1632
beds, E0271–E0280, E0300–E0316, E0328–E0329
bed board, E0273
bed, board/table, E0315
bed cradle, E0280
bed pan, standard, E0275
bed side rails, E0305–E0310
bed-pan fracture, E0276
hospital bed, extra heavy duty, E0302, E0304
hospital bed, heavy duty, E0301–E0303
hospital bed, pediatric, electric, E0329
hospital bed, safety enclosure frame, E0316
mattress, foam rubber, E0272
mattress, innerspring, E0271
over-bed table, E0274
pediatric crib, E0300
powered pressure-reducing air mattress, E0277
wheelchairs, E0950–E1030, E1050–E1298, E2201–E2295, E2300–E2399, K0001–K0109
accessory tray, E0950
arm rest, E0994
back upholstery replacement, E0982
calf rest/pad, E0995
commode seat, E0968
detachable armrest, E0973
elevating leg rest, E0990
headrest cushion, E0955
lateral trunk/hip support, E0956
loop-holder, E0951–E0952
manual swingaway, E1028
manual wheelchair, adapter, amputee, E0959
manual wheelchair, anti-rollback device, E0974
manual wheelchair, anti-tipping device, E0971
manual wheelchair, hand rim with projections, E0967
manual wheelchair, headrest extension, E0966
manual wheelchair, lever-activated, wheel drive, E0988
manual wheelchair, one-arm drive attachment, E0958
manual wheelchair, power add-on, E0983–E0984
manual wheelchair, push activated power assist, E0986
manual wheelchair, solid seat insert, E0992
medial thigh support, E0957
modification, pediatric size, E1011

◀ **New** ⟲ **Revised** ✔ **Reinstated** ~~deleted~~ **Deleted**

Accessories *(Continued)*
wheelchairs *(Continued)*
narrowing device, E0969
No. 2 footplates, E0970
oxygen related accessories, E1352–E1406
positioning belt/safety belt/pelvic strap, E0978
power-seating system, E1002–E1010
reclining back addition, pediatric size wheelchair, E1014
residual limb support system, E1020
safety vest, E0980
seat lift mechanism, E0985
seat upholstery replacement, E0981
shock absorber, E1015–E1018
shoulder harness strap, E0960
ventilator tray, E1029–E1030
wheel lock brake extension, manual, E0961
wheelchair, amputee, accessories, E1170–E1200
wheelchair, fully inclining, accessories, E1050–E1093
wheelchair, heavy duty, accessories, E1280–E1298
wheelchair, lightweight, accessories, E1240–E1270
wheelchair, semi-reclining, accessories, E1100–E1110
wheelchair, special size, E1220–E1239
wheelchair, standard, accessories, E1130–E1161
whirlpool equipment, E1300–E1310
Ace type, elastic bandage, *A6448–A6450*
Acetaminophen, J0131
Acetazolamide sodium, J1120
Acetylcysteine
inhalation solution, J7604, J7608
injection, J0132
Activity, therapy, *G0176*
Acyclovir, J0133
Adalimumab, J0135
Additions to
fracture orthosis, L2180–L2192
abduction bar, L2300–L2310
adjustable motion knee joint, L2186
anterior swing band, L2335
BK socket, PTB and AFO, L2350
disk or dial lock, knee flexion, L2425
dorsiflexion and plantar flexion, L2220
dorsiflexion assist, L2210
drop lock, L2405
drop lock knee joint, L2182
extended steel shank, L2360
foot plate, stirrup attachment, L2250
hip joint, pelvic band, thigh flange, pelvic belt, L2192
integrated release mechanism, L2515
lacer custom-fabricated, L2320–L2330
lift loop, drop lock ring, L2492
limited ankle motion, L2200
limited motion knee joint, L2184
long tongue stirrup, L2265
lower extremity orthrosis, L2200–L2397
molded inner boot, L2280

Additions to *(Continued)*
fracture orthosis (Continued)
offset knee joint, L2390
offset knee joint, heavy duty, L2395
Patten bottom, L2370
pelvic and thoracic control, L2570–L2680
plastic shoe insert with ankle joints, L2180
polycentric knee joint, L2387
pre-tibial shell, L2340
quadrilateral, L2188
ratchet lock knee extension, L2430
reinforced solid stirrup, L2260
rocker bottom, custom fabricated, L2232
round caliper/plate attachment, L2240
split flat caliper stirrups, L2230
straight knee joint, heavy duty, L2385
straight knee, or offset knee joints, L2405–L2492
suspension sleeve, L2397
thigh/weight bearing, L2500–L2550
torsion control, ankle joint, L2375
torsion control, straight knee joint, L2380
varus/valgus correction, L2270–L2275
waist belt, L2190
general additions, orthosis, L2750–L2999
lower extremity, above knee section, soft interface, L2830
lower extremity, concentric adjustable torsion style mechanism, L2861
lower extremity, drop lock retainer, L2785
lower extremity, extension, per extension, per bar, L2760
lower extremity, femoral length sock, L2850
lower extremity, full kneecap, L2795
lower extremity, high strength, lightweight material, hybrid lamination, L2755
lower extremity, knee control, condylar pad, L2810
lower extremity, knee control, knee cap, medial or lateral, L2800
lower extremity orthrosis, non-corrosive finish, per bar, L2780
lower extremity orthrosis, NOS, L2999
lower extremity, plating chrome or nickel, per bar, L2750
lower extremity, soft interface, below knee, L2820
lower extremity, tibial length sock, L2840
orthotic side bar, disconnect device, L2768
Adenosine, J0153
Adhesive, A4364
bandage, A6413
disc or foam pad, A5126
remover, A4455, A4456
support, breast prosthesis, A4280
wound, closure, G0168
Administration, chemotherapy, *Q0083–Q0085*
both infusion and other technique, Q0085
infusion technique only, Q0084
other than infusion technique, Q0083

Administration, Part D
vaccine, hepatitis B, G0010
vaccine, influenza, G0008
vaccine, pneumococcal, G0009
Administrative, Miscellaneous and Investigational, A9000–A9999
alert or alarm device, A9280
artificial saliva, A9155
DME delivery set-up, A9901
exercise equipment, A9300
external ambulatory insulin delivery system, A9274
foot pressure off loading/supportive device, A9283
helmets, A8000–A8004
home glucose disposable monitor, A9275
hot-water bottle, ice cap, heat wrap, A9273
miscellaneous DME, NOS, A9999
miscellaneous DME supply, A9900
monitoring feature/device, stand-alone or integrated, A9279
multiple vitamins, oral, per dose, A9153
non-covered item, A9270
non-prescription drugs, A9150
pediculosis treatment, topical, A9180
radiopharmaceuticals, A9500–A9700
reaching grabbing device, A9281
receiver, external, interstitial glucose monitoring system, A9278
sensor, invasive, interstitial continuous glucose monitoring, A9276
single vitamin/mineral trace element, A9152
spirometer, non-electronic, A9284
transmitter, interstitial continuous glucose monitoring system, A9277
wig, any type, A9282
wound suction, disposable, A9272
Admission, observation, *G0379*
Ado-trastuzumab, J9354
Adrenalin, J0171
Advanced life support, *A0390, A0426, A0427, A0433*
ALS2, A0433
ALS emergency transport, A0427
ALS mileage, A0390
ALS, non-emergency transport, A0426
Aerosol
compressor, E0571–E0572
compressor filter, *A7013–A7014*, K0178–K0179
mask, *A7015*, K0180
Aflibercept, J0178
AFO, E1815, E1830, L1900–L1990, L4392, L4396
Agalsidase beta, J0180
Aggrastat, J3245
A-hydroCort, J1710
Aid, hearing, *V5030–V5263*
Aide, home, health, *G0156, S9122, T1021*
home health aide/certified nurse assistant, in home, S9122
home health aide/certified nurse assistant, per visit, T1021
home health or hospital setting, G0156
Air bubble detector, dialysis, E1530
Air fluidized bed, E0194
Air pressure pad/mattress, E0186, E0197
Air travel and nonemergency transportation, A0140
Alarm
not otherwise classified, A9280
pressure, dialysis, E1540
Alatrofloxacin mesylate, J0200
Albumin, human, P9041, P9042
Albuterol
all formulations, inhalation solution, J7620
all formulations, inhalation solution, concentrated, J7610, J7611
all formulations, inhalation solution, unit dose, J7609, J7613
Alcohol, A4244
Alcohol/substance, assessment, *G0396, G0397, H0001, H0003, H0049*
alcohol abuse structured assessment, greater than 30 min., G0397
alcohol abuse structured assessment, 15–30 min., G0396
alcohol and/or drug assessment, Medicaid, H0001
alcohol and/or drug screening; laboratory analysis, Medicaid, H0003
alcohol and/or drug screening, Medicaid, H0049
Aldesleukin (IL2), J9015
Alcohol wipes, A4245
Alefacept, J0215
Alemtuzumab, J0202
Alert device, A9280
Alginate dressing, A6196–A6199
alginate, pad more than 48 sq. cm, A6198
alginate, pad size 16 sq. cm, A6196
alginate, pad size more than 16 sq. cm, A6197
alginate, wound filler, sterile, A6199
Alglucerase, J0205
Alglucosidase, J0220
Alglucosidase alfa, J0221
Alphanate, J7186
Alpha-1–proteinase inhibitor, human, J0256, J0257
Alprostadil
injection, J0270
urethral supposity, J0275
ALS mileage, *A0390*
Alteplase recombinant, J2997
Alternating pressure mattress/pad, A4640, E0180, E0181, E0277
overlay/pad, alternating, pump, heavy duty, E0181
powered pressure-reducing air mattress, E0277
replacement pad, owned by patient, A4640
Ambulance, A0021–A0999
air, A0430, A0431, A0435, A0436
conventional, transport, one way, fixed wing, A0430
conventional, transport, one way, rotary

◀ New ⮌ Revised ✔ Reinstated ~~deleted~~ Deleted

Ambulance *(Continued)*
air *(Continued)*
wing, A0431
fixed wing air mileage, A0435
rotary wing air mileage, A0436
disposable supplies, A0382–A0398
ALS routine disposable supplies, A0398
ALS specialized service disposable supplies, A0394
ALS specialized service, esophageal intubation, A0396
BLS routine disposable, A0832
BLS specialized service disposable supplies, defibrillation, A0384, A0392
non-emergency transport, fixed wing, S9960
non-emergency transport, rotary wing, S9961
oxygen, A0422
Ambulation device, E0100–E0159
brake attachment, wheeled walker replacement, E0159
cane, adjustable or fixed, with tip, E0100
cane, quad or three prong, adjustable or fixed, with tip, E0105
crutch attachment, walker, E0157
crutch forearm, each, with tips and handgrips, E0111
crutch substitute, lower leg platform, with or without wheels, each, E0118
crutch, underarm, articulating, spring assisted, each, E0117
crutches forearm, pair, tips and handgrips, E0110
crutches, underarm, other than wood, pair, with pads, tips and handgrips, E0114
crutches, underarm, other than wood, with pad, tip, handgrip, with or without shock absorber, each, E0116
crutches, underarm, wood, each, with pad, tip and handgrip, E0113
leg extensions, walker, set (4), E0158
platform attachment, forearm crutch, each, E0153
platform attachment, walker, E0154
seat attachment, walker, E0156
walker, enclosed, four-sided frame, wheeled, posterior seat, E0144
walker, folding, adjustable or fixed height, E0135
walker, folding, wheeled, adjustable or fixed height, E0143
walker, heavy duty, multiple braking system, variable wheel resistance, E0147
walker, heavy duty, wheeled, rigid or folding, E0149
walker, heavy duty, without wheels, rigid or folding, E0148
walker, rigid, adjustable or fixed height, E0130
walker, rigid, wheeled, adjustable or fixed height, E0141
walker, with trunk support, adjystable or fixed height, any, E0140
wheel attachment, rigid, pick up walker, per pair, E0155
Amikacin Sulfate, J0278
Aminolevulinate, J7309
Aminolevulinic acid HCl, J7308
Aminophylline, J0280
Amiodarone HCl, J0282
Amitriptyline HCl, J1320
Ammonia N-13, A9526
Ammonia test paper, A4774
Amniotic membrane, V2790
Amobarbital, J0300
Amphotericin B, J0285
Lipid Complex, J0287–J0289
Ampicillin
sodium, J0290
sodium/sulbactam sodium, J0295
Amputee
adapter, wheelchair, E0959
prosthesis, L5000–L7510, L7520, L7900, L8400–L8465
above knee, L5200–L5230
additions to exoskeletal knee-shin systems, L5710–L5782
additions to lower extremity, L5610–L5617
additions to socket insert and suspension, L5654–L5699
additions to socket variations, L5630–L5653
additions to test sockets, L5618–L5629
additions/replacements feet-ankle units, L5700–L5707
ankle, L5050–L5060
below knee, L5100–L5105
component modification, L5785–L5795
endoskeletal, L5810–L5999
endoskeleton, below knee, L5301–L5312
endoskeleton, hip disarticulation, L5331–L5341
fitting endoskeleton, above knee, L5321
fitting procedures, L5400–L5460
hemipelvectomy, L5280
hip disarticulation, L5250–L5270
initial prosthesis, L5500–L5505
knee disarticulation, L5150–L5160
male vacuum erection system, L7900
partial foot, L5000–L5020
preparatory prosthesis, L5510–L5600
prosthetic socks, L8400–L8485
repair, prosthetic device, L7520
tension ring, vacuum erection device, L7902
upper extremity, battery components, L7360–L7368
upper extremity, other/repair, L7400–L7510
upper extremity, preparatory, elbow, L6584–L6586
upper limb, above elbow, L6250
upper limb, additions, L6600–L6698
upper limb, below elbow, L6100–L6130
upper limb, elbow disarticulation, L6200–L6205
upper limb, endoskeletal, above elbow, L6500
upper limb, endoskeletal, below elbow, L6400
upper limb, endoskeletal, elbow disarticulation, L6450
upper limb, endoskeletal, interscapular thoracic, L6570

Amputee *(Continued)*
prosthesis *(Continued)*
upper limb, endoskeletal, shoulder disarticulation, L6550
upper limb, external power, device, L6920–L6975
upper limb, interscapular thoracic, L6350–L6370
upper limb, partial hand, L6000–L6025
upper limb, postsurgical procedures, L6380–L6388
upper limb, preparatory, shoulder, interscapular, L6588–L6590
upper limb, preparatory, wrist, L6580–L6582
upper limb, shoulder disarticulation, L6300–L6320
upper limb, terminal devices, L6703–L6915, L7007–L7261
upper limb, wrist disarticulation, L6050–L6055
stump sock, L8470–L8485
single ply, fitting above knee, L8480
single ply, fitting, below knee, L8470
single ply, fitting, upper limb, L8485
wheelchair, E1170–E1190, E1200, K0100
detachable arms, swing away detachable elevating footrests, E1190
detachable arms, swing away detachable footrests, E1180
detachable arms, without footrests or legrest, E1172
detachable elevating legrest, fixed full length arms, E1170
fixed full length arms, swing away detachable footrest, E1200
heavy duty wheelchair, swing away detachable elevating legrests, E1195
without footrests or legrest, fixed full length arms, E1171
Amygdalin, J3570
Anadulafungin, J0348
Analysis
semen, G0027
Angiography, iliac, artery, *G0278*
Angiography, renal, non-selective, *G0275*
non-ophthalmic fluorescent vascular, C9733
reconstruction, G0288
Anistreplase, J0350
Ankle splint, recumbent, K0126–K0130
Ankle-foot orthosis (AFO), L1900–L1990, L2106–L2116, L4361, L4392, L4396
ankle gauntlet, custom fabricated, L1904
ankle gauntlet, prefabricated, off-shelf, L1902
double upright free plantar dorsiflexion, olid stirrup, calf-band/cuff, custom, L1990
fracture orthrosis, tibial fracture, thermoplastic cast material, custom, L2106
multiligamentus ankle support, prefabricated, off-shelf, L1906
plastic or other material, custom fabricated, L1940
plastic or other material, prefabricated, fitting and adjustment, L1932, L1951
Ankle-foot orthosis (AFO) *(Continued)*
plastic or other material, with ankle joint, prefabricated, fitting and adjustment, L1971
plastic, rigid anterior tibial section, custom fabricated, L1945
plastic, with ankle joint, custom, L1970
posterior, single bar, clasp attachment to shoe, L1910
posterior, solid ankle, plastic, custom, L1960
replacement, soft interface material, static AFO, L4392
single upright free plantar dorsiflection, solid stirrup, calf-band/cuff, custom, L1980
single upright with static or adjustable stop, custom, L1920
spiral, plastic, custom fabricated, L1950
spring wire, dorsiflexion assist calf band, L1900
static or dynamic AFO, adjustable for fit, minimal ambulation, L4396
supramalleolar with straps, custom fabricated, L1907
tibial fracture cast orthrosis, custom, L2108
tibial fracture orthrosis, rigid, prefabricated, fitting and adjustment, L2116
tibial fracture orthrosis, semi-rigid, prefabricated, fitting and adjustment, L2114
tibial fracture orthrosis, soft prefabricated, fitting and adjustment, L2112
walking boot, prefabricated, off-the-shelf, L4361
Anterior-posterior-lateral orthosis, L0700, L0710
Antibiotic, *G8708–G8712*
antibiotic not prescribed or dispensed, G8712
patient not prescribed or dispensed antibiotic, G8708
patient prescribed antibiotic, documented condition, G8709
patient prescribed or dispensed antibiotic, G8710
prescribed or dispensed antibiotic, G8711
Antidepressant, documentation, *G8126–G8128*
Anti-emetic, oral, J8498, J8597, Q0163–Q0181
antiemetic drug, oral NOS, J8597
antiemetic drug, rectal suppository, NOS, J8498
diphenhydramine hydrochloride, 50 mg, oral, Q0163
dolasetron mesylate, 100 mg, oral, Q0180
dronabinol, 2.5 mg, Q0167
granisetron hydrochloride, 1 mg, oral, Q0166
hydroxyzine pomoate, 25 mg, oral, Q0177
perphenazine, 4 mg, oral, Q0175
prochlorperazine maleate, 5 mg, oral, Q0164
promethazine hydrochloride, 12.5 mg, oral, Q0169
thiethylperazine maleate, 10 mg, oral, Q0174
trimethobenzamide hydrochloride, 250 mg, oral, Q0173
unspecified oral dose, Q0181
Anti-hemophilic factor (Factor VIII), J7190–J7192
Anti-inhibitors, per I.U., J7198
Antimicrobial, prophylaxis, documentation, *G8201*
Anti-neoplastic drug, NOC, J9999
Antithrombin III, J7197
Antithrombin recombinant, J7196
Apomorphine, J0364

Appliance
cleaner, A5131
pneumatic, E0655–E0673
non-segmental pneumatic appliance, E0655, E0660, E0665, E0666
segmental gradient pressure, pneumatic appliance, E0671–E0673
segmental pneumatic appliance, E0656–E0657, E0667–E0670
Application, heat, cold, *E0200–E0239*
electric heat pad, moist, E0215
electric heat pad, standard, E0210
heat lamp with stand, E0205
heat lamp without stand, E0200
hydrocollator unit, pads, E0225
hydrocollator unit, portable, E0239
infrared heating pad system, E0221
non-contact wound warming device, E0231
paraffin bath unit, E0235
phototherapy (bilirubin), E0202
pump for water circulating pad, E0236
therapeutic lightbox, E0203
warming card, E0232
water circulating cold pad with pump, E0218
water circulating heat pad with pump, E0217
Aprotinin, J0365
Aqueous
shunt, L8612
sterile, J7051
ARB/ACE therapy, *G8473–G8475*
Arbutamine HCl, J0395
Arch support, L3040–L3100
hallus-valgus night dynamic splint, off-shelf, L3100
intralesional, J3302
non-removable, attached to shoe, longitudinal, L3070
non-removable, attached to shoe, longitudinal/metatarsal, each, L3090
non-removable, attached to shoe, metatarsal, L3080
removable, premolded, longitudinal, L3040
removable, premolded, longitudinal/metatarsal, each, L3060
removable, premolded, metatarsal, L3050
Arformoterol, J7605
Argatroban, J0883–J0884◀
Aripiprazole, J0400, J0401, J1942↩
Arm, wheelchair, E0973
Arsenic trioxide, J9017
Arthrography, injection, sacroiliac, joint, *G0259, G0260*
Arthroscopy, knee, surgical, *G0289, S2112*
chondroplasty, different compartment, knee, G0289
harvesting of cartilage, knee, S2112
Artificial
Cornea, L8609
kidney machines and accessories (*see also* Dialysis), E1510–E1699
larynx, L8500
saliva, A9155
Asparaginase, J9019–J9020
Aspiration, bone marrow, *G0364*
Aspirator, VABRA, *A4480*
Assessment
alcohol/substance (see also Alcohol/substance, assessment) G0396, G0397, H0001, H0003, H0049
assessment for hearing aid, V5010
audiologic, V5008–V5020
cardiac output, M0302
conformity evaluation, V5020
fitting/orientation, hearing aid, V5014
hearing screening, V5008
repair/modification hearing aid, V5014
speech, V5362–V5364
Assistive listening devices and accessories, V5281–V5290
FMlDM system, monaural, V5281
Astramorph,
Atherectomy, PTCA, *C9602, C9603*
Atropine
inhalation solution, concentrated, J7635
inhalation solution, unit dose, J7636
Atropine sulfate, J0461
Attachment, walker, *E0154–E0159*
brake attachment, wheeled walker, replacement, E0159
crutch attachment, walker, E0157
leg extension, walker, E0158
platform attachment, walker, E0154
seat attachment, walker, E0156
wheel attachment, rigid pick up walker, E0155
Audiologic assessment, V5008–V5020
Auditory osseointegrated device, L8690–L8693
Aurothioglucose, J2910
Azacitidine, J9025
Azathioprine, J7500, J7501
Azithromycin injection, J0456

B

Back supports, L0621–L0861, L0960
lumbar orthrosis, L0625–L0627
lumbar orthrosis, sagittal control, L0641–L0648
lumbar-sacral orthrosis, L0628–L0640
lumbar-sacral orthrosis, sagittal-coronal control, L0640, L0649–L0651
sacroiliac orthrosis, L0621–L0624
Baclofen, J0475, J0476
Bacterial sensitivity study, P7001
Bag
drainage, A4357
enema, A4458
irrigation supply, A4398
urinary, A4358, A5112
Bandage, conforming
elastic, <3", A6448
elastic, >3", <5", A6449

Bandage, conforming *(Continued)*
elastic, >5", A6450
elastic, load resistance <1.35 foot pounds, >3", <5", A6452
elastic, load resistance 1.25 to 1.34 foot pounds, >3", <5", A6451
non-elastic, non-sterile, >5", A6444
non-elastic, non-sterile, width <3 inches, A6442
non-elastic, non-sterile, width greater than or equal to 3 inches, <5 inches, A6443
non-elastic, sterile, >3" and <5", A6446
non-elastic, sterile, >5", A6447
Basiliximab, J0480
Bath, aid, *E0160–E0162, E0235, E0240–E0249*
bath tub rail, floor base, E0242
bath tub wall rail, E0241
bath/shower chair, with/without wheels, E0240
pad for water circulating heat unit, replacement, E0249
paraffin bath unit, portable, E0235
raised toilet seat, E0244
sitz bath chair, E0162
sitz type bath, portable, with faucet attachment, E0161
sitz type bath, portable, with/without commode, E0160
toilet rail, E0243
transfer bench, tub or toilet, E0248
transfer tub rail attachment, E0246
tub stool or bench, E0245
Bathtub
chair, E0240
stool or bench, E0245, E0247–E0248
transfer rail, E0246
wall rail, E0241–E0242
Battery, L7360, L7364–L7368
charger, E1066, L7362, L7366
replacement for blood glucose monitor, A4233–A4236
replacement for cochlear implant device, L8623–L8624
replacement for TENS, A4630
ventilator, A4611–A4613
BCG live, intravesical, J9031
Beclomethasone inhalation solution, J7622
Bed
accessories, E0271–E0280, E0300–E0326
bed board, E0273
bed cradle, E0280
bed pan, fracture, metal, E0276
bed pan, standard, metal, E0275
mattress, foam rubber, E0272
mattress innerspring, E0271
over-bed table, E0274
power pressure-reducing air mattress, E0277
air fluidized, E0194
cradle, any type, E0280
drainage bag, bottle, A4357, A5102
hospital, E0250–E0270, E0300–E0329
pan, E0275, E0276
Bed *(Continued)*
rail, E0305, E0310
safety enclosure frame/canopy, E0316
Behavioral, health, treatment services, *H0002–H2037 (Medicaid)*
activity therapy, H2032
alcohol/drug services, H0001, H0003, H0005–H0016, H0020–H0022, H0026–H0029, H0049–H0050, H2034–H2036
assertive community treatment, H0040
community based wrap-around services, H2021–H2022
comprehensive community support, H2015–H2016
comprehensive medication services, H2010
comprehensive multidisciplinary evaluation, H2000
crisis intervention, H2011
day treatment, per diem, H2013
day treatment, per hour, H2012
developmental delay prevention activities, dependent child of client, H2037
family assessment, H1011
foster care, child, H0041–H0042
health screening, H0002
hotline service, H0030
medication training, H0034
mental health clubhouse services, H2030–H2031
multisystemic therapy, juveniles, H2033
non-medical family planning, H1010
outreach service, H0023
partial hospitalization, H0035
plan development, non-physician, H0033
prenatal care, at risk, H1000–H1005
prevention, H0024–H0025
psychiatric supportive treatment, community, H0036–H0037
psychoeducational service, H2027
psychoscial rehabilitation, H2017–H2018
rehabilitation program, H2010
residential treatment program, H0017–H0019
respite care, not home, H0045
self-help/peer services, H0039
sexual offender treatment, H2028–H2029
skill training, H2014
supported employment, H2024–H2026
supported housing, H0043–H0044
therapeutic behavioral services, H2019–H2020
Behavioral therapy, cardiovascular disease, *G0446*
Belatacept, J0485
Belimumab, J0490
Belt
belt, strap, sleeve, garment, or covering, any type, A4467◀
extremity, E0945
ostomy, A4367
pelvic, E0944
safety, K0031
wheelchair, E0978, E0979

◀ New ⤻ Revised ✔ Reinstated ~~deleted~~ Deleted

Bench, bathtub (*see also* **Bathtub**)**,** E0245
Bendamustine HCl, J9033
Benesch boot, L3212–L3214
Benztropine, J0515
Beta-blocker therapy, *G9188–G9192*
Betadine, A4246, A4247
Betameth, J0704
Betamethasone
acetate and betamethasone sodium phosphate, J0702
inhalation solution, J7624
Bethanechol chloride, J0520
Bevacizumab, J9035, Q2024
Bifocal, glass or plastic, V2200–V2299
aniseikonic, bifocal, V2218
bifocal add-over 3.25 d, V2220
bifocal seg width over 28 mm, V2219
lenticular, bifocal, myodisc, V2215
lenticular lens, V2221
specialty bifocal, by report, V2200
sphere, bifocal, V2200–V2202
spherocylinder, bifocal, V2203–V2214
Bilirubin (phototherapy) light, E0202
Binder, A4465
Biofeedback device, E0746
Bioimpedance, electrical, cardiac output, M0302
Biosimilar (infliximab), Q5102◀
Biperiden lactate, J0190
Bitolterol mesylate, inhalation solution
concentrated, J7628
unit dose, J7629
Bivalirudin, J0583
Bivigam, 500 mg, *J1556*
Bladder calculi irrigation solution, Q2004
Bleomycin sulfate, J9040
Blood
count, G0306, G0307, S3630
complete CBC, automated, without platelet count, G0307
complete CBC, automated without platelet count, automated WBC differential, G0306
eosinophil count, blood, direct, S3630
fresh frozen plasma, P9017
glucose monitor, E0607, E2100, E2101, *S1030, S1031, S1034*
blood glucose monitor, integrated voice synthesizer, E2100
blood glucose monitor with integrated lancing/ blood sample, E2101
continuous noninvasive device, purchase, S1030
continuous noninvasive device, rental, S1031
home blood glucose monitor, E0607
glucose test, A4253
glucose, test strips, dialysis, A4772
granulocytes, pheresis, P9050
ketone test, A4252
leak detector, dialysis, E1560
leukocyte poor, P9016
Blood *(Continued)*
mucoprotein, P2038
platelets, P9019
platelets, irradiated, P9032
platelets, leukocytes reduced, P9031
platelets, leukocytes reduced, irradiated, P9033
platelets, pheresis, P9034
platelets, pheresis, irradiated, P9036
platelets, pheresis, leukocytes reduced, P9035
platelets, pheresis, leukocytes reduced, irradiated, P9037
pressure monitor, A4660, A4663, A4670
pump, dialysis, E1620
red blood cells, deglycerolized, P9039
red blood cells, irradiated, P9038
red blood cells, leukocytes reduced, P9016
red blood cells, leukocytes reduced, irradiated, P9040
red blood cells, washed, P9022
strips, A4253
supply, P9010–P9022
testing supplies, A4770
tubing, A4750, A4755
Blood collection devices accessory, A4257, E0620
BMI, *G8417–G8422*
Body jacket
scoliosis, L1300, L1310
Body, mass, index, *G8417–G8422*
Body sock, L0984
Bond or cement, ostomy skin, A4364
Bone
density, study, G0130
marrow, aspiration, G0364
Boot
pelvic, E0944
surgical, ambulatory, L3260
Bortezomib, J9041
Brachytherapy radioelements, Q3001
brachytherapy, LDR, prostate, G0458
brachytherapy planar source, C2645
brachytherapy, source, hospital outpatient, C1716–C1717, C1719
Breast prosthesis, L8000–L8035, L8600
adhesive skin support, A4280
custom breast prosthesis, post mastectomy, L8035
garment with mastectomy form, post mastectomy, L8015
implantable, silicone or equal, L8600
mastectomy bra, with integrated breast prosthesis form, unilateral, L8001
mastectomy bra, with prosthesis form, bilateral, L8002
mastectomy bra, without integrated breast prosthesis form, L8000
mastectomy form, L8020
mastectomy sleeve, L8010
nipple prosthesis, L8032
silicone or equal, with integral adhesive, L8031
silicone or equal, without integral adhesive, L8030

◀ New ↩ Revised ✔ Reinstated ~~deleted~~ Deleted

Breast pump
accessories, A4281–A4286
adapter, replacement, A4282
cap, breast pump bottle, replacement, A4283
locking ring, replacement, A4286
polycarbonate bottle, replacement, A4285
shield and splash protector, replacement, A4284
tubing, replacement, A4281
electric, any type, E0603
heavy duty, hospital grade, E0604
manual, any type, E0602
Breathing circuit, A4618
Brentuximab Vedotin, J9042
Brompheniramine maleate, J0945
Budesonide inhalation solution, J7626, J7627, J7633, J7634
Bulking agent, L8604, L8607
Buprenorphine hydrochlorides, J0592
Buprenorphine/Naloxone, J0571–J0575
Burn, compression garment, *A6501–A6513*
bodysuit, head-foot, A6501
burn mask, face and/or neck, A6513
chin strap, A6502
facial hood, A6503
foot to knee length, A6507
foot to thigh length, A6508
glove to axilla, A6506
glove to elbow, A6505
glove to wrist, A6504
lower trunk, including leg openings, A6511
trunk, including arms, down to leg openings, A6510
upper trunk to waist, including arm openings, A6509
Bus, nonemergency transportation, A0110
Busulfan, J0594, J8510
Butorphanol tartrate, J0595
Bypass, graft, coronary, artery
surgery, S2205–S2209

C

C-1 Esterase Inhibitor, J0596–J0598
Cabazitaxel, J9043
Cabergoline, oral, J8515
Cabinet/System, ultraviolet, *E0691–E0694*
multidirectional light system, 6 ft. cabinet, E0694
timer and eye protection, 4 foot, E0692
timer and eye protection, 6 foot, E0693
ultraviolet light therapy system, treatment area 2 sq ft., E0691
Caffeine citrate, J0706
Calcitonin-salmon, J0630
Calcitriol, J0636, *S0169*
Calcium
disodium edetate, J0600
gluconate, J0610
glycerophosphate and calcium lactate, J0620
Calcium *(Continued)*
lactate and calcium glycerophosphate, J0620
leucovorin, J0640
Calibrator solution, A4256
Canakinumab, J0638
Cancer, screening
cervical or vaginal, G0101
colorectal, G0104–G0106, G0120–G0122, G0328
alternative to screening colonoscopy, barium enema, G0120
alternative to screening sigmoidoscopy, barium enema, G0106
barium enema, G0122
colonoscopy, high risk, G0105
colonoscopy, not at high-risk, G0121
fecal occult blood test-1–3 simultaneous, G0328
flexible sigmoidoscopy, G0104
prostate, G0102, G0103
Cane, E0100, E0105
accessory, A4636, A4637
Canister
disposable, used with suction pump, A7000
non-disposable, used with suction pump, A7001
Cannula, nasal, A4615
Capecitabine, oral, J8520, J8521
Capsaicin patch, J7336
Carbidopa 5 mg/levodopa 20 mg enteral suspension, J7340
Carbon filter, A4680
Carboplatin, J9045
Cardia Event, recorder, implantable, E0616
Cardiokymography, Q0035
Cardiovascular services, M0300–M0301
Fabric wrapping abdominal aneurysm, M0301
IV chelation therapy, M0300
Cardioverter-defibrillator, *G0448*
Care, coordinated, *G9001–G9011, H1002*
coordinated care fee, home monitoring, G9006
coordinated care fee, initial rate, G9001
coordinated care fee, maintenance rate, G9002
coordinated care fee, physician coordinated care oversight, G9008
coordinated care fee, risk adjusted high, initial, G9003
coordinated care fee, risk adjusted low, initial, G9004
coordinated care fee, risk adjusted maintenance, G9005
coordinated care fee, risk adjusted maintenance, level 3, G9009
coordinated care fee, risk adjusted maintenance, level 4, G9010
coordinated care fee, risk adjusted maintenance, level 5, G9011
coordinated care fee, scheduled team conference, G9007
prenatal care, at-risk, enhanced service, care coordination, H1002
Care plan, *G0162*
Carfilzomib, J9047

◀ New ⤺ Revised ✔ Reinstated ~~deleted~~ Deleted

Carmustine, J9050
Case management, T1016, T1017
Caspofungin acetate, J0637
Cast
hand restoration, L6900–L6915
materials, special, A4590
supplies, A4580, A4590, Q4001–Q4051
body cast, adult, Q4001–Q4002
cast supplies, (e.g. plaster), A4580
cast supplies, unlisted types, Q4050
finger splint, static, Q4049
gauntlet cast, adult, Q4013–Q4014
gauntlet cast, pediatric, Q4015–Q4016
hip spica, adult, Q4025–Q4026
hip spica, pediatric, Q4027–Q4028
long arm cast, adult, Q4005–Q4006
long arm cast, pediatric, Q4007–Q4008
long arm splint, adult, Q4017–Q4018
long arm splint, pediatric, Q4019–Q4020
long leg cast, adult, Q4029–Q4030
long leg cast, pediatric, Q4031–Q4032
long leg cylinder cast, adult, Q4033–Q4034
long leg cylinder cast, pediatric, Q4035–Q4036
long leg splint, adult, Q4041–Q4042
long leg splint, pediatric, Q4043–Q4044
short arm cast, adult, Q4009–Q4010
short arm cast, pediatric, Q4011–Q4012
short arm splint, adult, Q4021–Q4022
short arm splint, pediatric, Q4023–Q4024
short leg cast, adult, Q4037–Q4038
short leg cast, pediatric, Q4039–Q4040
short leg splint, adult, Q4045–Q4046
short leg splint, pediatric, Q4047–Q4048
shoulder cast, adult, Q4003–Q4004
special casting material (fiberglass), A4590
splint supplies, miscellaneous, Q4051
thermoplastic, L2106, L2126
Caster
front, for power wheelchair, K0099
wheelchair, E0997, E0998
Catheter, A4300–A4355
anchoring device, A4333, A4334, A5200
cap, disposable (dialysis), A4860
external collection device, A4327–A4330, A4347–A7048
female external, A4327–A4328
indwelling, A4338–A4346
insertion tray, A4354
insulin infusion catheter, A4224◀
intermittent with insertion supplies, A4353
irrigation supplies, A4355
male external, A4324, A4325, *A4326*, A4348
oropharyngeal suction, A4628
starter set, A4329
trachea (suction), A4609, A4610, A4624
transluminal angioplasty, C2623
transtracheal oxygen, A4608
vascular, A4300–A4301
Catheterization, specimen collection, P9612, P9615
CBC, *G0306, G0307*
Cefazolin sodium, J0690
Cefepime HCl, J0692
Cefotaxime sodium, J0698
Ceftaroline fosamil, J0712
Ceftazidime, J0713, J0714
Ceftizoxime sodium, J0715
Ceftolozane 50 mg and tazobactam 25 mg, J0695
Ceftriaxone sodium, J0696
Cefuroxime sodium, J0697
CellCept, K0412
Cellular therapy, M0075
Cement, ostomy, A4364
Centrifuge, A4650
Centruroides Immune F(ab), J0716
Cephalin Floculation, blood, P2028
Cephalothin sodium, J1890
Cephapirin sodium, J0710
Certification, physician, home, health (per calendar month), *G0179–G0182*
Physician certification, home health, G0180
Physician recertification, home health, G0179
Physician supervision, home health, complex care, 30 min or more, G0181
Physician supervision, hospice 30 min or more, G0182
Certolizumab pegol, J0717
Cerumen, removal, *G0268*
Cervical
cancer, screening, G0101
cytopathology, G0123, G0124, G0141–G0148
screening, automated thin layer, manual rescreening, physician supervision, G0145
screening, automated thin layer preparation, cytotechnologist, physician interpretation, G0143
screening, automated thin layer preparation, physician supervision, G0144
screening, by cytotechnologist, physician supervision, G0123
screening, cytopathology smears, automated system, physician interpretation, G0141
screening, interpretation by physician, G0124
screening smears, automated system, manual rescreening, G0148
screening smears, automated system, physician supervision, G0147
halo, L0810–L0830
head harness/halter, E0942
orthosis, L0100–L0200
cervical collar molded to patient, L0170
cervical, flexible collar, L0120–L0130
cervical, multiple post collar, supports, L0180–L0200
cervical, semi-rigid collar, L0150–L0160, L0172, L0174
cranial cervical, L0112–L0113
traction, E0855, E0856

Cervical cap contraceptive, A4261
Cervical-thoracic-lumbar-sacral orthosis (CTLSO), L0700, L0710
Cetuximab, J9055
Chair
adjustable, dialysis, E1570
lift, E0627
rollabout, E1031
sitz bath, E0160–E0162
transport, E1035–E1039
chair, adult size, heavy duty, greater than 300 pounds, E1039
chair, adult size, up to 300 pounds, E1038
chair, pediatric, E1037
multi-positional patient transfer system, extra-wide, greater than 300 pounds, E1036
multi-positional patient transfer system, up to 300 pounds, E1035
Chelation therapy, M0300
Chemical endarterectomy, M0300
Chemistry and toxicology tests, P2028–P3001
Chemotherapy
administration (hospital reporting only), Q0083–Q0085
drug, oral, not otherwise classified, J8999
drugs (*see also* drug by name), J9000–J9999
Chest shell (cuirass), E0457
Chest Wall Oscillation System, E0483
hose, replacement, A7026
vest, replacement, A7025
Chest wrap, E0459
Chin cup, cervical, L0150
Chloramphenicol sodium succinate, J0720
Chlordiazepoxide HCl, J1990
Chloromycetin sodium succinate, J0720
Chloroprocaine HCl, J2400
Chloroquine HCl, J0390
Chlorothiazide sodium, J1205
Chlorpromazine HCl, J3230
Chlorpromazine HCL, 5 mg, oral, Q0161
Chorionic gonadotropin, J0725
Choroid, lesion, destruction, *G0186*
Chromic phosphate P32 suspension, A9564
Chromium CR-51 sodium chromate, A9553
Cidofovir, J0740
Cilastatin sodium, imipenem, J0743
Ciprofloxacin⮐
for intravenous infusion, J0744⮐
octic suspension, J7342◀
Cisplatin, J9060
Cladribine, J9065
Clamp
dialysis, A4918
external urethral, A4356
Cleanser, wound, A6260
Cleansing agent, dialysis equipment, A4790
Clofarabine, J9027
Clonidine, J0735
Closure, wound, adhesive, tissue, *G0168*
Clotting time tube, A4771
Clubfoot wedge, L3380
Cochlear prosthetic implant, L8614
accessories, L8615–L8617, *L8618*
batteries, L8621–L8624
replacement, L8619, L8627–L8629
external controller component, L8628
external speech processor and controller, integrated system, L8619
external speech processor, component, L8627
transmitting coil and cable, integrated, L8629
Codeine phosphate, J0745
~~**Colchicine**, J0760~~✖
Cold/Heat, application, *E0200–E0239*
bilirubin light, E0202
electric heat pad, moist, E0215
electric heat pad, standard, E0210
heat lamp with stand, E0205
heat lamp, without stand, E0200
hydrocollator unit, E0225
hydrocollator unit, portable, E0239
infrared heating pad system, E0221
non-contact wound warming device, E0231
paraffin bath unit, E0235
pump for water circulating pad, E0236
therapeutic lightbox, E0203
warming card, non-contact wound warming device, E0232
water circulating cold pad, with pump, E0218
water circulating heat pad, with pump, E0217
Colistimethate sodium, J0770
Collagen
meniscus implant procedure, G0428
skin test, G0025
urinary tract implant, L8603
wound dressing, A6020–A6024
Collagenase, Clostridium histolyticum, J0775
Collar, cervical
multiple post, L0180–L0200
nonadjust (foam), L0120
Colorectal, screening, cancer, *G0104–G0106, G0120–G0122, G0328*
Coly-Mycin M, J0770
Comfort items, A9190
Commode, E0160–E0175
chair, E0170–E0171
lift, E0172, E0625
pail, E0167
seat, wheelchair, E0968
Complete, blood, count, *G0306, G0307*
Composite dressing, A6200–A6205
Compressed gas system, E0424–E0446
oximeter device, E0445
portable gaseous oxygen system, purchase, E0430
portable gaseous oxygen system, rental, E0431
portable liquid oxygen, rental, container/ supplies, E0434

◀ New ⮐ Revised ✔ Reinstated ~~deleted~~ Deleted

Compressed gas system *(Continued)*
portable liquid oxygen, rental, home liquefier, E0433
portable liquid oxygen system, purchase, container/refill adapter, E0435
portable oxygen contents, gaseous, 1 month, E0443
portable oxygen contents, liquid, 1 month, E0444
stationary liquid oxygen system, purchase, use of reservoir, E0440
stationary liquid oxygen system, rental, container/supplies, E0439
stationary oxygen contents, gaseous, 1 month, E0441
stationary oxygen contents, liquid, 1 month, E0442
stationary purchase, compressed gas system, E0425
stationary rental, compressed gaseous oxygen system, E0424
topical oxygen delivery system, NOS, E0446
Compression
bandage, A4460
burn garment, A6501–A6512
stockings, A6530–A6549
Compressor, E0565, E0650–E0652, E0670–E0672
aerosol, E0572, E0575
air, E0565
nebulizer, E0570–E0585
pneumatic, E0650–E0676
Conductive gel/paste, *A4558*
Conductivity meter, bath, dialysis, E1550
Conference, team, *G0175, G9007, S0220, S0221*
coordinate care fee, scheduled team conference, G9007
medical conference /physician/interdisciplinary team, patient present, 30 min, S0220
medical conference physician/interdisciplinary team, patient present, 60 min, S0221
scheduled interdisciplinary team conference, patient present, G0175
Congo red, blood, P2029
Consultation, S0285, S0311, T1040, T1041◀
Telehealth, G0425–G0427
Contact layer, A6206–A6208
Contact lens, V2500–V2599
Continent device, A5082, A5083
Continuous glucose monitoring system
receiver, A9278, *S1037*
sensor, A9276, *S1035*
transmitter, A9277, *S1036*
Continuous passive motion exercise device, E0936
Continuous positive airway pressure (CPAP) device, E0601
compressor, K0269
Contraceptive
cervical cap, A4261
condoms, A4267, A4268
diaphragm, A4266
intratubal occlusion device, A4264
intrauterine, copper, J7300
intrauterine, levonorgestrel releasing, J7297, J7298, J7301
Contraceptive *(Continued)*
~~levonorgestrel, implants and supplies~~, ~~A4260~~✖
patch, J7304
spermicide, A4269
supply, A4267–A4269
vaginal ring, J7303
Contracts, maintenance, ESRD, A4890
Contrast, *Q9951–Q9969*
HOCM, Q9958–Q9964
injection, iron based magnetic resonance, per ml, Q9953
Injection, non-radioactive, non-contrast, visualization adjunct, Q9968
injection, octafluoropropane microspheres, per ml, Q9956
injection, perflexane lipid microspheres, per ml, Q9955
injection, perflutren lipid microspheres, per ml, Q9957
LOCM, Q9965–Q9967
LOCM, 400 or greater mg/ml iodine, per ml, Q9951
oral magnetic resonance contrast, Q9954
Tc-99m per study dose, Q9969
Contrast material
injection during MRI, A4643
low osmolar, A4644–A4646
Coordinated, care, *G9001–G9011*
CORF, registered nurse- face-face, G0128
Corneal tissue processing, V2785
Corset, spinal orthosis, L0970–L0976
LSO, corset front, L0972
LSO, full corset, L0976
TLSO, corset front, L0970
TLSO, full corset, L0974
Corticorelin ovine triflutate, J0795
Corticotropin, J0800
Corvert, *see* **Ibutilide fumarate**
Cosyntropin, J0833, J0834
Cough stimulating device, A7020, E0482
Counseling
alcohol misuse, G0443
cardiovascular disease, G0448
obesity, G0447
sexually transmitted infection, G0445
Count, blood, *G0306, G0307*
Counterpulsation, external, *G0166*
Cover, wound
alginate dressing, A6196–A6198
foam dressing, A6209–A6214
hydrogel dressing, A6242–A6248
non-contact wound warming cover, and accessory, A6000, E0231, E0232
specialty absorptive dressing, A6251–A6256
CPAP (continuous positive airway pressure) device, E0601
headgear, K0185
humidifier, A7046
intermittent assist, E0452

◀ **New** ⤾ **Revised** ✔ **Reinstated** ~~deleted~~ **Deleted**

Cradle, bed, E0280
Crib, E0300
Cromolyn sodium, inhalation solution, unit dose, J7631, J7632
Crotalidae polyvalent immune fab, J0840
Crutches, E0110–E0118
accessories, A4635–A4637, K0102
crutch substitute, lower leg, E0118
forearm, E0110–E0111
underarm, E0112–E0117
Cryoprecipitate, each unit, P9012
CTLSO, L0700, L0710, L1000–L1120
addition, axilla sling, L1010
addition, cover for upright, each, L1120
addition, kyphosis pad, L1020
addition, kyphosis pad, floating, L1025
addition, lumbar bolster pad, L1030
addition, lumbar rib pad, L1040
addition, lumbar sling, L1090
addition, outrigger, L1080
addition, outrigger bilateral, vertical extensions, L1085
addition, ring flange, L1100
addition, ring flange, molded to patient model, L1110
addition, sternal pad, L1050
addition, thoracic pad, L1060
addition, trapezius sling, L1070
anterior-posterior-lateral control, molded to patient model (CTLSO), L0710
cervical, thoracic, lumbar, sacral orthrosis (CTLSO), L0700
furnishing initial orthrosis, L1000
immobilizer, infant size, L1001
tension based scoliosis orthosis, fitting, L1005
Cuirass, E0457
Culture sensitivity study, P7001
Cushion, wheelchair, E0977
Cyanocobalamin Cobalt C057, A9559
Cycler dialysis machine, E1594
Cyclophosphamide, J9070
oral, J8530
Cyclosporine, J7502, J7515, J7516
Cytarabine, J9100
liposome, J9098
Cytomegalovirus immune globulin (human), J0850
Cytopathology, cervical or vaginal, *G0123, G0124,* G0141–G0148

D

Dacarbazine, J9130
Daclizumab, J7513
Dactinomycin, J9120
Dalalone, J1100
Dalbavancin, 5mg, J0875
Dalteparin sodium, J1645
Daptomycin, J0878
Daratumumab, J9145◄
Darbepoetin Alfa, J0881–J0882
Daunorubicin
Citrate, J9151
HCl, J9150
DaunoXome, *see* **Daunorubicin citrate**
Decitabine, J0894
Decubitus care equipment, E0181–E0199
air fluidized bed, E0194
air pressure mattress, E0186
air pressure pad, standard mattress, E0197
dry pressure mattress, E0184
dry pressure pad, standard mattress, E0199
gel or gel-like pressure pad mattress, standard, E0185
gel pressure mattress, E0196
heel or elbow protector, E0191
positioning cushion, E0190
power pressure reducing mattress overlay, with pump, E0181
powered air flotation bed, E0193
pump, alternating pressure pad, replacement, E0182
synthetic sheepskin pad, E0189
water pressure mattress, E0187
water pressure pad, standard mattress, E0198
Deferoxamine mesylate, J0895
Defibrillator, external, E0617, K0606
battery, K0607
electrode, K0609
garment, K0608
Degarelix, J9155
Deionizer, water purification system, E1615
Delivery/set-up/dispensing, A9901
Denileukin diftitox, J9160
Denosumab, J0897
Density, bone, study, *G0130*
Depo-estradiol cypionate, J1000
Dermal filler injection, *G0429*
Desmopressin acetate, J2597
Destruction, lesion, choroid, *G0186*
Detector, blood leak, dialysis, E1560
Developmental testing, *G0451*
Devices, other orthopedic, *E1800–E1841*
assistive listening device, V5267–V5290
Dexamethasone
acetate, J1094
inhalation solution, concentrated, J7637
inhalation solution, unit dose, J7638
intravitreal implant, J7312
oral, J8540
sodium phosphate, J1100
Dextran, J7100
Dextrose
saline (normal), J7042
water, J7060, J7070
Dextrose, 5% in lactated ringers infusion, J7121
Dextrostick, A4772
Diabetes
evaluation, G0245, G0246
shoes (fitting/modifications), A5500–A5508

◄ New ⮌ Revised ✔ Reinstated ~~deleted~~ Deleted

Diabetes *(Continued)*
deluxe feature, depth-inlay shoe, A5508
depth inlay shoe, A5500
molded from cast patient's foot, A5501
shoe with metatarsal bar, A5505
shoe with off-set heel(s), A5506
shoe with rocker or rigid-bottom rocker, A5503
shoe with wedge(s), A5504
specified modification NOS, depth-inlay shoe, A5507
training, outpatient, G0108, G0109
Diagnostic
florbetaben, Q9983◀
flutemetamol f18, Q9982◀
mammography, digital image, bilateral, G0204, G0206
radiology services, R0070–R0076
Dialysate
concentrate additives, peritoneal dialysis, A4765
solution, *A4720*–A4728
testing solution, test kit, peritoneal, A4760
Dialysis
air bubble detector, E1530
bath conductivity, meter, E1550
chemicals/antiseptics solution, A4674
disposable cycler set, A4671
emergency, G0257
equipment, E1510–E1702
extension line, A4672–A4673
filter, A4680
fluid barrier, E1575
home, S9335, S9339
kit, A4820
pressure alarm, E1540
shunt, A4740
supplies, A4650–A4927
tourniquet, A4929
unipuncture control system, E1580
unscheduled, G0257
venous pressure clamp, A4918
Dialyzer, A4690
Diaper, T1500, T4521–T4540, T4543, T4544
adult incontinence garment, A4520, A4553⮌
incontinence supply, rectal insert, any type, each, A4337
Diazepam, J3360
Diazoxide, J1730
Diclofenac, J1130◀
Dicyclomine HCl, J0500
Diethylstilbestrol diphosphate, J9165
Digoxin, J1160
Digoxin immune fab (ovine), J1162
Dihydroergotamine mesylate, J1110
Dimenhydrinate, J1240
Dimercaprol, J0470
Dimethyl sulfoxide (DMSO), J1212
Diphenhydramine HCl, J1200
Dipyridamole, J1245
Disarticulation
lower extremities, prosthesis, L5000–L5999
above knee, L5200–L5230
additions exoskeletal-knee-shin system, L5710–L5782
additions to lower extremities, L5610–L5617
additions to socket insert, L5654–L5699
additions to socket variations, L5630–L5653
additions to test sockets, L5618–L5629
additions/replacements, feet-ankle units, L5700–L5707
ankle, L5050–L5060
below knee, L5100–L5105
component modification, L5785–L5795
endoskeletal, L5810–L5999
endoskeletal, above knee, L5321
endoskeletal, hip disarticulation, L5331–L5341
endoskeleton, below knee, L5301–L5312
hemipelvectomy, L5280
hip disarticulation, L5250–L5270
immediate postsurgical fitting, L5400–L5460
initial prosthesis, L5500–L5505
knee disarticulation, L5150–L5160
partial foot, L5000–L5020
preparatory prosthesis, L5510–L5600
upper extremities, prosthesis, L6000–L6692
above elbow, L6250
additions to upper limb, L6600–L6698
below elbow, L6100–L6130
elbow disarticulation, L6200–L6205
endoskeletal, below elbow, L6400
endoskeletal, interscapular thoracic, L6570–L6590
endoskeletal, shoulder disarticulation, L6550
immediate postsurgical procedures, L6380–L6388
interscapular/thoracic, L6350–L6370
partial hand, L6000–L6026
shoulder disarticulation, L6300–L6320
wrist disarticulation, L6050–L6055
Disease
status, oncology, G9063–G9139
Dispensing, fee, pharmacy, *G0333*, *Q0510–Q0514*, *S9430*
dispensing fee inhalation drug(s), 30 days, Q0513
dispensing fee inhalation drug(s), 90 days, Q0514
inhalation drugs, 30 days, as a beneficiary, G0333
initial immunosuppressive drug(s), post transplanr, G0510
oral anti-cancer, oral anti-emetic, immunosuppressive, first prescription, Q0511
oral anti-cancer, oral anti-emetic, immunosuppressive, subsequent preparation, Q0512
Disposable supplies, ambulance, A0382, A0384, A0392–A0398
DME
miscellaneous, A9900–A9999
DME delivery, set up, A9901
DME supple, NOS, A9999
DME supplies, A9900
DMSO, J1212
Dobutamine HCl, J1250

◀ New ⮌ Revised ✔ Reinstated ~~deleted~~ Deleted

D

Docetaxel, J9171
Documentation
antidepressant, G8126–G8128
blood pressure, G8476–G8478
bypass, graft, coronary, artery, documentation, G8160–G8163
CABG, G8160–G8163
dysphagia, G8232
dysphagia, screening, G8232, V5364
ECG, 12-lead, G8705, G8706
eye, functions, G8315–G8333
influenza, immunization, G8482–G8484
pharmacologic therapy for osteoporosis, G8635
physician for DME, G0454
prophylactic antibiotic, G8702, G8703
prophylactic parenteral antibiotic, G8629–G8632
prophylaxis, DVT, G8218
prophylaxis, thrombosis, deep, vein, G8218
urinary, incontinence, G8063, G8267
Dolasetron mesylate, J1260
Dome and mouthpiece (for nebulizer), A7016
Dopamine HCl, J1265
Doripenem, J1267
Dornase alpha, inhalation solution, unit dose form, J7639
Doxercalciferol, J1270
Doxil, J9001
Doxorubicin HCl, J9000
Drainage
bag, A4357, A4358
board, postural, E0606
bottle, A5102
Dressing (*see also* **Bandage**), A6020–A6406
alginate, A6196–A6199
collagen, A6020–A6024
composite, A6200–A6205
contact layer, A6206–A6208
foam, A6209–A6215
gauze, A6216–A6230, A6402–A6406
holder/binder, A4462
hydrocolloid, A6234–A6241
hydrogel, A6242–A6248
specialty absorptive, A6251–A6256
transparent film, A6257–A6259
tubular, A6457
wound, K0744–K0746
Droperidol, J1790
and fentanyl citrate, J1810
Dropper, A4649
Drugs (*see also* **Table of Drugs**)
administered through a metered dose inhaler, J3535
antiemetic, J8498, J8597, Q0163–Q0181
chemotherapy, J8500–J9999
disposable delivery system, 50 ml or greater per hour, A4305
disposable delivery system, 5 ml or less per hour, A4306
Drugs *(Continued)*
immunosuppressive, J7500–J7599
infusion supplies, A4221, A4222, A4230–A4232
inhalation solutions, J7608–J7699
non-prescription, A9150
not otherwise classified, J3490, J7599, J7699, J7799, J7999, J8499, J8999, J9999
oral, NOS, J8499
prescription, oral, J8499, J8999
Dry pressure pad/mattress, E0179, E0184, E0199
Durable medical equipment (DME), E0100–E1830, K Codes
additional oxygen related equipment, E1352–E1406
arm support, wheelchair, E2626–E2633
artificial kidney machines/accessories, E1500–E1699
attachments, E0156–E0159
bath and toilet aides, E0240–E0249
canes, E0100–E0105
commodes, E0160–E0175
crutches, E0110–E0118
decubitus care equipment, E0181–E0199
DME, respiratory, inexpensive, purchased, A7000–A7509
gait trainer, E8000–E8002
heat/cold application, E0200–E0239
hospital beds and accessories, E0250–E0373
humidifiers/nebulizers/compressors, oxygen IPPB, E0550–E0585
infusion supplies, E0776–E0791
IPPB machines, E0500
jaw motion rehabilitation system, E1700–E1702
miscellaneous, E1902–E2120
monitoring equipment, home glucose, E0607
negative pressure, E2402
other orthopedic devices, E1800–E1841
oxygen/respiratory equipment, E0424–E0487
pacemaker monitor, E0610–E0620
patient lifts, E0621–E0642
pneumatic compressor, E0650–E0676
rollout chair/transfer system, E1031–E1039
safety equipment, E0700–E0705
speech device, E2500–E2599
suction pump/room vaporizers, E0600–E0606
temporary DME codes, regional carriers, K0000–K9999
TENS/stimulation device(s), E0720–E0770
traction equipment, E0830–E0900
trapeze equipment, fracture frame, E0910–E0948
walkers, E0130–E0155
wheelchair accessories, E2201–E2397
wheelchair, accessories, E0950–E1030
wheelchair, amputee, E1170–E1200
wheelchair cusion/protection, E2601–E2621
wheelchair, fully reclining, E1050–E1093
wheelchair, heavy duty, E1280–E1298
wheelchair, lightweight, E1240–E1270
wheelchair, semi-reclining, E1100–E1110

◀ New ⤻ Revised ✔ Reinstated ~~deleted~~ Deleted

Durable medical equipment (DME) *(Continued)*
wheelchair, skin protection, E2622–E2625
wheelchair, special size, E1220–E1239
wheelchair, standard, E1130–E1161
whirlpool equipment, E1300–E1310
Duraclon, *see* **Clonidine**
Dyphylline, J1180
Dysphagia, screening, documentation, *G8232, V5364*
Dystrophic, nails, trimming, *G0127*

E

Ear mold, V5264, *V5265*
Ecallantide, J1290
Echocardiography injectable contrast material, A9700
ECG, 12-lead, G8704
Eculizumab, J1300
ED, visit, *G0380–G0384*
Edetate
calcium disodium, J0600
disodium, J3520
Educational Services
chronic kidney disease, G0420, G0421
Eggcrate dry pressure pad/mattress, E0184, E0199
EKG, *G0403–G0405*
~~**Elastic garments**~~, ~~A4466~~✖
Elbow
disarticulation, endoskeletal, L6450
orthosis (EO), E1800, L3702–L3740, L3760
dynamic adjustable elbow flexion device, *E1800*
elbow arthrosis, *L3702–L3766*
protector, E0191
Electric hand, *L7007–L7008*
Electric, nerve, stimulator, transcutaneous, *A4595, E0720–E0749*
conductive garment, E0731
electric joint stimulation device, E0762
electrical stimulator supplies, A4595
electromagnetic wound treatment device, E0769
electronic salivary reflex stimulator, E0755
EMG, biofeedback device, E0746
functional electrical stimulator, nerve and/or muscle groups, E0770
functional stimulator sequential muscle groups, E0764
incontinence treatment system, E0740
nerve stimulator (FDA), treatment nausea and vomiting, E0765
osteogenesis stimulator, electrical, surgically implanted, E0749
osteogenesis stimulator, low-intensity ultrasound, E0760
osteogenesis stimulator, non-invasive, not spinal, E0747
osteogenesis stimulator, non-invasive, spinal, E0748
radiowaves, non-thermal, high frequency, E0761
Electric, nerve, stimulator, transcutaneous, *(Continued)*
stimulator, electrical shock unit, E0745
stimulator for scoliosis, E0744
TENS, four or more leads, E0730
TENS, two lead, E0720
Electrical stimulation device used for cancer treatment, E0766
Electrical work, dialysis equipment, A4870
Electrodes, per pair, A4555, A4556
Electromagnetic, therapy, *G0295, G0329*
Electronic medication compliance, *T1505*
Elevating leg rest, K0195
Elliotts b solution, J9175
Elotuzumab, J9176◀
Emergency department, visit, *G0380–G0384*
EMG, E0746
Eminase, J0350
Endarterectomy, chemical, M0300
Endoscope sheath, A4270
Endoskeletal system, addition, L5848, L5856–L5857, L5925, *L5961*, L5969
Enema, bag, *A4458*
Enfuvirtide, J1324
Enoxaparin sodium, J1650
Enteral
feeding supply kit (syringe) (pump) (gravity), B4034–B4036
formulae, B4149–B4156, *B4157–B4162*
nutrition infusion pump (with alarm) (without), B9002
therapy, supplies, B4000–B9999
enteral and parenteral pumps, B9002–B9999
enteral formula/medical supplies, B0434–B4162
parenteral solutions/supplies, B4164–B5200
Epinephrine, J0171
Epirubicin HCl, J9178
Epoetin alpha, J0885, Q4081
Epoetin beta, J0887–J0888
Epoprostenol, J1325
Equipment
decubitus, E0181–E0199
exercise, A9300, E0935, E0936
orthopedic, E0910–E0948, E1800–E8002
oxygen, E0424–E0486, E1353–E1406
pump, E0781, E0784, E0791
respiratory, E0424–E0601
safety, E0700, E0705
traction, E0830–E0900
transfer, E0705
trapeze, E0910–E0912, E0940
whirlpool, E1300, E1310
Erection device, tension ring, *L7902*
Ergonovine maleate, J1330
Eribulin mesylate, J9179
Ertapenem sodium, J1335
Erythromycin lactobionate, J1364

ESRD (End-Stage Renal Disease; *see also* **Dialysis)**
machines and accessories, E1500–E1699
adjustable chair, ESRD, E1570
centrifuge, dialysis, E1500
dialysis equipment, NOS, E1699
hemodialysis, air bubble detector, replacement, E1530
hemodialysis, bath conductivity meter, E1550
hemodialysis, blood leak detector, replacement, E1560
hemodialysis, blood pump, replacement, E1620
hemodialysis equipment, delivery/instillation charges, E1600
hemodialysis, heparin infusion pump, E1520
hemodialysis machine, E1590
hemodialysis, portable travel hemodialyzer system, E1635
hemodialysis, pressure alarm, E1540
hemodialysis, reverse osmosis water system, E1615
hemodialysis, sorbent cartridges, E1636
hemodialysis, transducer protectors, E1575
hemodialysis, unipuncture control system, E1580
hemodialysis, water softening system, E1625
hemostats, E1637
peritoneal dialysis, automatic intermittent system, E1592
peritoneal dialysis clamps, E1634
peritoneal dialysis, cycler dialysis machine, E1594
peritoneal dialysis, reciprocating system, E1630
scale, E1639
wearable artificial kidney, E1632
plumbing, A4870
supplies, A4653–A4932
acetate concentrate solution, hemodialysis, A4708
acid concentrate solution, hemodialysis, A4709
activated carbon filters, hemodialysis, A4680
ammonia test strip, dialysis, A4774
automatic blood pressure monitor, A4670
bicarbonate concentrate, powder, hemodialysis, A4707
bicarbonate concentrate, solution, A4706
blood collection tube, vaccum, dialysis, A4770
blood glucose test strip, dialysis, A4772
blood pressure cuff only, A4663
blood tubing, arterial and venous, hemodialysis, A4755
blood tubing, arterial or venous, hemodialysis, A4750
chemicals/antiseptics solution, clean dialysis equipment, A4674
dialysate solution, non-dextrose, A4728
dialysate solution, peritoneal dialysis, A4720–A4726, A4760–A4766
dialyzers, hemodialysis, A4690
disposable catheter tips, peritoneal dialysis, A4860
disposable cycler set, dialysis machine, A4671
drainage extension line, dialysis, sterile, A4672
extension line easy lock connectors, dialysis, A4673

ESRD (End-Stage Renal Disease) *(Continued)*
supplies *(Continued)*
fistula cannulation set, hemodialysis, A4730
injectable anesthetic, dialysis, A4737
occult blood test strips, dialysis, A4773
peritoneal dialysis, catheter anchoring device, A4653
protamine sulfate, hemodialysis, A4802
serum clotting timetube, dialysis, A4771
shunt accessory, hemodialysis, A4740
sphygmomanometer, cuff and stethoscope, A4660
syringes, A4657
topical anesthetic, dialysis, A4736
treated water, peritoneal dialysis, A4714
"Y set" tubing, peritoneal dialysis, A4719
Estrogen conjugated, J1410
Estrone (5, Aqueous), J1435
Ethanolamine oleate, J1430
Etidronate disodium, J1436
Etonogestrel implant system, J7307
Etoposide, J9181
oral, J8560
Euflexxa, J7323
Evaluation
conformity, V5020
contact lens, S0592
diabetic, G0245, G0246
footwear, G8410–G8416
hearing, S0618, V5008, V5010
hospice, G0337
multidisciplinary, H2000
nursing, T1001
ocularist, S9150
performance measurement, S3005
resident, T2011
speech, S9152
team, T1024
Everolimus, J7527
Examination
gynecological, S0610–S0613
ophthalmological, S0620, S0621
pinworm, Q0113
Exercise
class, S9451
equipment, A9300, E0935, E0936
External
ambulatory infusion pump, E0781, E0784
ambulatory insulin delivery system, A9274
power, battery components, L7360–L7368
power, elbow, L7160–L7191
urinary supplies, A4356–A4359
Extremity
belt/harness, E0945
traction, E0870–E0880
Eye
case, V2756
functions, documentation, G8315–G8333
lens (contact) (spectacle), V2100–V2615
pad, patch, A6410–A6412

Eye *(Continued)*
prosthetic, V2623, V2629
service (miscellaneous), V2700–V2799

F

Face tent, oxygen, A4619
Faceplate, ostomy, A4361
Factor VIIA coagulation factor, recombinant, J7189, J7205
Factor VIII, anti-hemophilic factor, J7182, J7185, J7190–J7192, J7207, J7209↩
Factor IX, J7193, J7194, J7195, J7200–J7202↩
Factor X, J7179◀
Factor XIII, anti-hemophilic factor, J7180, J7188
Factor XIII, A-subunit, J7181
Family Planning Education, H1010
Fee
coordinated care, G9001–G9011
dispensing, pharmacy, G0333, Q0510–Q0514, S9430
Fentanyl citrate, J3010
and droperidol, J1810
Fern test, Q0114
Ferumoxytol, Q0138, Q0139
Filgrastim (G-CSF & TBO), J1442, J1447, Q5101
Filler, wound
alginate dressing, A6199
foam dressing, A6215
hydrocolloid dressing, A6240, A6241
hydrogel dressing, A6248
not elsewhere classified, A6261, A6262
Film, transparent (for dressing), A6257–A6259
Filter
aerosol compressor, A7014
dialysis carbon, A4680
ostomy, A4368
tracheostoma, A4481
ultrasonic generator, A7014
Fistula cannulation set, A4730
Flebogamma, J1572
Florbetapir F18, A9586
Flowmeter, E0440, E0555, E0580
Floxuridine, J9200
Fluconazole, injection, J1450
Fludarabine phosphate, J8562, J9185
Fluid barrier, dialysis, E1575
Flunisolide inhalation solution, J7641
Fluocinolone, J7311, J7313
Fluorodeoxyglucose F-18 FDG, A9552
Fluorouracil, J9190
Fluphenazine decanoate, *J2680*
Foam
dressing, A6209–A6215
pad adhesive, A5126
Folding walker, E0135, E0143
Foley catheter, A4312–A4316, A4338–A4346
indwelling catheter, specialty type, A4340
Foley catheter *(Continued)*
indwelling catheter, three-way, continuous irrigation, A4346
indwelling catheter, two-way, all silicone, A4344
indwelling catheter, two-way latex, A4338
insertion tray with drainage bag, A4312
insertion tray with drainage bag, three-way, continuous irrigation, A4316
insertion tray with drainage bag, two-way latex, A4314
insertion tray with drainage bag, two-way, silicone, A4315
insertion tray without drainage bag, A4313
Fomepizole, J1451
Fomivirsen sodium intraocular, J1452
Fondaparinux sodium, J1652
Foot care, *G0247*
Footdrop splint, L4398
Footplate, E0175, E0970, L3031
Footwear, orthopedic, L3201–L3265
additional charge for split size, L3257
Benesch boot, pair, child, L3213
Benesch boot, pair, infant, L3212
Benesch boot, pair, junior, L3214
custom molded shoe, prosthetic shoe, L3250
custom shoe, depth inlay, L3230
ladies shoe, hightop, L3217
ladies shoe, oxford, L3216
ladies shoe, oxford/brace, L3224
mens shoe, depth inlay, L3221
mens shoe, hightop, L3222
mens shoe, oxford, L3219
mens shoe, oxford/brace, L3225
molded shoe, custom fitted, Plastazote, L3253
non-standard size or length, L3255
non-standard size or width, L3254
Plastazote sandal, L3265
shoe, hightop, child, L3206
shoe, hightop, infant, L3204
shoe, hightop, junior, L3207
shoe molded/patient model, Plastazote, L3252
shoe, molded/patient model, silicone, L3251
shoe, oxford, child, L3202
shoe, oxford, infant, L3201
shoe, oxford, junior, L3203
surgical boot, child, L3209
surgical boot, infant, L3208
surgical boot, junior, L3211
surgical boot/shoe, L3260
Forearm crutches, E0110, E0111
Formoterol, J7640
fumarate, J7606
Fosaprepitant, J1453
Foscarnet sodium, J1455
Fosphenytoin, Q2009
Fracture
bedpan, E0276
frame, E0920, E0930, E0946–E0948
attached to bed/weights, E0920
attachments for complex cervical traction, E0948

Fracture *(Continued)*
frame *(Continued)*
attachments for complex pelvic traction, E0947
dual, cross bars, attached to bed, E0946
free standing/weights, E0930
orthosis, L2106–L2136, L3980–L3984
ankle/foot orthosis, fracture, L2106–L2128
KAFO, fracture orthosis, L2132–L2136
upper extremity, fracture orthosis, L3980–L3984
orthotic additions, L2180–L2192, L3995
addition to upper extremity orthosis, sock, fracture, L3995
additions lower extremity fracture, L2180–L2192
Fragmin, *see* **Dalteparin sodium,** *J1645*
Frames (spectacles), V2020, V2025
Deluxe frame, V2025
Purchases, V2020
Fulvestrant, J9395
Furosemide, J1940

G

Gadobutrol, A9585
Gadofosveset trisodium, A9583
Gadoxetate disodium, A9581
Gait trainer, E8000–E8002
Gallium Ga67, A9556
Gallium nitrate, J1457
Galsulfase, J1458
Gamma globulin, J1460, J1560
injection, gamma globulin (IM), 1cc, J1460
injection, gamma globulin, (IM), over 10cc, J1560
Gammagard liquid, J1569
Gammaplex, J1557
Gamunex, J1561
Ganciclovir
implant, J7310
sodium, J1570
Garamycin, J1580
Gas system
compressed, E0424, E0425
gaseous, E0430, E0431, E0441, E0443
liquid, E0434–E0440, E0442, E0444
Gastric freezing, hypothermia, *M0100*
Gatifloxacin, J1590
Gauze (*see also* **Bandage**)
impregnated, A6222–A6233, A6266
non-impregnated, A6402–A6404
Gefitinib, J8565
Gel
conductive, A4558
pressure pad, E0185, E0196
Gemcitabine HCl, J9201
Gemtuzumab ozogamicin, J9300
Generator
neurostimulator (implantable), high frequency, C1822
ultrasonic with nebulizer, E0574
Gentamicin (Sulfate), J1580
Glasses
air conduction, V5070
binaural, V5120–V5150
behind the ear, V5140
body, V5120
glasses, V5150
in the ear, V5130
bone conduction, V5080
frames, V2020, V2025
hearing aid, V5230
Glaucoma
screening, G0117, G0118
Gloves, A4927
Glucagon HCl, J1610
Glucose
monitor with integrated lancing/blood sample collection, E2101
monitor with integrated voice synthesizer, E2100
test strips, A4253, A4772
Gluteal pad, L2650
Glycopyrrolate, inhalation solution, concentrated, J7642
Glycopyrrolate, inhalation solution, unit dose, J7643
Gold
sodium thiomalate, J1600
Golimumab, J1602
Gomco drain bottle, A4912
Gonadorelin HCl, J1620
Goserelin acetate implant (*see also* **Implant**), J9202
Grab bar, trapeze, E0910, E0940
Grade-aid, wheelchair, E0974
Gradient, compression stockings, *A6530–A6549*
below knee, 18–30 mmHg, A6530
below knee, 30–40 mmHg, A6531
below knee, thigh length, 18–30 mmHg, A6533
full length/chap style, 18–30 mmHg, A6536
full length/chap style, 30–40 mmHg, A6537
full length/chap style, 40–50 mmHg, A6538
garter belt, A6544
non-elastic below knee, 30–50 mmhg, A6545
sleeve, NOS, A6549
thigh length, 30–40 mmHg, A6534
thigh length, 40–50 mmHg, A6535
waist length, 18–30 mmHg, A6539
waist length, 30–40 mmHg, A6540
waist length, 40–50 mmHg, A6541
Granisetron HCl, J1626
Gravity traction device, E0941
Gravlee jet washer, A4470
Guidelines, practice, oncology, *G9056–G9062*

H

Hair analysis (excluding arsenic), P2031
Halaven, Injection, eribulin mesylate, 0.1 mg, J9179
Hallus-Valgus dynamic splint, L3100

Hallux prosthetic implant, L8642
Halo procedures, L0810–L0861
addition HALO procedure, MRI compatible systems, L0859
addition HALO procedure, replacement liner, L0861
cervical halo/jacket vest, L0810
cervical halo/Milwaukee type orthosis, L0830
cervical halo/plaster body jacket, L0820
Haloperidol, J1630
decanoate, J1631
Halter, cervical head, E0942
Hand finger orthosis, prefabricated, L3923
Hand restoration, L6900–L6915
orthosis (WHFO), E1805, E1825, L3800–L3805, L3900–L3954
partial prosthesis, L6000–L6020
partial hand, little and/or ring finger remaining, L6010
partial hand, no finger, L6020
partial hand, thumb remaining, L6000
transcarpal/metacarpal or partial hand disarticulation prosthesis, L6025
rims, wheelchair, E0967
Handgrip (cane, crutch, walker), A4636
Harness, E0942, E0944, E0945
Headgear (for positive airway pressure device), K0185
Hearing
aid, V5030–V5267, V5298
aid-body worn, V5100
assistive listening device, V5268–V5274, V5281–V5290
battery, use in hearing device, V5266
dispensing fee, binaural, V5160
dispensing fee, monaural hearing aid, any type, V5241
dispensing fee, unspecified hearing aid, V5090
ear impression, each, V5275
ear mold/insert, disposable, any type, V5265
ear mold/insert, not disposable, V5264
glasses, air conduction, V5070
glasses, bone conduction, V5080
hearing aid, analog, binaural, CIC, V5248
hearing aid, analog, binaural, ITC, V5249
hearing aid, analog, monaural, CIC, V5242
hearing aid, analog, monaural, ITC, V5243
hearing aid, BICROS, V5210–V5240
hearing aid, binaural, V5120–V5150
hearing aid, CROS, V5170–V5200
hearing aid, digital, V5254–V5261
hearing aid, digitally programmable, V5244–V5247, V5250–V5253
hearing aid, disposable, any type, binaural, V5263
hearing aid, disposable, any type, monaural, V5262
hearing aid, monaural, V5030–V5060
hearing aid, NOC, V5298
hearing aid or assistive listening device/supplies/ accessories, NOS, V5267
Hearing *(Continued)*
aid (Continued)
hearing service, miscellaneous, V5299
semi-implantable, middle ear, V5095
assessment, S0618, V5008, V5010
devices, L8614, V5000–V5299
services, V5000–V5999
Heat
application, E0200–E0239
infrared heating pad system, A4639, E0221
lamp, E0200, E0205
pad, A9273, E0210, E0215, E0237, E0249
Heater (nebulizer), E1372
Heavy duty, wheelchair, *E1280–E1298, K0006, K0007, K0801–K0886*
detachable arms, elevating legrests, E1280
detachable arms, swing away detachable footrest, E1290
extra heavy duty wheelchair, K0007
fixed full length arms, elevating legrest, E1295
fixed full length arms, swing away detachable footrest, E1285
heavy duty wheelchair, K0006
power mobility device, not coded by DME PDAC or no criteria, K0900
power operated vehicle, group 2, K0806–K0808
power operated vehicle, NOC, K0812
power wheelchair, group 1, K0813–K0816
power wheelchair, group 2, K0820–K0843
power wheelchair, group 3, K0848–K0864
power wheelchair, group 4, K0868–K0886
power wheelchair, group 5, pediatric, K0890–K0891
power wheelchair, NOC, K0898
power-operated vehicle, group 1, K0800–K0802
special wheelchair seat depth and/or width, by construction, E1298
special wheelchair seat depth, by upholstery, E1297
special wheelchair seat height from floor, E1296
Heel
elevator, air, E0370
protector, E0191
shoe, L3430–L3485
stabilizer, L3170
Helicopter, ambulance (*see also* **Ambulance**)
Helmet
cervical, L0100, L0110
head, A8000–A8004
Hemin, J1640
Hemipelvectomy prosthesis, L5280
Hemi-wheelchair, E1083–E1086
Hemodialysis machine, E1590
Hemodialysis, vessel mapping, *G0365*
Hemodialyzer, portable, E1635
Hemofil M, J7190
Hemophilia clotting factor, J7190–J7198
anti-inhibitor, per IU, J7198
anti-thrombin III, human, per IU, J7197
Factor IX, complex, per IU, J7194

◀ New ⮌ Revised ✔ Reinstated ~~deleted~~ Deleted

Hemophilia clotting factor *(Continued)*
Factor IX, purified, non-recombinant, per IU, J7193
Factor IX, recombinant, J7195
Factor VIII, human, per IU, J7190
Factor VIII, porcine, per IU, J7191
Factor VIII, recombinant, per IU, NOS, J7192
injection, antithrombin recombinant, 50 i.u., J7196
NOC, J7199
Hemostats, A4850, *E1637*
Hemostix, A4773
Hepagam B
IM, J1571
IV, J1573
Heparin
infusion pump, dialysis, E1520
lock flush, J1642
sodium, J1644
Hepatitis B, vaccine, administration, *G0010*
Hep-Lock (U/P), J1642
Hexalite, A4590
High osmolar contrast material, Q9958–Q9964
HOCM, 150–199 mg/ml iodine, Q9959
HOCM, 200–249 mg/ml iodine, Q9960
HOCM, 250–299 mg/ml iodine, Q9961
HOCM, 300–349 mg/ml iodine, Q9962
HOCM, 350–399 mg/ml iodine, Q9963
HOCM, 400 or greater mg/ml iodine, Q9964
HOCM, up to 149 mg/ml iodine, Q9958
Hip
disarticulation prosthesis, L5250, L5270
orthosis (HO), L1600–L1690
Hip-knee-ankle-foot orthosis (HKAFO), L2040–L2090
Histrelin
acetate, J1675
implant, J9225
HKAFO, L2040–L2090
Home
certification, home health, G0180
glucose, monitor, E0607, E2100, E2101, S1030, S1031
health, aide, G0156, S9122, T1021
health, aide, in home, per hour, S9122
health, aide, per visit, T1021
health, clinical, social worker, G0155
health, hospice, each 15 min, G0156
health, occupational, therapist, G0152
health, physical therapist, G0151
health, physician, certification, G0179–G0182
health, respiratory therapy, S5180, S5181
recerticication, home health, G0179
supervision, home health, G0181
supervision, hospice, G0182
therapist, speech, S9128
Home Health Agency Services, T0221, *T1022*
care improvement home visit assessment, G9187
Home sleep study test, *G0398–G0400*
HOPPS, *C1000–C9999*
Hospice care
assisted living facility, Q5002
hospice facility, Q5010
inpatient hospice facility, Q5006
inpatient hospital, Q5005
inpatient psychiatric facility, Q5008
long term care facility, Q5007
nursing long-term facility, Q5003
patient's home, Q5001
skilled nursing facility, Q5004
Hospice, evaluation, pre-election, *G0337*
Hospice physician supervision, *G0182*
Hospital
bed, E0250–E0304, E0328, E0329
observation, G0378, G0379
outpatient clinic visit, assessment, G0463
Hospital Outpatient Payment System, *C1000–C9999*
Hot water bottle, A9273
Human fibrinogen concentrate, J7178
Humidifier, A7046, E0550–E0563
durable, diring IPPB treatment, E0560
durable, extensive, IPPB, E0550
durable glass bottle type, for regulator, E0555
heated, used with positive airway pressure device, E0562
non-heated, used with positive airway pressure, E0561
water chamber, humidifier, replacement, positive airway device, A7046
Hyalgan, J7321
Hyalomatrix, *Q4117*
Hyaluronan, J7326, J7327⮐
gel-Syn, J7328◀
genvisc, J7320◀
hymovis, *J7322*◀
Hyaluronate, sodium, J7317
Hyaluronidase, J3470
ovine, J3471–J3473
Hydralazine HCl, J0360
Hydraulic patient lift, E0630
Hydrocollator, E0225, E0239
Hydrocolloid dressing, A6234–A6241
Hydrocortisone
acetate, J1700
sodium phosphate, J1710
sodium succinate, J1720
Hydrogel dressing, A6231–A6233, A6242–A6248
Hydromorphone, J1170
Hydroxyprogesterone caproate, J1725
Hydroxyzine HCl, J3410
Hygienic item or device, disposable or non-disposable, any type, each, A9286◀
Hylan G-F 20, J7322
Hyoscyamine Sulfate, J1980
Hyperbaric oxygen chamber, topical, A4575
Hypertonic saline solution, J7130, *J7131*

◀ New ⮐ Revised ✔ Reinstated ~~deleted~~ Deleted

I

Ibandronate sodium, J1740
Ibuprofen, J1741
Ibutilide Fumarate, J1742
Icatibant, J1744
Ice
cap, E0230
collar, E0230
Idarubicin HCl, J9211
Idursulfase, J1743
Ifosfamide, J9208
Iliac, artery, angiography, *G0278*
Iloprost, Q4074
Imaging, PET, *G0219, G0235*
any site, NOS, G0235
whole body, melanoma, non-covered indications, G0219
Imiglucerase, J1786
Immune globulin, J1575
Bivigam, 500 mg, J1556
Flebogamma, J1572
Gammagard liquid, J1569
Gammaplex, J1557
Gamunex, J1561
HepaGam B, J1571
Hizentra, J1559
Intravenous services, supplies and accessories, Q2052
NOS, J1566
Octagam, J1568
Privigen, J1459
Rho(D), J2788, J2790, *J2791*
Rhophylac, J2791
Subcutaneous, J1562
Immunosuppressive drug, not otherwise classified, J7599
Implant
access system, A4301
aqueous shunt, L8612
breast, L8600
buprenorphine implant, J0570◀
cochlear, L8614, L8619
collagen, urinary tract, L8603
dextranomer/hyaluronic acid copolymer, L8604
ganciclovir, J7310
hallux, L8642
infusion pump, programmable, E0783, E0786
implantable, programmable, E0783
implantable, programmable, replacement, E0786
joint, L8630, L8641, L8658
interphalangeal joint spacer, silicone or equal, L8658
metacarpophalangeal joint implant, L8630
metatarsal joint implant, L8641
lacrimal duct, A4262, A4263
metacarpophalangeal joint, L8630
metatarsal joint, L8641
Implant *(Continued)*
neurostimulator pulse generator, L8679, L8681–L8688
not otherwise specified, L8699
ocular, L8610
ossicular, L8613
osteogenesis stimulator, E0749
percutaneous access system, A4301
replacement implantable intraspinal catheter, E0785
synthetic, urinary, L8606
urinary tract, L8603, L8606
vascular graft, L8670
Implantable radiation dosimeter, A4650
Impregnated gauze dressing, A6222–A6230, *A6231–A6233*
Incobotulinumtoxin a, J0588
Incontinence
appliances and supplies, A4310, A4331, A4332, A4360, A5071–A5075, *A5081–A5093*, A5102–A5114↩
garment, A4520, T4521–T4543
adult sized disposable incontinence product, T4522–T4528
any type, e.g., brief, diaper, A4520
pediatric sized disposable incontinence product, T4529–T4532
youth sized disposable incontinence product, T4533–T4534
supply, A4335, A4356–A4360
bedside drainage bag, A4357
disposable external urethral clamp/compression device, A4360
external urethral clamp or compression device, A4356
incontinence supply, miscellaneous, A4335
urinary drainage bag, leg or abdomen, A4358
treatment system, E0740
Indium IN-111
carpromab pendetide, A9507
ibritumomab tiuxetan, A9542
labeled autologous platelets, A9571
labeled autologous white blood cells, A9570
oxyquinoline, A9547
pentetate, A9548
pentetreotide, A9572
satumomab, A4642
Infliximab injection, J1745
Influenza
afluria, Q2035
agriflu, Q2034
flulaval, Q2036
fluvirin, Q2037
fluzone, Q2038
immunization, documentation, G8482–G8484
not otherwise specified, Q2039
vaccine, administration, G0008
virus vaccine, Q2034–Q2039

Infusion
pump, ambulatory, with administrative equipment, E0781
pump, heparin, dialysis, E1520
pump, implantable, E0782, E0783
pump, implantable, refill kit, A4220
pump, insulin, E0784
pump, mechanical, reusable, E0779, E0780
pump, uninterrupted infusion of Epiprostenol, K0455
replacement battery, A4602
saline, J7030–J7060
supplies, A4219, A4221, A4222, A4225, A4230–A4232, E0776–E0791↩
therapy, other than chemotherapeutic drugs, Q0081

Inhalation solution (*see also* **drug name**), J7608–J7699, Q4074

Injection device, needle-free, *A4210*

Injections (*see also* **drug name**), J0120–J7320, *J7321–J7330*, J9032, J9039, J9271, J9299, J9308, Q9950
ado-trastuzumab emtansine, 1 mg, J9354
aripiprazole, extended release, J0401
arthrography, sacroiliac, joint, G0259, G0260
carfilzomib, 1 mg, J9047
certolizumab pegol, J0717
dermal filler (LDS), G0429
filgrastim, J1442
interferon beta-1a, IM, Q3027
interferon beta-1a, SC, Q3028
omacetaxtine mepesuccinate, 0.01 mg, J9262
pertuzumb, 1 mg, J9306
sculptra, 0.5 mg, Q2028
supplies for self-administered, A4211
vincristine, 1 mg, J9371
ziv-aflibercept, 1 mg, J9400

INR, monitoring, *G0248–G0250*
demonstration prior to initiation, home INR, G0248
physician review and interpretation, home INR, G0250
provision of test materials, home INR, G0249

Insertion tray, A4310–A4316

Insulin, J1815, J1817, *S5550–S5571*
ambulatory, external, system, A9274
treatment, outpatient, G9147

Integra flowable wound matrix, *Q4114*

Interferon
Alpha, J9212–J9215
Beta-1a, J1826, Q3027, Q3028
Beta-1b, J1830
Gamma, J9216

Intermittent
assist device with continuous positive airway pressure device, E0470–E0472
limb compression device, E0676
peritoneal dialysis system, E1592
positive pressure breathing (IPPB) machine, E0500

Interphalangeal joint, prosthetic implant, L8658, L8659

Interscapular thoracic prosthesis
endoskeletal, L6570
upper limb, L6350–L6370

Intervention, alcohol/substance (not tobacco), *G0396–G0397*

Intervention, tobacco, *G9016*

Intraconazole, J1835

Intraocular
lenses, V2630–V2632

Intrapulmonary percussive ventilation system, E0481

Intrauterine copper contraceptive, J7300

Inversion/eversion correction device, A9285◀

Iodine I-123
iobenguane, A9582
ioflupane, A9584
sodium iodide, A9509, A9516

Iodine I-125
serum albumin, A9532
sodium iodide, A9527
sodium iothalamate, A9554

Iodine I-131
iodinated serum albumin, A9524
sodium iodide capsule, A9517, A9528
sodium iodide solution, A9529–A9531
~~tositumomab, A9544–A9545~~✖

Iodine Iobenguane sulfate I-131, A9508

Iodine swabs/wipes, A4247

IPD
system, E1592

Ipilimumab, J9228

IPPB machine, E0500

Ipratropium bromide, inhalation solution, unit dose, J7644, J7645

Irinotecan, J9205, J9206↩

Iron
Dextran, J1750
sucrose, J1756

Irrigation solution for bladder calculi, Q2004

Irrigation supplies, A4320–A4322, A4355, A4397–A4400
irrigation supply, sleeve, each, A4397
irrigation syringe, bulb, or piston, each, A4320
irrigation tubing set, bladder irrigation, A4355
ostomy irrigation set, A4400
ostomy irrigation supply, bag, A4398
ostomy irrigation supply, cone/catheter, A4399

Irrigation/evacuation system, bowel
control unit, E0350
disposable supplies for, E0352
manual pump enema, A4459

Isavuconazonium, J1833

Islet, transplant, *G0341–G0343, S2102*

Isoetharine HCl, inhalation solution
concentrated, J7647, J7648
unit dose, J7649, J7650

Isolates, B4150, B4152

◀ New ↩ Revised ✔ Reinstated ~~deleted~~ Deleted

Isoproterenol HCl, inhalation solution
concentrated, J7657, J7658
unit dose, J7659, J7660
Isosulfan blue, Q9968
Item, non-covered, *A9270*
IUD, *J7300, S4989*
IV pole, each, E0776, K0105
Ixabepilone, J9207

J

Jacket
scoliosis, L1300, L1310
Jaw, motion, rehabilitation system, *E1700–E1702*
Jenamicin, J1580
Jetria, (ocriplasmin), *J7316*

K

Kadcyla, ado-trastuzumab emtansine, 1 mg, *J9354*
Kanamycin sulfate, J1840, J1850
Kartop patient lift, toilet or bathroom (*see also* **Lift**), E0625
Ketorolac thomethamine, J1885
Kidney
ESRD supply, A4650–A4927
machine, E1500–E1699
machine, accessories, E1500–E1699
system, E1510
wearable artificial, E1632
Kits
enteral feeding supply (syringe) (pump) (gravity), B4034–B4036
fistula cannulation (set), A4730
parenteral nutrition, B4220–B4224
administration kit, per day, B4224
supply kit, home mix, per day, B4222
supply kit, premix, per day, B4220
surgical dressing (tray), A4550
tracheostomy, A4625
Knee
arthroscopy, surgical, G0289, S2112, S2300
knee, surgical, harvesting cartilage, S2112
knee, surgical, removal loose body, chondroplasty, different compartment, G0289
shoulder, surgical, thermally-induced, capsulorraphy, S2300
disarticulation, prosthesis, L5150, L5160
joint, miniature, L5826
orthosis (KO), E1810, L1800–L1885↩
dynamic adjustable elbow entension/flexion device, *E1800*
dynamic adjustable knee extension/flexion device, *E1810*
static-progressive devices, *E1801, E1806, E1811, E1816–E1818, E1831, E1841*
Knee-ankle-foot orthosis (KAFO), L2000–L2039, L2126–L2136
addition, high strength, lightweight material, L2755
base procedure, used with any knee joint, double upright, double bar, L2020
base procedure, used with any knee joint, full plastic double upright, L2036
base procedure, used with any knee joint, single upright, single bar, L2000
foot orthrosis, double upright, double bar, without knee joint, L2030
foot orthrosis, single upright, single bar, without knee joint, L2010
Kyphosis pad, L1020, L1025

L

Laboratory
services, P0000–P9999
Laboratory tests
chemistry, P2028–P2038
cephalin flocculation, blood, P2028
congo red, blood, P2029
hair analysis, excluding arsenic, P2031
mucoprotein, blood, P2038
thymol turbidity, blood, P2033
microbiology, P7001
miscellaneous, P9010–P9615, Q0111–Q0115
blood, split unit, P9011
blood, whole, transfusion, unit, P9010
catheterization, collection specimen, multiple patients, P9615
catheterization, collection specimen, single patient, P9612
cryoprecipitate, each unit, P9012
fern test, Q0114
fresh frozen plasma, donor retested, each unit, P9060
fresh frozen plasma (single donor), frozen within 8 hours, P9017
fresh frozen plasma, within 8–24 hours of collection, each unit, P9059
granulocytes, pheresis, each unit, P9050
infusion, albumin (human), 25%, 20 ml, P9046
infusion, albumin (human), 25%, 50 ml, P9047
infusion, albumin (human), 5%, 250 ml, P9045
infusion, albumin (human), 5%, 50 ml, P9041
infusion, plasma protein fraction, human, 5%, 250 ml, P9048
infusion, plasma protein fraction, human, 5%, 50 ml, P9043
KOH preparation, Q0112
pinworm examinations, Q0113
plasma, cryoprecipitate reduced, each unit, P9044
plasma, pooled, multiple donor, frozen, P9023
platelet rich plasma, each unit, P9020

Laboratory tests *(Continued)*
miscellaneous *(Continued)*
platelets, each unit, P9019
platelets, HLA-matched leukocytes reduced, apheresis/pheresis, each unit, P9052
platelets, irradiated, each unit, P9032
platelets, leukocytes reduced, CMV-neg, aphresis/pheresis, each unit, P9055
platelets, leukocytes reduced, each unit, P9031
platelets, leukocytes reduced, irradiated, each unit, P9033
platelets, pheresis, each unit, P9034
platelets, pheresis, irradiated, each unit, P9036
platelets, pheresis, leukocytes reduced, CMV-neg, irradiated, each unit, P9053
platelets, pheresis, leukocytes reduced, each unit, P9035
platelets, pheresis, leukocytes reduced, irradiated, each unit, P9037
post-coital, direct qualitative, vaginal or cervical mucous, Q0115
red blood cells, deglycerolized, each unit, P9039
red blood cells, each unit, P9021
red blood cells, frozen/deglycerolized/washed, leukocytes reduced, irradiated, each unit, P9057
red blood cells, irradiated, each unit, P9038
red blood cells, leukocytes reduced, CMV-neg, irradiated, each unit, P9058
red blood cells, leukocytes reduced, each unit, P9016
red blood cells, leukocytes reduced, irradiated, each unit, P9040
red blood cells, washed, each unit, P9022
travel allowance, one way, specimen collection, home/nursing home, P9603, P9604
wet mounts, vaginal, cervical, or skin, Q0111
whole blood, leukocytes reduced, irradiated, each unit, P9056
whole blood or red blood cells, leukocytes reduced, CMV-neg, each unit, P9051
whole blood or red blood cells, leukocytes reduced, frozen, deglycerol, washed, each unit, P9054
toxicology, P3000–P3001, Q0091
Lacrimal duct, implant
permanent, A4263
temporary, A4262
Lactated Ringer's infusion, J7120
Laetrile, J3570
Lancet, A4258, A4259
Language, screening, *V5363*
Lanreotide, J1930
Laronidase, J1931
Larynx, artificial, L8500
Laser blood collection device and accessory, A4257, E0620
LASIK, *S0800*
Lead investigation, T1029
Lead wires, per pair, A4557
Leg
bag, A4358, A5105, A5112
leg or abdomen, vinyl, with/without tubes, straps, each, A4358
urinary drainage bag, leg bag, leg/abdomen, latex, with/without tube, straps, A5112
urinary suspensory, leg bag, with/without tube, each, A5105
extensions for walker, E0158
rest, elevating, K0195
rest, wheelchair, E0990
strap, replacement, A5113–A5114
Legg Perthes orthosis, L1700–L1755
Newington type, L1710
Patten bottom type, L1755
Scottish Rite type, L1730
Tachdjian type, L1720
Toronto type, L1700
Lens
aniseikonic, V2118, V2318
contact, V2500–V2599
gas permeable, V2510–V2513
hydrophilic, V2520–V2523
other type, V2599
PMMA, V2500–V2503
scleral, gas, V2530–V2531
eye, V2100–V2615, V2700–V2799
bifocal, glass or plastic, V2200–V2299
contact lenses, V2500–V2599
low vision aids, V2600–V2615
miscellaneous, V2700–V2799
single vision, glass or plastic, V2100–V2199
trifocal, glass or plastic, V2300–V2399
variable asphericity, V2410–V2499
intraocular, C1840, Q1004–Q1005, V2630–V2632
anterior chamber, V2630
iris supported, V2631
new technology, category 4, IOL, Q1004
new technology, category 5, IOL, Q1005
posterior chamber, V2632
telescopic lens, C1840
low vision, V2600–V2615
hand held vision aids, V2600
single lens spectacle mounted, V2610
telescopic and other compound lens system, V2615
progressive, V2781
Lepirudin, J1945
Lesion, destruction, choroid, *G0186*
Leucovorin calcium, J0640
Leukocyte poor blood, each unit, P9016
Leuprolide acetate, J1950, J9217, J9218, J9219
for depot suspension, 7.5 mg, J9217
implant, 65 mg, J9219
injection, for depot suspension, per 3.75 mg, J1950
per 1 mg, J9218
Levalbuterol, all formulations, inhalation solution
concentrated, J7607, J7612
unit dose, J7614, J7615

Levetiracetam, J1953
Levocarnitine, J1955
Levofloxacin, J1956
Levoleucovorin, J0641
Levonorgestrel, (contraceptive), implants and supplies, J7306
Levorphanol tartrate, J1960
Lexidronam, A9604
Lidocaine HCl, J2001
Lift
patient (includes seat lift), E0621–E0635
bathroom or toilet, E0625
mechanism incorporated into a combination lift-chair, E0627
patient lift, electric, E0635
patient lift, hydraulic or mechanical, E0630
separate seat lift mechanism, patient owned furniture, non-electric, E0629
sling or seat, canvas or nylon, E0621
shoe, L3300–L3334
lift, elevation, heel, L3334
lift, elevation, heel and sole, cork, L3320
lift, elevation, heel and sole, Neoprene, L3310
lift, elevation, heel, tapered to metatarsals, L3300
lift, elevation, inside shoe, L3332
lift, elevation, metal extension, L3330
***Lightweight, wheelchair,** E1087–E1090, E1240–E1270*
detachable arms, swing away detachable, elevating leg rests, E1240
detachable arms, swing away detachable footrest, E1260
fixed full length arms, swing away detachable elevating legrests, E1270
fixed full length arms, swing away detachable footrest, E1250
high strength, detachable arms desk, E1088
high strength, detachable arms desk or full length, E1090
high strength, fixed full length arms, E1087
high strength, fixed length arms swing away footrest, E1089
Lincomycin HCl, J2010
Linezolid, J2020
Liquid barrier, ostomy, A4363
***Listening devices, assistive,** V5281–V5290*
personal blue tooth FM/DM, V5286
personal FM/DM adapter/boot coupling device for receiver, V5289
personal FM/DM binaural, 2 receivers, V5282
personal FM/DM, direct audio input, V5285
personal FM/DM, ear level receiver, V5284
personal FM/DM monaural, 1 receiver, V5281
personal FM/DM neck, loop induction receiver, V5283
personal FM/DM transmitter assistive listening device, V5288
transmitter microphone, V5290
Lodging, recipient, escort nonemergency transport, A0180, A0200
***LOPS,** G0245–G0247*
follow-up evaluation and management, G0246
initial evaluation and management, G0245
routine foot care, G0247
Lorazepam, J2060
***Loss of protective sensation,** G0245–G0247*
Low osmolar contrast material, Q9965–Q9967
LSO, L0621–L0640
Lubricant, A4332, A4402
Lumbar flexion, L0540
Lumbar-sacral orthosis (LSO), L0621–L0640
***LVRS, services,** G0302–G0305*
Lymphocyte immune globulin, J7504, J7511

M

Machine
IPPB, E0500
kidney, E1500–E1699
Magnesium sulphate, J3475
Maintenance contract, ESRD, A4890
***Mammography, screening,** G0202*
Mannitol, J2150, J7665
***Mapping, vessel, for hemodialysis access,** G0365*
***Marker, tissue,** A4648*
Mask
aerosol, K0180
oxygen, A4620
Mastectomy
bra, L8000
form, L8020
prosthesis, L8030, L8600
sleeve, L8010
***Matristem,** Q4118*
micromatrix, 1 mg, Q4118
Mattress
air pressure, E0186
alternating pressure, E0277
dry pressure, E0184
gel pressure, E0196
hospital bed, E0271, E0272
non-powered, pressure reducing, E0373
overlay, E0371–E0372
powered, pressure reducing, E0277
water pressure, E0187
Measurement period
left ventricular function testing, G8682
Mecasermin, J2170
Mechlorethamine HCl, J9230
***Medicaid, codes,** T1000–T9999*
Medical and surgical supplies, A4206–A8999
***Medical nutritional therapy,** G0270, G0271*

◀ New ⮌ Revised ✔ Reinstated ~~deleted~~ Deleted

Medical services, other, *M0000–M9999*
Medroxyprogesterone acetate, J1050
Melphalan
HCl, J9245
oral, J8600
Mental, health, training services, *G0177*
Meperidine, J2175
and promethazine, J2180
Mepivacaine HCl, J0670
Mepolizumab, J2182◀
Meropenem, J2185
Mesna, J9209
Metacarpophalangeal joint, prosthetic implant, L8630, L8631
Metaproterenol sulfate, inhalation solution
concentrated, J7667, J7668
unit dose, J7669, J7670
Metaraminol bitartrate, J0380
Metatarsal joint, prosthetic implant, L8641
Meter, bath conductivity, dialysis, E1550
Methacholine chloride, J7674
Methadone HCl, J1230
Methergine, *J2210*
Methocarbamol, J2800
Methotrexate
oral, J8610
sodium, J9250, J9260
Methyldopate HCl, J0210
Methylene blue, Q9968
Methylnaltrexone, J2212
Methylprednisolone
acetate, J1020–J1040
injection, 20 mg, J1020
injection, 40 mg, J1030
injection, 80 mg, J1040
oral, J7509
sodium succinate, J2920, J2930
Metoclopramide HCl, J2765
Micafungin sodium, J2248
Microbiology test, P7001
Midazolam HCl, J2250
Mileage
ALS, A0390
ambulance, A0380, A0390
Milrinone lactate, J2260
Mini-bus, nonemergency transportation, A0120
Minocycline hydrochloride, J2265
Miscellaneous and investigational, *A9000–A9999*
Mitomycin, J7315, J9280
Mitoxantrone HCl, J9293
MNT, *G0270, G0271*
Mobility device, physician, service, *G0372*
Modalities, with office visit, M0005–M0008
Moisture exchanger for use with invasive mechanical ventilation, A4483
Moisturizer, skin, A6250
Molecular pathology procedure, *G0452*
Monitor
blood glucose, home, E0607
blood pressure, A4670
pacemaker, E0610, E0615
Monitoring feature/device, A9279
Monitoring, INR, *G0248–G0250*
demonstration prior to initiation, G0248
physician review and interpretation, G0250
provision of test materials, G0249
Monoclonal antibodies, J7505
Morphine sulfate, J2270
epidural or intrathecal use, J2274
Motion, jaw, rehabilitation system, *E1700–E1702*
motion rehabilitation system, E1700
replacement cushions, E1701
replacement measuring scales, E1702
Mouthpiece (for respiratory equipment), A4617
Moxifloxacin, J2280
Mucoprotein, blood, P2038
Multiaxial ankle, L5986
Multidisciplinary services, H2000–H2001, T1023–T1028
Multiple post collar, cervical, L0180–L0200
occipital/mandibular supports, adjustable, L0180
occipital/mandibular supports, adjustable cervical bars, L0200
SQMI, Guilford, Taylor types, L0190
Multi-Podus type AFO, L4396
Muromonab-CD3, J7505
Mycophenolate mofetil, J7517
Mycophenolic acid, J7518

N

Nabilone, J8650
Nails, trimming, dystrophic, *G0127*
Nalbuphine HCl, J2300
Naloxone HCl, J2310
Naltrexone, J2315
Nandrolone
decanoate, J2320
Narrowing device, wheelchair, E0969
Nasal
application device, K0183
pillows/seals (for nasal application device), K0184
vaccine inhalation, J3530
Nasogastric tubing, B4081, B4082
Natalizumab, J2323
Nebulizer, E0570–E0585
aerosol compressor, E0571, *E0572*
aerosol mask, A7015
corrugated tubing, disposable, A7010
filter, disposable, A7013
filter, non-disposable, A7014
heater, E1372
large volume, disposable, prefilled, A7008
large volume, disposable, unfilled, A7007
not used with oxygen, durable, glass, A7017

◀ New ⤺ Revised ✔ Reinstated ~~deleted~~ Deleted

Nebulizer *(Continued)*
pneumatic, administration set, A7003, A7005, A7006
pneumatic, nonfiltered, A7004
portable, E0570
small volume, A7003–A7005
ultrasonic, E0575
ultrasonic, dome and mouthpiece, A7016
ultrasonic, reservoir bottle, non-disposable, A7009
water collection device, large volume nebulizer, A7012
Necitumumab, J9295◀
Needle, A4215
bone marrow biopsy, C1830
non-coring, A4212
with syringe, A4206–A4209
Negative pressure wound therapy pump, E2402
accessories, A6550
Nelarabine, J9261
Neonatal transport, ambulance, base rate, A0225
Neostigmine methylsulfate, J2710
Nerve, conduction, sensory, test, *G0255*
Nerve stimulator with batteries, E0765
Nesiritide injection, J2324, *J2325*
Neupogen, injection, filgrastim, 1 mcg, *J1442*
Neuromuscular stimulator, E0745
Neurophysiology, intraoperative, monitoring, *G0453*
Neurostimulator
battery recharging system, L8695
external antenna, L8696
implantable pulse generator, L8679
pulse generator, L8681–L8688
dual array, non-rechargeable, with extension, L8688
dual array, rechargeable, with extension, L8687
patient programmer (external), replacement only, L8681
radiofrequency receiver, L8682
radiofrequency transmitter (external), sacral root receiver, bowel and bladder management, L8684
radiofrequency transmitter (external), with implantable receiver, L8683
single array, rechargeable, with extension, L8686
Nitrogen N-13 ammonia, A9526
NMES, *E0720–E0749*
Nonchemotherapy drug, oral, NOS, J8499
Noncovered services, A9270
Nonemergency transportation, A0080–A0210
Nonimpregnated gauze dressing, A6216–A6221, A6402–A6404
Nonprescription drug, A9150
Not otherwise classified drug, J3490, J7599, J7699, J7799, J8499, J8999, J9999, Q0181
NPH, J1820
NPWT, pump, *E2402*
NTIOL category 3, Q1003
NTIOL category 4, Q1004
NTIOL category 5, Q1005
Nursing care, T1030–T1031
Nursing service, direct, skilled, outpatient, *G0128*
Nutrition
enteral infusion pump, B9002↩
parenteral infusion pump, B9004, B9006
parenteral solution, B4164–B5200
therapy, medical, G0270, G0271

O

O & P supply/accessory/service, L9900
Observation
admission, G0379
hospital, G0378
Occipital/mandibular support, cervical, L0160
Occlusive device, placement, *G0269*
Occupational, therapy, *G0129, S9129*
Ocriplasmin, J7316
Octafluoropropane, Q9956
Octagam, J1568
Octreotide acetate, J2353, J2354
Ocular prosthetic implant, L8610
Ofatumumab, J9302
Olanzapine, J2358
Omacetaxine Mepesuccinate, J9262
Omalizumab, J2357
OnabotulinumtoxinA, J0585
Oncology
disease status, G9063–G9139
practice guidelines, G9056–G9062
visit, G9050–G9055
Ondansetron HCl, J2405
Ondansetron oral, Q0162
One arm, drive attachment, K0101
Ophthalmological examination, refraction, *S0621*
Oprelvekin, J2355
Oral device/appliance, E0485–E0486
Oral interface, A7047
Oral, NOS, drug, *J8499*
Oral/nasal mask, A7027
nasal pillows, A7029
oral cushion, A7028
Oritavancin, J2407
Oropharyngeal suction catheter, A4628
Orphenadrine, J2360
Orthopedic shoes
arch support, L3040–L3100
footwear, *L3000–L3649*, L3201–L3265
insert, L3000–L3030
lift, L3300–L3334
miscellaneous additions, L3500–L3595
positioning device, L3140–L3170
transfer, L3600–L3649
wedge, L3340–L3420

Orthotic additions
carbon graphite lamination, L2755
fracture, L2180–L2192, L3995
halo, L0860
lower extremity, L2200–L2999, L4320
ratchet lock, L2430
scoliosis, L1010–L1120, L1210–L1290
shoe, L3300–L3595, L3649
spinal, L0970–L0984
upper limb, L3810–L3890, *L3900*, *L3901*, L3970–L3974, *L3975–L3978*, L3995

Orthotic devices
ankle-foot (AFO) (*see also* Orthopedic shoes), E1815, E1816, E1830, L1900–L1990, L2102–L2116, L3160, L4361, *L4397*
anterior-posterior-lateral, L0700, L0710
cervical, L0100–L0200
cervical-thoracic-lumbar-sacral (CTLSO), L0700, L0710
elbow (EO), E1800, E1801, L3700–L3740, *L3760–L3762*
fracture, L2102–L2136, L3980–L3986
halo, L0810–L0830
hand, (WHFO), E1805, E1825, L3807, L3900–L3954, *L3956*
hand, finger, prefabricated, L3923
hip (HO), L1600–L1690
hip-knee-ankle-foot (HKAFO), L2040–L2090
interface material, E1820
knee (KO), E1810, E1811, L1800–L1885
knee-ankle-foot (KAFO) (*see also* Orthopedic shoes), L2000–L2038, L2126–L2136
Legg Perthes, L1700–L1755
lumbar, L0625–L0651
multiple post collar, L0180–L0200
not otherwise specified, L0999, L1499, L2999, L3999, L5999, L7499, L8039, L8239
pneumatic splint, L4350–L4380
pronation/supination, E1818
repair or replacement, L4000–L4210
replace soft interface material, L4390–L4394
sacroiliac, L0600–L0620, *L0621–L0624*
scoliosis, L1000–L1499
shoe, *see* Orthopedic shoes
shoulder (SO), L1840, L3650, L3674, *L3678*
shoulder-elbow-wrist-hand (SEWHO), L3960–L3978
side bar disconnect, L2768
spinal, cervical, L0100–L0200
spinal, DME, K0112–K0116
thoracic, L0210, *L0220*
thoracic-hip-knee-ankle (THKO), L1500–L1520
toe, E1830
wrist-hand-finger (WHFO), E1805, E1806, E1825, *L3806–L3809*, L3900–L3954, *L3956*

Orthovisc, J7324
Ossicula prosthetic implant, L8613
Osteogenesis stimulator, E0747–E0749, E0760
Ostomy
accessories, A5093
belt, A4396
pouches, A4416–A4435, *A5056*, *A5057*
skin barrier, A4401–A4449, *A4462*
supplies, A4361–A4434, A5051–A5131, *A5200*
Otto Bock, prosthesis, *L7007*
Outpatient payment system, hospital, *C1000–C9999*
Overdoor, traction, *E0860*
Oxacillin sodium, J2700
Oxaliplatin, J9263
Oxygen
ambulance, A0422
battery charger, E1357
battery pack/cartridge, E1356
catheter, transtracheal, A7018
chamber, hyperbaric, topical, A4575
concentrator, E1390–E1391
DC power adapter, E1358
delivery system, topical NOS, E0446
equipment, E0424–E0486, E1353–E1406
Liquid oxygen system, E0433
mask, A4620
medication supplies, A4611–A4627
rack/stand, E1355
regulator, E1352, E1353
respiratory equipment/supplies, A4611–A4627, E0424–E0480, *E0481*
supplies and equipment, E0425–E0444, E0455
tent, E0455
tubing, A4616
water vapor enriching system, E1405, E1406
wheeled cart, E1354

Oxymorphone HCl, J2410
Oxytetracycline HCl, J2460
Oxytocin, J2590

P

Pacemaker monitor, E0610, E0615
Paclitaxel, J9267
Paclitaxel protein-bound particles, J9264
Pad
correction, CTLSO, L1020–L1060
gel pressure, E0185, E0196
heat, *A9273*, E0210, E0215, E0217, E0249
electric heat pad, moist, E0215
electric heat pad, standard, E0210
hot water bottle, ice cap or collar, heat and/or cold wrap, A9273
pad for water circulating heat unit, replacement only, E0249
water circulating heat pad with pump, E0217
orthotic device interface, E1820
sheepskin, E0188, E0189

Pad *(Continued)*
water circulating cold with pump, E0218
water circulating heat unit, E0249
water circulating heat with pump, E0217
Pail, for use with commode chair, E0167
Pain assessment, *G8730–G8732*
Palate, prosthetic implant, L8618
Palifermin, J2425
Paliperidone palmitate, J2426
Palonosetron, J2469, J8655
Pamidronate disodium, J2430
Pan, for use with commode chair, E0167
Panitumumab, J9303
Papanicolaou (Pap) screening smear, P3000, P3001, Q0091
cervical or vaginal, up to 3 smears, by technician, P3000
cervical or vaginal, up to 3 smears, physician interpretation, P3001
obtaining, preparing and conveyance, Q0091
Papaverine HCl, J2440
Paraffin, A4265
bath unit, E0235
Parenteral nutrition
administration kit, B4224
pump, B9004, B9006
solution, B4164–B5200
compounded amino acid and carbohydrates, with electrolytes, B4189–B4199, B5000–B5200
nutrition additives, homemix, B4216
nutrition administration kit, B4224
nutrition solution, amino acid, B4168–B4178
nutrition solution, carbohydrates, B4164, B4180
nutrition solution, per 10 grams, liquid, B4185
nutrition supply kit, homemix, B4222
supply kit, B4220, B4222
Paricalcitol, J2501
Parking fee, nonemergency transport, A0170
Partial Hospitalization, OT, *G0129*
Pasireotide long acting, J2502
Paste, conductive, A4558
Pathology and laboratory tests, miscellaneous, P9010–P9615
Pathology, surgical, *G0416*
Patient support system, E0636
Patient transfer system, E1035–E1036
Pediculosis (lice) treatment, *A9180*
PEFR, peak expiratory flow rate meter, A4614
Pegademase bovine, J2504
Pegaptanib, J2503
Pegaspargase, J9266
Pegfilgrastim, J2505
Peginesatide, J0890
Pegloticase, J2507
Pelvic
belt/harness/boot, E0944
traction, E0890, E0900, E0947
Pemetrexed, J9305
Penicillin
G benzathine/G benzathine and penicillin G procaine, J0558, J0561
G potassium, J2540
G procaine, aqueous, J2510
Pentamidine isethionate, J2545, J7676
Pentastarch, 10% solution, J2513
Pentazocine HCl, J3070
Pentobarbital sodium, J2515
Pentostatin, J9268
Peramivir, J2547
Percussor, E0480
Percutaneous access system, A4301
Perflexane lipid microspheres, Q9955
Perflutren lipid microspheres, Q9957
Peroneal strap, L0980
Peroxide, A4244
Perphenazine, J3310
Personal care services, T1019–T1021
home health aide or CAN, per visit, T1021
per diem, T1020
provided by home health aide or CAN, per 15 minutes, T1019
Pertuzumab, J9306
Pessary, A4561, A4562
PET, *G0219, G0235, G0252*
Pharmacologic therapy, *G8633*
Pharmacy, fee, *G0333*
Phenobarbital sodium, J2560
Phentolamine mesylate, J2760
Phenylephrine HCl, J2370
Phenytoin sodium, J1165
Phisohex solution, A4246
Photofrin, *see* **Porfimer sodium**
Photorefraction keratectomy, (PRK), *S0810*
Phototherapeutic keratectomy, (PTK), *S0812*
Phototherapy light, E0202
Phytonadione, J3430
Pillow, cervical, E0943
Pinworm examination, Q0113
Plasma
multiple donor, pooled, frozen, P9023, P9070
single donor, fresh frozen, P9017, P9071
Plastazote, L3002, L3252, L3253, L3265, L5654–L5658
addition to lower extremity socket insert, L5654
addition to lower extremity socket insert, above knee, L5658
addition to lower extremity socket insert, below knee, L5655
addition to lower extremity socket insert, knee disarticulation, L5656
foot insert, removable, plastazote, L3002
foot, molded shoe, custom fitted, plastazote, L3253
foot, shoe molded to patient model, plastazote, L3252
plastazote sandal, L3265

◄ New ⤺ Revised ✔ Reinstated ~~deleted~~ Deleted

Platelet, P9072
concentrate, each unit, P9019
rich plasma, each unit, P9020
Platelets, *P9031–P9037, P9052–P9053, P9055*
Platform attachment
forearm crutch, E0153
walker, E0154
Plerixafor, J2562
Plicamycin, J9270
Plumbing, for home ESRD equipment, A4870
Pneumatic
appliance, E0655–E0673, L4350–L4380
compressor, E0650–E0652
splint, L4350–L4380
ventricular assist device, Q0480–Q0504
Pneumatic nebulizer
administration set, small volume, filtered, A7006
administration set, small volume, nonfiltered, A7003
administration set, small volume, nonfiltered, non-disposable, A7005
small volume, disposable, A7004
Pneumococcal
vaccine, administration, G0009
Porfimer, J9600
Portable
equipment transfer, R0070–R0076
gaseous oxygen, K0741, K0742
hemodialyzer system, E1635
liquid oxygen system, E0433
x-ray equipment, Q0092
Positioning seat, T5001
Positive airway pressure device, accessories, A7030–A7039, E0561–E0562
Positive expiratory pressure device, E0484
Post-coital examination, Q0115
Postural drainage board, E0606
Potassium
chloride, J3480
hydroxide (KOH) preparation, Q0112
Pouch
fecal collection, A4330
ostomy, A4375–A4378, A5051–A5054, A5061–A5065
urinary, A4379–A4383, A5071–A5075
Practice, guidelines, oncology, *G9056–G9062*
Pralatrexate, J9307
Pralidoxime chloride, J2730
Prednisolone
acetate, J2650
oral, J7510
Prednisone, J7512
Preparation kits, dialysis, A4914
Preparatory prosthesis, L5510–L5595
chemotherapy, J8999
nonchemotherapy, J8499
Pressure
alarm, dialysis, E1540
pad, A4640, E0180–E0199
Privigen, J1459
Procainamide HCl, J2690
Procedure
HALO, L0810–L0861
noncovered, G0293, G0294
scoliosis, L1000–L1499
Prochlorperazine, J0780
Prolotherapy, M0076
Promazine HCl, J2950
Promethazine
and meperdine, J2180
HCl, J2550
Propranolol HCl, J1800
Prostate, cancer, screening, *G0102, G0103*
Prosthesis
artificial larynx battery/accessory, L8505
breast, L8000–L8035, L8600
eye, L8610, L8613, V2623–V2629
fitting, L5400–L5460, L6380–L6388
foot/ankle one piece system, L5979
hand, L6000–L6020, L6026
implants, L8600–L8690
larynx, L8500
lower extremity, L5700–L5999, L8640–L8642
mandible, L8617
maxilla, L8616
maxillofacial, provided by a non-physician, L8040–L8048
miscellaneous service, L8499
ocular, V2623–V2629
repair of, L7520, L8049
socks (shrinker, sheath, stump sock), L8400–L8485
taxes, orthotic/prosthetic/other, L9999
tracheo-esophageal, L8507–L8509
upper extremity, L6000–L6999
vacuum erection system, L7900
Prosthetic additions
lower extremity, L5610–L5999
upper extremity, L6600–L7405
Prosthetic, eye, *V2623*
Prosthodontic procedure
Protamine sulfate, J2720
Protectant, skin, A6250
Protector, heel or elbow, E0191
Protein C Concentrate, J2724
Protirelin, J2725
Psychotherapy, group, partial hospitalization, *G0410–G0411*
Pulse generator, E2120
Pump
alternating pressure pad, E0182
ambulatory infusion, E0781
ambulatory insulin, E0784
blood, dialysis, E1620
breast, E0602–E0604
enteral infusion, B9000, B9002
external infusion, E0779

Pump *(Continued)*
heparin infusion, E1520
implantable infusion, E0782, E0783
implantable infusion, refill kit, A4220
infusion, supplies, A4230, A4232
negative pressure wound therapy, E2402
parenteral infusion, B9004, B9006
suction, portable, E0600
water circulating pad, E0236
wound, negative, pressure, E2402
Purification system, E1610, E1615
Pyridoxine HCl, J3415

Q

Quad cane, E0105
Quinupristin/dalfopristin, J2770

R

Rack/stand, oxygen, E1355
Radiesse, Q2026
Radioelements for brachytherapy, Q3001
***Radiological, supplies,** A4641, A4642*
Radiology service, R0070–R0076
Radiopharmaceutical diagnostic and therapeutic imaging agent, A4641, A4642, A9500–A9699
***Radiosurgery, robotic,** G0339–G0340*
***Radiosurgery, stereotactic,** G0339, G0340*
Rail
bathtub, E0241, E0242, E0246
bed, E0305, E0310
toilet, E0243
Ranibizumab, J2778
Rasburicase, J2783
Reaching/grabbing device, A9281
Reagent strip, A4252
Reciprocating peritoneal dialysis system, E1630
Reclast, J3488, *J3489*
***Reclining, wheelchair,** E1014, E1050–E1070, E1100–E1110*
***Reconstruction, angiography,** G0288*
Red blood cells, P9021, P9022
Regadenoson, J2785
Regular insulin, *J1815*, J1820
Regulator, oxygen, E1353
Rehabilitation
cardiac, S9472
program, H2001
psychosocial, H2017, H2018
pulmonary, S9473
system, jaw, motion, E1700–E1702
vestibular, S9476
***Removal, cerumen,** G0268*
Repair
contract, ESRD, A4890
durable medical equipment, E1340
maxillofacial prosthesis, L8049
orthosis, L4000–L4130
prosthetic, L7500, L7510
Replacement
battery, A4630
pad (alternating pressure), A4640
tanks, dialysis, A4880
tip for cane, crutches, walker, A4637
underarm pad for crutches, A4635
Reslizumab, J2786◄
RespiGam, *see* **Respiratory syncytial virus immune globulin**
Respiratory
DME, A7000–A7527
equipment, E0424–E0601
function, therapeutic, procedure, G0237–G0239, S5180–S5181
supplies, A4604–A4629
Restraint, any type, E0710
Reteplase, J2993
***Revascularization,** C9603–C9608*
Rho(D) immune globulin, human, J2788, J2790, J2791, J2792
Rib belt, thoracic, A4572, L0220
Rilanocept, J2793
RimabotulinumtoxinB, J0587
Ring, ostomy, A4404
Ringers lactate infusion, J7120
Risk-adjusted functional status
elbow, wrist or hand, G8667–G8670
hip, G8651–G8654
lower leg, foot or ankle, G8655–G8658
lumbar spine, G8659–G8662
neck, cranium, mandible, thoracic spine, ribs, or other, G8671–G8674
shoulder, G8663–G8666
Risperidone, J2794
Rituximab, J9310
Robin-Aids, L6000, L6010, L6020, L6855, L6860
Rocking bed, E0462
Rolapitant, J8670◄
Rollabout chair, E1031
Romidepsin, J9315
Romiplostim, J2796
Ropivacaine HCl, J2795
Rubidium Rb-82, A9555

S

Sacral nerve stimulation test lead, A4290
Safety equipment, E0700
vest, wheelchair, E0980

Saline
hypertonic, *J7131*
infusion, J7030–J7060
solution, A4216–A4218, J7030–J7050
Saliva
artificial, A9155
Samarium SM 153 Lexidronamm, A9605
Sargramostim (GM-CSF), J2820
Scoliosis, L1000–L1499
additions, L1010–L1120, L1210–L1290
Screening
alcohol misuse, G0442
cancer, cervical or vaginal, G0101
colorectal, cancer, G0104–G0106, G0120–G0122, G0328
cytopathology cervical or vaginal, G0123, G0124, G0141–G0148
depression, G0444
dysphagia, documentation, V5364
enzyme immunoassay, G0432
glaucoma, G0117, G0118
infectious agent antibody detection, G0433, G0435
language, V5363
mammography, digital image, G0202
prostate, cancer, G0102, G0103
speech, V5362
Sculptra, Q2028
Sealant
skin, A6250
Seat
attachment, walker, E0156
insert, wheelchair, E0992
lift (patient), E0621, E0627–E0629
upholstery, wheelchair, E0975, *E0981*
Sebelipase alfa, J2840◄
Secretin, J2850
Semen analysis, G0027
Semi-reclining, wheelchair, *E1100, E1110*
Sensitivity study, P7001
Sensory nerve conduction test, *G0255*
Sermorelin acetate, Q0515
Serum clotting time tube, A4771
Service
Allied Health, home health, hospice, G0151–G0161
behavioral health and/or substance abuse, H0001–H9999
hearing, V5000–V5999
laboratory, P0000–P9999
mental, health, training, G0177
non-covered, A9270
physician, for mobility device, G0372
pulmonary, for LVRS, G0302–G0305
skilled, RN/LPN, home health, hospice, G0162
social, psychological, G0409–G0411
speech-language, V5336–V5364
vision, V2020–V2799
SEWHO, L3960–L3974, *L3975–L3978*
SEXA, *G0130*
Sheepskin pad, E0188, E0189
Shoes
arch support, L3040–L3100
for diabetics, A5500–A5508
insert, L3000–L3030, *L3031*
lift, L3300–L3334
miscellaneous additions, L3500–L3595
orthopedic, L3201–L3265
positioning device, L3140–L3170
transfer, L3600–L3649
wedge, L3340–L3485
Shoulder
disarticulation, prosthetic, L6300–L6320, L6550
orthosis (SO), L3650–L3674
spinal, cervical, L0100–L0200
Shoulder sling, A4566
Shoulder-elbow-wrist-hand orthosis (SEWHO), L3960–L3969, *L3971–L3978*
Shunt accessory for dialysis, A4740
aqueous, L8612
Sigmoidoscopy, cancer screening, G0104, G0106
Siltuximab, J2860
Sincalide, J2805
Sipuleucel-T, Q2043
Sirolimus, J7520
Sitz bath, E0160–E0162
Skin
barrier, ostomy, A4362, A4363, A4369–A4373, A4385, A5120
bond or cement, ostomy, A4364
sealant, protectant, moisturizer, A6250
substitute, Q4100–Q4175↩
Skyla, 13.5 mg, *J7301*
Sling, A4565
patient lift, E0621, E0630, E0635
Smear, Papanicolaou, screening, *P3000, P3001, Q0091*
SNCT, *G0255*
Social worker, clinical, home, health, *G0155*
Social worker, nonemergency transport, A0160
Social work/psychological services, CORF, *G0409*
Sock
body sock, L0984
prosthetic sock, *L8417*, L8420–L8435, L8470, L8480, L8485
stump sock, L8470–L8485
Sodium
chloride injection, J2912
ferric gluconate complex in sucrose, J2916
fluoride F-18, A9580
hyaluronate
Euflexxa, J7323
Hyalgan, J7321
Orthovisc, J7324
Supartz, J7321
Synvisc and Synvisc-One, J7325
phosphate P32, A9563
pyrophosphate, J1443
succinate, J1720

◄ New ↩ Revised ✔ Reinstated ~~deleted~~ Deleted

Solution
calibrator, A4256
dialysate, A4760
elliotts b, J9175
enteral formulae, B4149–B4156, *B4157–B4162*
parenteral nutrition, B4164–B5200
Solvent, adhesive remover, *A4455*
Somatrem, J2940
Somatropin, J2941
Sorbent cartridge, ESRD, E1636
Special size, wheelchair, *E1220–E1239*
Specialty absorptive dressing, A6251–A6256
Spectacle lenses, *V2100–V2199*
Spectinomycin HCl, J3320
Speech assessment, V5362–V5364
Speech generating device, E2500–E2599
Speech, pathologist, *G0153*
Speech-Language pathology, services, *V5336–V5364*
Spherocylinder, single vision, *V2100–V2114*
bifocal, V2203–V2214
trifocal, V2303–V2314
Spinal orthosis
cervical, L0100–L0200
cervical-thoracic-lumbar-sacral (CTLSO), L0700, L0710
DME, K0112–K0116
halo, L0810–L0830
multiple post collar, L0180–L0200
scoliosis, L1000–L1499
torso supports, L0960
Splint, A4570, L3100, L4350–L4380
ankle, L4390–L4398
dynamic, E1800, E1805, E1810, E1815, E1825, E1830, E1840
footdrop, L4398
supplies, miscellaneous, Q4051
Standard, wheelchair, *E1130, K0001*
Static progressive stretch, E1801, E1806, E1811, E1816, E1818, E1821
Status
disease, oncology, G9063–G9139
STELARA, ustekinumab, 1 mg, *J3357*
Stent, transcatheter, placement, *C9600, C9601*
Stereotactic, radiosurgery, *G0339, G0340*
Sterile cefuroxime sodium, J0697
Sterile water, A4216–A4217
Stimulation, electrical, non-attended, *G0281–G0283*
Stimulators
neuromuscular, E0744, E0745
osteogenesis, electrical, E0747–E0749
salivary reflex, E0755
stoma absorptive cover, A5083
transcutaneous, electric, nerve, A4595, E0720–E0749
ultrasound, E0760
Stockings
gradient, compression, A6530–A6549
surgical, A4490–A4510
Stoma, plug or seal, *A5081*
Stomach tube, B4083
Streptokinase, J2995
Streptomycin, J3000
Streptozocin, J9320
Strip, blood glucose test, A4253–A4772
urine reagent, A4250
Strontium-89 chloride, supply of, A9600
Study, bone density, *G0130*
Stump sock, L8470–L8485
Stylet, A4212
Substance/Alcohol, assessment, *G0396, G0397, H0001, H0003, H0049*
Succinylcholine chloride, J0330
Suction pump
gastric, home model, E2000
portable, E0600
respiratory, home model, E0600
Sumatriptan succinate, J3030
Supartz, J7321
Supplies
battery, A4233–A4236, A4601, A4611–A4613, A4638
cast, A4580, A4590, Q4001–Q4051
catheters, A4300–A4306
contraceptive, A4267–A4269
diabetic shoes, A5500–A5513
dialysis, A4653–A4928
DME, other, A4630–A4640
dressings, A6000–A6513
enteral, therapy, B4000–B9999
incontinence, A4310–A4355, A5102–A5200
infusion, A4221, A4222, A4230–A4232, E0776–E0791
needle, A4212, A4215
needle-free device, A4210
ostomy, A4361–A4434, A5051–A5093, A5120–A5200
parenteral, therapy, B4000–B9999
radiological, A4641, A4642
refill kit, infusion pump, A4220
respiratory, A4604–A4629
self-administered injections, A4211
splint, Q4051
sterile water/saline and/or dextrose, A4216–A4218
surgical, miscellaneous, A4649
syringe, A4206–A4209, A4213, A4232
syringe with needle, A4206–A4209
urinary, external, A4356–A4360
Supply/accessory/service, A9900
Support
arch, L3040–L3090
cervical, L0100–L0200
spinal, L0960
stockings, L8100–L8239
Surgical
arthroscopy, knee, G0289, S2112
boot, L3208–L3211
dressing, A6196–A6406

◀ New ⮌ Revised ✔ Reinstated ~~deleted~~ Deleted

Surgical *(Continued)*
procedure, noncovered, G0293, G0294
stocking, A4490–A4510
supplies, A4649
tray, A4550
Swabs, betadine or iodine, A4247
Synvisc and Synvisc-One, J7325
Syringe, A4213
with needle, A4206–A4209
System
external, ambulatory insulin, A9274
rehabilitation, jaw, motion, E1700–E1702
transport, E1035–E1039

T

Tables, bed, E0274, E0315
Tacrolimus
oral, J7503, J7507, J7508
parenteral, J7525
Taliglucerace, J3060
Talimogene laheroareovec, J9325◀
Tape, *A4450–A4452*
Taxi, non emergency transportation, A0100
Team, conference, *G0175, G9007, S0220, S0221*
Technetium TC 99M
Arcitumomab, A9568
Bicisate, A9557
Depreotide, A9536
Disofenin, A9510
Exametazine, A9521
Exametazine labeled autologous white blood cells, A9569
Fanolesomab, A9566
Glucepatate, A9550
Labeled red blood cells, A9560
Macroaggregated albumin, A9540
Mebrofenin, A9537
Mertiatide, A9562
Oxidronate, A9561
Pentetate, A9539, A9567
Pertechnetate, A9512
Pyrophosphate, A9538
Sestamibi, A9500
Succimer, A9551
Sulfur colloid, A9541
Teboroxime, A9501
Tetrofosmin, A9502
Tilmanocept, A9520
Tedizolid phosphate, J3090
TEEV, J0900
Telavancin, J3095
Telehealth, Q3014
Telehealth transmission, T1014
Temozolomide
injection, J9328
oral, J8700
Temporary codes, *Q0000–Q9999*, S0009–S9999
Temsirolimus, J9330
Tenecteplase, J3101
Teniposide, Q2017
TENS, A4595, E0720–E0749
Tent, oxygen, E0455
Terbutaline sulfate, J3105
inhalation solution, concentrated, J7680
inhalation solution, unit dose, J7681
Teriparatide, J3110
Terminal devices, L6700–L6895
Test
sensory, nerve, conduction, G0255
Testosterone
cypionate and estradiol cypionate, J1071
enanthate, J3121
undecanoate, J3145
Tetanus immune globulin, human, J1670
Tetracycline, J0120
Thallous Chloride TL 201, A9505
Theophylline, J2810
Therapeutic lightbox, A4634, E0203
Therapy
activity, G0176
electromagnetic, G0295, G0329
enteral, supplies, B4000–B9999
medical, nutritional, G0270, G0271
occupational, *G0129*, H5300, *S9129*
occupational, health, G0152
parenteral, supplies, B4000–B9999
respiratory, function, procedure, G0237–S0239, S5180, S5181
speech, home, G0153, S9128
wound, negative, pressure, pump, E2402
Theraskin, *Q4121*
Thermometer, A4931–A4932
dialysis, A4910
Thiamine HCl, J3411
Thiethylperazine maleate, J3280
Thiotepa, J9340
Thoracic orthosis, L0210
Thoracic-hip-knee-ankle (THKAO), L1500–L1520
Thoracic-lumbar-sacral orthosis (TLSO)
scoliosis, L1200–L1290
spinal, L0450–L0492
Thymol turbidity, blood, P2033
Thyrotropin Alfa, J3240
Tigecycline, J3243
Tinzarparin sodium, J1655
Tip (cane, crutch, walker) replacement, A4637
Tire, wheelchair, *E2211–E2225, E2381–E2395*↩
Tirofiban, J3246
Tissue marker, A4648
TLSO, L0450–L0492, L1200–L1290
Tobacco
intervention, G9016

Tobramycin
inhalation solution, unit dose, J7682, J7685
sulfate, J3260
Tocilizumab, J2362
Toe device, *E1831*
Toilet accessories, E0167–E0179, E0243, E0244, E0625
Tolazoline HCl, J2670
Toll, non emergency transport, A0170
Topical hyperbaric oxygen chamber, A4575
Topotecan, J8705, J9351
Torsemide, J3265
Trabectedin, J9352◀
Tracheostoma heat moisture exchange system, A7501–A7509
Tracheostomy
care kit, A4629
filter, A4481
speaking valve, L8501
supplies, A4623, A4629, A7523–A7524
tube, A7520–A7522
Tracheotomy mask or collar, A7525–A7526
Traction
cervical, E0855, E0856
device, ambulatory, E0830
equipment, E0840–E0948
extremity, E0870–E0880
pelvic, E0890, E0900, E0947
Training
diabetes, outpatient, G0108, G0109
home health or hospice, G0162
services, mental, health, G0177
Transcutaneous electrical nerve stimulator (TENS), E0720–E0770
Transducer protector, dialysis, E1575
Transfer (shoe orthosis), L3600–L3640
Transfer system with seat, E1035
Transparent film (for dressing), A6257–A6259
Transplant
islet, G0341–G0343, S2102
Transport
chair, E1035–E1039
system, E1035–E1039
x-ray, R0070–R0076
Transportation
ambulance, A0021–A0999, Q3019, Q3020
corneal tissue, V2785
EKG (portable), R0076
handicapped, A0130
non emergency, A0080–A0210, T2001–T2005
service, including ambulance, A0021, A0999, T2006
taxi, non emergency, A0100
toll, non emergency, A0170
volunteer, non emergency, A0080, A0090
x-ray (portable), R0070, R0075, *R0076*
Transportation services
air services, A0430, A0431, A0435, A0436
ALS disposable supplies, A0398
Transportation services *(Continued)*
ALS mileage, A0390
ALS specialized service, A0392, A0394, A0396
ambulance, ALS, A0426, A0427, A0433
ambulance, outside state, Medicaid, A0021
ambulance oxygen, A0422
ambulance, waiting time, A0420
ancillary, lodging, escort, A0200
ancillary, lodging, recipient, A0180
ancillary, meals, escort, A0210
ancillary, meals, recipient, A0190
ancillary, parking fees, tolls, A0170
BLS disposable supplies, A0382
BLS mileage, A0380
BLS specialized service, A0384
emergency, neonatal, one-way, A0225
extra ambulance attendant, A0424
ground mileage, A0425
non-emergency, air travel, A0140
non-emergency, bus, A0110
non-emergency, case worker, A0160
non-emergency, mini-bus, A0120
non-emergency, no vested interest, A0080
non-emergency, taxi, A0100
non-emergency, wheelchair van, A0130
non-emergency, with vested interest, A0090
paramedic intercept, A0432
response and treat, no transport, A0998
specialty transport, A0434
Transtracheal oxygen catheter, A7018
Trapeze bar, E0910–E0912, E0940
Trauma, response, team, *G0390*
Tray
insertion, A4310–A4316
irrigation, A4320
surgical (*see also* kits), A4550
wheelchair, E0950
Treatment
bone, G0412–G0415
pediculosis (lice), A9180
services, behavioral health, H0002–H2037
Treprostinil, J3285
Triamcinolone, J3301–J3303
acetonide, J3300, J3301
diacetate, J3302
hexacetonide, J3303
inhalation solution, concentrated, J7683
inhalation solution, unit dose, J7684
Triflupromazine HCl, J3400
Trifocal, glass or plastic, V2300–V2399
aniseikonic, V2318
lenticular, V2315, V2321
specialty trifocal, by report, V2399
sphere, plus or minus, V2300–V2302
spherocylinder, V2303–V2314
trifocal add-over 3.25d, V2320
trifocal, seg width over 28 mm, V2319

◀ New   ↩ Revised   ✔ Reinstated   ~~deleted~~ Deleted

Trimethobenzamide HCl, J3250
Trimetrexate glucuoronate, J3305
Trimming, nails, dystrophic, *G0127*
Triptorelin pamoate, J3315
Truss, L8300–L8330
addition to standard pad, scrotal pad, L8330
addition to standard pad, water pad, L8320
double, standard pads, L8310
single, standard pad, L8300
Tube/Tubing
anchoring device, A5200
blood, A4750, A4755
corrugated tubing, non-disposable, used with large volume nebulizer,10 feet, A4337
drainage extension, A4331
gastrostomy, B4087, B4088
irrigation, A4355
larynectomy, A4622
nasogastric, B4081, B4082
oxygen, A4616
serum clotting time, A4771
stomach, B4083
suction pump, each, A7002
tire, K0091, K0093, K0095, K0097
tracheostomy, A4622
urinary drainage, K0280

U

Ultrasonic nebulizer, E0575
Ultrasound, *S8055, S9024*
paranasal sinus ultrasound, S9024
ultrasound guidance, multifetal pregnancy reduction, technical component, S8055
Ultraviolet, cabinet/system, *E0691, E0694*
Ultraviolet light therapy system, A4633, E0691–E0694
light therapy system in 6 foot cabinet, E0694
replacement bulb/lamp, A4633
therapy system panel, 4 foot, E0692
therapy system panel, 6 foot, E0693
treatment area 2 sq feet or less, E0691
Unclassified drug, J3490
Underpads, disposable, *A4554*
Unipuncture control system, dialysis, E1580
Upper extremity addition, locking elbow, L6693
Upper extremity fracture orthosis, L3980–L3999
Upper limb prosthesis, L6000–L7499
Urea, J3350
Ureterostomy supplies, A4454–A4590
Urethral suppository, Alprostadil, J0275
Urinal, E0325, E0326
Urinary
catheter, A4338–A4346, A4351–A4353
indwelling catheter, A4338–A4346
intermittent urinary catheter, A4351–A4353
male external catheter, A4349
Urinary *(Continued)*
collection and retention (supplies), A4310–A4360
bedside drainage bag, A4357
disposable external urethral clamp, A4360
external urethral clamp, A4356
female external urinary collection device, A4328
insertion trays, A4310–A4316, A4354–A4355
irrigation syringe, A4322
irrigation tray, A4320
male external catheter/integral collection chamber, A4326
perianal fecal collection pouch, A4330
therapeutic agent urinary catheter irrigation, A4321
urinary drainage bag, leg/abdomen, A4358
supplies, external, A4335, A4356–A4358
bedside drainage bag, A4357
external urethral clamp/compression device, A4356
incontinence supply, A4335
urinary drainage bag, leg or abdomen, A4358
tract implant, collagen, L8603
tract implant, synthetic, L8606
Urine
sensitivity study, P7001
tests, A4250
Urofollitropin, J3355
Urokinase, J3364, J3365
Ustekinumab, J3357
U-V lens, V2755

V

Vabra aspirator, A4480
Vaccination, administration
flublok, Q2033
hepatitis B, G0010
influenza virus, G0008
pneumococcal, G0009
Vaccine
administration, influenza, G0008
administration, pneumococcal, G0009
hepatitis B, administration, G0010
Vaginal
cancer, screening, G0101
cytopathologist, G0123
cytopathology, G0123, G0124, G0141–G0148
screening, cervical/vaginal, thin-layer, cytopathologist, G0123
screening, cervical/vaginal, thin-layer, physician interpretation, G0124
screening cytopathology smears, automated, G0141–G0148
Vancomycin HCl, J3370
Vaporizer, E0605
Vascular
catheter (appliances and supplies), A4300–A4306
disposable drug delivery system, >50 ml/hr, *A4305*
disposable drug delivery system, <50 ml/hr, *A4306*

Vascular *(Continued)*
catheter (appliances and supplies) *(Continued)*
implantable access catheter, external, *A4300*
implantable access total, catheter, *A4301*
graft material, synthetic, L8670
Vasoxyl, J3390
Vedolizumab, J3380
Vehicle, power-operated, *K0800–K0899*
Velaglucerase alfa, J3385
Venous pressure clamp, dialysis, A4918
Ventilator
battery, A4611–A4613
home ventilator, any type, E0465, E0466
used with invasive interface, (e.g., tracheostomy tube), E0465
used with non-invasive interface, (e.g., mask, chest shell), E0466
moisture exchanger, disposable, A4483
Ventricular assist device, Q0478–Q0509
battery clips, electric or electric/pneumatic, replacement, Q0497
battery, lithium-ion, electric or electric/pneumatic, replacement, Q0506
battery, other than lithium-ion, electric or electric/pneumatic, replacement, Q0496
battery, pneumatic, replacement, Q0503
battery/power-pack charger, electric or electric/pneumatic, replacement, Q0495
belt/vest/bag, carry external components, replacement, Q0499
driver, replacement, Q0480
emergency hand pump, electric or electric/pneumatic, replacement, Q0494
emergency power source, electric, replacement, Q0490
emergency power source, electric/pneumatic, replacement, Q0491
emergency power supply cable, electric, replacement, Q0492
emergency power supply cable, electric/pneumatic, replacement, Q0493
filters, electric or electric/pneumatic, replacement, Q0500
holster, electric or electric/pneumatic, replacement, Q0498
leads (pneumatic/electrical), replacement, Q0487
microprocessor control unit, electric/pneumatic combination, replacement, Q0482
microprocessor control unit, pneumatic, replacement, Q0481
miscellaneous supply, external VAD, Q0507
miscellaneous supply, implanted device, Q0508
miscellaneous supply, implanted device, payment not made under Medicare Part A, Q0509
mobility cart, replacement, Q0502
monitor control cable, electric, replacement, Q0485
monitor control cable, electric/pneumatic, Q0486
monitor/display module, electric, replacement, Q0483

Ventricular assist device *(Continued)*
monitor/display module, electric/electric pneumatic, replacement, Q0484
power adapter, pneumatic, replacement, vehicle type, Q0504
power adapter, vehicle type, Q0478
power module, replacement, Q0479
power-pack base, electric, replacement, Q0488
power-pack base, electric/pneumatic, replacement, Q0489
shower cover, electric or electric/pneumatic, replacement, Q0501
Verteporfin, J3396
Vest, safety, wheelchair, E0980
Vinblastine sulfate, J9360
Vincristine sulfate, J9370, J9371
Vinorelbine tartrate, J9390
Vision service, V2020–V2799
bifocal, glass or plastic, V2200–V2299
contact lenses, V2500–V2599
frames, V2020–V2025
intraocular lenses, V2630–V2632
low-vision aids, V2600–V2615
miscellaneous, V2700–V2799
prosthetic eye, V2623–V2629
spectacle lenses, V2100–V2199
trifocal, glass or plastic, V2300–V2399
variable asphericity, V2410–V2499
Visit, emergency department, *G0380–G0384*
Visual, function, postoperative cataract surgery, *G0915–G0918*
Vitamin B-12 cyanocobalamin, J3420
Vitamin K, J3430
Voice
amplifier, L8510
prosthesis, L8511–L8514
Von Willebrand Factor Complex, human, J7179, J7183, J7187↩
Voriconazole, J3465

W

Waiver, T2012–T2050
assessment/plan of care development, T2024
case management, per month, T2022
day habilitation, per 15 minutes, T2021
day habilitation, per diem, T2020
habilitation, educational, per diem, T2012
habilitation, educational, per hour, T2013
habilitation, prevocational, per diem, T2014
habilitation, prevocational, per hour, T2015
habilitation, residential, 15 minutes, T2017
habilitation, residential, per diem, T2016
habilitation, supported employment, 15 minutes, T2019
habilitation, supported employment, per diem, T2018
targeted case management, per month, T2023
waiver services NOS, T2025

X

Y

Z

◀ New ↩ Revised ✔ Reinstated ~~deleted~~ Deleted

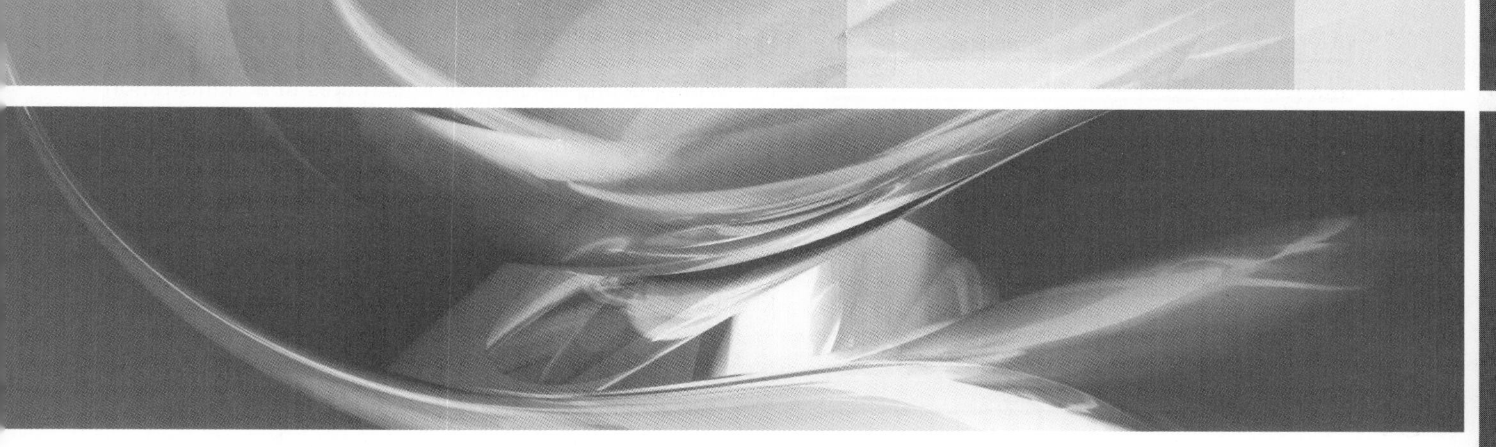

2017 TABLE OF DRUGS

IA	Intra-arterial administration
IU	International unit
IV	Intravenous administration
IM	Intramuscular administration
IT	Intrathecal
SC	Subcutaneous administration
INH	Administration by inhaled solution
VAR	Various routes of administration
OTH	Other routes of administration
ORAL	Administered orally

Intravenous administration includes all methods, such as gravity infusion, injections, and timed pushes. The "VAR" posting denotes various routes of administration and is used for drugs that are commonly administered into joints, cavities, tissues, or topical applications, in addition to other parenteral administrations. Listings posted with "OTH" indicate other administration methods, such as suppositories or catheter injections.

Questions regarding coding and billing guidance should be submitted to the insurer in whose jurisdiction a claim would be filed. For private sector health insurance systems, please contact the individual private insurance entity. For Medicaid systems, please contact the Medicaid Agency in the state in which the claim is being filed. For Medicare, contact the Medicare contractor.

Blue typeface terms are added by publisher.

DRUG NAME	DOSAGE	METHOD OF ADMINISTRATION	HCPCS CODE
A			
Abatacept	10 mg	IV	**J0129**
Abbokinase	5,000 IU vial	IV	J3364
	250,000 IU vial	IV	J3365
Abbokinase, Open Cath	5,000 IU vial	IV	J3364
Abciximab	10 mg	IV	**J0130**
Abelcet	10 mg	IV	J0287-J0289
Abilify	0.25 mg		J0400
	1 mg		J0401
Ablavar	1 ml		A9583
ABLC	50 mg	IV	J0285
AbobotulinumtoxintypeA	5 units	IM	**J0586**
Abraxane	1 mg		J9264
Accuneb	1 mg		J7613
Acetadote	100 mg		J0132
Acetaminophen	10 mg	IV	**J0131**
Acetazolamide sodium	up to 500 mg	IM, IV	**J1120**
Acetylcysteine			
injection	100 mg	IV	**J0132**
unit dose form	per gram	INH	**J7604, J7608**
Achromycin	up to 250 mg	IM, IV	J0120
Actemra	1 mg		J3262
ACTH	up to 40 units	IV, IM, SC	J0800
Acthar	up to 40 units	IV, IM, SC	J0800
Acthib			J3490
Acthrel	1 mcg		J0795
Actimmune	0.25 mg	SC	J1830
	3 million units	SC	J9216
Activase	1 mg	IV	J2997

▶ New ⤾ Revised ✔ Reinstated ~~deleted~~ Deleted

DRUG NAME	DOSAGE	METHOD OF ADMINISTRATION	HCPCS CODE
Acyclovir	5 mg		**J0133**
			J8499
Adagen	25 IU		**J2504**
Adalimumab	20 mg	SC	**J0135**
Adcetris	1 mg	IV	**J9042**
Adenocard	1 mg	IV	**J0153**
Adenoscan	1 mg	IV	**J0153**
Adenosine	1 mg	IV	**J0153**
Ado-trastuzumab Emtansine	1 mg	IV	**J9354**
Adrenalin Chloride	up to 1 ml ampule	SC, IM	**J0171**
Adrenalin, epinephrine	0.1 mg	SC, IM	**J0171**
Adriamycin, PFS, RDF	10 mg	IV	**J9000**
Adrucil	500 mg	IV	**J9190**
Advate	per IU		**J7192**
Aflibercept	1 mg	OTH	**J0178**
Agalsidase beta	1 mg	IV	**J0180**
Aggrastat	0.25 mg	IM, IV	**J3246**
A-hydroCort	up to 50 mg	IV, IM, SC	**J1710**
	up to 100 mg		**J1720**
Akineton	per 5 mg	IM, IV	**J0190**
Akynzeo	300 mg and 0.5 mg		**J8655**
Alatrofloxacin mesylate, Injection	100 mg	IV	**J0200**
Albumin			**P9041, P9045, P9046, P9047**
Albuterol	0.5 mg	INH	**J7620**
concentrated form	1 mg	INH	**J7610, J7611**
unit dose form	1 mg	INH	**J7609, J7613**
Aldesleukin	per single use vial	IM, IV	**J9015**
Aldomet	up to 250 mg	IV	**J0210**
Aldurazyme	0.1 mg		**J1931**
Alefacept	0.5 mg	IM, IV	**J0215**
Alemtuzumab	1 mg		**J0202**
Alferon N	250,000 IU	IM	**J9215**
Alglucerase	per 10 units	IV	**J0205**
Alglucosidase alfa	10 mg	IV	**J0220, J0221**
Alimta	10 mg		**J9305**
Alkaban-AQ	1 mg	IV	**J9360**
Alkeran	2 mg	ORAL	**J8600**
	50 mg	IV	**J9245**
Aloxi	25 mcg		**J2469**
Alpha 1-proteinase inhibitor, human	10 mg	IV	**J0256, J0257**
Alphanate			**J7186**
AlphaNine SD	per IU		**J7193**

▶ **New** ↩ **Revised** ✔ **Reinstated** ~~deleted~~ **Deleted**

DRUG NAME	DOSAGE	METHOD OF ADMINISTRATION	HCPCS CODE
Alprolix	per IU		J7201
Alprostadil			
injection	1.25 mcg	OTH	**J0270**
urethral suppository	each	OTH	**J0275**
Alteplase recombinant	1 mg	IV	**J2997**
Alupent	per 10 mg	INH	**J7667, J7668**
noncompounded, unit dose	10 mg	INH	J7669
unit does	10 mg	INH	J7670
AmBisome	10 mg	IV	J0289
Amcort	per 5 mg	IM	J3302
A-methaPred	up to 40 mg	IM, IV	J2920
	up to 125 mg	IM, IV	J2930
Amevive	0.5 mg		J0215
Amgen	1 mcg	SC	J9212
Amifostine	500 mg	IV	**J0207**
Amikacin sulfate	100 mg	IM, IV	**J0278**
Amikin	100 mg	IM, IV	J0278
Aminocaproic Acid			J3490
Aminolevalinic acid HCl	unit dose (354 mg)	OTH	**J7308**
Aminolevulinate	1 g	OTH	**J7309**
Aminophylline	up to 250 mg	IV	**J0280**
Amiodarone HCl	30 mg	IV	**J0282**
Amitriptyline HCl	up to 20 mg	IM	**J1320**
Amobarbital	up to 125 mg	IM, IV	**J0300**
Amphocin	50 mg	IV	J0285
Amphotericin B	50 mg	IV	**J0285**
Amphotericin B, lipid complex	10 mg	IV	**J0287-J0289**
Ampicillin			
sodium	up to 500 mg	IM, IV	**J0290**
sodium/sulbactam sodium	per 1.5 g	IM, IV	**J0295**
Amygdalin			J3570
Amytal	up to 125 mg	IM, IV	J0300
Anabolin LA 100	up to 50 mg	IM	J2320
Anadulafungin	1 mg	IV	**J0348**
Anascorp	up to 120 mg	IV	J0716
Ancef	500 mg	IV, IM	J0690
Andrest 90-4	1 mg	IM	J3121
Andro-Cyp	1 mg		J1071
Andro-Cyp 200	1 mg		J1071
Andro L.A. 200	1 mg	IM	J3121
Andro-Estro 90-4	1 mg	IM	J3121
Andro/Fem	1 mg		J1071
Androgyn L.A	1 mg	IM	J3121

▶ New ⤺ Revised ✔ Reinstated ~~deleted~~ Deleted

DRUG NAME	DOSAGE	METHOD OF ADMINISTRATION	HCPCS CODE
Androlone-50	up to 50 mg		J2320
Androlone-D 100	up to 50 mg	IM	J2320
Andronaq-50	up to 50 mg	IM	J3140
Andronaq-LA	1 mg		J1071
Andronate-100	1 mg		J1071
Andronate-200	1 mg		J1071
Andropository 100	1 mg		J3121
Andryl 200	1 mg		J3121
Anectine	up to 20 mg	IM, IV	J0330
Anergan 25	up to 50 mg	IM, IV	J2550
	12.5 mg	ORAL	Q0169
Anergan 50	up to 50 mg	IM, IV	J2550
	12.5 mg	ORAL	Q0169
Anestacaine	10 mg		J2001
Angiomax	1 mg		J0583
Anidulafungin	1 mg	IV	J0348
Anistreplase	30 units	IV	J0350
Antiflex	up to 60 mg		J2360
Anti-Inhibitor	per IU	IV	J7198
Antispas	up to 20 mg	IM	J0500
Antithrombin III (human)	per IU	IV	J7197
Antithrombin recombinant	50 IU	IV	J7196
Anzemet	10 mg	IV	J1260
	50 mg	ORAL	S0174
	100 mg	ORAL	Q0180
Apidra Solostar	per 50 units		J1817
A.P.L.	per 1,000 USP units	IM	J0725
Apomorphine Hydrochloride	1 mg	SC	J0364
Aprepitant	5 mg	ORAL	J8501
Apresoline	up to 20 mg	IV, IM	J0360
Aprotinin	10,000 kiu		J0365
AquaMEPHYTON	per 1 mg	IM, SC, IV	J3430
Aralast	10 mg	IV	J0256
Aralen	up to 250 mg	IM	J0390
Aramine	per 10 mg	IV, IM, SC	J0380
Aranesp			
ESRD use	1 mcg		J0882
Non-ESRD use	1 mcg		J0881
Arbutamine	1 mg	IV	J0395
Arcalyst	1 mg		J2793
Aredia	per 30 mg	IV	J2430
Arfonad, *see* Trimethaphan camsylate			
Arformoterol tartrate	15 mcg	INH	J7605

▶ New ↩ Revised ✔ Reinstated ~~deleted~~ Deleted

DRUG NAME	DOSAGE	METHOD OF ADMINISTRATION	HCPCS CODE
Argatroban			◀
(for non-ESRD use)	1 mg	IV	**J0883** ◀
(for ESRD use)	1 mg	IV	**J0884** ◀
Aridol	25% in 50 ml	IV	J2150
	5 mg	INH	J7665
Arimidex			J8999
Aripiprazole	0.25 mg	IM	**J0400**
Aripiprazole, extended release	1 mg	IV	**J0401** ⮌
Aripiprazole lauroxil	1 mg	IV	**J1942** ◀
Aristocort Forte	per 5 mg	IM	J3302
Aristocort Intralesional	per 5 mg	IM	J3302
Aristopan	per 5 mg		J3303
Aristospan Intra-Articular	per 5 mg	VAR	J3303
Aristospan Intralesional	per 5 mg	VAR	J3303
Arixtra	per 0.5 m		J1652
Aromasin			J8999
Arranon	50 mg		J9261
Arrestin	up to 200 mg	IM	J3250
	250 mg	ORAL	Q0173
Arsenic trioxide	1 mg	IV	**J9017**
Arzerra	10 mg		J9302
Asparaginase	1,000 units	IV, IM	**J9019**
	10,000 units	IV, IM	**J9020**
Astagraf XL	0.1 mg		J7508
Astramorph PF	up to 10 mg	IM, IV, SC	J2270
Atgam	250 mg	IV	J7504
Ativan	2 mg	IM, IV	J2060
Atropine			
concentrated form	per mg	INH	**J7635**
unit dose form	per mg	INH	**J7636**
sulfate	0.01 mg, per mg	IV, IM, SC	J0461, J7636
Atrovent	per mg	INH	J7644, J7645
Atryn	50 IU		J7196
Aurothioglucose	up to 50 mg	IM	**J2910**
Autologous cultured chondrocytes implant		OTH	**J7330**
Autoplex T	per IU	IV	J7198, J7199
Avastin	10 mg		J9035
Avelox	100 mg		J2280
Avonex	30 mcg	IM	J1826
	1 mcg	IM	Q3027
	1 mcg	SC	Q3028
Azacitidine	1 mg	SC	**J9025**
Azasan	50 mg		J7500

▶ New ⮌ Revised ✔ Reinstated ~~deleted~~ Deleted

DRUG NAME	DOSAGE	METHOD OF ADMINISTRATION	HCPCS CODE
Azathioprine	50 mg	ORAL	**J7500**
Azathioprine, parenteral	100 mg	IV	**J7501**
Azithromycin, dihydrate	1 gram	ORAL	**Q0144**
Azithromycin, Injection	500 mg	IV	**J0456**
B			
Baciim			**J3490**
Baci-RX			**J3490**
Bacitracin			**J3490**
Baclofen	10 mg	IT	**J0475**
Baclofen for intrathecal trial	50 mcg	OTH	**J0476**
Bactocill	up to 250 mg	IM, IV	**J2700**
BAL in oil	per 100 mg	IM	**J0470**
Banflex	up to 60 mg	IV, IM	**J2360**
Basiliximab	20 mg	IV	**J0480**
Bayhep B			**J3590**
BayRho-D	50 mcg		**J2788**
BCG (Bacillus Calmette and Guerin), live	per vial	IV	**J9031**
Bebulin VH	per IU		**J7194**
Beclomethasone inhalation solution, unit dose form	per mg	INH	**J7622, J7624**
Belatacept	1 mg	IV	**J0485**
Beleodaq	10 mg		**J9032**
Belimumab	10 mg	IV	**J0490**
Belinostat	10 mg	IV	**J9032**
Bena-D 10	up to 50 mg	IV, IM	**J1200**
Bena-D 50	up to 50 mg	IV, IM	**J1200**
Benadryl	up to 50 mg	IV, IM	**J1200**
Benahist 10	up to 50 mg	IV, IM	**J1200**
Benahist 50	up to 50 mg	IV, IM	**J1200**
Ben-Allergin-50	up to 50 mg	IV, IM	**J1200**
	50 mg	ORAL	**Q0163**
Bendamustine HCl	1 mg	IV	**J9033**
Benefix	per IU	IV	**J7195**
Benlysta	10 mg		**J0490**
Benoject-10	up to 50 mg	IV, IM	**J1200**
Benoject-50	up to 50 mg	IV, IM	**J1200**
Bentyl	up to 20 mg	IM	**J0500**
Benzocaine			**J3490**
Benztropine mesylate	per 1 mg	IM, IV	**J0515**
Berinert, *see* C-1 esterase inhibitor			
Berubigen	up to 1,000 mcg	IM, SC	**J3420**
Beta amyloid	per study dose	OTH	**A9599**
Betalin 12	up to 1,000 mcg	IM, SC	**J3420**
Betameth	per 3 mg	IM, IV	**J0702**

▶ **New** ⤾ **Revised** ✔ **Reinstated** ~~deleted~~ **Deleted**

DRUG NAME	DOSAGE	METHOD OF ADMINISTRATION	HCPCS CODE
Betamethasone acetate & betamethasone sodium phosphate	per 3 mg	IM	**J0702**
Betamethasone inhalation solution, unit dose form	per mg	INH	**J7624**
Betaseron	0.25 mg	SC	J1830
Bethanechol chloride	up to 5 mg	SC	**J0520**
Bethkis	300 mg		J7682
Bevacizumab	10 mg	IV	**J9035**
Bicillin C-R	100,000 units		J0558
Bicillin C-R 900/300	100,000 units	IM	J0558, J0561
Bicillin L-A	100,000 units	IM	J0561
BiCNU	100 mg	IV	J9050
Biperiden lactate	per 5 mg	IM, IV	**J0190**
Bitolterol mesylate			
concentrated form	per mg	INH	**J7628**
unit dose form	per mg	INH	**J7629**
Bivalirudin	1 mg	IV	**J0583**
Blenoxane	15 units	IM, IV, SC	J9040
Bleomycin sulfate	15 units	IM, IV, SC	**J9040**
Blinatumomab	1 microgram	IV	**J9039**
Boniva	1 mg		J1740
Bortezomib	0.1 mg	IV	**J9041**
Botox	1 unit		J0585
Bravelle	75 IU		J3355
Brentuximab Vedotin	1 mg	IV	**J9042**
Brethine			
concentrated form	per 1 mg	INH	J7680
unit dose	per 1 mg	INH	J7681
	up to 1 mg	SC, IV	J3105
Brevital Sodium			J3490
Bricanyl Subcutaneous	up to 1 mg	SC, IV	J3105
Brompheniramine maleate	per 10 mg	IM, SC, IV	**J0945**
Broncho Saline	10 ml		A4216
Bronkephrine, *see* Ethylnorepinephrine HCl			
Bronkosol			
concentrated form	per mg	INH	J7647, J7648
unit dose form	per mg	INH	J7649, J7650
Brovana			J7605, J7699
Budesonide inhalation solution			
concentrated form	0.25 mg	INH	**J7633, J7634**
unit dose form	0.5 mg	INH	**J7626, J7627**
Bumetanide			J3490
Bupivacaine			J3490
Buprenorphine Hydrochloride	0.1 mg	IM	**J0592**

▶ **New** ↩ **Revised** ✔ **Reinstated** ~~deleted~~ **Deleted**

DRUG NAME	DOSAGE	METHOD OF ADMINISTRATION	HCPCS CODE
Buprenorphine/Naloxone	1 mg	ORAL	**J0571**
	< = 3 mg	ORAL	**J0572**
	> 3 mg but < = 6 mg	ORAL	**J0573**
	> 6 mg but < = 10 mg	ORAL	**J0574**
	> 10 mg	ORAL	**J0575**
Busulfan	1 mg	IV	**J0594**
	2 mg	ORAL	**J8510**
Butorphanol tartrate	1 mg		**J0595**
C			
C1 Esterase Inhibitor	10 units	IV	**J0596-J0598**
Cabazitaxel	1 mg	IV	**J9043**
Cabergoline	0.25 mg	ORAL	**J8515**
Cafcit	5 mg	IV	J0706
Caffeine citrate	5 mg	IV	**J0706**
Caine-1	10 mg	IV	J2001
Caine-2	10 mg	IV	J2001
Calcijex	0.1 mcg	IM	J0636
Calcimar	up to 400 units	SC, IM	J0630
Calcitonin-salmon	up to 400 units	SC, IM	**J0630**
Calcitriol	0.1 mcg	IM	**J0636**
Calcium Disodium Versenate	up to 1,000 mg	IV, SC, IM	J0600
Calcium folinate (Hungarian import)	per 50 mg		J0640
Calcium gluconate	per 10 ml	IV	**J0610**
Calcium glycerophosphate and calcium lactate	per 10 ml	IM, SC	**J0620**
Caldolor	100 mg	IV	J1741
Calphosan	per 10 ml	IM, SC	J0620
Camptosar	20 mg	IV	J9206
Canakinumab	1 mg	SC	**J0638**
Cancidas	5 mg		J0637
Capecitabine	150 mg	ORAL	**J8520**
	500 mg	ORAL	**J8521**
Capsaicin patch	per sq cm	OTH	**J7336**
Carbidopa 5 mg/levodopa 20 mg enteral suspension		IV	**J7340**
Carbocaine	per 10 ml	VAR	J0670
Carbocaine with Neo-Cobefrin	per 10 ml	VAR	J0670
Carboplatin	50 mg	IV	**J9045**
Carfilzomib	1 mg	IV	**J9047**
Carimune	500 mg		J1566
Carmustine	100 mg	IV	**J9050**
Carnitor	per 1 g	IV	J1955
Carticel			J7330
Caspofungin acetate	5 mg	IV	**J0637**
Cathflo Activase	1 mg		J2997

▶ New ⮐ Revised ✔ Reinstated ~~deleted~~ Deleted

DRUG NAME	DOSAGE	METHOD OF ADMINISTRATION	HCPCS CODE
Caverject	per 1.25 mcg		J0270
Cayston	500 mg		S0073
Cefadyl	up to 1 g	IV, IM	J0710
Cefazolin sodium	500 mg	IV, IM	J0690
Cefepime hydrochloride	500 mg	IV	J0692
Cefizox	per 500 mg	IM, IV	J0715
Cefotaxime sodium	per 1 g	IV, IM	J0698
Cefotetan			J3490
Cefoxitin sodium	1 g	IV, IM	J0694
Ceftaroline fosamil	1 mg		J0712
Ceftazidime	per 500 mg	IM, IV	J0713
Ceftazidime and avibactam	0.5 g/0.125 g	IV	J0714
Ceftizoxime sodium	per 500 mg	IV, IM	J0715
Ceftolozane 50 mg and tazobactam 25 mg		IV	J0695
Ceftriaxone sodium	per 250 mg	IV, IM	J0696
Cefuroxime sodium, sterile	per 750 mg	IM, IV	J0697
Celestone Soluspan	per 3 mg	IM	J0702
	per mg	ORAL	J7624
CellCept	250 mg	ORAL	J7517
Cel-U-Jec	per 4 mg	IM, IV	Q0511
Cenacort A-40	1 mg		J3300
	per 5 mg		J3302
	per 10 mg	IM	J3301
Cenacort Forte	per 5 mg	IM	J3302
Centruroides Immune F(ab)	up to 120 mg	IV	J0716
Cephalothin sodium	up to 1 g	IM, IV	J1890
Cephapirin sodium	up to 1 g	IV, IM	J0710
Ceprotin	10 IU		J2724
Ceredase	per 10 units	IV	J0205
Cerezyme	10 units		J1786
Certolizumab pegol	1 mg	SC	J0717
Cerubidine	10 mg	IV	J9150
Cetuximab	10 mg	IV	J9055
Chealamide	per 150 mg	IV	J3520
Chirhostim	1 mcg	IV	J2850
Chloramphenicol sodium succinate	up to 1 g	IV	J0720
Chlordiazepoxide HCl	up to 100 mg	IM, IV	J1990
Chloromycetin Sodium Succinate	up to 1 g	IV	J0720
Chloroprocaine HCl	per 30 ml	VAR	J2400
	10 mg	ORAL	Q0171
	25 mg	ORAL	Q0172
	up to 50 mg	IM, IV	J3230
Chloroquine HCl	up to 250 mg	IM	J0390

▶ New ↩ Revised ✔ Reinstated ~~deleted~~ Deleted

DRUG NAME	DOSAGE	METHOD OF ADMINISTRATION	HCPCS CODE
Chlorothiazide sodium	per 500 mg	IV	**J1205**
Chlorpromazine	5 mg	ORAL	**Q0161**
Chlorpromazine HCl	up to 50 mg	IM, IV	**J3230**
Cholografin Meglumine	per ml		**Q9961**
Chorex-5	per 1,000 USP units	IM	**J0725**
Chorex-10	per 1,000 USP units	IM	**J0725**
Chorignon	per 1,000 USP units	IM	**J0725**
Chorionic gonadotropin	per 1,000 USP units	IM	**J0725**
Choron 10	per 1,000 USP units	IM	**J0725**
Cidofovir	375 mg	IV	**J0740**
Cilastatin sodium, imipenem	per 250 mg	IV, IM	**J0743**
Cimzia	1 mg	SC	**J0717**
Cinryze	10 units		**J0598**
Cipro IV	200 mg	IV	**J0706**
Ciprofloxacin	200 mg	IV	**J0706**
octic suspension	6 mg	OTH	**J7342** ◀
			J3490
Cisplatin, powder or solution	per 10 mg	IV	**J9060**
Cladribine	per mg	IV	**J9065**
Claforan	per 1 gm	IM, IV	**J0698**
Cleocin Phosphate			**J3490**
Clinacort	per 5 mg		**J3302**
Clindamycin			**J3490**
Clofarabine	1 mg	IV	**J9027**
Clolar	1 mg		**J9027**
Clonidine Hydrochloride	1 mg	Epidural	**J0735**
Cobex	up to 1,000 mcg	IM, SC	**J3420**
Cobolin-M	up to 1,000 mcg		**J3420**
Codeine phosphate	per 30 mg	IM, IV, SC	**J0745**
Codimal-A	per 10 mg	IM, SC, IV	**J0945**
Cogentin	per 1 mg	IM, IV	**J0515**
~~Colchicine~~	~~per 1 mg~~	~~IV~~	~~**J0760**~~ ✖
Colistimethate sodium	up to 150 mg	IM, IV	**J0770, S0142**
Collagenase, Clostridium Histolyticum	0.01 mg	OTH	**J0775**
Coly-Mycin M	up to 150 mg	IM, IV	**J0770**
Compa-Z	up to 10 mg	IM, IV	**J0780**
Compazine	up to 10 mg	IM, IV	**J0780**
	5 mg	ORAL	**Q0164**
			J8498
Compounded drug, not otherwise classified			**J7999**
Compro			**J8498**
Comptosar	20 mg		**J9206**
Conray	per ml		**Q9961**

▶ **New** ⤾ **Revised** ✔ **Reinstated** ~~deleted~~ **Deleted**

DRUG NAME	DOSAGE	METHOD OF ADMINISTRATION	HCPCS CODE
Conray 30	per ml		Q9958
Conray 43	per ml		Q9960
Copaxone	20 mg		J1595
Cophene-B	per 10 mg	IM, SC, IV	J0945
Copper contraceptive, intrauterine		OTH	J7300
Cordarone	30 mg	IV	J0282
Corgonject-5	per 1,000 USP units	IM	J0725
Corifact	1 IU		J7180
Corticorelin ovine triflutate	1 mcg		J0795
Corticotropin	up to 40 units	IV, IM, SC	J0800
Cortrosyn	per 0.25 mg	IM, IV	J0835
Corvert	1 mg		J1742
Cosmegen	0.5 mg	IV	J9120
Cosyntropin	per 0.25 mg	IM, IV	J0833, J0834
Cotolone	up to 1 ml		J2650
	per 5 mg		J7510
Cotranzine	up to 10 mg	IM, IV	J0780
Crofab	up to 1 gram		J0840
Cromolyn sodium, unit dose form	per 10 mg	INH	J7631, J7632
Crotalidae Polyvalent Immune Fab	up to 1 gram	IV	J0840
Crysticillin 300 A.S.	up to 600,000 units	IM, IV	J2510
Crysticillin 600 A.S.	up to 600,000 units	IM, IV	J2510
Cubicin	1 mg		J0878
Cyanocobalamin	up to 1,000 mcg		J3420
Cyclophosphamide	100 mg	IV	J9070
oral	25 mg	ORAL	J8530
Cyclosporine	25 mg	ORAL	J7515
	100 mg	ORAL	J7502
parenteral	250 mg	IV	J7516
	1 mg	ORAL	J7512
Cymetra	1 cc		Q4112
Cyomin	up to 1,000 mcg		J3420
Cyramza	5 mg		J9308
Cysto-Cornray LI	per ml		Q9958
Cystografin	per ml		Q9958
Cystografin-Dilute	per ml		Q9958
Cytarabine	100 mg	SC, IV	J9100
Cytarabine liposome	10 mg	IT	J9098
CytoGam	per vial		J0850
Cytomegalovirus immune globulin intravenous (human)	per vial	IV	J0850
Cytosar-U	100 mg	SC, IV	J9100
Cytovene	500 mg	IV	J1570
Cytoxan	100 mg	IV	J8530, J9070

▶ New ⤾ Revised ✔ Reinstated ~~deleted~~ Deleted

DRUG NAME	DOSAGE	METHOD OF ADMINISTRATION	HCPCS CODE
D			
D-5-W, infusion	1000 cc	IV	**J7070**
Dacarbazine	100 mg	IV	**J9130**
Daclizumab	25 mg	IV	**J7513**
Dacogen	1 mg		J0894
Dactinomycin	0.5 mg	IV	**J9120**
Dalalone	1 mg	IM, IV, OTH	J1100
Dalalone L.A	1 mg	IM	J1094
Dalbavancin	5 mg	IV	**J0875**
Dalteparin sodium	per 2500 IU	SC	**J1645**
Dalvance	5 mg		J0875
Daptomycin	1 mg	IV	**J0878**
Daratumumab	10 mg	IV	**J9145** ◀
Darbepoetin Alfa	1 mcg	IV, SC	**J0881, J0882**
Daunorubicin citrate, liposomal formulation	10 mg	IV	**J9151**
Daunorubicin HCl	10 mg	IV	**J9150**
Daunoxome	10 mg	IV	J9151
DDAVP	1 mcg	IV, SC	J2597
Decadron	1 mg	IM, IV, OTH	J1100
	0.25 mg		J8540
Decadron Phosphate	1 mg	IM, IV, OTH	J1100
Decadron-LA	1 mg	IM	J1094
Deca-Durabolin	up to 50 mg	IM	J2320
Decaject	1 mg	IM, IV, OTH	J1100
Decaject-L.A.	1 mg	IM	J1094
Decitabine	1 mg	IV	**J0894**
Decolone-50	up to 50 mg	IM	J2320
Decolone-100	up to 50 mg	IM	J2320
De-Comberol	1 mg		J1071
Deferoxamine mesylate	500 mg	IM, SC, IV	**J0895**
Definity	per ml		J3490, Q9957
Degarelix	1 mg	SC	**J9155**
Dehist	per 10 mg	IM, SC, IV	J0945
Deladumone	1 mg		J3121
Deladumone OB	1 mg		J3121
Delatest	1 mg		J3121
Delatestadiol	1 mg		J3121
Delatestryl	1 mg		J3121
Delestrogen	up to 10 mg	IM	J1380
Delta-Cortef	5 mg	ORAL	J7510
Demadex	10 mg/ml	IV	J3265
Demerol HCl	per 100 mg	IM, IV, SC	J2175
Denileukin diftitox	300 mcg	IV	**J9160**

▶ New ↩ Revised ✔ Reinstated ~~deleted~~ Deleted

DRUG NAME	DOSAGE	METHOD OF ADMINISTRATION	HCPCS CODE
Denosumab	1 mg	SC	**J0897**
DepAndro 100	1 mg		**J1071**
DepAndro 200	1 mg		**J1071**
DepAndrogyn	1 mg		**J1071**
DepGynogen	up to 5 mg	IM	**J1000**
DepMedalone 40	20 mg	IM	**J1020**
	40 mg	IM	**J1030**
	80 mg	IM	**J1040**
DepMedalone 80	20 mg	IM	**J1020**
	40 mg	IM	**J1030**
	80 mg	IM	**J1040**
DepoCyt	10 mg		**J9098**
Depo-estradiol cypionate	up to 5 mg	IM	**J1000**
Depogen	up to 5 mg	IM	**J1000**
Depoject	20 mg	IM	**J1020**
	40 mg	IM	**J1030**
	80 mg	IM	**J1040**
Depo-Medrol	20 mg	IM	**J1020**
	40 mg	IM	**J1030**
	80 mg	IM	**J1040**
Depopred-40	20 mg	IM	**J1020**
	40 mg	IM	**J1030**
	80 mg	IM	**J1040**
Depopred-80	20 mg	IM	**J1020**
	40 mg	IM	**J1030**
	80 mg	IM	**J1040**
Depo-Provera Contraceptive	1 mg		**J1050**
Depotest	1 mg		**J1071**
Depo-Testadiol	1 mg		**J1071**
Depo-Testosterone	1 mg		**J1071**
Depotestrogen	1 mg		**J1071**
Dermagraft	per square centimeter		**Q4106**
Desferal Mesylate	500 mg	IM, SC, IV	**J0895**
Desmopressin acetate	1 mcg	IV, SC	**J2597**
Dexacen-4	1 mg	IM, IV, OTH	**J1100**
Dexacen LA-8	1 mg	IM	**J1094**
Dexamethasone			
acetate	1 mg	IM	**J1094**
concentrated form	per mg	INH	**J7637**
intravitreal implant	0.1 mg	OTH	**J7312**
oral	0.25 mg	ORAL	**J8540**
sodium phosphate	1 mg	IM, IV, OTH	**J1100, J7638**
unit form	per mg	INH	**J7638**

▶ **New** ⤺ **Revised** ✔ **Reinstated** ~~deleted~~ **Deleted**

DRUG NAME	DOSAGE	METHOD OF ADMINISTRATION	HCPCS CODE
Dexasone	1 mg	IM, IV, OTH	**J1100**
Dexasone L.A.	1 mg	IM	**J1094**
Dexferrum	50 mg		**J1750**
Dexone	0.25 mg	ORAL	**J8540**
	1 mg	IM, IV, OTH	**J1100**
Dexone LA	1 mg	IM	**J1094**
Dexpak	0.25 mg	ORAL	**J8540**
Dexrazoxane hydrochloride	250 mg	IV	**J1190**
Dextran 40	500 ml	IV	**J7100**
Dextran 75	500 ml	IV	**J7110**
Dextrose 5%/normal saline solution	500 ml = 1 unit	IV	**J7042**
Dextrose/water (5%)	500 ml = 1 unit	IV	**J7060**
D.H.E. 45	per 1 mg		**J1110**
Diamox	up to 500 mg	IM, IV	**J1120**
Diazepam	up to 5 mg	IM, IV	**J3360**
Diazoxide	up to 300 mg	IV	**J1730**
Dibent	up to 20 mg	IM	**J0500**
Diclofenac sodium	37.5	IV	**J1130** ◄
Dicyclocot	up to 20 mg		**J0500**
Dicyclomine HCl	up to 20 mg	IM	**J0500**
Didronel	per 300 mg	IV	**J1436**
Diethylstilbestrol diphosphate	250 mg	IV	**J9165**
Diflucan	200 mg	IV	**J1450**
Digibind	per vial		**J1162**
DigiFab	per vial		**J1162**
Digoxin	up to 0.5 mg	IM, IV	**J1160**
Digoxin immune fab (ovine)	per vial		**J1162**
Dihydrex	up to 50 mg	IV, IM	**J1200**
	50 mg	ORAL	**Q0163**
Dihydroergotamine mesylate	per 1 mg	IM, IV	**J1110**
Dilantin	per 50 mg	IM, IV	**J1165**
Dilaudid	up to 4 mg	SC, IM, IV	**J1170**
	250 mg	OTH	**S0092**
Dilocaine	10 mg	IV	**J2001**
Dilomine	up to 20 mg	IM	**J0500**
Dilor	up to 500 mg	IM	**J1180**
Dimenhydrinate	up to 50 mg	IM, IV	**J1240**
Dimercaprol	per 100 mg	IM	**J0470**
Dimethyl sulfoxide	50%, 50 ml	OTH	**J1212**
Dinate	up to 50 mg	IM, IV	**J1240**
Dioval	up to 10 mg	IM	**J1380**
Dioval 40	up to 10 mg	IM	**J1380**

▶ **New** ⤺ **Revised** ✔ **Reinstated** ~~deleted~~ **Deleted**

DRUG NAME	DOSAGE	METHOD OF ADMINISTRATION	HCPCS CODE
Dioval XX	up to 10 mg	IM	J1380
Diphenacen-50	up to 50 mg	IV, IM	J1200
	50 mg	ORAL	Q0163
Diphenhydramine HCl			
injection	up to 50 mg	IV, IM	J1200
oral	50 mg	ORAL	Q0163
Diprivan	10 mg		J2704
			J3490
Dipyridamole	per 10 mg	IV	J1245
Diruril	per 500 mg	IV	J1205
Disotate	per 150 mg	IV	J3520
Di-Spaz	up to 20 mg	IM	J0500
Ditate-DS	1 mg		J3121
Diuril Sodium	per 500 mg	IV	J1205
D-Med 80	20 mg	IM	J1020
	40 mg	IM	J1030
	80 mg	IM	J1040
DMSO, Dimethyl sulfoxide 50%	50 ml	OTH	J1212
Dobutamine HCl	per 250 mg	IV	J1250
Dobutrex	per 250 mg	IV	J1250
Docefrez	1 mg		J9171
Docetaxel	20 mg	IV	J9171
Dolasetron mesylate			
injection	10 mg	IV	J1260
tablets	100 mg	ORAL	Q0180
Dolophine HCl	up to 10 mg	IM, SC	J1230
Dommanate	up to 50 mg	IM, IV	J1240
Donbax	10 mg		J1267
Dopamine	40 mg		J1265
Dopamine HCl	40 mg		J1265
Doribax	10 mg		J1267
Doripenem	10 mg	IV	J1267
Dornase alpha, unit dose form	per mg	INH	J7639
Dotarem	0.1 ml		A9575
Doxercalciferol	1 mcg	IV	J1270
Doxil	10 mg	IV	Q2048
Doxorubicin HCL	10 mg	IV	J9000
Dramamine	up to 50 mg	IM, IV	J1240
Dramanate	up to 50 mg	IM, IV	J1240
Dramilin	up to 50 mg	IM, IV	J1240
Dramocen	up to 50 mg	IM, IV	J1240
Dramoject	up to 50 mg	IM, IV	J1240
Dronabinol	2.5 mg	ORAL	Q0167

▶ New ↩ Revised ✔ Reinstated ~~deleted~~ Deleted

DRUG NAME	DOSAGE	METHOD OF ADMINISTRATION	HCPCS CODE
Droperidol	up to 5 mg	IM, IV	**J1790**
Droperidol and fentanyl citrate	up to 2 ml ampule	IM, IV	**J1810**
Droxia		ORAL	**J8999**
Drug administered through a metered dose inhaler		INH	**J3535**
DTIC-Dome	100 mg	IV	**J9130**
Dua-Gen L.A.	1 mg		**J3121**
DuoNeb	up to 2.5 mg		**J7620**
	up to 0.5 mg		**J7620**
Duoval P.A.	1 mg		**J3121**
Durabolin	up to 50 mg	IM	**J2320**
Duracillin A.S.	up to 600,000 units	IM, IV	**J2510**
Duraclon	1 mg	Epidural	**J0735**
Dura-Estrin	up to 5 mg	IM	**J1000**
Duragen-10	up to 10 mg	IM	**J1380**
Duragen-20	up to 10 mg	IM	**J1380**
Duragen-40	up to 10 mg	IM	**J1380**
Duralone-40	20 mg	IM	**J1020**
	40 mg	IM	**J1030**
	80 mg	IM	**J1040**
Duralone-80	20 mg	IM	**J1020**
	40 mg	IM	**J1030**
	80 mg	IM	**J1040**
Duralutin, *see* Hydroxyprogesterone Caproate			
Duramorph	up to 10 mg	IM, IV, SC	**J2270, J2274**
Duratest-100	1 mg		**J1071**
Duratest-200	1 mg		**J1071**
Duratestrin	1 mg		**J1071**
Durathate-200	1 mg		**J3121**
Dymenate	up to 50 mg	IM, IV	**J1240**
Dyphylline	up to 500 mg	IM	**J1180**
Dysport	5 units		**J0586**
Dalvance	5 mg		**J0875**
E			
Ecallantide	1 mg	SC	**J1290**
Eculizumab	10 mg	IV	**J1300**
Edetate calcium disodium	up to 1,000 mg	IV, SC, IM	**J0600**
Edetate disodium	per 150 mg	IV	**J3520**
Elaprase	1 mg		**J1743**
Elavil	up to 20 mg	IM	**J1320**
Elelyso	10 units		**J3060**
Eligard	7.5 mg		**J9217**
Elitek	0.5 mg		**J2783**
Ellence	2 mg		**J9178**

▶ **New** ⤾ **Revised** ✔ **Reinstated** ~~deleted~~ **Deleted**

DRUG NAME	DOSAGE	METHOD OF ADMINISTRATION	HCPCS CODE	
Elliotts B solution	1 ml	OTH	**J9175**	
Eloctate	per IU		**J7205**	
Elosulfase alfa	1 mg	IV	**J1322**	
Elotuzuman	1 mg	IV	**J9176**	◀
Eloxatin	0.5 mg		**J9263**	
Elspar	10,000 units	IV, IM	**J9020**	
Emend			**J1453, J8501**	
Emete-Con, *see* Benzquinamide				
Eminase	30 units	IV	**J0350**	
Enbrel	25 mg	IM, IV	**J1438**	
Endrate ethylenediamine-tetra-acetic acid	per 150 mg	IV	**J3520**	
Enfuvirtide	1 mg	SC	**J1324**	
Engerix-B			**J3490**	
Enovil	up to 20 mg	IM	**J1320**	
Enoxaparin sodium	10 mg	SC	**J1650**	
Eovist	1 ml		**A9581**	
Epinephrine			**J7799**	
Epinephrine, adrenalin	0.1 mg	SC, IM	**J0171**	
Epirubicin hydrochloride	2 mg		**J7799, J9178**	
Epoetin alfa	100 units	IV, SC	**Q4081**	↩
Epoetin alfa, non-ESRD use	1000 units	IV	**J0885**	◀
Epoetin beta, ESRD use	1 mcg	IV	**J0887**	
Epoetin beta, non-ESRD use	1 mcg	IV	**J0888**	
Epogen	1,000 units		**J0885**	
			Q4081	
Epoprostenol	0.5 mg	IV	**J1325**	
Eptifibatide, Injection	5 mg	IM, IV	**J1327**	
Eraxis	1 mg	IV	**J0348**	
Erbitux	10 mg		**J9055**	
Ergonovine maleate	up to 0.2 mg	IM, IV	**J1330**	
Eribulin mesylate	0.1 mg	IV	**J9179**	
Ertapenem sodium	500 mg	IM, IV	**J1335**	
Erwinase	1,000 units	IV, IM	**J9019**	
	10,000 units	IV, IM	**J9020**	
Erythromycin lactobionate	500 mg	IV	**J1364**	
Estra-D	up to 5 mg	IM	**J1000**	
Estradiol				
L.A.	up to 10 mg	IM	**J1380**	
L.A. 20	up to 10 mg	IM	**J1380**	
L.A. 40	up to 10 mg	IM	**J1380**	
Estradiol Cypionate	up to 5 mg	IM	**J1000**	
Estradiol valerate	up to 10 mg	IM	**J1380**	
Estragyn 5	per 1 mg		**J1435**	

▶ New ↩ Revised ✔ Reinstated ~~deleted~~ Deleted

DRUG NAME	DOSAGE	METHOD OF ADMINISTRATION	HCPCS CODE
Estra-L 20	up to 10 mg	IM	J1380
Estra-L 40	up to 10 mg	IM	J1380
Estra-Testrin	1 mg		J3121
Estro-Cyp	up to 5 mg	IM	J1000
Estrogen, conjugated	per 25 mg	IV, IM	J1410
Estroject L.A.	up to 5 mg	IM	J1000
Estrone	per 1 mg	IM	J1435
Estrone 5	per 1 mg	IM	J1435
Estrone Aqueous	per 1 mg	IM	J1435
Estronol	per 1 mg	IM	J1435
Estronol-L.A.	up to 5 mg	IM	J1000
Etanercept, Injection	25 mg	IM, IV	J1438
Ethamolin	100 mg		J1430
Ethanolamine	100 mg		J1430, J3490
Ethyol	500 mg	IV	J0207
Etidronate disodium	per 300 mg	IV	J1436
Etonogestrel implant			J7307
Etopophos	10 mg	IV	J9181
Etoposide	10 mg	IV	J9181
oral	50 mg	ORAL	J8560
Euflexxa	per dose	OTH	J7323
Everolimus	0.25 mg	ORAL	J7527
Everone	1 mg		J3121
Evomela	50 mg		J9245
Eylea	1 mg		J0178
Eylen	1 mg	OTH	J0178
F			
Fabrazyme	1 mg	IV	J0180
Factor IX			
anti-hemophilic factor, purified, non-recombinant	per IU	IV	J7193
anti-hemophilic factor, recombinant	per IU	IV	J7195, J7200-J7201
complex	per IU	IV	J7194
Factor X (human)	per IU	IV	J7175 ◀
Factor XIII A-subunit (recombinant)	per IU	IV	J7181
Factor VIIa (coagulation factor, recombinant)	1 mcg	IV	J7189
Factor VIII (anti-hemophilic factor)			
human	per IU	IV	J7190
porcine	per IU	IV	J7191
recombinant	per IU	IV	J7182, J7185, J7192, J7188
Factor VIII Fc fusion (recombinant)	per iu	IV	J7205, J7207, J7209 ↩
Factors, other hemophilia clotting	per IU	IV	J7196

▶ New ↩ Revised ✔ Reinstated ~~deleted~~ Deleted

DRUG NAME	DOSAGE	METHOD OF ADMINISTRATION	HCPCS CODE
Factrel	per 100 mcg	SC, IV	J1620
Famotidine			J3490
Faslodex	25 mg		J9395
Feiba VH Immuno	per IU	IV	J7196
Fentanyl citrate	0.1 mg	IM, IV	**J3010**
Feraheme	1 mg		Q0138, Q0139
Ferric carboxymaltose	1 mg	IV	**J1439**
Ferric pyrophosphate citrate solution	0.1 mg of iron	IV	**J1443**
Ferrlecit	12.5 mg		J2916
Ferumoxytol	1 mg		**Q0138, Q0139**
Filgrastim			
(G-CSF)	1 mcg	SC, IV	**J1442, Q5101**
(TBO)	1 mcg	IV	**J1447**
Firazyr	1 mg	SC	J1744
Firmagon	1 mg		J9155
Flebogamma	500 mg	IV	**J1572**
	1 cc		J1460
Flexoject	up to 60 mg	IV, IM	J2360
Flexon	up to 60 mg	IV, IM	J2360
Flolan	0.5 mg	IV	J1325
Flo-Pred	5 mg		J7510
Florbetaben f18, diagnostic	per study dose	IV	**Q9983** ◀
Floxuridine	500 mg	IV	**J9200**
Fluconazole	200 mg	IV	**J1450**
Fludara	1 mg	ORAL	**J8562**
	50 mg	IV	J9185
Fludarabine phosphate	50 mg	IV	**J9185**
Flunisolide inhalation solution, unit dose form	per mg	INH	**J7641**
Fluocinolone		OTH	**J7311, J7313**
Fluorouracil	500 mg	IV	**J9190**
Fluphenazine decanoate	up to 25 mg		J2680
Flutamide			J8999
Flutemetamol f18, diagnostic	per study dose	IV	**Q9982** ◀
Folex	5 mg	IA, IM, IT, IV	J9250
	50 mg	IA, IM, IT, IV	J9260
Folex PFS	5 mg	IA, IM, IT, IV	J9250
	50 mg	IA, IM, IT, IV	J9260
Follutein	per 1,000 USP units	IM	J0725
Folotyn	1 mg		J9307
Fomepizole	15 mg		**J1451**
Fomivirsen sodium	1.65 mg	Intraocular	**J1452**
Fondaparinux sodium	0.5 mg	SC	**J1652**

▶ New ⤼ Revised ✔ Reinstated ~~deleted~~ Deleted

DRUG NAME	DOSAGE	METHOD OF ADMINISTRATION	HCPCS CODE
Formoterol	12 mcg	INH	**J7640**
Formoterol fumarate	20 mcg	INH	**J7606**
	12 mcg		J7640
Fortaz	per 500 mg	IM, IV	J0713
Forteo	10 mcg		J3110
Fosaprepitant	1 mg	IV	**J1453**
Foscarnet sodium	per 1,000 mg	IV	**J1455**
Foscavir	per 1,000 mg	IV	J1455
Fosphenytoin	50 mg	IV	**Q2009**
Fragmin	per 2,500 IU		J1645
FUDR	500 mg	IV	J9200
Fulvestrant	25 mg	IM	**J9395**
Fungizone intravenous	50 mg	IV	J0285
Furomide M.D.	up to 20 mg	IM, IV	J1940
Furosemide	up to 20 mg	IM, IV	**J1940**
Fuzeon	1 mg		J1324
G			
Gablofen	10 mg		J0475
	50 mcg		J0476
Gadavist	0.1 ml		A9585
Gadoxetate disodium	1 ml	IV	**A9581**
Gallium nitrate	1 mg	IV	**J1457**
Galsulfase	1 mg	IV	**J1458**
Gamastan	1 cc	IM	J1460
	over 10 cc	IM	J1560
Gamma globulin	1 cc	IM	**J1460**
	over 10 cc	IM	**J1560**
Gammagard Liquid	500 mg	IV	**J1569**
Gammagard S/D			J1566
GammaGraft	per square centimeter		Q4111
Gammaplex	500 mg	IV	**J1557**
Gammar	1 cc	IM	J1460
	over 10 cc	IM	J1560
Gammar-IV, *see* Immune globin intravenous (human)			
Gamulin RH			
immune globulin, human	100 IU		J2791
	1 dose package, 300 mcg	IM	J2790
immune globulin, human, solvent detergent	100 IU	IV	J2792
Gamunex	500 mg	IV	**J1561**
Ganciclovir, implant	4.5 mg	OTH	**J7310**
Ganciclovir sodium	500 mg	IV	**J1570**
Ganirelix			J3490

▶ New ↩ Revised ✔ Reinstated ~~deleted~~ Deleted

DRUG NAME	DOSAGE	METHOD OF ADMINISTRATION	HCPCS CODE
Garamycin, gentamicin	up to 80 mg	IM, IV	J1580
Gastrografin	per ml		Q9963
Gatifloxacin	10 mg	IV	J1590
Gazyva	10 mg		J9301
Gefitinib	250 mg	ORAL	J8565
Gel-One	per dose	OTH	J7326
Gemcitabine HCl	200 mg	IV	J9201
Gemsar	200 mg	IV	J9201
Gemtuzumab ozogamicin	5 mg	IV	J9300
Gengraf	100 mg		J7502
	25 mg	ORAL	J7515
	250 mg		J7516
Genotropin	1 mg		J2941
Gentamicin Sulfate	up to 80 mg	IM, IV	J1580, J7699
Gentran	500 ml	IV	J7100
Gentran 75	500 ml	IV	J7110
Geodon	10 mg		J3486
Gesterol 50	per 50 mg		J2675
Glassia	10 mg	IV	J0257
Glatiramer Acetate	20 mg	SC	J1595
GlucaGen	per 1 mg		J1610
Glucagon HCl	per 1 mg	SC, IM, IV	J1610
Glukor	per 1,000 USP units	IM	J0725
Glycopyrrolate			
concentrated form	per 1 mg	INH	J7642
unit dose form	per 1 mg	INH	J7643
Gold sodium thiomalate	up to 50 mg	IM	J1600
Golimumab	1 mg	IV	J1602
Gonadorelin HCl	per 100 mcg	SC, IV	J1620
Gonal-F			J3490
Gonic	per 1,000 USP units	IM	J0725
Goserelin acetate implant	per 3.6 mg	SC	J9202
Graftjacket	per square centimeter		Q4107
Graftjacket express	1 cc		Q4113
Granisetron HCl			
injection	100 mcg	IV	J1626
oral	1 mg	ORAL	Q0166
Gynogen L.A. A10	up to 10 mg	IM	J1380
Gynogen L.A. A20	up to 10 mg	IM	J1380
Gynogen L.A. A40	up to 10 mg	IM	J1380
H			
Halaven	0.1 mg		J9179
Haldol	up to 5 mg	IM, IV	J1630

▶ New ⮐ Revised ✔ Reinstated ~~deleted~~ Deleted

DRUG NAME	DOSAGE	METHOD OF ADMINISTRATION	HCPCS CODE
Haloperidol	up to 5 mg	IM, IV	**J1630**
Haloperidol decanoate	per 50 mg	IM	**J1631**
Haloperidol Lactate	up to 5 mg		**J1630**
Hectoral	1 mcg	IV	**J1270**
Helixate FS	per IU		**J7192**
Hemin	1 mg		**J1640**
Hemofil M	per IU	IV	**J7190**
Hemophilia clotting factors (e.g., anti-inhibitors)	per IU	IV	**J7198**
NOC	per IU	IV	**J7199**
Hepagam B	0.5 ml	IM	**J1571**
	0.5 ml	IV	**J1573**
Heparin (Procine)	per 1,000 units		**J1644**
Heparin (Procine) Lock Flush	per 10 units		**J1642**
Heparin sodium	1,000 units	IV, SC	**J1644**
Heparin Sodium (Bovine)	per 1,000 units		**J1644**
Heparin Sodium Flush	per 10 units		**J1642**
Heparin sodium (heparin lock flush)	10 units	IV	**J1642**
Heparin Sodium (Procine)	per 1,000 units		**J1644**
Hep-Lock	10 units	IV	**J1642**
Hep-Lock U/P	10 units	IV	**J1642**
Herceptin	10 mg	IV	**J9355**
Hexabrix 320	per ml		**Q9967**
Hexadrol Phosphate	1 mg	IM, IV, OTH	**J1100**
Histaject	per 10 mg	IM, SC, IV	**J0945**
Histerone 50	up to 50 mg	IM	**J3140**
Histerone 100	up to 50 mg	IM	**J3140**
Histrelin			
acetate	10 mcg		**J1675**
implant	50 mg	OTH	**J9225, J9226**
Hizentra, *see* Immune globulin			
Humalog	per 5 units		**J1815**
	per 50 units		**J1817**
Human fibrinogen concentrate	100 mg	IV	**J7178**
Humate-P	per IU		**J7187**
Humatrope	1 mg		**J2941**
Humira	20 mg		**J0135**
Humulin	per 5 units		**J1815**
	per 50 units		**J1817**
Hyalgan		OTH	**J7321**
Hyaluronan or derivative	per dose	IV	**J7327**
Gel-Syn	0.1 mg	IA	**J7328** ↩
Gen Visc 850	1 mg	IA	**J7320** ↩
Hyaluronic Acid			**J3490**

▶ **New** ↩ **Revised** ✔ **Reinstated** ~~deleted~~ **Deleted**

DRUG NAME	DOSAGE	METHOD OF ADMINISTRATION	HCPCS CODE
Hyaluronidase	up to 150 units	SC, IV	**J3470**
Hyaluronidase			
ovine	up to 999 units	VAR	**J3471**
ovine	per 1000 units	VAR	**J3472**
recombinant	1 usp	SC	**J3473**
Hyate:C	per IU	IV	J7191
Hybolin Decanoate	up to 50 mg	IM	J2320
Hybolin Improved, *see* Nandrolone phenpropionate			
Hycamtin	0.25 mg	ORAL	J8705
	4 mg	IV	J9351
Hydralazine HCl	up to 20 mg	IV, IM	**J0360**
Hydrate	up to 50 mg	IM, IV	J1240
Hydrea			J8999
Hydrocortisone acetate	up to 25 mg	IV, IM, SC	**J1700**
Hydrocortisone sodium phosphate	up to 50 mg	IV, IM, SC	**J1710**
Hydrocortisone succinate sodium	up to 100 mg	IV, IM, SC	**J1720**
Hydrocortone Acetate	up to 25 mg	IV, IM, SC	J1700
Hydrocortone Phosphate	up to 50 mg	IM, IV, SC	J1710
Hydromorphone HCl	up to 4 mg	SC, IM, IV	**J1170**
Hydroxocobalamin	up to 1,000 mcg		J3420
Hydroxyprogesterone Caproate	1 mg	IM	**J1725**
Hydroxyurea			J8999
Hydroxyzine HCl	up to 25 mg	IM	**J3410**
Hydroxyzine Pamoate	25 mg	ORAL	**Q0177**
Hylan G-F 20		OTH	J7325
Hylenex	1 USP unit		J3473
Hymovis	1 mg	IA	**J7322** ◀
Hyoscyamine sulfate	up to 0.25 mg	SC, IM, IV	**J1980**
Hyperhep B			J3590
Hyperrho S/D	300 mcg		J2790
	100 IU		J2792
Hyperstat IV	up to 300 mg	IV	J1730
Hyper-Tet	up to 250 units	IM	J1670
HypRho-D	300 mcg	IM	J2790
			J2791
	50 mcg		J2788
Hyrexin-50	up to 50 mg	IV, IM	J1200
Hyzine-50	up to 25 mg	IM	J3410
I			
Ibandronate sodium	1 mg	IV	**J1740**
Ibuprofen	100 mg	IV	**J1741**
Ibutilide fumarate	1 mg	IV	**J1742**
Icatibant	1 mg	SC	**J1744**

▶ **New** ⤻ **Revised** ✔ **Reinstated** ~~deleted~~ **Deleted**

DRUG NAME	DOSAGE	METHOD OF ADMINISTRATION	HCPCS CODE
Idamycin	5 mg	IV	J9211
Idarubicin HCl	5 mg	IV	**J9211**
Idursulfase	1 mg	IV	**J1743**
Ifex	1 g	IV	J9208
Ifosfamide	1 g	IV	**J9208**
Ifosfamide/Mesna			J9999
Ilaris	1 mg		**J0638**
Iloprost	20 mcg	INH	**Q4074**
Ilotycin, *see* Erythromycin gluceptate			
Iluvien	0.01 mg		J7313
Imferon	50 mg		J1750, J1752
Imiglucerase	10 units	IV	**J1786**
Imitrex	6 mg	SC	J3030
Immune globulin			
Bivigam	500 mg	IV	**J1556**
Flebogamma	500 mg	IV	**J1572**
Gammagard Liquid	500 mg	IV	**J1569**
Gammaplex	500 mg	IV	**J1557**
Gamunex	500 mg	IV	**J1561**
HepaGam B	0.5 ml	IM	**J1571**
	0.5 ml	IV	**J1573**
Hizentra	100 mg	SC	**J1559**
Hyaluronidase, (HYQVIA)	100 mg	IV	**J1575**
NOS	500 mg	IV	**J1566, J1599**
Octagam	500 mg	IV	**J1568**
Privigen	500 mg	IV	**J1459**
Rhophylac	100 IU	IM	**J2791**
Subcutaneous	100 mg	SC	**J1562**
Immunosuppressive drug, not otherwise classified			**J7599**
Imuran	50 mg	ORAL	J7500
	100 mg		J7501
Inapsine	up to 5 mg	IM, IV	J1790
Incobotulinumtoxin type A	1 unit	IM	**J0588**
Increlex	1 mg		J2170
Inderal	up to 1 mg	IV	J1800
Infed	50 mg		J1750
Infergen	1 mcg	SC	J9212
Infliximab, Injection	10 mg	IM, IV	**J1745, Q5102** ↩
Infumorph	10 mg		J2274
Injectafer	1 mg		J1439
Innohep	1,000 iu	SC	J1655
Innovar	up to 2 ml ampule	IM, IV	J1810
Insulin	5 units	SC	**J1815**

▶ **New** ↩ **Revised** ✔ **Reinstated** ~~deleted~~ **Deleted**

DRUG NAME	DOSAGE	METHOD OF ADMINISTRATION	HCPCS CODE
Insulin-Humalog	per 50 units		J1817
Insulin lispro	50 units	SC	**J1817**
Intal	per 10 mg	INH	J7631, J7632
Integra			
Bilayer Matrix Wound Dressing (BMWD)	per square centimeter		Q4104
Dermal Regeneration Template (DRT)	per square centimeter		Q4105
Flowable Wound Matrix	1 cc		Q4114
Matrix	per square centimeter		Q4108
Integrilin	5 mg	IM, IV	J1327
Interferon alfa-2a, recombinant	3 million units	SC, IM	**J9213**
Interferon alfa-2b, recombinant	1 million units	SC, IM	**J9214**
Interferon alfa-n3 (human leukocyte derived)	250,000 IU	IM	**J9215**
Interferon alphacon-1, recombinant	1 mcg	SC	**J9212**
Interferon beta-1a	30 mcg	IM	**J1826**
	1 mcg	IM	**Q3027**
	1 mcg	SC	**Q3028**
Interferon beta-1b	0.25 mg	SC	**J1830**
Interferon gamma-1b	3 million units	SC	**J9216**
Intrauterine copper contraceptive		OTH	J7300
Intron-A	1 million units		J9214
Invanz	500 mg		J1335
Invega Sustenna	1 mg		J2426
Ipilimumab	1 mg	IV	**J9228**
Ipratropium bromide, unit dose form	per mg	INH	J3535, J7620, J7644, J7645
Irinotecan	20 mg	IV	**J9205, J9206** ↩
Iron dextran	50 mg	IV, IM	**J1750**
Iron sucrose	1 mg	IV	**J1756**
Irrigation solution for Tx of bladder calculi	per 50 ml	OTH	**Q2004**
Isavuconazonium	1 mg	IV	**J1833**
Isocaine HCl	per 10 ml	VAR	J0670
Isoetharine HCl			
concentrated form	per mg	INH	**J7647, J7648**
unit dose form	per mg	INH	**J7649, J7650**
Isoproterenol HCl			
concentrated form	per mg	INH	**J7657, J7658**
unit dose form	per mg	INH	**J7659, J7660**
Isovue-200	per ml		Q9966, Q9967
Istodax	1 mg		J9315
Isuprel			
concentrated form	per mg	INH	J7657, J7658
unit dose form	per mg	INH	J7659, J7660

▶ **New** ↩ **Revised** ✔ **Reinstated** ~~deleted~~ **Deleted**

DRUG NAME	DOSAGE	METHOD OF ADMINISTRATION	HCPCS CODE
Itraconazole	50 mg	IV	**J1835**
Ixabepilone	1 mg	IV	**J9207**
Ixempra	1 mg		**J9207**
J			
Jenamicin	up to 80 mg	IM, IV	**J1580**
Jetrea	0.125 mg		**J7316**
Jevtana	1 mg		**J9043**
K			
Kabikinase	per 250,000 IU	IV	**J2995**
Kadcyla	1 mg		**J9354**
Kalbitor	1 mg		**J1290**
Kaleinate	per 10 ml	IV	**J0610**
Kanamycin sulfate	up to 75 mg	IM, IV	**J1850**
	up to 500 mg	IM, IV	**J1840**
Kantrex	up to 75 mg	IM, IV	**J1850**
	up to 500 mg	IM, IV	**J1840**
Kay-Pred	up to 1 ml		**J2650**
Keflin	up to 1 g	IM, IV	**J1890**
Kefurox	per 750 mg		**J0697**
Kefzol	500 mg	IV, IM	**J0690**
Kenaject-40	per 10 mg	IM	**J3301**
	1 mg		**J3300**
Kenalog-10	per 10 mg	IM	**J3301**
	1 mg		**J3300**
Kenalog-40	per 10 mg	IM	**J3301**
	1 mg		**J3300**
Kepivance	50 mcg		**J2425**
Keppra	10 mg		**J1953**
Kestrone 5	per 1 mg	IM	**J1435**
Ketorolac tromethamine	per 15 mg	IM, IV	**J1885**
Key-Pred 25	up to 1 ml	IM	**J2650**
Key-Pred 50	up to 1 ml	IM	**J2650**
Key-Pred-SP, *see* Prednisolone sodium phosphate			
Keytruda	1 mg		**J9271**
K-Flex	up to 60 mg	IV, IM	**J2360**
Kitabis PAK	per 300 mg		**J7682**
Klebcil	up to 75 mg	IM, IV	**J1850**
	up to 500 mg	IM, IV	**J1840**
Koate-HP (anti-hemophilic factor)			
human	per IU	IV	**J7190**
porcine	per IU	IV	**J7191**
recombinant	per IU	IV	**J7192**

▶ **New** ⤾ **Revised** ✔ **Reinstated** ~~deleted~~ **Deleted**

DRUG NAME	DOSAGE	METHOD OF ADMINISTRATION	HCPCS CODE
Kogenate			
human	per IU	IV	**J7190**
porcine	per IU	IV	**J7191**
recombinant	per IU	IV	**J7192**
Konakion	per 1 mg	IM, SC, IV	**J3430**
Konyne-80	per IU	IV	**J7194, J7195**
Krystexxa	1 mg		**J2507**
Kyprolis	1 mg		**J9047**
Kytril	1 mg	ORAL	**Q0166**
	1 mg	IV	**S0091**
	100 mcg	IV	**J1626**
L			
Lactated Ringers	up to 1,000 cc		**J7120**
L.A.E. 20	up to 10 mg	IM	**J1380**
Laetrile, Amygdalin, vitamin B-17			**J3570**
Lanoxin	up to 0.5 mg	IM, IV	**J1160**
Lanreotide	1 mg	SC	**J1930**
Lantus	per 5 units		**J1815**
Largon, *see* Propiomazine HCl			
Laronidase	0.1 mg	IV	**J1931**
Lasix	up to 20 mg	IM, IV	**J1940**
L-Caine	10 mg	IV	**J2001**
LEMTRADA	1 mg		**J0202**
Lepirudin	50 mg		**J1945**
Leucovorin calcium	per 50 mg	IM, IV	**J0640**
Leukeran			**J8999**
Leukine	50mcg	IV	**J2820**
Leuprolide acetate	per 1 mg	IM	**J9218**
Leuprolide acetate (for depot suspension)	per 3.75 mg	IM	**J1950**
	7.5 mg	IM	**J9217**
Leuprolide acetate implant	65 mg	OTH	**J9219**
Leustatin	per mg	IV	**J9065**
Levalbuterol HCl			
concentrated form	0.5 mg	INH	**J7607, J7612**
unit dose form	0.5 mg	INH	**J7614, J7615**
Levaquin I.U.	250 mg	IV	**J1956**
Levemir	per 5 units		**J1815**
Levetiracetam	10 mg	IV	**J1953**
Levocarnitine	per 1 gm	IV	**J1955**
Levo-Dromoran	up to 2 mg	SC, IV	**J1960**
Levofloxacin	250 mg	IV	**J1956**
Levoleucovorin calcium	0.5 mg	IV	**J0641**
Levonorgestrel implant		OTH	**J7306**

▶ **New** ⮐ **Revised** ✔ **Reinstated** ~~deleted~~ **Deleted**

DRUG NAME	DOSAGE	METHOD OF ADMINISTRATION	HCPCS CODE
Levonorgestrel-releasing intrauterine contraceptive system	52 mg	OTH	J7297, J7298
Levorphanol tartrate	up to 2 mg	SC, IV	J1960
Levsin	up to 0.25 mg	SC, IM, IV	J1980
Levulan Kerastick	unit dose (354 mg)	OTH	J7308
Lexiscan	0.1 mg		J2785
Librium	up to 100 mg	IM, IV	J1990
Lidocaine HCl	10 mg	IV	J2001
Lidoject-1	10 mg	IV	J2001
Lidoject-2	10 mg	IV	J2001
Lincocin	up to 300 mg	IV	J2010
Lincomycin HCl	up to 300 mg	IV	J2010
Linezolid	200 mg	IV	J2020
Lioresal	10 mg	IT	J0475
			J0476
Lipodox			Q2049
Liquaemin Sodium	1,000 units	IV, SC	J1644
LMD (10%)	500 ml	IV	J7100
Lorazepam	2 mg	IM, IV	J2060
Lovenox	10 mg	SC	J1650
Lucentis	0.1 mg		J2778
Lufyllin	up to 500 mg	IM	J1180
Lumason	per ml		Q9950
Luminal Sodium	up to 120 mg	IM, IV	J2560
Lumizyme	10 mg		J0221
Lupon Depot	7.5 mg		J9217
	3.75 mg		J1950
Lupron	per 1 mg	IM	J9218
	per 3.75 mg	IM	J1950
	7.5 mg	IM	J9217
~~Lymphocyte immune globulin~~			
Lyophilized			J1566
M			
Macugen	0.3 mg		J2503
Magnesium sulfate	500 mg		J3475
Magnevist	per ml		A9579
Makena	1 mg		J1725
Mannitol	25% in 50 ml	IV	J2150
	5 mg	INH	J7665, J7799
Marcaine			J3490
Marinol	2.5 mg	ORAL	Q0167
Marmine	up to 50 mg	IM, IV	J1240
Maxipime	500 mg	IV	J0692
MD-76R	per ml		Q9963

▶ New ⤺ Revised ✔ Reinstated ~~deleted~~ Deleted

DRUG NAME	DOSAGE	METHOD OF ADMINISTRATION	HCPCS CODE
MD Gastroview	per ml		Q9963
Mecasermin	1 mg	SC	**J2170**
Mechlorethamine HCl (nitrogen mustard), HN2	10 mg	IV	**J9230**
Medralone 40	20 mg	IM	J1020
	40 mg	IM	J1030
	80 mg	IM	J1040
Medralone 80	20 mg	IM	J1020
	40 mg	IM	J1030
	80 mg	IM	J1040
Medrol	per 4 mg	ORAL	J7509
Medroxyprogesterone acetate	1 mg	IM	**J1050**
Mefoxin	1 g	IV, IM	J0694
Megace			J8999
Megestrol Acetate			J8999
Melphalan HCl	50 mg	IV	**J9245**
Melphalan, oral	2 mg	ORAL	**J8600**
Menoject LA	1 mg		J1071
Mepergan Injection	up to 50 mg	IM, IV	J2180
Meperidine and promethazine HCl	up to 50 mg	IM, IV	**J2180**
Meperidine HCl	per 100 mg	IM, IV, SC	**J2175**
Mepivacaine HCl	per 10 ml	VAR	**J0670**
Mepolizumab	1 mg	IV	**J2182** ◀
Mercaptopurine			J8999
Meropenem	100 mg	IV	**J2185**
Merrem	100 mg		J2185
Mesna	200 mg	IV	**J9209**
Mesnex	200 mg	IV	J9209
Metaprel			
concentrated form	per 10 mg	INH	J7667, J7668
unit dose form	per 10 mg	INH	J7669, J7670
Metaproterenol sulfate			
concentrated form	per 10 mg	INH	**J7667, J7668**
unit dose form	per 10 mg	INH	**J7669, J7670**
Metaraminol bitartrate	per 10 mg	IV, IM, SC	**J0380**
Metastron	per millicurie		A9600
Methacholine chloride	1 mg	INH	**J7674**
Methadone HCl	up to 10 mg	IM, SC	**J1230**
Methergine	up to 0.2 mg		J2210
Methocarbamol	up to 10 ml	IV, IM	**J2800**
Methotrexate LPF	5 mg	IV, IM, IT, IA	J9250
	50 mg	IV, IM, IT, IA	J9260
Methotrexate, oral	2.5 mg	ORAL	**J8610**

▶ New ↩ Revised ✔ Reinstated ~~deleted~~ Deleted

DRUG NAME	DOSAGE	METHOD OF ADMINISTRATION	HCPCS CODE
Methotrexate sodium	5 mg	IV, IM, IT, IA	**J9250**
	50 mg	IV, IM, IT, IA	**J9260**
Methyldopate HCl	up to 250 mg	IV	**J0210**
Methylergonovine maleate	up to 0.2 mg		**J2210**
Methylnaltrexone	0.1 mg	SC	**J2212**
Methylpred	20 mg		**J1020**
Methylprednisolone acetate	20 mg	IM	**J1020**
	40 mg	IM	**J1030**
	80 mg	IM	**J1040**
Methylprednisolone, oral	per 4 mg	ORAL	**J7509**
Methylprednisolone sodium succinate	up to 40 mg	IM, IV	**J2920**
	up to 125 mg	IM, IV	**J2930**
Metoclopramide HCl	up to 10 mg	IV	**J2765**
Metrodin	75 IU		**J3355**
Metronidazole			**J3490**
Metvixia	1 g	OTH	**J7309**
Miacalcin	up to 400 units	SC, IM	**J0630**
Micafungin sodium	1 mg		**J2248**
MicRhoGAM	50 mcg		**J2788**
Midazolam HCl	per 1 mg	IM, IV	**J2250**
Milrinone lactate	5 mg	IV	**J2260**
Minocine	1 mg		**J2265**
Minocycline Hydrochloride	1 mg	IV	**J2265**
Mio-Rel	up to 60 mg		**J2360**
Mircera	1 mcg		**J0887, J0888**
Mirena	52 mg	OTH	**J7297, J7298**
Mithracin	2,500 mcg	IV	**J9270**
Mitomycin	0.2 mg	Ophthalmic	**J7315**
	5 mg	IV	**J9280**
Mitosol	0.2 mg	Ophthalmic	**J7315**
	5 mg	IV	**J9280**
Mitoxantrone HCl	per 5 mg	IV	**J9293**
Monocid, *see* Cefonicic sodium			
Monoclate-P			
human	per IU	IV	**J7190**
porcine	per IU	IV	**J7191**
Monoclonal antibodies, parenteral	5 mg	IV	**J7505**
Mononine	per IU	IV	**J7193**
Morphine sulfate	up to 10 mg	IM, IV, SC	**J2270**
preservative-free	10 mg	SC, IM, IV	**J1174**
Moxifloxacin	100 mg	IV	**J2280**
Mozobil	1 mg		**J2562**

▶ **New** ⤾ **Revised** ✔ **Reinstated** ~~deleted~~ **Deleted**

DRUG NAME	DOSAGE	METHOD OF ADMINISTRATION	HCPCS CODE
M-Prednisol-40	20 mg	IM	J1020
	40 mg	IM	J1030
	80 mg	IM	J1040
M-Prednisol-80	20 mg	IM	J1020
	40 mg	IM	J1030
	80 mg	IM	J1040
Mucomyst			
unit dose form	per gram	INH	J7604, J7608
Mucosol			
injection	100 mg	IV	J0132
unit dose	per gram	INH	J7604, J7608
MultiHance	per ml		A9577
MultiHance Multipack	per ml		A9578
Muromonab-CD3	5 mg	IV	J7505
Muse		OTH	J0275
	1.25 mcg	OTH	J0270
Mustargen	10 mg	IV	J9230
Mutamycin	5 mg	IV	J9280
Mycamine	1 mg		J2248
Mycophenolate Mofetil	250 mg	ORAL	J7517
Mycophenolic acid	180 mg	ORAL	J7518
Myfortic	180 mg		J7518
Myleran	1 mg		J0594
	2 mg	ORAL	J8510
Mylotarg	5 mg	IV	J9300
Myobloc	per 100 units	IM	J0587
Myochrysine	up to 50 mg	IM	J1600
Myolin	up to 60 mg	IV, IM	J2360
N			
Nabi-HB			J3590
Nabilone	1 mg	ORAL	J8650
Nafcillin			J3490
Naglazyme	1 mg		J1458
Nalbuphine HCl	per 10 mg	IM, IV, SC	J2300
Nalojix	1 mg		J0485
Naloxone HCl	per 1 mg	IM, IV, SC	J2310, J3490
Naltrexone			J3490
Naltrexone, depot form	1 mg	IM	J2315
Nandrobolic L.A.	up to 50 mg	IM	J2320
Nandrolone decanoate	up to 50 mg	IM	J2320
Narcan	1 mg	IM, IV, SC	J2310

▶ New ↩ Revised ✔ Reinstated ~~deleted~~ Deleted

DRUG NAME	DOSAGE	METHOD OF ADMINISTRATION	HCPCS CODE
Naropin	1 mg		J2795
Nasahist B	per 10 mg	IM, SC, IV	J0945
Nasal vaccine inhalation		INH	J3530
Natalizumab	1 mg	IV	J2323
Natrecor	0.1 mg		J2325
Navane, *see* Thiothixene			
Navelbine	per 10 mg	IV	J9390
ND Stat	per 10 mg	IM, SC, IV	J0945
Nebcin	up to 80 mg	IM, IV	J3260
	per 300 mg		J7682
NebuPent	per 300 mg	INH	J2545, J7676
Necitumumab	1 mg	IV	J9295 ◀
Nelarabine	50 mg	IV	J9261
Nembutal Sodium Solution	per 50 mg	IM, IV, OTH	J2515
Neocyten	up to 60 mg	IV, IM	J2360
Neo-Durabolic	up to 50 mg	IM	J2320
Neoquess	up to 20 mg	IM	J0500
Neoral	100 mg		J7502
	25 mg		J7515
Neosar	100 mg	IV	J9070
Neostigmine methylsulfate	up to 0.5 mg	IM, IV, SC	J2710
Neo-Synephrine	up to 1 ml	SC, IM, IV	J2370
Nervocaine 1%	10 mg	IV	J2001
Nervocaine 2%	10 mg	IV	J2001
Nesacaine	per 30 ml	VAR	J2400
Nesacaine-MPF	per 30 ml	VAR	J2400
Nesiritide	0.1 mg	IV	J2325
Netupitant 300 mg and palonosetron 0.5 mg		ORAL	J8655
Neulasta	6 mg		J2505
Neumega	5 mg	SC	J2355
Neupogen			
(G-CSF)	1 mcg	SC, IV	J1442
Neuroforte-R	up to 1,000 mcg		J3420
Neutrexin	per 25 mg	IV	J3305
Nipent	per 10 mg	IV	J9268
Nivolumab	1 mg	IV	J9299
Nolvadex			J8999
Nordryl	up to 50 mg	IV, IM	J1200
	50 mg	ORAL	Q0163
Norflex	up to 60 mg	IV, IM	J2360
Norzine	up to 10 mg	IM	J3280

▶ New ↩ Revised ✔ Reinstated ~~deleted~~ Deleted

DRUG NAME	DOSAGE	METHOD OF ADMINISTRATION	HCPCS CODE
Not otherwise classified drugs			J3490
other than inhalation solution administered through DME			J7799
inhalation solution administered through DME			J7699
anti-neoplastic			J9999
chemotherapeutic		ORAL	J8999
immunosuppressive			J7599
nonchemotherapeutic		ORAL	J8499
Novantrone	per 5 mg	IV	J9293
Novarel	per 1,000 USP Units		J0725
Novolin	per 5 units		J1815
	per 50 units		J1817
Novolog	per 5 units		J1815
	per 50 units		J1817
Novo Seven	1 mcg	IV	J7189
NPH	5 units	SC	J1815
Nplate	100 units		J0587
	10 mcg		J2796
Nubain	per 10 mg	IM, IV, SC	J2300
Nulecit	12.5 mg		J2916
Nulicaine	10 mg	IV	J2001
Nulojix	1 mg	IV	J0485
Numorphan	up to 1 mg	IV, SC, IM	J2410
Numorphan H.P.	up to 1 mg	IV, SC, IM	J2410
Nutropin	1 mg		J2941
O			
Oasis Burn Matrix	per square centimeter		Q4103
Oasis Wound Matrix	per square centimeter		Q4102
Obinutuzumab	10 mg		J9301
Ocriplasmin	0.125 mg	IV	J7316
Octagam	500 mg	IV	J1568
Octreotide Acetate, Injection	1 mg	IM	J2353
	25 mcg	IV, SQ	J2354
Oculinum	per unit	IM	J0585
Ofatumumab	10 mg		J9302
Ofirmev	10 mg	IV	J0131
O-Flex	up to 60 mg	IV, IM	J2360
Oforta	10 mg		J8562
Olanzapine	1 mg	IM	J2358
Omacetaxine Mepesuccinate	0.01 mg	IV	J9262
Omalizumab	5 mg	SC	J2357
Omnipaque	per ml		Q9965, Q9966, Q9967

▶ New ↩ Revised ✔ Reinstated ~~deleted~~ Deleted

DRUG NAME	DOSAGE	METHOD OF ADMINISTRATION	HCPCS CODE
Omnipen-N	up to 500 mg	IM, IV	J0290
	per 1.5 gm	IM, IV	J0295
Omniscan	per ml		A9579
Omnitrope	1 mg		J2941
Omontys	0.1 mg	IV, SC	J0890
OnabotulinumtoxinA	1 unit	IM	J0585
Oncaspar	per single dose vial	IM, IV	J9266
Oncovin	1 mg	IV	J9370
Ondansetron HCl	1 mg	IV	J2405
	1 mg	ORAL	Q0162
Opana	up to 1 mg		J2410
Opdivo	1 mg		J9299
Oprelvekin	5 mg	SC	J2355
Optimark	per ml		A9579
Optiray	per ml		Q9966, Q9967
Optison	per ml		Q9956
Oraminic II	per 10 mg	IM, SC, IV	J0945
Orapred	per 5 mg	ORAL	J7510
Orbactiv	10 mg		J2407
Orencia	10 mg		J0129
Orfro	up to 60 mg		J2360
Oritavancin	10 mg	IV	J2407
Ormazine	up to 50 mg	IM, IV	J3230
Orphenadrine citrate	up to 60 mg	IV, IM	J2360
Orphenate	up to 60 mg	IV, IM	J2360
Orthovisc		OTH	J7324
Or-Tyl	up to 20 mg	IM	J0500
Osmitrol			J7799
Ovidrel			J3490
Oxacillin sodium	up to 250 mg	IM, IV	J2700
Oxaliplatin	0.5 mg	IV	J9263
Oxilan	per ml		Q9967
Oxymorphone HCl	up to 1 mg	IV, SC, IM	J2410
Oxytetracycline HCl	up to 50 mg	IM	J2460
Oxytocin	up to 10 units	IV, IM	J2590
Ozurdex	0.1 mg		J7312
P			
Paclitaxel	1 mg	IV	J9267
Paclitaxel protein-bound particles	1 mg	IV	J9264
Palifermin	50 mcg	IV	J2425
Paliperidone Palmitate	1 mg	IM	J2426
Palonosetron HCl	25 mcg	IV	J2469
Pamidronate disodium	per 30 mg	IV	J2430

▶ New ⤺ Revised ✔ Reinstated ~~deleted~~ Deleted

DRUG NAME	DOSAGE	METHOD OF ADMINISTRATION	HCPCS CODE
Panhematin	1 mg		J1640
Panitumumab	10 mg	IV	J9303
Papaverine HCl	up to 60 mg	IV, IM	J2440
Paragard T 380 A		OTH	J7300
Paraplatin	50 mg	IV	J9045
Paricalcitol, Injection	1 mcg	IV, IM	J2501
Pasireotide, long acting	1 mg	IV	J2502
Pediapred	per 5 mg	ORAL	J7510
Peforomist	20 mcg		J7606
Pegademase bovine	25 IU		J2504
Pegaptinib	0.3 mg	OTH	J2503
Pegaspargase	per single dose vial	IM, IV	J9266
Pegasys			J3490
Pegfilgrastim	6 mg	SC	J2505
Peginesatide	0.1 mg	IV, SC	J0890
Peg-Intron			J3490
Pegloticase	1 mg	IV	J2507
Pembrolizumab	1 mg	IV	J9271
Pemetrexed	10 mg	IV	J9305
Penicillin G benzathine	up to 100,000 units	IM	J0561
Penicillin G benzathine and penicillin G procaine	100,000 units	IM	J0558
Penicillin G potassium	up to 600,000 units	IM, IV	J2540
Penicillin G procaine, aqueous	up to 600,000 units	IM, IV	J2510
Penicillin G Sodium			J3490
Pentam	per 300 mg		J7676
Pentamidine isethionate	per 300 mg	INH, IM	J2545, J7676
Pentastarch, 10%	100 ml		J2513
Pentazocine HCl	30 mg	IM, SC, IV	J3070
Pentobarbital sodium	per 50 mg	IM, IV, OTH	J2515
Pentostatin	per 10 mg	IV	J9268
Peramivir	1 mg	IV	J2547
Perjeta	1 mg		J9306
Permapen	up to 600,000	IM	J0561
Perphenazine			
injection	up to 5 mg	IM, IV	J3310
tablets	4 mg	ORAL	Q0175
Persantine IV	per 10 mg	IV	J1245
Pertuzumab	1 mg	IV	J9306
Pet Imaging ◀			
Gallium Ga-68, dotatate, diagnostic ◀	0.1 millicurie	IV	A9587
Fluciclovine F-18, diagnostic ◀	1 millcurie	IV	A9588

▶ New ↩ Revised ✔ Reinstated ~~deleted~~ Deleted

DRUG NAME	DOSAGE	METHOD OF ADMINISTRATION	HCPCS CODE	
Pfizerpen	up to 600,000 units	IM, IV	**J2540**	
Pfizerpen A.S.	up to 600,000 units	IM, IV	**J2510**	
Phenadoz			**J8498**	
Phenazine 25	up to 50 mg	IM, IV	**J2550**	
	12.5 mg	ORAL	**Q0169**	
Phenazine 50	up to 50 mg	IM, IV	**J2550**	
	12.5 mg	ORAL	**Q0169**	
Phenergan	12.5 mg	ORAL	**Q0169**	
	up to 50 mg	IM, IV	**J2550**	
			J8498	
Phenobarbital sodium	up to 120 mg	IM, IV	**J2560**	
Phentolamine mesylate	up to 5 mg	IM, IV	**J2760**	
Phenylephrine HCl	up to 1 ml	SC, IM, IV	**J2370, J7799**	
Phenytoin sodium	per 50 mg	IM, IV	**J1165**	
Photofrin	75 mg	IV	**J9600**	
Phytonadione (Vitamin K)	per 1 mg	IM, SC, IV	**J3430**	
Piperacillin/Tazobactam Sodium, Injection	1.125 g	IV	**J2543, J3490**	
Pitocin	up to 10 units	IV, IM	**J2590**	
Plantinol AQ	10 mg	IV	**J9060**	
Plasma				
cryoprecipitate reduced	each unit	IV	**P9044**	
pooled multiple donor, frozen	each unit	IV	**P9023, P9070**	
(single donor), pathogen reduced, frozen	each unit	IV	**P9071**	
Plas+SD	each unit	IV	**P9023**	
Platelets, pheresis, pathogen reduced	each unit	IV	**P9072**	
Platinol	10 mg	IV, IM	**J9060**	
Plerixafor	1 mg	SC	**J2562**	
Plicamycin	2,500 mcg	IV	**J9270**	
Polocaine	per 10 ml	VAR	**J0670**	
Polycillin-N	up to 500 mg	IM, IV	**J0290**	
	per 1.5 gm	IM, IV	**J0295**	
Polygam	500 mg		**J1566**	
Porfimer Sodium	75 mg	IV	**J9600**	
Positron emission tomography radiopharmaceutical, diagnostic				◀
for non-tumor identification, NOC		IV	**A9598**	◀
for tumor identification, NOC		IV	**A9597**	◀
Potassium chloride	per 2 mEq	IV	**J3480**	
Pralatrexate	1 mg	IV	**J9307**	
Pralidoxime chloride	up to 1 g	IV, IM, SC	**J2730**	
Predalone-50	up to 1 ml	IM	**J2650**	
Predcor-25	up to 1 ml	IM	**J2650**	
Predcor-50	up to 1 ml	IM	**J2650**	
Predicort-50	up to 1 ml	IM	**J2650**	

▶ New ↻ Revised ✔ Reinstated ~~deleted~~ Deleted

DRUG NAME	DOSAGE	METHOD OF ADMINISTRATION	HCPCS CODE
Prednisolone acetate	up to 1 ml	IM	**J2650**
Prednisolone, oral	5 mg	ORAL	**J7510**
Prednisone, immediate release or delayed release	1 mg	ORAL	**J7512**
Predoject-50	up to 1 ml	IM	J2650
Pregnyl	per 1,000 USP units	IM	J0725
Prelone	5 mg		J7510
Premarin Intravenous	per 25 mg	IV, IM	J1410
Prescription, chemotherapeutic, not otherwise specified		ORAL	**J8999**
Prescription, nonchemotherapeutic, not otherwise specified		ORAL	**J8499**
Prialt	1 mcg		J2278
Primacor	5 mg	IV	J2260
Primatrix	per square centimeter		Q4110
Primaxin	per 250 mg	IV, IM	J0743
Priscoline HCl	up to 25 mg	IV	J2670
Privigen	500 mg	IV	**J1459**
Procainamide HCl	up to 1 g	IM, IV	**J2690**
Prochlorperazine	up to 10 mg	IM, IV	**J0780**
			J8498
Prochlorperazine maleate	5 mg	ORAL	**Q0164**
			S0183
Procrit			J0885
			Q4081
Pro-Depo, *see* Hydroxyprogesterone Caproate			
Profasi HP	per 1,000 USP units	IM	J0725
Profilnine Heat-Treated	per IU	IV	J7194
Profilnine-SD	per IU		J7193, J7194, J7195
Progestaject	per 50 mg		J2675
Progesterone	per 50 mg	IM	**J2675**
Prograf			
oral	1 mg	ORAL	J7507
parenteral	5 mg		J7525
Prohance Multipack	per ml		A9576
Prokine	50 mcg	IV	J2820
Prolastin	10 mg	IV	J0256
Proleukin	per single use vial	IM, IV	J9015
Prolia	1 mg		J0897
Prolixin Decanoate	up to 25 mg	IM, SC	J2680
Promazine HCl	up to 25 mg	IM	**J2950**
Promethazine			J8498
Promethazine HCl			
injection	up to 50 mg	IM, IV	**J2550**
oral	12.5 mg	ORAL	**Q0169**

▶ New ↩ Revised ✔ Reinstated ~~deleted~~ Deleted

DRUG NAME	DOSAGE	METHOD OF ADMINISTRATION	HCPCS CODE
Promethegan			J8498
Pronestyl	up to 1 g	IM, IV	J2690
Proplex SX-T			
non-recombinant	per IU	IV	J7193
recombinant	per IU	IV	J7195
complex	per IU	IV	J7194
Proplex T			
complex	per IU	IV	J7194
non-recombinant	per IU	IV	J7193
recombinant	per IU	IV	J7195
Propofol	10 mg	IV	J2704
Propranolol HCl	up to 1 mg	IV	J1800
Prorex-25			
	up to 50 mg	IM, IV	J2550
	12.5 mg	ORAL	Q0169
Prorex-50	up to 50 mg	IM, IV	J2550
	12.5 mg	ORAL	Q0169
Prostaglandin E1	per 1.25 mcg		J0270
Prostaphlin	up to 1 g	IM, IV	J2690
Prostigmin	up to 0.5 mg	IM, IV, SC	J2710
Protamine sulfate	per 10 mg	IV	J2720
Protein C Concentrate	10 IU	IV	J2724
Prothazine	up to 50 mg	IM, IV	J2550
	12.5 mg	ORAL	Q0169
Protirelin	per 250 mcg	IV	J2725
Protonix			J3490
Protopam Chloride	up to 1 g	IV, IM, SC	J2730
Proventil			
concentrated form	1 mg	INH	J7610, J7611
unit dose form	1 mg	INH	J7609, J7613
Provocholine	per 1 mg		J7674
Prozine-50	up to 25 mg	IM	J2950
Pulmicort	0.25 mg	INH	J7633
Pulmicort Respules	0.5 mg	INH	J7626, J7627
	per 0.25 mg		J7633
noncompounded, concentrated	up to 0.5 mg	INH	J7626
Pulmozyme	per mg		J7639
Pyridoxine HCl	100 mg		J3415
Q			
Quelicin	up to 20 mg	IV, IM	J0330
Quinupristin/dalfopristin	500 mg (150/350)	IV	J2770
Qutenza	per square cm		J7336

▶ New ⤾ Revised ✔ Reinstated ~~deleted~~ Deleted

DRUG NAME	DOSAGE	METHOD OF ADMINISTRATION	HCPCS CODE
R			
Ramucirumab	5 mg	IV	**J9308**
Ranibizumab	0.1 mg	OTH	**J2778**
Ranitidine HCl, Injection	25 mg	IV, IM	**J2780**
Rapamune	1 mg	ORAL	**J7520**
Rasburicase	0.5 mg	IV	**J2783**
Rebif	11 mcg		**Q3026**
Reclast	1 mg		**J3489**
Recombinate anti-hemophilic factor			
human	per IU	IV	**J7190**
porcine	per IU	IV	**J7191**
recombinant	per IU	IV	**J7192**
Recombivax			**J3490**
Redisol	up to 1,000 mcg	IM, SC	**J3420**
Refacto	per IU		**J7192**
Refludan	50 mg		**J1945**
Regadenoson	0.1 mg	IV	**J2785**
Regitine	up to 5 mg	IM, IV	**J2760**
Reglan	up to 10 mg	IV	**J2765**
Regular	5 units	SC	**J1815**
Relefact TRH	per 250 mcg	IV	**J2725**
Relistor	0.1 mg	SC	**J2212**
Remicade	10 mg	IM, IV	**J1745**
Remodulin	1 mg		**J3285**
Reno-60	per ml		**Q9961**
Reno-Dip	per ml		**Q9958**
ReoPro	10 mg	IV	**J0130**
Rep-Pred 40	20 mg	IM	**J1020**
	40 mg	IM	**J1030**
	80 mg	IM	**J1040**
Rep-Pred 80	20 mg	IM	**J1020**
	40 mg	IM	**J1030**
	80 mg	IM	**J1040**
Resectisol			**J7799**
Reslizumab	1 mg	IV	**J2786** ◄
Retavase	18.1 mg	IV	**J2993**
Reteplase	18.1 mg	IV	**J2993**
Retisert			**J7311**
Retrovir	10 mg	IV	**J3485**
Rheomacrodex	500 ml	IV	**J7100**
Rhesonativ	300 mcg	IM	**J2790**
	50 mg		**J2788**
Rheumatrex Dose Pack	2.5 mg	ORAL	**J8610**

► **New** ⤾ **Revised** ✔ **Reinstated** ~~deleted~~ **Deleted**

DRUG NAME	DOSAGE	METHOD OF ADMINISTRATION	HCPCS CODE
Rho(D)			
immune globulin		IM, IV	**J2791**
immune globulin, human	1 dose package/ 300 mcg	IM	**J2790**
	50 mg	IM	**J2788**
immune globulin, human, solvent detergent	100 IU	IU, IV	**J2792**
RhoGAM	300 mcg	IM	J2790
	50 mg		J2788
Rhophylac	100 IU	IM, IV	**J2791**
Riastap	100 mg		**J7178**
Rifadin			J3490
Rifampin			J3490
Rilonacept	1 mg	SC	**J2793**
RimabotulinumtoxinB	100 units	IM	**J0587**
Rimso-50	50 ml		J1212
Ringers lactate infusion	up to 1,000 cc	IV	**J7120, J7121**
Risperdal Costa	0.5 mg		J2794
Risperidone	0.5 mg	IM	**J2794**
Rituxan	100 mg	IV	J9310
Rituximab	100 mg	IV	**J9310**
Robaxin	up to 10 ml	IV, IM	J2800
Robinul	per mg		J7643
Rocephin	per 250 mg	IV, IM	J0696
Rodex	100 mg		J3415
Roferon-A	3 million units	SC, IM	J9213
Rolapitant, oral, 1 mg	1 mg	ORAL	**J8670** ◀
Romidepsin	1 mg	IV	**J9315**
Romiplostim	10 mcg	SC	**J2796**
Ropivacaine Hydrochloride	1 mg	OTH	**J2795**
Rubex	10 mg	IV	J9000
Rubramin PC	up to 1,000 mcg	IM, SC	J3420
S			
Saizen	1 mg		J2941
Saline solution	10 ml		A4216
5% dextrose	500 ml	IV	**J7042**
infusion	250 cc	IV	**J7050**
	1,000 cc	IV	**J7030**
sterile	500 ml = 1 unit	IV, OTH	**J7040**
Sandimmune	25 mg	ORAL	J7515
	100 mg	ORAL	J7502
	250 mg	OTH	J7516
Sandoglobulin, *see* Immune globin intravenous (human)			

▶ **New** ⮌ **Revised** ✔ **Reinstated** ~~deleted~~ **Deleted**

DRUG NAME	DOSAGE	METHOD OF ADMINISTRATION	HCPCS CODE
Sandostatin, Lar Depot	25 mcg		J2354
	1 mg	IM	J2353
Sargramostim (GM-CSF)	50 mcg	IV	**J2820**
Sculptra	0.5 mg	IV	**Q2028**
Sebelelipase alfa	1 mg	IV	**J2840** ◀
Selestoject	per 4 mg	IM, IV	J0702
Sensorcaine MPF			J3490
Sermorelin acetate	1 mcg	SC	**Q0515**
Serostim	1 mg		J2941
Siltuximab	10 mg	IV	**J2860**
Simponi Aria	1 mg		J1602
Simulect	20 mg		J0480
Sincalide	5 mcg	IV	**J2805**
Sinografin	per ml		Q9963
Sinusol-B	per 10 mg	IM, SC, IV	J0945
Sirolimus	1 mg	ORAL	**J7520**
Sivextro	1 mg		J3090
Skyla	13.5 mg	OTH	**J7301**
Smz-TMP			J3490
Sodium Chloride	1,000 cc		J7030
	10 ml		A4216
	500 ml = 1 unit		J7040
	500 ml		A4217
	250 cc		J7050
inhalation solution			J7699
Sodium Chloride Bacteriostatic	10 ml		A4216
Sodium Chloride Concentrate			J7799
Sodium ferricgluconate in sucrose	12.5 mg		**J2916**
Sodium Hyaluronate			J3490
Euflexxa			**J7323**
Hyalgan			**J7321**
Orthovisc			**J7324**
Supartz			**J7321**
Solganal	up to 50 mg	IM	J2910
Soliris	10 mg		J1300
Solu-Cortef	up to 50 mg	IV, IM, SC	J1710
	100 mg		J1720
Solu-Medrol	up to 40 mg	IM, IV	J2920
	up to 125 mg	IM, IV	J2930
Solurex	1 mg	IM, IV, OTH	J1100
Solurex LA	1 mg	IM	J1094
Somatrem	1 mg	SC	**J2940**
Somatropin	1 mg	SC	**J2941**

▶ **New** ⤾ **Revised** ✔ **Reinstated** ~~deleted~~ **Deleted**

DRUG NAME	DOSAGE	METHOD OF ADMINISTRATION	HCPCS CODE
Somatulin Depot	1 mg		**J1930**
Sparine	up to 25 mg	IM	J2950
Spasmoject	up to 20 mg	IM	J0500
Spectinomycin HCl	up to 2 g	IM	**J3320**
Sporanox	50 mg	IV	**J1835**
Stadol	1 mg		J0595
Staphcillin, *see* Methicillin sodium			
Stelara	1 mg		J3357
Stilphostrol	250 mg	IV	J9165
Streptase	250,000 IU	IV	J2995
Streptokinase	per 250,000	IU, IV	**J2995**
Streptomycin	up to 1 g	IM	**J3000**
Streptomycin Sulfate	up to 1 g	IM	J3000
Streptozocin	1 gm	IV	**J9320**
Strontium-89 chloride	per millicurie		**A9600**
Sublimaze	0.1 mg	IM, IV	J3010
Succinylcholine chloride	up to 20 mg	IV, IM	**J0330**
Infection, sulfur hexafluoride lipid microspheres	per ml	IV	**Q9950**
Sufentanil Citrate			J3490
Sumarel Dosepro	6 mg		J3030
Sumatriptan succinate	6 mg	SC	**J3030**
Supartz		OTH	**J7321**
Surostrin	up to 20 mg	IV, IM	**J0330**
Sus-Phrine	up to 1 ml ampule	SC, IM	J0171
Synercid	500 mg (150/350)	IV	J2770
Synkavite	per 1 mg	IM, SC, IV	J3430
Syntocinon	up to 10 units	IV, IM	J2590
Synvisc and Synvisc-One	1 mg	OTH	**J7325**
Syrex	10 ml		A4216
Sytobex	1,000 mcg	IM, SC	J3420
T			
Tacrolimus			
(Envarsus XR)	0.25 mg	ORAL	**J7503**
oral, extended release	0.1 mg	ORAL	**J7508**
oral, immediate release	1 mg	ORAL	**J7507**
parenteral	5 mg	IV	**J7525**
Taliglucerace Alfa	10 units	IV	**J3060**
Talimogene laherparepvec	per 1 million plaque forming units	IV	**J9325**
Talwin	30 mg	IM, SC, IV	J3070
Tamoxifen Citrate			J8999
Taractan, *see* Chlorprothixene			
Taxol	1 mg	IV	J9267

▶ New ↩ Revised ✔ Reinstated ~~deleted~~ Deleted

DRUG NAME	DOSAGE	METHOD OF ADMINISTRATION	HCPCS CODE
Taxotere	20 mg	IV	J9171
Tazicef	per 500 mg		J0713
Tazidime, *see* Ceftazidime Technetium TC Sestambi	per dose		**A9500**
			J0713
Tedizolid phosphate	1 mg	IV	**J3090**
TEEV	1 mg		J3121
Teflaro	1 mg		J0712
Telavancin	10 mg	IV	**J3095**
Temodar	5 mg	ORAL	J8700, J9328
Temozolomide	1 mg	IV	**J9328**
	5 mg	ORAL	**J8700**
Temsirolimus	1 mg	IV	**J9330**
Tenecteplase	1 mg	IV	**J3101**
Teniposide	50 mg		**Q2017**
Tequin	10 mg	IV	J1590
Terbutaline sulfate	up to 1 mg	SC, IV	**J3105**
concentrated form	per 1 mg	INH	**J7680**
unit dose form	per 1 mg	INH	**J7681**
Teriparatide	10 mcg	SC	**J3110**
Terramycin IM	up to 50 mg	IM	J2460
Testa-C	1 mg		J1071
Testadiate	1 mg		J3121
Testadiate-Depo	1 mg		J1071
Testaject-LA	1 mg		J1071
Testaqua	up to 50 mg	IM	J3140
Test-Estro Cypionates	1 mg		J1071
Test-Estro-C	1 mg		J1071
Testex	up to 100 mg	IM	J3150
Testo AQ	up to 50 mg		J3140
Testoject-50	up to 50 mg	IM	J3140
Testoject-LA	1 mg		J1071
Testone			
LA 200	1 mg		J3121
LA 100	1 mg		J3121
Testosterone Aqueous	up to 50 mg	IM	J3140
Testosterone cypionate	1 mg	IM	**J1071**
Testosterone enanthate	1 mg	IM	**J3121**
Testosterone undecanoate	1 mg	IM	**J3145**
Testradiol 90/4	1 mg		J3121
Testrin PA	1 mg		J3121
Testro AQ	up to 50 mg		J3140
Tetanus immune globulin, human	up to 250 units	IM	**J1670**
Tetracycline	up to 250 mg	IM, IV	**J0120**

▶ **New** ↩ **Revised** ✔ **Reinstated** ~~deleted~~ **Deleted**

DRUG NAME	DOSAGE	METHOD OF ADMINISTRATION	HCPCS CODE
Tev-Tropin	1 mg		J2941
Thallous Chloride TI-201	per MCI		A9505
Theelin Aqueous	per 1 mg	IM	J1435
Theophylline	per 40 mg	IV	J2810
TheraCys	per vial	IV	J9031
Thiamine HCl	100 mg		J3411
Thiethylperazine maleate			
injection	up to 10 mg	IM	J3280
oral	10 mg	ORAL	Q0174
Thiotepa	15 mg	IV	J9340
Thorazine	up to 50 mg	IM, IV	J3230
Thrombate III	per IU		J7197
Thymoglobulin (*see also* Immune globin)			
anti-thymocyte globulin, equine	250 mg	IV	J7504
anti-thymocyte globulin, rabbit	25 mg	IV	J7511
Thypinone	per 250 mcg	IV	J2725
Thyrogen	0.9 mg	IM, SC	J3240
Thyrotropin Alfa, injection	0.9 mg	IM, SC	J3240
Tice BCG	per vial	IV	J9031
Ticon			
injection	up to 200 mg	IM	J3250
oral	250 mg	ORAL	Q0173
Tigan			
injection	up to 200 mg	IM	J3250
oral	250 mg	ORAL	Q0173
Tigecycline	1 mg	IV	J3243
Tiject-20	up to 200 mg	IM	J3250
	250 mg	ORAL	Q0173
Tinzaparin	1,000 IU	SC	J1655
Tirofiban Hydrochloride, injection	0.25 mg	IM, IV	J3246
TNKase	1 mg		J3101
Tobi	300 mg	INH	J7682, J7685
Tobramycin, inhalation solution	300 mg	INH	J7682, J7685
Tobramycin sulfate	up to 80 mg	IM, IV	J3260, J7685
Tocilizumab	1 mg	IV	J3262
Tofranil, *see* Imipramine HCl			
Tolazoline HCl	up to 25 mg	IV	J2670
Toposar	10 mg		J1981
Topotecan	0.25 mg	ORAL	J8705
	0.1 mg	IV	J9351
Toradol	per 15 mg	IM, IV	J1885
Torecan	10 mg	ORAL	Q0174
	up to 10 mg	IM	J3280

▶ New ⮌ Revised ✔ Reinstated ~~deleted~~ Deleted

DRUG NAME	DOSAGE	METHOD OF ADMINISTRATION	HCPCS CODE
Torisel	1 mg		**J9330**
Tornalate			
concentrated form	per mg	INH	**J7628**
unit dose	per mg	INH	**J7629**
Torsemide	10 mg/ml	IV	**J3265**
Totacillin-N	up to 500 mg	IM, IV	**J0290**
	per 1.5 gm	IM, IV	**J0295**
Trabectedin	0.1 mg	IV	**J9352** ▶
Trastuzumab	10 mg	IV	**J9355**
Trasylol	10,000 KIU		**J0365**
Treanda	1 mg		**J9033, J3490**
Trelstar Depot	3.75 mg		**J3315**
Trelstar LA	3.75 mg		**J3315**
Treprostinil	1 mg		**J3285, J7686**
Trexall	2.5 mg	ORAL	**J8610**
Triam-A	1 mg		**J3300**
	per 10 mg	IM	**J3301**
Triamcinolone			
concentrated form	per 1 mg	INH	**J7683**
unit dose	per 1 mg	INH	**J7684**
Triamcinolone acetonide	1 mg		**J3300, J7684**
	per 10 mg	IM	**J3301**
Triamcinolone diacetate	per 5 mg	IM	**J3302**
Triamcinolone hexacetonide	per 5 mg	VAR	**J3303**
Triamcot	per 5 mg		**J3302**
Triesence	1 mg		**J3300**
	per 10 mg	IM	**J3301**
Triethylene thio Phosphoramide/T	15 mg		**J9340**
Triethylenethosphoramide	15 mg		**J9340**
Triflupromazine HCl	up to 20 mg	IM, IV	**J3400**
Tri-Kort	1 mg		**J3300**
	per 10 mg	IM	**J3301**
Trilafon	4 mg	ORAL	**Q0175**
	8 mg	ORAL	**Q0176**
	up to 5 mg	IM, IV	**J3310**
Trilog	1 mg		**J3300**
	per 10 mg	IM	**J3301**
Trilone	per 5 mg		**J3302**
Trimethobenzamide HCl			
injection	up to 200 mg	IM	**J3250**
oral	250 mg	ORAL	**Q0173**
Trimetrexate glucuronate	per 25 mg	IV	**J3305**
Triptorelin Pamoate	3.75 mg	SC	**J3315**

▶ New ↩ Revised ✔ Reinstated ~~deleted~~ Deleted

DRUG NAME	DOSAGE	METHOD OF ADMINISTRATION	HCPCS CODE
Trisenox	1 mg	IV	J9017
Trobicin	up to 2 g	IM	J3320
Trovan	100 mg	IV	J0200
Truxadryl	50 mg		J1200
Twinrix			J3490
Tysabri	1 mg		J2323
Tyvaso	1.74 mg		J7686
U			
Ultravist 150	per ml		Q9965
Ultravist 240	per ml		Q9966
Ultravist 300	per ml		Q9967
Ultravist 370	per ml		Q9967
Ultrazine-10	up to 10 mg	IM, IV	J0780
Unasyn	per 1.5 gm	IM, IV	J0295
Unclassified drugs (*see also* Not elsewhere classified)			J3490
Unspecified oral antiemetic			Q0181
Urea	up to 40 g	IV	J3350
Ureaphil	up to 40 g	IV	J3350
Urecholine	up to 5 mg	SC	J0520
Urofollitropin	75 IU		J3355
Urokinase	5,000 IU vial	IV	J3364
	250,000 IU vial	IV	J3365
Ustekinumab	1 mg	SC	J3357
V			
Valcyte			J3490
Valergen 10	10 mg	IM	J1380
Valergen 20	10 mg	IM	J1380
Valergen 40	up to 10 mg	IM	J1380
Valertest No. 1	1 mg		J3121
Valertest No. 2	1 mg		J3121
Valium	up to 5 mg	IM, IV	J3360
Valrubicin, intravesical	200 mg	OTH	J9357
Valstar	200 mg	OTH	J9357
Vancocin	500 mg	IV, IM	J3370
Vancoled	500 mg	IV, IM	J3370
Vancomycin HCl	500 mg	IV, IM	J3370
Vantas	50 mg		J9226
Vasceze	per 10 mg		J1642
Vasceze Sodium Chloride	10 ml		A4216
Vasoxyl, *see* Methoxamine HCl			
Vectibix	10 mg		J9303
Vedolizumab	1 mg	IV	J3380
Velaglucerase alfa	100 units	IV	J3385

▶ New ⤾ Revised ✔ Reinstated ~~deleted~~ Deleted

DRUG NAME	DOSAGE	METHOD OF ADMINISTRATION	HCPCS CODE
Velban	1 mg	IV	J9360
Velcade	0.1 mg		J9041
Veletri	0.5 mg		J1325
Velsar	1 mg	IV	J9360
Venofer	1 mg	IV	J1756
Ventavis	20 mcg		Q4074
Ventolin	0.5 mg	INH	J7620
concentrated form	1 mg	INH	J7610, J7611
unit dose form	1 mg	INH	J7609, J7613
VePesid			
	10 mg	IV	J9181
	50 mg	ORAL	J8560
Veritas Collagen Matrix			J3490
Versed	per 1 mg	IM, IV	J2250
Verteporfin	0.1 mg	IV	J3396
Vesprin	up to 20 mg	IM, IV	J3400
VFEND IV	10 mg		J3465
V-Gan 25	up to 50 mg	IM, IV	J2550
	12.5 mg	ORAL	Q0169
V-Gan 50	up to 50 mg	IM, IV	J2550
	12.5 mg	ORAL	Q0169
Viadur	65 mg		J9219
Vibativ	10 mg		J3095
Vidaza	1 mg		J9025
Vinblastine sulfate	1 mg	IV	J9360
Vincasar PFS	1 mg	IV	J9370
Vincristine sulfate	1 mg	IV	J9370
Vincristine sulfate Liposome	1 mg	IV	J9371
Vinorelbine tartrate	per 10 mg	IV	J9390
Vispaque	per ml		Q9966, Q9967
Vistacot	up to 25 mg		J3410
Vistaject-25	up to 25 mg	IM	J3410
Vistaril	up to 25 mg	IM	J3410
	25 mg	ORAL	Q0177
Vistide	375 mg	IV	J0740
Visudyne	0.1 mg	IV	J3396
Vita #12	up to 1,000 mcg		J3420
Vitamin B-12 cyanocobalamin	up to 1,000 mcg	IM, SC	J3420
Vitamin K, phytonadione, menadione, menadiol sodium diphosphate	per 1 mg	IM, SC, IV	J3430
Vitrase	per 1 USP unit		J3471
Vivaglobin	100 mg		J1562
Vivitrol	1 mg		J2315

▶ New ⤾ Revised ✔ Reinstated ~~deleted~~ Deleted

DRUG NAME	DOSAGE	METHOD OF ADMINISTRATION	HCPCS CODE
Von Willebrand Factor Complex, human	per IU VWF:RCo	IV	**J7187**
Wilate	per IU VWF	IV	**J7183**
Vonvendi	per IU VWF:RCp	IV	**J7179** ◄
Voriconazole	10 mg	IV	**J3465**
Vpriv	100 units		**J3385**
W			
Wehamine	up to 50 mg	IM, IV	**J1240**
Wehdryl	up to 50 mg	IM, IV	**J1200**
	50 mg	ORAL	**Q0163**
Wellcovorin	per 50 mg	IM, IV	**J0640**
Wilate	per IU	IV	**J7187**
Win Rho SD	100 IU	IV	**J2792**
Wyamine Sulfate, *see* Mephentermine sulfate			
Wycillin	up to 600,000 units	IM, IV	**J2510**
Wydase	up to 150 units	SC, IV	**J3470**
X			
Xeloda	150 mg	ORAL	**J8520**
	500 mg	ORAL	**J8521**
Xeomin	1 unit		**J0588**
Xgera	1 mg		**J0987**
Xgeva	1 mg		**J0897**
Xiaflex	0.01 mg		**J0775**
Xolair	5 mg		**J2357**
Xopenex	0.5 mg	INH	**J7620**
concentrated form	1 mg	INH	**J7610, J7611, J7612**
unit dose form	1 mg	INH	**J7609, J7613, J7614**
Xylocaine HCl	10 mg	IV	**J2001**
Xyntha	per IU IV		**J7185, J7192**
Y			
Yervoy	1 mg		**J9228**
Z			
Zaltrap	1 mg		**J9400**
Zanosar	1 g	IV	**J9320**
Zantac	25 mg	IV, IM	**J2780**
Zarxio	1 mcg		**Q5101**
Zemaira	10 mg	IV	**J0256**
Zemplar	1 mcg	IM, IV	**J2501**
Zenapax	25 mg	IV	**J7513**
Zetran	up to 5 mg	IM, IV	**J3360**
Ziconotide	1 mcg	OTH	**J2278**
Zidovudine	10 mg	IV	**J3485**

▶ **New** ↩ **Revised** ✔ **Reinstated** ~~deleted~~ **Deleted**

DRUG NAME	DOSAGE	METHOD OF ADMINISTRATION	HCPCS CODE
Zinacef	per 750 mg	IM, IV	J0697
Zinecard	per 250 mg		J1190
Ziprasidone Mesylate	10 mg	IM	J3486
Zithromax	1 gm	ORAL	Q0144
injection	500 mg	IV	J0456
Ziv-Aflibercept	1 mg	IV	J9400
Zmax	1 g		Q0144
Zofran	1 mg	IV	J2405
	1 mg	ORAL	Q0162
Zoladex	per 3.6 mg	SC	J9202
Zoledronic Acid	1 mg	IV	J3489
Zolicef	500 mg	IV, IM	J0690
Zometra	1 mg		J3489
Zorbtive	1 mg		J2941
Zortress	0.25 mg	ORAL	J7527
Zosyn	1.125 g	IV	J2543
Zovirax	5 mg		J8499
Zyprexa Relprevv	1 mg		J2358
Zyvox	200 mg	IV	J2020

▶ New ⤺ Revised ✔ Reinstated ~~deleted~~ Deleted

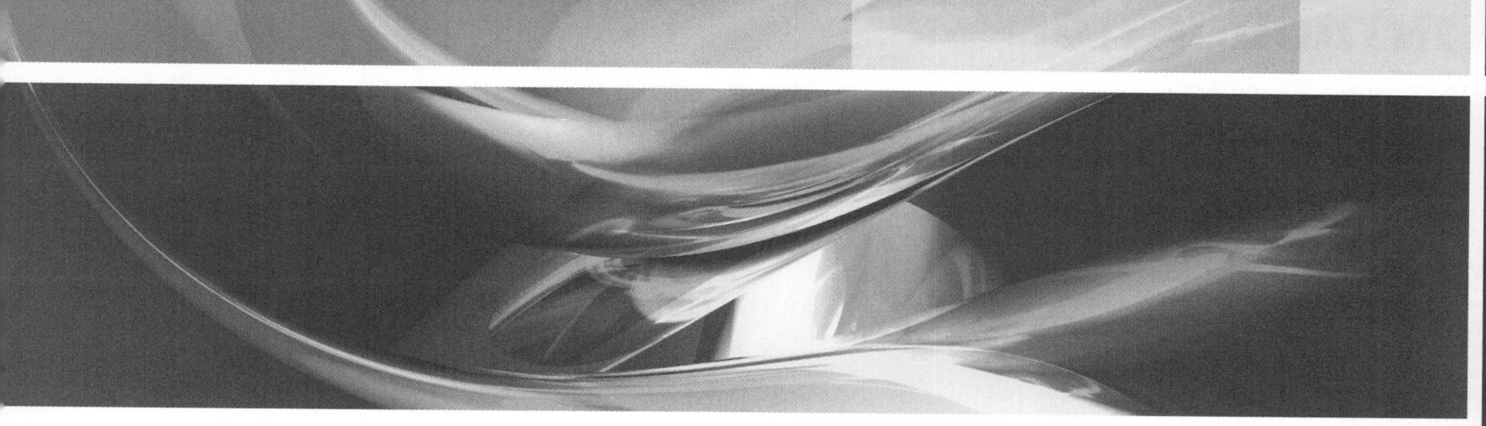

HCPCS 2017 LEVEL II NATIONAL CODES

2017 HCPCS quarterly updates available on the companion website at: http://www.codingupdates.com

DISCLAIMER

Every effort has been made to make this text complete and accurate, but no guarantee, warranty, or representation is made for its accuracy or completeness. This text is based on the Centers for Medicare and Medicaid Services Healthcare Common Procedure Coding System (HCPCS).

INTRODUCTION

2017 HCPCS quarterly updates available on the companion website at: www.codingupdates.com

The Centers for Medicare and Medicaid Services (CMS) (formerly Health Care Financing Administration [HCFA]) Healthcare Common Procedure Coding System (HCPCS) is a collection of codes and descriptors that represent procedures, supplies, products, and services that may be provided to Medicare beneficiaries and to individuals enrolled in private health insurance programs. The codes are divided as follows:

Level I Codes and descriptors copyrighted by the American Medical Association's (AMA's) Current Procedural Terminology, ed. 4 (CPT-4). These are 5 position numeric codes representing physician and nonphysician services.

Level II Includes codes and descriptors copyrighted by the American Dental Association's current dental terminology, seventh edition (CDT-7/8). These are 5 position alpha-numeric codes comprising the D series. All other Level II codes and descriptors are approved and maintained jointly by the alpha-numeric editorial panel (consisting of CMS, the Health Insurance Association of America, and the Blue Cross and Blue Shield Association). These are 5 position alpha-numeric codes representing primarily items and nonphysician services that are not represented in the Level I codes.

Level III The CMS eliminated Level III local codes., *see Program Memorandum AB-02-113*

Headings are provided as a means of grouping similar or closely related items. The placement of a code under a heading does not indicate additional means of classification, nor does it relate to any health insurance coverage categories.

HCPCS also contains modifiers, which are two-position codes and descriptors used to indicate that a service or procedure that has been performed has been altered by some specific circumstance but not changed in its definition or code. Modifiers are grouped by the levels. Level I modifiers and descriptors are copyrighted by the AMA. Level II modifiers are HCPCS modifiers. Modifiers in the D series are copyrighted by the ADA.

HCPCS is designed to promote uniform reporting and statistical data collection of medical procedures, supplies, products, and services.

HCPCS Disclaimer

Inclusion or exclusion of a procedure, supply, product, or service does not imply any health insurance coverage or reimbursement policy.

HCPCS makes as much use as possible of generic descriptions, but the inclusion of brand names to describe devices or drugs is intended only for indexing purposes; it is not meant to convey endorsement of any particular product or drug.

Updating HCPCS

The primary updates are made annually. Quarterly updates are also issued by CMS.

Do not report HCPCS modifiers with PQRI CPT Category II codes, rather use Category II modifiers (i.e., 1P, 2P, 3P, or 8P) or the claim may be returned or denied.

LEVEL II NATIONAL MODIFERS

* ✻ **A1** Dressing for one wound
* ✻ **A2** Dressing for two wounds
* ✻ **A3** Dressing for three wounds
* ✻ **A4** Dressing for four wounds
* ✻ **A5** Dressing for five wounds
* ✻ **A6** Dressing for six wounds
* ✻ **A7** Dressing for seven wounds
* ✻ **A8** Dressing for eight wounds
* ✻ **A9** Dressing for nine or more wounds
* ✪ **AA** Anesthesia services performed personally by anesthesiologist
  IOM: 100-04, 12, 90.4
* ✪ **AD** Medical supervision by a physician: more than four concurrent anesthesia procedures
  IOM: 100-04, 12, 90.4
* ✻ **AE** Registered dietician
* ✻ **AF** Specialty physician
* ✻ **AG** Primary physician
* ✪ **AH** Clinical psychologist
  IOM: 100-04, 12, 170
* ✻ **AI** Principal physician of record
* ✪ **AJ** Clinical social worker
  IOM: 100-04, 12, 170; 100-04, 12, 150
* ✻ **AK** Nonparticipating physician
* ✪ **AM** Physician, team member service
  Not assigned for Medicare
  Cross Reference QM
* ✻ **AO** Alternate payment method declined by provider of service
* ✻ **AP** Determination of refractive state was not performed in the course of diagnostic ophthalmological examination
* ✻ **AQ** Physician providing a service in an unlisted health professional shortage area (HPSA)
* ✻ **AR** Physician provider services in a physician scarcity area
* ✻ **AS** Physician assistant, nurse practitioner, or clinical nurse specialist services for assistant at surgery
* ✻ **AT** Acute treatment (this modifier should be used when reporting service 98940, 98941, 98942)
* ✻ **AU** Item furnished in conjunction with a urological, ostomy, or tracheostomy supply
* ✻ **AV** Item furnished in conjunction with a prosthetic device, prosthetic or orthotic
* ✻ **AW** Item furnished in conjunction with a surgical dressing
* ✻ **AX** Item furnished in conjunction with dialysis services
* ✻ **AY** Item or service furnished to an ESRD patient that is not for the treatment of ESRD
* ⃠ **AZ** Physician providing a service in a dental health professional shortage area for the purpose of an electronic health record incentive payment
* ✻ **BA** Item furnished in conjunction with parenteral enteral nutrition (PEN) services
* ✻ **BL** Special acquisition of blood and blood products
* ✻ **BO** Orally administered nutrition, not by feeding tube
* ✻ **BP** The beneficiary has been informed of the purchase and rental options and has elected to purchase the item
* ✻ **BR** The beneficiary has been informed of the purchase and rental options and has elected to rent the item
* ✻ **BU** The beneficiary has been informed of the purchase and rental options and after 30 days has not informed the supplier of his/her decision
* ✻ **CA** Procedure payable only in the inpatient setting when performed emergently on an outpatient who expires prior to admission
* ✻ **CB** Service ordered by a renal dialysis facility (RDF) physician as part of the ESRD beneficiary's dialysis benefit, is not part of the composite rate, and is separately reimbursable
* ✻ **CC** Procedure code change (Use CC when the procedure code submitted was changed either for administrative reasons or because an incorrect code was filed)
* ✪ **CD** AMCC test has been ordered by an ESRD facility or MCP physician that is part of the composite rate and is not separately billable

⊕ **CE** AMCC test has been ordered by an ESRD facility or MCP physician that is a composite rate test but is beyond the normal frequency covered under the rate and is separately reimbursable based on medical necessity

⊕ **CF** AMCC test has been ordered by an ESRD facility or MCP physician that is not part of the composite rate and is separately billable

* **CG** Policy criteria applied

⊕ **CH** 0 percent impaired, limited or restricted

⊕ **CI** At least 1 percent but less than 20 percent impaired, limited or restricted

⊕ **CJ** At least 20 percent but less than 40 percent impaired, limited or restricted

⊕ **CK** At least 40 percent but less than 60 percent impaired, limited or restricted

⊕ **CL** At least 60 percent but less than 80 percent impaired, limited or restricted

⊕ **CM** At least 80 percent but less than 100 percent impaired, limited or restricted

⊕ **CN** 100 percent impaired, limited or restricted

* **CP** Adjunctive service related to a procedure assigned to a comprehensive ambulatory payment classification (C-APC) procedure, but reported on a different claim

* **CR** Catastrophe/Disaster related

* **CS** Item or service related, in whole or in part, to an illness, injury, or condition that was caused by or exacerbated by the effects, direct or indirect, of the 2010 oil spill in the Gulf of Mexico, including but not limited to subsequent clean-up activities

* **CT** Computed tomography services furnished using equipment that does not meet each of the attributes of the national electrical manufacturers association (NEMA) XR-29-2013 standard

* **DA** Oral health assessment by a licensed health professional other than a dentist

* **E1** Upper left, eyelid

* **E2** Lower left, eyelid

* **E3** Upper right, eyelid

* **E4** Lower right, eyelid

⊕ **EA** Erythropoetic stimulating agent (ESA) administered to treat anemia due to anti-cancer chemotherapy

CMS requires claims for non-ESRD ESAs (J0881 and J0885) to include one of three modifiers: EA, EB, EC.

⊕ **EB** Erythropoetic stimulating agent (ESA) administered to treat anemia due to anti-cancer radiotherapy

CMS requires claims for non-ESRD ESAs (J0881 and J0885) to include one of three modifiers: EA, EB, EC.

⊕ **EC** Erythropoetic stimulating agent (ESA) administered to treat anemia not due to anti-cancer radiotherapy or anti-cancer chemotherapy

CMS requires claims for non-ESRD ESAs (J0881 and J0885) to include one of three modifiers: EA, EB, EC.

⊕ **ED** Hematocrit level has exceeded 39% (or hemoglobin level has exceeded 13.0 g/dl) for 3 or more consecutive billing cycles immediately prior to and including the current cycle

⊕ **EE** Hematocrit level has not exceeded 39% (or hemoglobin level has not exceeded 13.0 g/dl) for 3 or more consecutive billing cycles immediately prior to and including the current cycle

⊕ **EJ** Subsequent claims for a defined course of therapy, e.g., EPO, sodium hyaluronate, infliximab

⊕ **EM** Emergency reserve supply (for ESRD benefit only)

* **EP** Service provided as part of Medicaid early periodic screening diagnosis and treatment (EPSDT) program

* **ET** Emergency services

* **EX** Expatriate beneficiary

* **EY** No physician or other licensed health care provider order for this item or service

Items billed before a signed and dated order has been received by the supplier must be submitted with an EY modifier added to each related HCPCS code.

* **F1** Left hand, second digit

* **F2** Left hand, third digit

* **F3** Left hand, fourth digit

* **F4** Left hand, fifth digit

* **F5** Right hand, thumb

* **F6** Right hand, second digit

* **F7** Right hand, third digit

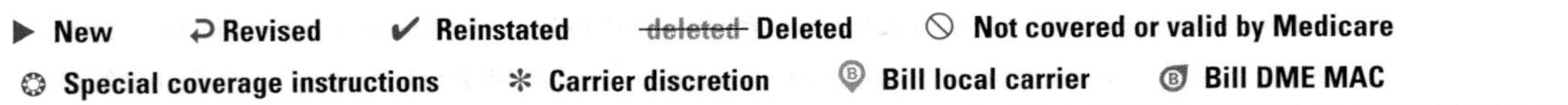

✻ **F8** Right hand, fourth digit

✻ **F9** Right hand, fifth digit

✻ **FA** Left hand, thumb

⃠ **FB** Item provided without cost to provider, supplier or practitioner, or full credit received for replaced device (examples, but not limited to, covered under warranty, replaced due to defect, free samples)

✪ **FC** Partial credit received for replaced device

✻ **FP** Service provided as part of family planning program

▶✻ **FX** X-ray taken using film

✻ **G1** Most recent URR reading of less than 60

IOM: 100-04, 8, 50.9

✻ **G2** Most recent URR reading of 60 to 64.9

IOM: 100-04, 8, 50.9

✻ **G3** Most recent URR reading of 65 to 69.9

IOM: 100-04, 8, 50.9

✻ **G4** Most recent URR reading of 70 to 74.9

IOM: 100-04, 8, 50.9

✻ **G5** Most recent URR reading of 75 or greater

IOM: 100-04, 8, 50.9

✻ **G6** ESRD patient for whom less than six dialysis sessions have been provided in a month

IOM: 100-04, 8, 50.9

✪ **G7** Pregnancy resulted from rape or incest or pregnancy certified by physician as life threatening

IOM: 100-02, 15, 20.1; 100-03, 3, 170.3

anest. ✻ **G8** Monitored anesthesia care (MAC) for deep complex, complicated, or markedly invasive surgical procedure

anest. ✻ **G9** Monitored anesthesia care for patient who has history of severe cardiopulmonary condition

✻ **GA** Waiver of liability statement issued as required by payer policy, individual case

An item/service is expected to be denied as not reasonable and necessary and an ABN is on file. Modifier GA can be used on either a specific or a miscellaneous HCPCS code. Modifiers GA and GY should never be reported together on the same line for the same HCPCS code.

✻ **GB** Claim being resubmitted for payment because it is no longer covered under a global payment demonstration

✪ **GC** This service has been performed in part by a resident under the direction of a teaching physician.

IOM: 100-04, 12, 90.4, 100

✻ **GD** Units of service exceeds medically unlikely edit value and represents reasonable and necessary services

✪ **GE** This service has been performed by a resident without the presence of a teaching physician under the primary care exception

✻ **GF** Non-physician (e.g., nurse practitioner (NP), certified registered nurse anesthetist (CRNA), certified registered nurse (CRN), clinical nurse specialist (CNS), physician assistant (PA)) services in a critical access hospital

✻ **GG** Performance and payment of a screening mammogram and diagnostic mammogram on the same patient, same day

✻ **GH** Diagnostic mammogram converted from screening mammogram on same day

✻ **GJ** "Opt out" physician or practitioner emergency or urgent service

✻ **GK** Reasonable and necessary item/service associated with a GA or GZ modifier

An upgrade is defined as an item that goes beyond what is medically necessary under Medicare's coverage requirements. An item can be considered an upgrade even if the physician has signed an order for it. When suppliers know that an item will not be paid in full because it does not meet the coverage criteria stated in the LCD, the supplier can still obtain partial payment at the time of initial determination if the claim is billed using one of the upgrade modifiers (GK or GL). (https://www.cms.gov/manuals/downloads/clm104c01.pdf)

✻ **GL** Medically unnecessary upgrade provided instead of non-upgraded item, no charge, no Advance Beneficiary Notice (ABN)

✻ **GM** Multiple patients on one ambulance trip

✻ **GN** Services delivered under an outpatient speech language pathology plan of care

✻ **GO** Services delivered under an outpatient occupational therapy plan of care

▶ New ↻ Revised ✔ Reinstated ~~deleted~~ Deleted ⃠ Not covered or valid by Medicare
✪ Special coverage instructions ✻ Carrier discretion Ⓑ Bill local carrier Ⓓ Bill DME MAC

✻ **GP** Services delivered under an outpatient physical therapy plan of care

✻ **GQ** Via asynchronous telecommunications system

✻ **GR** This service was performed in whole or in part by a resident in a department of Veterans Affairs medical center or clinic, supervised in accordance with VA policy

☼ **GS** Dosage of erythropoietin-stimulating agent has been reduced and maintained in response to hematocrit or hemoglobin level

☼ **GT** Via interactive audio and video telecommunication systems

✻ **GU** Waiver of liability statement issued as required by payer policy, routine notice

☼ **GV** Attending physician not employed or paid under arrangement by the patient's hospice provider

☼ **GW** Service not related to the hospice patient's terminal condition

✻ **GX** Notice of liability issued, voluntary under payer policy

GX modifier must be submitted with non-covered charges only. This modifier differentiates from the required uses in conjunction with ABN. (https://www.cms.gov/manuals/downloads/clm104c01.pdf)

⃠ **GY** Item or service statutorily excluded, does not meet the definition of any Medicare benefit or, for non-Medicare insurers, is not a contract benefit

Examples of "statutorily excluded" include: Infusion drug not administered using a durable infusion pump, a wheelchair that is for use for mobility outside the home or hearing aids. GA and GY should never be coded together on the same line for the same HCPCS code. (https://www.cms.gov/manuals/downloads/clm104c01.pdf)

⃠ **GZ** Item or service expected to be denied as not reasonable or necessary

Used when an ABN is not on file and can be used on either a specific or a miscellaneous HCPCS code. It would never be correct to place any combination of GY, GZ or GA modifiers on the same claim line and will result in rejected or denied claim for invalid coding. (https://www.cms.gov/manuals/downloads/clm104c01.pdf)

⃠ **H9** Court-ordered

⃠ **HA** Child/adolescent program

⃠ **HB** Adult program, nongeriatric

⃠ **HC** Adult program, geriatric

⃠ **HD** Pregnant/parenting women's program

⃠ **HE** Mental health program

⃠ **HF** Substance abuse program

⃠ **HG** Opioid addiction treatment program

⃠ **HH** Integrated mental health/substance abuse program

⃠ **HI** Integrated mental health and intellectual disability/developmental disabilities program

⃠ **HJ** Employee assistance program

⃠ **HK** Specialized mental health programs for high-risk populations

⃠ **HL** Intern

⃠ **HM** Less than bachelor degree level

⃠ **HN** Bachelors degree level

⃠ **HO** Masters degree level

⃠ **HP** Doctoral level

⃠ **HQ** Group setting

⃠ **HR** Family/couple with client present

⃠ **HS** Family/couple without client present

⃠ **HT** Multi-disciplinary team

⃠ **HU** Funded by child welfare agency

⃠ **HV** Funded by state addictions agency

⃠ **HW** Funded by state mental health agency

⃠ **HX** Funded by county/local agency

⃠ **HY** Funded by juvenile justice agency

⃠ **HZ** Funded by criminal justice agency

✻ **J1** Competitive acquisition program no-pay submission for a prescription number

✻ **J2** Competitive acquisition program, restocking of emergency drugs after emergency administration

✻ **J3** Competitive acquisition program (CAP), drug not available through CAP as written, reimbursed under average sales price methodology

✻ **J4** DMEPOS item subject to DMEPOS competitive bidding program that is furnished by a hospital upon discharge

✻ **JA** Administered intravenously

This modifier is informational only (not a payment modifier) and may be submitted with all injection codes. According to Medicare, reporting this modifier is voluntary. (CMS Pub. 100-04, chapter 8, section 60.2.3.1 and Pub. 100-04, chapter 17, section 80.11)

✻ **JB** Administered subcutaneously

▶ New ⤺ Revised ✔ Reinstated ~~deleted~~ Deleted ⃠ Not covered or valid by Medicare
☼ Special coverage instructions ✻ Carrier discretion Ⓑ Bill local carrier Ⓑ Bill DME MAC

✻ **JC** Skin substitute used as a graft

✻ **JD** Skin substitute not used as a graft

✻ **JE** Administered via dialysate

✻ **JW** Drug amount discarded/not administered to any patient

Use JW to identify unused drugs or biologicals from single use vial/package that are appropriately discarded. Bill on separate line for payment of discarded drug/biological.

IOM: 100-4, 17, 40

✻ **K0** Lower extremity prosthesis functional Level 0 - does not have the ability or potential to ambulate or transfer safely with or without assistance and a prosthesis does not enhance their quality of life or mobility.

✻ **K1** Lower extremity prosthesis functional Level 1 - has the ability or potential to use a prosthesis for transfers or ambulation on level surfaces at fixed cadence. Typical of the limited and unlimited household ambulator.

✻ **K2** Lower extremity prosthesis functional Level 2 - has the ability or potential for ambulation with the ability to traverse low level environmental barriers such as curbs, stairs or uneven surfaces. Typical of the limited community ambulator.

✻ **K3** Lower extremity prosthesis functional Level 3 - has the ability or potential for ambulation with variable cadence. Typical of the community ambulator who has the ability to traverse most environmental barriers and may have vocational, therapeutic, or exercise activity that demands prosthetic utilization beyond simple locomotion.

✻ **K4** Lower extremity prosthesis functional Level 4 - has the ability or potential for prosthetic ambulation that exceeds the basic ambulation skills, exhibiting high impact, stress, or energy levels, typical of the prosthetic demands of the child, active adult, or athlete.

✻ **KA** Add on option/accessory for wheelchair

✻ **KB** Beneficiary requested upgrade for ABN, more than 4 modifiers identified on claim

✻ **KC** Replacement of special power wheelchair interface

✻ **KD** Drug or biological infused through DME

✻ **KE** Bid under round one of the DMEPOS competitive bidding program for use with non-competitive bid base equipment

✻ **KF** Item designated by FDA as Class III device

✻ **KG** DMEPOS item subject to DMEPOS competitive bidding program number 1

✻ **KH** DMEPOS item, initial claim, purchase or first month rental

✻ **KI** DMEPOS item, second or third month rental

✻ **KJ** DMEPOS item, parenteral enteral nutrition (PEN) pump or capped rental, months four to fifteen

✻ **KK** DMEPOS item subject to DMEPOS competitive bidding program number 2

✻ **KL** DMEPOS item delivered via mail

✻ **KM** Replacement of facial prosthesis including new impression/moulage

✻ **KN** Replacement of facial prosthesis using previous master model

✻ **KO** Single drug unit dose formulation

✻ **KP** First drug of a multiple drug unit dose formulation

✻ **KQ** Second or subsequent drug of a multiple drug unit dose formulation

✻ **KR** Rental item, billing for partial month

✪ **KS** Glucose monitor supply for diabetic beneficiary not treated with insulin

✻ **KT** Beneficiary resides in a competitive bidding area and travels outside that competitive bidding area and receives a competitive bid item

✻ **KU** DMEPOS item subject to DMEPOS competitive bidding program number 3

✻ **KV** DMEPOS item subject to DMEPOS competitive bidding program that is furnished as part of a professional service

✻ **KW** DMEPOS item subject to DMEPOS competitive bidding program number 4

✻ **KX** Requirements specified in the medical policy have been met

Used for physical, occupational, or speech-language therapy to request an exception to therapy payment caps and indicate the services are reasonable and necessary and that there is documentation of medical necessity in the patient's medical record. (Pub 100-04 Attachment - Business Requirements Centers for Medicare and Medicaid Services, Transmittal 2457, April 27, 2012)

Medicare requires modifier KX for implanted permanent cardiac pacemakers, single chamber or duel chamber, for one of the following CPT codes: 33206, 33207, 33208.

▶ New ⮌ Revised ✔ Reinstated ~~deleted~~ Deleted ⊘ Not covered or valid by Medicare
✪ Special coverage instructions ✻ Carrier discretion Ⓑ Bill local carrier Ⓓ Bill DME MAC

✻	**KY**	DMEPOS item subject to DMEPOS competitive bidding program number 5
✻	**KZ**	New coverage not implemented by managed care
	~~L1~~	~~Provider attestation that the hospital laboratory test(s) is not packaged under the hospital OPPS~~ ✖
✻	**LC**	Left circumflex coronary artery
✻	**LD**	Left anterior descending coronary artery
✻	**LL**	Lease/rental (use the LL modifier when DME equipment rental is to be applied against the purchase price)
✻	**LM**	Left main coronary artery
✻	**LR**	Laboratory round trip
✪	**LS**	FDA-monitored intraocular lens implant
✻	**LT**	Left side (used to identify procedures performed on the left side of the body) Modifiers LT and RT identify procedures which can be performed on paired organs. Used for procedures performed on one side only. Should also be used when the procedures are similar but not identical and are performed on paired body parts.
✻	**M2**	Medicare secondary payer (MSP)
✻	**MS**	Six month maintenance and servicing fee for reasonable and necessary parts and labor which are not covered under any manufacturer or supplier warranty
✻	**NB**	Nebulizer system, any type, FDA-cleared for use with specific drug
✻	**NR**	New when rented (use the NR modifier when DME which was new at the time of rental is subsequently purchased)
✻	**NU**	New equipment
✻	**P1**	A normal healthy patient
✻	**P2**	A patient with mild systemic disease
✻	**P3**	A patient with severe systemic disease
✻	**P4**	A patient with severe systemic disease that is a constant threat to life
✻	**P5**	A moribund patient who is not expected to survive without the operation
✻	**P6**	A declared brain-dead patient whose organs are being removed for donor purposes
⃠	**PA**	Surgical or other invasive procedure on wrong body part
⃠	**PB**	Surgical or other invasive procedure on wrong patient
⃠	**PC**	Wrong surgery or other invasive procedure on patient
✻	**PD**	Diagnostic or related non diagnostic item or service provided in a wholly owned or operated entity to a patient who is admitted as an inpatient within 3 days
✻	**PI**	Positron emission tomography (PET) or PET/computed tomography (CT) to inform the initial treatment strategy of tumors that are biopsy proven or strongly suspected of being cancerous based on other diagnostic testing
✻	**PL**	Progressive addition lenses
✻	**PM**	Post mortem
▶ ✻	**PN**	Non-excepted service provided at an off-campus, outpatient, provider-based department of a hospital
⮌ ✻	**PO**	Expected services provided at off-campus, outpatient, provider-based department of a hospital
✻	**PS**	Positron emission tomography (PET) or PET/computed tomography (CT) to inform the subsequent treatment strategy of cancerous tumors when the beneficiary's treating physician determines that the PET study is needed to inform subsequent anti-tumor strategy
✻	**PT**	Colorectal cancer screening test; converted to diagnostic text or other procedure Assign this modifier with the appropriate CPT procedure code for colonoscopy, flexible sigmoidoscopy, or barium enema when the service is initiated as a colorectal cancer screening service but then becomes a diagnostic service. (MLN Matters article MM7012 (PDF, 75 KB) Reference Medicare Transmittal 3232 April 3, 2015.
✪	**Q0**	Investigational clinical service provided in a clinical research study that is in an approved clinical research study
✪	**Q1**	Routine clinical service provided in a clinical research study that is in an approved clinical research study
⮌ ✻	**Q2**	Demonstration procedure/service
✻	**Q3**	Live kidney donor surgery and related services
✻	**Q4**	Service for ordering/referring physician qualifies as a service exemption

▶ New ⮌ Revised ✔ Reinstated ~~deleted~~ Deleted ⃠ Not covered or valid by Medicare
✪ Special coverage instructions ✻ Carrier discretion Ⓑ Bill local carrier Ⓑ Bill DME MAC

⊙ **Q5** Service furnished by a substitute physician under a reciprocal billing arrangement

IOM: 100-04, 1, 30.2.10

⊙ **Q6** Service furnished by a locum tenens physician

IOM: 100-04, 1, 30.2.11

* **Q7** One Class A finding

* **Q8** Two Class B findings

* **Q9** One Class B and two Class C findings

* **QC** Single channel monitoring

* **QD** Recording and storage in solid state memory by a digital recorder

* **QE** Prescribed amount of oxygen is less than 1 liter per minute (LPM)

* **QF** Prescribed amount of oxygen exceeds 4 liters per minute (LPM) and portable oxygen is prescribed

* **QG** Prescribed amount of oxygen is greater than 4 liters per minute (LPM)

* **QH** Oxygen conserving device is being used with an oxygen delivery system

⊙ **QJ** Services/items provided to a prisoner or patient in state or local custody, however, the state or local government, as applicable, meets the requirements in 42 CFR 411.4 (B)

⊙ **QK** Medical direction of two, three, or four concurrent anesthesia procedures involving qualified individuals

IOM: 100-04, 12, 50K, 90

* **QL** Patient pronounced dead after ambulance called

* **QM** Ambulance service provided under arrangement by a provider of services

* **QN** Ambulance service furnished directly by a provider of services

⊙ **QP** Documentation is on file showing that the laboratory test(s) was ordered individually or ordered as a CPT-recognized panel other than automated profile codes 80002-80019, G0058, G0059, and G0060.

⊙ **QS** Monitored anesthesia care service

IOM: 100-04, 12, 30.6, 501

* **QT** Recording and storage on tape by an analog tape recorder

* **QW** CLIA-waived test

* **QX** CRNA service: with medical direction by a physician

⊙ **QY** Medical direction of one certified registered nurse anesthetist (CRNA) by an anesthesiologist

IOM: 100-04, 12, 50K, 90

* **QZ** CRNA service: without medical direction by a physician

* **RA** Replacement of a DME, orthotic or prosthetic item

Contractors will deny claims for replacement parts when furnished in conjunction with the repair of a capped rental item and billed with modifier RB, including claims for parts submitted using code E1399, that are billed during the capped rental period (i.e., the last day of the 13th month of continuous use or before). Repair includes all maintenance, servicing, and repair of capped rental DME because it is included in the allowed rental payment amounts. (Pub 100-20 One-Time Notification Centers for Medicare & Medicaid Services, Transmittal: 901, May 13, 2011)

* **RB** Replacement of a part of a DME, orthotic or prosthetic item furnished as part of a repair

* **RC** Right coronary artery

* **RD** Drug provided to beneficiary, but not administered "incident-to"

* **RE** Furnished in full compliance with FDA-mandated risk evaluation and mitigation strategy (REMS)

* **RI** Ramus intermedius coronary artery

* **RR** Rental (use the "RR" modifier when DME is to be rented)

* **RT** Right side (used to identify procedures performed on the right side of the body)

Modifiers LT and RT identify procedures which can be performed on paired organs. Used for procedures performed on one side only. Should also be used when the procedures are similar but not identical and are performed on paired body parts.

⊘ **SA** Nurse practitioner rendering service in collaboration with a physician

⊘ **SB** Nurse midwife

* **SC** Medically necessary service or supply

⊘ **SD** Services provided by registered nurse with specialized, highly technical home infusion training

⊘ **SE** State and/or federally funded programs/services

▶ New ↻ Revised ✔ Reinstated ~~deleted~~ Deleted ⊘ Not covered or valid by Medicare
⊙ Special coverage instructions * Carrier discretion Ⓑ Bill local carrier Ⓓ Bill DME MAC

Report when

	Code	Description
✻	**SF**	Second opinion ordered by a professional review organization (PRO) per Section 9401, P.L. 99-272 (100% reimbursement - no Medicare deductible or coinsurance)
✻	**SG**	Ambulatory surgical center (ASC) facility service Only valid for surgical codes. After 1/1/08 not required for ASC facility charges.
⃠	**SH**	Second concurrently administered infusion therapy
⃠	**SJ**	Third or more concurrently administered infusion therapy
⃠	**SK**	Member of high risk population (use only with codes for immunization)
⃠	**SL**	State supplied vaccine
⃠	**SM**	Second surgical opinion
⃠	**SN**	Third surgical opinion
⃠	**SQ**	Item ordered by home health
⃠	**SS**	Home infusion services provided in the infusion suite of the IV therapy provider
⃠	**ST**	Related to trauma or injury
⃠	**SU**	Procedure performed in physician's office (to denote use of facility and equipment)
⃠	**SV**	Pharmaceuticals delivered to patient's home but not utilized
✻	**SW**	Services provided by a certified diabetic educator
⃠	**SY**	Persons who are in close contact with member of high-risk population (use only with codes for immunization)
✻	**SZ**	Habilitative services
✻	**T1**	Left foot, second digit
✻	**T2**	Left foot, third digit
✻	**T3**	Left foot, fourth digit
✻	**T4**	Left foot, fifth digit
✻	**T5**	Right foot, great toe
✻	**T6**	Right foot, second digit
✻	**T7**	Right foot, third digit
✻	**T8**	Right foot, fourth digit
✻	**T9**	Right foot, fifth digit
✻	**TA**	Left foot, great toe
✻	**TC**	Technical component; Under certain circumstances, a charge may be made for the technical component alone; under those circumstances the technical component charge is identified by adding modifier TC to the usual procedure number; technical component charges are institutional charges and not billed separately by physicians; however, portable x-ray suppliers only bill for technical component and should utilize modifier TC; the charge data from portable x-ray suppliers will then be used to build customary and prevailing profiles.
⃠	**TD**	RN
⃠	**TE**	LPN/LVN
⃠	**TF**	Intermediate level of care
⃠	**TG**	Complex/high tech level of care
⃠	**TH**	Obstetrical treatment/services, prenatal or postpartum
⃠	**TJ**	Program group, child and/or adolescent
⃠	**TK**	Extra patient or passenger, non-ambulance
⃠	**TL**	Early intervention/individualized family service plan (IFSP)
⃠	**TM**	Individualized education program (IEP)
⃠	**TN**	Rural/outside providers' customary service area
⃠	**TP**	Medical transport, unloaded vehicle
⃠	**TQ**	Basic life support transport by a volunteer ambulance provider
⃠	**TR**	School-based individual education program (IEP) services provided outside the public school district responsible for the student
✻	**TS**	Follow-up service
⃠	**TT**	Individualized service provided to more than one patient in same setting
⃠	**TU**	Special payment rate, overtime
⃠	**TV**	Special payment rates, holidays/ weekends
⃠	**TW**	Back-up equipment
⃠	**U1**	Medicaid Level of Care 1, as defined by each State
⃠	**U2**	Medicaid Level of Care 2, as defined by each State
⃠	**U3**	Medicaid Level of Care 3, as defined by each State
⃠	**U4**	Medicaid Level of Care 4, as defined by each State

▶ New ⟲ Revised ✔ Reinstated ~~deleted~~ Deleted ⃠ Not covered or valid by Medicare
Special coverage instructions ✻ Carrier discretion Bill local carrier Bill DME MAC

⃠	**U5**	Medicaid Level of Care 5, as defined by each State
⃠	**U6**	Medicaid Level of Care 6, as defined by each State
⃠	**U7**	Medicaid Level of Care 7, as defined by each State
⃠	**U8**	Medicaid Level of Care 8, as defined by each State
⃠	**U9**	Medicaid Level of Care 9, as defined by each State
⃠	**UA**	Medicaid Level of Care 10, as defined by each State
⃠	**UB**	Medicaid Level of Care 11, as defined by each State
⃠	**UC**	Medicaid Level of Care 12, as defined by each State
⃠	**UD**	Medicaid Level of Care 13, as defined by each State
✻	**UE**	Used durable medical equipment
⃠	**UF**	Services provided in the morning
⃠	**UG**	Services provided in the afternoon
⃠	**UH**	Services provided in the evening
⮐ ✻	**UJ**	Services provided at night
⃠	**UK**	Services provided on behalf of the client to someone other than the client (collateral relationship)
✻	**UN**	Two patients served
✻	**UP**	Three patients served
✻	**UQ**	Four patients served
✻	**UR**	Five patients served
✻	**US**	Six or more patients served
▶ ✻	**V1**	Demonstration Modifier 1
▶ ✻	**V2**	Demonstration Modifier 2
▶ ✻	**V3**	Demonstration Modifier 3
✻	**V5**	Vascular catheter (alone or with any other vascular access)
✻	**V6**	Arteriovenous graft (or other vascular access not including a vascular catheter)
✻	**V7**	Arteriovenous fistula only (in use with two needles)
✻	**VP**	Aphakic patient
✻	**XE**	Separate encounter, a service that is distinct because it occurred during a separate encounter
✻	**XP**	Separate practitioner, a service that is distinct because it was performed by a different practitioner
✻	**XS**	Separate structure, a service that is distinct because it was performed on a separate organ/structure
✻	**XU**	Unusual non-overlapping service, the use of a service that is distinct because it does not overlap usual components of the main service
✻	**ZA**	Novartis/Sandoz
▶ ✻	**ZB**	Pfizer/Hospira

Ambulance Modifiers

Modifiers that are used on claims for ambulance services are created by combining two alpha characters. Each alpha character, with the exception of X, represents an origin (source) code or a destination code. The pair of alpha codes creates one modifier. The first position alpha-code = origin; the second position alpha-code = destination. On form CMS-1491, used to report ambulance services, Item 12 should contain the origin code and Item 13 should contain the destination code. Origin and destination codes and their descriptions are as follows:

D	Diagnostic or therapeutic site other than P or H when these are used as origin codes
E	Residential, domiciliary, custodial facility (other than an 1819 facility)
G	Hospital-based dialysis facility (hospital or hospital related)
H	Hospital
I	Site of transfer (e.g., airport or helicopter pad) between modes of ambulance transport
J	Non-hospital-based dialysis facility
N	Skilled nursing facility (SNF) (1819 facility)
P	Physician's office (includes HMO non-hospital facility, clinic, etc.)
R	Residence
S	Scene of accident or acute event
X	Destination code only. Intermediate stop at physician's office en route to the hospital (includes non-hospital facility, clinic, etc.)

TRANSPORT SERVICES INCLUDING AMBULANCE (A0000-A0999)

⃠ **A0021** Ambulance service, outside state per mile, transport (Medicaid only) Ⓑ

Cross Reference A0030

⃠ **A0080** Non-emergency transportation, per mile - vehicle provided by volunteer (individual or organization), with no vested interest Ⓑ

⃠ **A0090** Non-emergency transportation, per mile - vehicle provided by individual (family member, self, neighbor) with vested interest Ⓑ

⃠ **A0100** Non-emergency transportation; taxi Ⓑ

⃠ **A0110** Non-emergency transportation and bus, intra or inter state carrier Ⓑ

⃠ **A0120** Non-emergency transportation: mini-bus, mountain area transports, or other transportation systems Ⓑ

⃠ **A0130** Non-emergency transportation: wheelchair van Ⓑ

⃠ **A0140** Non-emergency transportation and air travel (private or commercial), intra or inter state Ⓑ

⃠ **A0160** Non-emergency transportation: per mile - caseworker or social worker Ⓑ

⃠ **A0170** Transportation: ancillary: parking fees, tolls, other Ⓑ

⃠ **A0180** Non-emergency transportation: ancillary: lodging - recipient Ⓑ

⃠ **A0190** Non-emergency transportation: ancillary: meals - recipient Ⓑ

⃠ **A0200** Non-emergency transportation: ancillary: lodging - escort Ⓑ

⃠ **A0210** Non-emergency transportation: ancillary: meals - escort Ⓑ

⃠ **A0225** Ambulance service, neonatal transport, base rate, emergency transport, one way Ⓑ

⃠ **A0380** BLS mileage (per mile) Ⓑ

Cross Reference A0425

⃠ **A0382** BLS routine disposable supplies Ⓑ

⃠ **A0384** BLS specialized service disposable supplies; defibrillation (used by ALS ambulances and BLS ambulances in jurisdictions where defibrillation is permitted in BLS ambulances) Ⓑ

⃠ **A0390** ALS mileage (per mile) Ⓑ

Cross Reference A0425

⃠ **A0392** ALS specialized service disposable supplies; defibrillation (to be used only in jurisdictions where defibrillation cannot be performed in BLS ambulances) Ⓑ

⃠ **A0394** ALS specialized service disposable supplies; IV drug therapy Ⓑ

⃠ **A0396** ALS specialized service disposable supplies; esophageal intubation Ⓑ

⃠ **A0398** ALS routine disposable supplies Ⓑ

⃠ **A0420** Ambulance waiting time (ALS or BLS), one half (½) hour increments Ⓑ

Waiting Time Table

UNITS	TIME	UNITS	TIME
1	½ to 1 hr.	6	3 to 3½ hrs.
2	1 to 1½ hrs.	7	3½ to 4 hrs.
3	1½ to 2 hrs.	8	4 to 4½ hrs.
4	2 to 2½ hrs.	9	4½ to 5 hrs.
5	2½ to 3 hrs.	10	5 to 5½ hrs.

⃠ **A0422** Ambulance (ALS or BLS) oxygen and oxygen supplies, life-sustaining situation Ⓑ

⃠ **A0424** Extra ambulance attendant, ground (ALS or BLS) or air (fixed or rotary winged); (requires medical review) Ⓑ

✻ **A0425** Ground mileage, per statute mile Ⓑ

✻ **A0426** Ambulance service, advanced life support, non-emergency transport, Level 1 (ALS 1) Ⓑ

✻ **A0427** Ambulance service, advanced life support, emergency transport, Level 1 (ALS 1-Emergency) Ⓑ

✻ **A0428** Ambulance service, basic life support, non-emergency transport (BLS) Ⓑ

✻ **A0429** Ambulance service, basic life support, emergency transport (BLS-Emergency) Ⓑ

✻ **A0430** Ambulance service, conventional air services, transport, one way (fixed wing) Ⓑ

✻ **A0431** Ambulance service, conventional air services, transport, one way (rotary wing) Ⓑ

✻ **A0432** Paramedic intercept (PI), rural area, transport furnished by a volunteer ambulance company, which is prohibited by state law from billing third party payers Ⓑ

✻ **A0433** Advanced life support, Level 2 (ALS2) Ⓑ

✻ **A0434** Specialty care transport (SCT) Ⓑ

* A0435 Fixed wing air mileage, per statute mile

* A0436 Rotary wing air mileage, per statute mile

⊘ A0888 Noncovered ambulance mileage, per mile (e.g., for miles traveled beyond closest appropriate facility)

MCM: 2125

⊘ A0998 Ambulance response and treatment, no transport

IOM: 100-02, 10, 20

A0999 Unlisted ambulance service

IOM: 100-02, 10, 20

MEDICAL AND SURGICAL SUPPLIES (A4000-A6513)

* A4206 Syringe with needle, sterile 1 cc or less, each

Bill Local Carrier if incident to a physician's service (not separately payable). If other, bill DME MAC.

* A4207 Syringe with needle, sterile 2 cc, each

Bill Local Carrier if incident to a physician's service (not separately payable). If other, bill DME MAC.

* A4208 Syringe with needle, sterile 3 cc, each

Bill Local Carrier if incident to a physician's service (not separately payable). If other, bill DME MAC.

* A4209 Syringe with needle, sterile 5 cc or greater, each

Bill Local Carrier if incident to a physician's service (not separately payable). If other, bill DME MAC.

⊘ A4210 Needle-free injection device, each

IOM: 100-03, 4, 280.1

A4211 Supplies for self-administered injections

Bill Local Carrier if incident to a physician's service (not separately payable). If other, bill DME MAC.

IOM: 100-02, 15, 50

* A4212 Non-coring needle or stylet with or without catheter

* A4213 Syringe, sterile, 20 cc or greater, each

Bill Local Carrier if incident to a physician's service (not separately payable). If other, bill DME MAC.

* A4215 Needle, sterile, any size, each

Bill Local Carrier if incident to a physician's service (not separately payable). If other, bill DME MAC.

A4216 Sterile water, saline and/or dextrose diluent/flush, 10 ml

Bill Local Carrier if incident to a physician's service (not separately payable). If other, bill DME MAC.

Other: Broncho Saline, Monoject Prefill advanced, Sodium Chloride, Sodium Chloride Bacteriostatic, Syrex, Vasceze Sodium Chloride

IOM: 100-02, 15, 50

A4217 Sterile water/saline, 500 ml

Bill Local Carrier if incident to a physician's service (not separately payable). If other, bill DME MAC.

Other: Sodium Chloride

IOM: 100-02, 15, 50

A4218 Sterile saline or water, metered dose dispenser, 10 ml

Bill Local Carrier if incident to a physician's service (not separately payable). If other, bill DME MAC.

Other: Sodium Chloride

A4220 Refill kit for implantable infusion pump

Do not report with 95990 or 95991 since Medicare payment for these codes includes the refill kit.

IOM: 100-03, 4, 280.1

* A4221 Supplies for maintenance of non-insulin drug infusion catheter, per week (list drugs separately)

Bill Local Carrier if incident to a physician's service (not separately payable). If other, bill DME MAC.

Includes dressings for catheter site and flush solutions not directly related to drug infusion.

* A4222 Infusion supplies for external drug infusion pump, per cassette or bag (list drug separately)

Bill Local Carrier if incident to a physician's service (not separately payable). If other, bill DME MAC.

Includes cassette or bag, diluting solutions, tubing and/or administration supplies, port cap changes, compounding charges, and preparation charges.

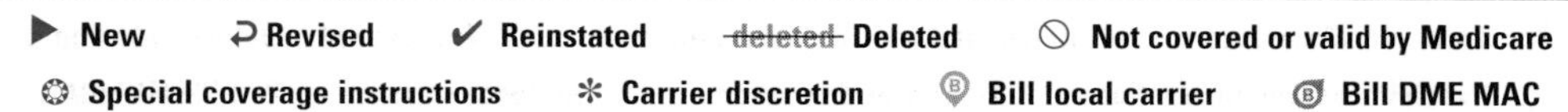

✻ **A4223** Infusion supplies not used with external infusion pump, per cassette or bag (list drugs separately) Ⓑ Ⓑ

Bill Local Carrier if incident to a physician's service (not separately payable). If other, bill DME MAC.

IOM: 100-03, 4, 280.1

▶ ✻ **A4224** Supplies for maintenance of insulin infusion catheter, per week

▶ ✪ **A4225** Supplies for external insulin infusion pump, syringe type cartridge, sterile, each

IOM: 100-03, 1, 50.3

✪ **A4230** Infusion set for external insulin pump, non-needle cannula type Ⓑ Ⓑ

Bill Local Carrier if incident to a physician's service (not separately payable). If other, bill DME MAC.

Requires prior authorization and copy of invoice.

IOM: 100-03, 4, 280.1

✪ **A4231** Infusion set for external insulin pump, needle type Ⓑ Ⓑ

Bill Local Carrier if incident to a physician's service (not separately payable). If other, bill DME MAC.

Requires prior authorization and copy of invoice.

IOM: 100-03, 4, 280.1

⦸ **A4232** Syringe with needle for external insulin pump, sterile, 3 cc Ⓑ Ⓑ

Bill Local Carrier if incident to a physician's service (not separately payable). If other, bill DME MAC.

Reports insulin reservoir for use with external insulin infusion pump (E0784); may be glass or plastic; includes needle for drawing up insulin. Does not include insulin for use in reservoir.

IOM: 100-03, 4, 280.1

✻ **A4233** Replacement battery, alkaline (other than J cell), for use with medically necessary home blood glucose monitor owned by patient, each Ⓑ Ⓑ

Bill Local Carrier if incident to a physician's service (not separately payable). If other, bill DME MAC.

✻ **A4234** Replacement battery, alkaline, J cell, for use with medically necessary home blood glucose monitor owned by patient, each Ⓑ Ⓑ

Bill Local Carrier if incident to a physician's service (not separately payable). If other, bill DME MAC.

✻ **A4235** Replacement battery, lithium, for use with medically necessary home blood glucose monitor owned by patient, each Ⓑ Ⓑ

Bill Local Carrier if incident to a physician's service (not separately payable). If other, bill DME MAC.

✻ **A4236** Replacement battery, silver oxide, for use with medically necessary home blood glucose monitor owned by patient, each Ⓑ Ⓑ

Bill Local Carrier if incident to a physician's service (not separately payable). If other, bill DME MAC.

✻ **A4244** Alcohol or peroxide, per pint Ⓑ Ⓑ

Local carrier if incident to a physician's service (not separately payable). If other, bill DME MAC.

✻ **A4245** Alcohol wipes, per box Ⓑ Ⓑ

Local carrier if incident to a physician's service (not separately payable). If other, bill DME MAC.

✻ **A4246** Betadine or pHisoHex solution, per pint Ⓑ Ⓑ

Bill Local Carrier if incident to a physician's service (not separately payable). If other, bill DME MAC.

✻ **A4247** Betadine or iodine swabs/wipes, per box Ⓑ Ⓑ

Bill Local Carrier if incident to a physician's service (not separately payable). If other, bill DME MAC.

✻ **A4248** Chlorhexidine containing antiseptic, 1 ml Ⓑ Ⓑ

Bill Local Carrier if incident to a physician's service (not separately payable). If other, bill DME MAC.

⦸ **A4250** Urine test or reagent strips or tablets (100 tablets or strips) Ⓑ Ⓑ

Bill Local Carrier if incident to a physician's service (not separately payable). If other, bill DME MAC.

IOM: 100-02, 15, 110

⦸ **A4252** Blood ketone test or reagent strip, each Ⓑ

Medicare Statute 1861(n)

✪ **A4253** Blood glucose test or reagent strips for home blood glucose monitor, per 50 strips Ⓑ

Test strips (1 unit = 50 strips); non-insulin treated (every 3 months) 100 test strips (1×/day testing), 100 lancets (1×/day testing); modifier KS

IOM: 100-03, 1, 40.2

⊕ **A4255** Platforms for home blood glucose monitor, 50 per box

IOM: 100-03, 1, 40.2

⊕ **A4256** Normal, low and high calibrator solution/chips

IOM: 100-03, 1, 40.2

✻ **A4257** Replacement lens shield cartridge for use with laser skin piercing device, each

⊕ **A4258** Spring-powered device for lancet, each

IOM: 100-03, 1, 40.2

⊕ **A4259** Lancets, per box of 100

IOM: 100-03, 1, 40.2

⊘ **A4261** Cervical cap for contraceptive use

Medicare Statute 1862A1

⊕ **A4262** Temporary, absorbable lacrimal duct implant, each

IOM: 100-04, 12, 20.3, 30.4

⊕ **A4263** Permanent, long term, non-dissolvable lacrimal duct implant, each

Bundled with insertion if performed in physician office.

IOM: 100-04, 12, 30.4

⊘ **A4264** Permanent implantable contraceptive intratubal occlusion device(s) and delivery system

Reports the Essure device.

⊕ **A4265** Paraffin, per pound

Bill Local Carrier if incident to a physician's service (not separately payable). If other, bill DME MAC.

IOM: 100-03, 4, 280.1

⊘ **A4266** Diaphragm for contraceptive use

⊘ **A4267** Contraceptive supply, condom, male, each

⊘ **A4268** Contraceptive supply, condom, female, each

⊘ **A4269** Contraceptive supply, spermicide (e.g., foam, gel), each

✻ **A4270** Disposable endoscope sheath, each

✻ **A4280** Adhesive skin support attachment for use with external breast prosthesis, each

✻ **A4281** Tubing for breast pump, replacement

✻ **A4282** Adapter for breast pump, replacement

✻ **A4283** Cap for breast pump bottle, replacement

✻ **A4284** Breast shield and splash protector for use with breast pump, replacement

✻ **A4285** Polycarbonate bottle for use with breast pump, replacement

✻ **A4286** Locking ring for breast pump, replacement

✻ **A4290** Sacral nerve stimulation test lead, each

Service not separately priced by Part B (e.g., services not covered, bundled, used by Part A only)

Implantable Catheters

⊕ **A4300** Implantable access catheter, (e.g., venous, arterial, epidural subarachnoid, or peritoneal, etc.) external access

IOM: 100-02, 15, 120

✻ **A4301** Implantable access total; catheter, port/reservoir (e.g., venous, arterial, epidural, subarachnoid, peritoneal, etc.)

Disposable Drug Delivery System

A4305-A4306: Bill Local Carrier if incident to a physician's service (not separately payable). If other, bill DME MAC.

✻ **A4305** Disposable drug delivery system, flow rate of 50 ml or greater per hour

✻ **A4306** Disposable drug delivery system, flow rate of less than 50 ml per hour

Incontinence Appliances and Care Supplies

A4310-A4355: If provided in the physician's office for a temporary condition, the item is incident to the physician's service and billed to the Local Carrier. If provided in the physician's office or other place of service for a permanent condition, the item is a prosthetic device and billed to the DME MAC.

⊕ **A4310** Insertion tray without drainage bag and without catheter (accessories only)

IOM: 100-02, 15, 120

⊕ **A4311** Insertion tray without drainage bag with indwelling catheter, Foley type, two-way latex with coating (Teflon, silicone, silicone elastomer, or hydrophilic, etc.)

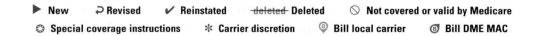

A4312 Insertion tray without drainage bag with indwelling catheter, Foley type, two-way, all silicone

Must meet criteria for indwelling catheter and medical record must justify need for:

- Recurrent encrustation
- Inability to pass a straight catheter
- Sensitivity to latex

Must be medically necessary.

IOM: 100-02, 15, 120

A4313 Insertion tray without drainage bag with indwelling catheter, Foley type, three-way, for continuous irrigation

Must meet criteria for indwelling catheter and medical record must justify need for:

- Recurrent encrustation
- Inability to pass a straight catheter
- Sensitivity to latex

Must be medically necessary.

IOM: 100-02, 15, 120

A4314 Insertion tray with drainage bag with indwelling catheter, Foley type, two-way latex with coating (Teflon, silicone, silicone elastomer or hydrophilic, etc.)

IOM: 100-02, 15, 120

A4315 Insertion tray with drainage bag with indwelling catheter, Foley type, two-way, all silicone

IOM: 100-02, 15, 120

A4316 Insertion tray with drainage bag with indwelling catheter, Foley type, three-way, for continuous irrigation

IOM: 100-02, 15, 120

A4320 Irrigation tray with bulb or piston syringe, any purpose

IOM: 100-02, 15, 120

A4321 Therapeutic agent for urinary catheter irrigation

IOM: 100-02, 15, 120

A4322 Irrigation syringe, bulb, or piston, each

IOM: 100-02, 15, 120

A4326 Male external catheter with integral collection chamber, any type, each

IOM: 100-02, 15, 120

A4327 Female external urinary collection device; metal cup, each

IOM: 100-02, 15, 120

A4328 Female external urinary collection device; pouch, each

IOM: 100-02, 15, 120

A4330 Perianal fecal collection pouch with adhesive, each

IOM: 100-02, 15, 120

A4331 Extension drainage tubing, any type, any length, with connector/adaptor, for use with urinary leg bag or urostomy pouch, each

IOM: 100-02, 15, 120

A4332 Lubricant, individual sterile packet, each

IOM: 100-02, 15, 120

A4333 Urinary catheter anchoring device, adhesive skin attachment, each

IOM: 100-02, 15, 120

A4334 Urinary catheter anchoring device, leg strap, each

IOM: 100-02, 15, 120

A4335 Incontinence supply; miscellaneous

IOM: 100-02, 15, 120

A4336 Incontinence supply, urethral insert, any type, each

IOM: 100-02, 15, 120

A4337 Incontinence supply, rectal insert, any type, each

IOM: 100-02, 15, 120

A4338 Indwelling catheter; Foley type, two-way latex with coating (Teflon, silicone, silicone elastomer, or hydrophilic, etc.), each

IOM: 100-02, 15, 120

A4340 Indwelling catheter; specialty type (e.g., coude, mushroom, wing, etc.), each

IOM: 100-02, 15, 120

Must meet criteria for indwelling catheter and medical record must justify need for:

- Recurrent encrustation
- Inability to pass a straight catheter
- Sensitivity to latex

Must be medically necessary.

IOM: 100-02, 15, 120

⊕ **A4344** Indwelling catheter, Foley type, two-way, all silicone, each Ⓑ Ⓑ

Must meet criteria for indwelling catheter and medical record must justify need for:

- Recurrent encrustation
- Inability to pass a straight catheter
- Sensitivity to latex

Must be medically necessary.

IOM: 100-02, 15, 120

⊕ **A4346** Indwelling catheter; Foley type, three way for continuous irrigation, each Ⓑ Ⓑ

IOM: 100-02, 15, 120

⊕ **A4349** Male external catheter, with or without adhesive, disposable, each Ⓑ Ⓑ

IOM: 100-02, 15, 120

⊕ **A4351** Intermittent urinary catheter; straight tip, with or without coating (Teflon, silicone, silicone elastomer, or hydrophilic, etc.), each Ⓑ Ⓑ

IOM: 100-02, 15, 120

⊕ **A4352** Intermittent urinary catheter; coude (curved) tip, with or without coating (Teflon, silicone, silicone elastomeric, or hydrophilic, etc.), each Ⓑ Ⓑ

IOM: 100-02, 15, 120

⊕ **A4353** Intermittent urinary catheter, with insertion supplies Ⓑ Ⓑ

IOM: 100-02, 15, 120

⊕ **A4354** Insertion tray with drainage bag but without catheter Ⓑ Ⓑ

IOM: 100-02, 15, 120

⊕ **A4355** Irrigation tubing set for continuous bladder irrigation through a three-way indwelling Foley catheter, each Ⓑ Ⓑ

IOM: 100-02, 15, 120

External Urinary Supplies

A4356-A4360: If provided in the physician's office for a temporary condition, the item is incident to the physician's service and billed to the Local Carrier. If provided in the physician's office or other place of service for a permanent condition, the item is a prosthetic device and billed to the DME MAC.

⊕ **A4356** External urethral clamp or compression device (not to be used for catheter clamp), each Ⓑ Ⓑ

IOM: 100-02, 15, 120

⊕ **A4357** Bedside drainage bag, day or night, with or without anti-reflux device, with or without tube, each Ⓑ Ⓑ

IOM: 100-02, 15, 120

⊕ **A4358** Urinary drainage bag, leg or abdomen, vinyl, with or without tube, with straps, each Ⓑ Ⓑ

IOM: 100-02, 15, 120

⊕ **A4360** Disposable external urethral clamp or compression device, with pad and/or pouch, each Ⓑ Ⓑ

Ostomy Supplies

A4361-A4435: If provided in the physician's office for a temporary condition, the item is incident to the physician's service and billed to the Local Carrier. If provided in the physician's office or other place of service for a permanent condition, the item is a prosthetic device and billed to the DME MAC.

⊕ **A4361** Ostomy faceplate, each Ⓑ Ⓑ

IOM: 100-02, 15, 120

⊕ **A4362** Skin barrier; solid, 4 × 4 or equivalent; each Ⓑ Ⓑ

IOM: 100-02, 15, 120

⊕ **A4363** Ostomy clamp, any type, replacement only, each Ⓑ Ⓑ

⊕ **A4364** Adhesive, liquid or equal, any type, per oz Ⓑ Ⓑ

Fee schedule category: Ostomy, tracheostomy, and urologicals items.

IOM: 100-02, 15, 120

* **A4366** Ostomy vent, any type, each Ⓑ Ⓑ

⊕ **A4367** Ostomy belt, each Ⓑ Ⓑ

IOM: 100-02, 15, 120

* **A4368** Ostomy filter, any type, each Ⓑ Ⓑ

⊕ **A4369** Ostomy skin barrier, liquid (spray, brush, etc.), per oz Ⓑ Ⓑ

IOM: 100-02, 15, 120

⊕ **A4371** Ostomy skin barrier, powder, per oz Ⓑ Ⓑ

IOM: 100-02, 15, 120

⊕ **A4372** Ostomy skin barrier, solid 4 × 4 or equivalent, standard wear, with built-in convexity, each Ⓑ Ⓑ

IOM: 100-02, 15, 120

⊕ **A4373** Ostomy skin barrier, with flange (solid, flexible, or accordion), with built-in convexity, any size, each Ⓑ Ⓑ

A4375 Ostomy pouch, drainable, with faceplate attached, plastic, each
IOM: 100-02, 15, 120

A4376 Ostomy pouch, drainable, with faceplate attached, rubber, each
IOM: 100-02, 15, 120

A4377 Ostomy pouch, drainable, for use on faceplate, plastic, each
IOM: 100-02, 15, 120

A4378 Ostomy pouch, drainable, for use on faceplate, rubber, each
IOM: 100-02, 15, 120

A4379 Ostomy pouch, urinary, with faceplate attached, plastic, each
IOM: 100-02, 15, 120

A4380 Ostomy pouch, urinary, with faceplate attached, rubber, each
IOM: 100-02, 15, 120

A4381 Ostomy pouch, urinary, for use on faceplate, plastic, each
IOM: 100-02, 15, 120

A4382 Ostomy pouch, urinary, for use on faceplate, heavy plastic, each
IOM: 100-02, 15, 120

A4383 Ostomy pouch, urinary, for use on faceplate, rubber, each
IOM: 100-02, 15, 120

A4384 Ostomy faceplate equivalent, silicone ring, each
IOM: 100-02, 15, 120

A4385 Ostomy skin barrier, solid 4 × 4 or equivalent, extended wear, without built-in convexity, each
IOM: 100-02, 15, 120

A4387 Ostomy pouch closed, with barrier attached, with built-in convexity (1 piece), each
IOM: 100-02, 15, 120

A4388 Ostomy pouch, drainable, with extended wear barrier attached (1 piece), each
IOM: 100-02, 15, 120

A4389 Ostomy pouch, drainable, with barrier attached, with built-in convexity (1 piece), each
IOM: 100-02, 15, 120

A4390 Ostomy pouch, drainable, with extended wear barrier attached, with built-in convexity (1 piece), each
IOM: 100-02, 15, 120

A4391 Ostomy pouch, urinary, with extended wear barrier attached (1 piece), each
IOM: 100-02, 15, 120

A4392 Ostomy pouch, urinary, with standard wear barrier attached, with built-in convexity (1 piece), each
IOM: 100-02, 15, 120

A4393 Ostomy pouch, urinary, with extended wear barrier attached, with built-in convexity (1 piece), each
IOM: 100-02, 15, 120

A4394 Ostomy deodorant, with or without lubricant, for use in ostomy pouch, per fluid ounce
IOM: 100-02, 15, 20

A4395 Ostomy deodorant for use in ostomy pouch, solid, per tablet
IOM: 100-02, 15, 20

A4396 Ostomy belt with peristomal hernia support
IOM: 100-02, 15, 120

A4397 Irrigation supply; sleeve, each
IOM: 100-02, 15, 120

A4398 Ostomy irrigation supply; bag, each
IOM: 100-02, 15, 120

A4399 Ostomy irrigation supply; cone/catheter, with or without brush
IOM: 100-02, 15, 120

A4400 Ostomy irrigation set
IOM: 100-02, 15, 120

A4402 Lubricant, per ounce
IOM: 100-02, 15, 120

A4404 Ostomy ring, each
IOM: 100-02, 15, 120

A4405 Ostomy skin barrier, non-pectin based, paste, per ounce
IOM: 100-02, 15, 120

A4406 Ostomy skin barrier, pectin-based, paste, per ounce
IOM: 100-02, 15, 120

A4407 Ostomy skin barrier, with flange (solid, flexible, or accordion), extended wear, with built-in convexity, 4 × 4 inches or smaller, each
IOM: 100-02, 15, 120

❂ **A4408** Ostomy skin barrier, with flange (solid, flexible, or accordion), extended wear, with built-in convexity, larger than 4 × 4 inches, each Ⓑ Ⓑ

IOM: 100-02, 15, 120

❂ **A4409** Ostomy skin barrier, with flange (solid, flexible, or accordion), extended wear, without built-in convexity, 4 × 4 inches or smaller, each Ⓑ Ⓑ

IOM: 100-02, 15, 120

❂ **A4410** Ostomy skin barrier, with flange (solid, flexible, or accordion), extended wear, without built-in convexity, larger than 4 × 4 inches, each Ⓑ Ⓑ

IOM: 100-02, 15, 120

❂ **A4411** Ostomy skin barrier, solid 4 × 4 or equivalent, extended wear, with built-in convexity, each Ⓑ Ⓑ

❂ **A4412** Ostomy pouch, drainable, high output, for use on a barrier with flange (2 piece system), without filter, each Ⓑ Ⓑ

IOM: 100-02, 15, 120

❂ **A4413** Ostomy pouch, drainable, high output, for use on a barrier with flange (2 piece system), with filter, each Ⓑ Ⓑ

IOM: 100-02, 15, 120

❂ **A4414** Ostomy skin barrier, with flange (solid, flexible, or accordion), without built-in convexity, 4 × 4 inches or smaller, each Ⓑ Ⓑ

IOM: 100-02, 15, 120

❂ **A4415** Ostomy skin barrier, with flange (solid, flexible, or accordion), without built-in convexity, larger than 4 × 4 inches, each Ⓑ Ⓑ

IOM: 100-02, 15, 120

✻ **A4416** Ostomy pouch, closed, with barrier attached, with filter (1 piece), each Ⓑ Ⓑ

✻ **A4417** Ostomy pouch, closed, with barrier attached, with built-in convexity, with filter (1 piece), each Ⓑ Ⓑ

✻ **A4418** Ostomy pouch, closed; without barrier attached, with filter (1 piece), each Ⓑ Ⓑ

✻ **A4419** Ostomy pouch, closed; for use on barrier with non-locking flange, with filter (2 piece), each Ⓑ Ⓑ

✻ **A4420** Ostomy pouch, closed; for use on barrier with locking flange (2 piece), each Ⓑ Ⓑ

✻ **A4421** Ostomy supply; miscellaneous Ⓑ Ⓑ

❂ **A4422** Ostomy absorbent material (sheet/pad/crystal packet) for use in ostomy pouch to thicken liquid stomal output, each Ⓑ Ⓑ

IOM: 100-02, 15, 120

✻ **A4423** Ostomy pouch, closed; for use on barrier with locking flange, with filter (2 piece), each Ⓑ Ⓑ

✻ **A4424** Ostomy pouch, drainable, with barrier attached, with filter (1 piece), each Ⓑ Ⓑ

✻ **A4425** Ostomy pouch, drainable; for use on barrier with non-locking flange, with filter (2-piece system), each Ⓑ Ⓑ

✻ **A4426** Ostomy pouch, drainable; for use on barrier with locking flange (2 piece system), each Ⓑ Ⓑ

✻ **A4427** Ostomy pouch, drainable; for use on barrier with locking flange, with filter (2-piece system), each Ⓑ Ⓑ

✻ **A4428** Ostomy pouch, urinary, with extended wear barrier attached, with faucet-type tap with valve (1 piece), each Ⓑ Ⓑ

✻ **A4429** Ostomy pouch, urinary, with barrier attached, with built-in convexity, with faucet-type tap with valve (1 piece), each Ⓑ Ⓑ

✻ **A4430** Ostomy pouch, urinary, with extended wear barrier attached, with built-in convexity, with faucet-type tap with valve (1 piece), each Ⓑ Ⓑ

✻ **A4431** Ostomy pouch, urinary; with barrier attached, with faucet-type tap with valve (1 piece), each Ⓑ Ⓑ

✻ **A4432** Ostomy pouch, urinary; for use on barrier with non-locking flange, with faucet-type tap with valve (2 piece), each Ⓑ Ⓑ

✻ **A4433** Ostomy pouch, urinary; for use on barrier with locking flange (2 piece), each Ⓑ Ⓑ

✻ **A4434** Ostomy pouch, urinary; for use on barrier with locking flange, with faucet-type tap with valve (2 piece), each Ⓑ Ⓑ

✻ **A4435** Ostomy pouch, drainable, high output, with extended wear barrier (one-piece system), with or without filter, each Ⓑ Ⓑ

Miscellaneous Supplies

A4450 Tape, non-waterproof, per 18 square inches

Bill Local Carrier if incident to a physician's service (not separately payable) or if supply for implanted prosthetic device. If other, bill DME MAC.

If used with surgical dressings, billed with AW modifier (in addition to appropriate A1-A9 modifier).

IOM: 100-02, 15, 120

A4452 Tape, waterproof, per 18 square inches

Bill Local Carrier if incident to a physician's service (not separately payable) or if supply for implanted prosthetic device. If other, bill DME MAC.

If used with surgical dressings, billed with AW modifier (in addition to appropriate A1-A9 modifier).

IOM: 100-02, 15, 120

A4455 Adhesive remover or solvent (for tape, cement or other adhesive), per ounce

Bill Local Carrier if incident to a physician's service (not separately payable) or if supply for implanted prosthetic device. If other, bill DME MAC.

IOM: 100-02, 15, 120

A4456 Adhesive remover, wipes, any type, each

Bill Local Carrier if incident to a physician's service (not separately payable) or if supply for implanted prosthetic device. If other, bill DME MAC.

May be reimbursed for male or female clients to home health DME providers and DME medical suppliers in the home setting.

IOM: 100-02, 15, 120

* **A4458** Enema bag with tubing, reusable

* **A4459** Manual pump-operated enema system, includes balloon, catheter and all accessories, reusable, any type

* **A4461** Surgical dressing holder, non-reusable, each

Bill Local Carrier if incident to a physician's service (not separately payable). If other, bill DME MAC.

* **A4463** Surgical dressing holder, reusable, each

Bill Local Carrier if incident to a physician's service (not separately payable). If other, bill DME MAC.

* **A4465** Non-elastic binder for extremity

~~A4466 Garment, belt, sleeve or other covering, elastic or similar stretchable material, any type, each~~ ✖

▶ **A4467** Belt, strap, sleeve, garment, or covering, any type

A4470 Gravlee jet washer

Symptoms suggestive of endometrial disease must be present for this disposable diagnostic tool to be covered.

IOM: 100-02, 16, 90; 100-03, 4, 230.5

A4480 VABRA aspirator

Symptoms suggestive of endometrial disease must be present for this disposable diagnostic tool to be covered.

IOM: 100-02, 16, 90; 100-03, 4, 230.6

A4481 Tracheostoma filter, any type, any size, each

Bill Local Carrier if incident to a physician's service (not separately payable). If other, bill DME MAC.

IOM: 100-02, 15, 120

A4483 Moisture exchanger, disposable, for use with invasive mechanical ventilation

IOM: 100-02, 15, 120

A4490 Surgical stockings above knee length, each

IOM: 100-02, 15, 100; 100-02, 15, 110; 100-03, 4, 280.1

A4495 Surgical stockings thigh length, each

IOM: 100-02, 15, 100; 100-02, 15, 110; 100-03, 4, 280.1

A4500 Surgical stockings below knee length, each

IOM: 100-02, 15, 100; 100-02, 15, 110; 100-03, 4, 280.1

A4510 Surgical stockings full length, each

IOM: 100-02, 15, 100; 100-02, 15, 110; 100-03, 4, 280.1

A4520 Incontinence garment, any type, (e.g., brief, diaper), each

IOM: 100-03, 4, 280.1

▶ New ↩ Revised ✔ Reinstated ~~deleted~~ Deleted ⃠ Not covered or valid by Medicare
Special coverage instructions * Carrier discretion Bill local carrier Bill DME MAC

✪ **A4550** Surgical trays

No longer payable by Medicare; included in practice expense for procedures. Some private payers may pay, most private payers follow Medicare guidelines

IOM: 100-04, 12, 20.3, 30.4

▶ ⊘ **A4553** Non-disposable underpads, all sizes

IOM: 100-03, 4, 280.1

⊘ **A4554** Disposable underpads, all sizes

IOM: 100-03, 4, 280.1

⊘ **A4555** Electrode/transducer for use with electrical stimulation device used for cancer treatment, replacement only

Bill Local Carrier if incident to a physician's service (not separately payable). If other, bill DME MAC.

✱ **A4556** Electrodes, (e.g., apnea monitor), per pair

Bill Local Carrier if incident to a physician's service (not separately payable). If other, bill DME MAC.

✱ **A4557** Lead wires, (e.g., apnea monitor), per pair

Bill Local Carrier if incident to a physician's service (not separately payable). If other, bill DME MAC.

✱ **A4558** Conductive gel or paste, for use with electrical device (e.g., TENS, NMES), per oz

Bill Local Carrier if incident to a physician's service (not separately payable). If other, bill DME MAC.

✱ **A4559** Coupling gel or paste, for use with ultrasound device, per oz

Bill Local Carrier if incident to a physician's service (not separately payable). If other, bill DME MAC.

✱ **A4561** Pessary, rubber, any type

✱ **A4562** Pessary, non rubber, any type

✱ **A4565** Slings

⊘ **A4566** Shoulder sling or vest design, abduction restrainer, with or without swathe control, prefabricated, includes fitting and adjustment

⊘ **A4570** Splint

IOM: 100-02, 6, 10; 100-02, 15, 100; 100-04, 4, 240

⊘ **A4575** Topical hyperbaric oxygen chamber, disposable

IOM: 100-03, 1, 20.29

⊘ **A4580** Cast supplies (e.g., plaster)

IOM: 100-02, 6, 10; 100-02, 15, 100; 100-04, 4, 240

⊘ **A4590** Special casting material (e.g., fiberglass)

IOM: 100-02, 6, 10; 100-02, 15, 100; 100-04, 4, 240

✪ **A4595** Electrical stimulator supplies, 2 lead, per month (e.g., TENS, NMES)

Bill Local Carrier if incident to a physician's service (not separately payable). If other, bill DME MAC.

IOM: 100-03, 2, 160.13

✱ **A4600** Sleeve for intermittent limb compression device, replacement only, each

✱ **A4601** Lithium ion battery, rechargeable, for non-prosthetic use, replacement

✱ **A4602** Replacement battery for external infusion pump owned by patient, lithium, 1.5 volt, each

✱ **A4604** Tubing with integrated heating element for use with positive airway pressure device

✱ **A4605** Tracheal suction catheter, closed system, each

✱ **A4606** Oxygen probe for use with oximeter device, replacement

✱ **A4608** Transtracheal oxygen catheter, each

Supplies for Respiratory and Oxygen Equipment

A4614-A4629: Bill Local Carrier if incident to a physician's service (not separately payable). If other, bill DME MAC.

⊘ **A4611** Battery, heavy duty; replacement for patient owned ventilator

Medicare Statute 1834(a)(3)(a)

⊘ **A4612** Battery cables; replacement for patient-owned ventilator

Medicare Statute 1834(a)(3)(a)

⊘ **A4613** Battery charger; replacement for patient-owned ventilator

Medicare Statute 1834(a)(3)(a)

✱ **A4614** Peak expiratory flow rate meter, hand held

✪ **A4615** Cannula, nasal

IOM: 100-03, 2, 160.6; 100-04, 20, 100.2

✪ **A4616** Tubing (oxygen), per foot

IOM: 100-03, 2, 160.6; 100-04, 20, 100.2

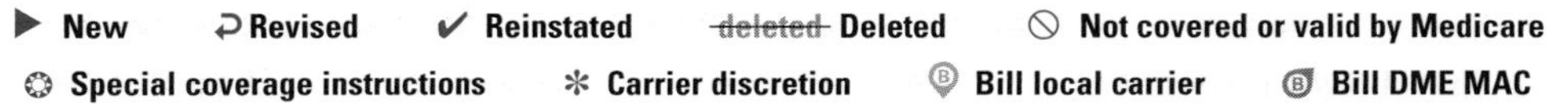

A4617 Mouth piece
IOM: 100-03, 2, 160.6; 100-04, 20, 100.2

A4618 Breathing circuits
IOM: 100-03, 2, 160.6; 100-04, 20, 100.2

A4619 Face tent
IOM: 100-03, 2, 160.6; 100-04, 20, 100.2

A4620 Variable concentration mask
IOM: 100-03, 2, 160.6; 100-04, 20, 100.2

A4623 Tracheostomy, inner cannula
IOM: 100-02, 15, 120; 100-03, 1, 20.9

* **A4624** Tracheal suction catheter, any type, other than closed system, each

Sterile suction catheters are medically necessary only for tracheostomy suctioning. Limitations include three suction catheters per day when covered for medically necessary tracheostomy suctioning. Assign DX Z43.0 or Z93.0 on the claim form. (CMS Manual System, Pub. 100-3, NCD manual, Chapter 1, Section 280-1)

A4625 Tracheostomy care kit for new tracheostomy

Dressings used with tracheostomies are included in the allowance for the code. This starter kit is covered after a surgical tracheostomy. (https://www.noridianmedicare.com/dme/coverage/docs/lcds/current_lcds/tracheostomy_care_supplies.htm)

IOM: 100-02, 15, 120

A4626 Tracheostomy cleaning brush, each
IOM: 100-02, 15, 120

⊘ **A4627** Spacer, bag, or reservoir, with or without mask, for use with metered dose inhaler
IOM: 100-02, 15, 110

* **A4628** Oropharyngeal suction catheter, each

No more than three catheters per week are covered for medically necessary oropharyngeal suctioning because the catheters can be reused if cleansed and disinfected. (MS Manual System, Pub. 100-3, NCD manual, Chapter 1, Section 280-1)

A4629 Tracheostomy care kit for established tracheostomy
IOM: 100-02, 15, 120

Supplies for Other Durable Medical Equipment

A4630 Replacement batteries, medically necessary, transcutaneous electrical stimulator, owned by patient
IOM: 100-03, 3, 160.7

* **A4633** Replacement bulb/lamp for ultraviolet light therapy system, each

* **A4634** Replacement bulb for therapeutic light box, tabletop model

A4635 Underarm pad, crutch, replacement, each
IOM: 100-03, 4, 280.1

A4636 Replacement, handgrip, cane, crutch, or walker, each
IOM: 100-03, 4, 280.1

A4637 Replacement, tip, cane, crutch, walker, each
IOM: 100-03, 4, 280.1

* **A4638** Replacement battery for patient-owned ear pulse generator, each

* **A4639** Replacement pad for infrared heating pad system, each

A4640 Replacement pad for use with medically necessary alternating pressure pad owned by patient
IOM: 100-03, 4, 280.1; 100-08, 5, 5.2.3

Supplies for Radiological Procedures

* **A4641** Radiopharmaceutical, diagnostic, not otherwise classified

Is not an applicable tracer for PET scans

* **A4642** Indium In-111 satumomab pendetide, diagnostic, per study dose, up to 6 millicuries

Miscellaneous Supplies

* **A4648** Tissue marker, implantable, any type, each

* **A4649** Surgical supply miscellaneous

Bill Local Carrier if incident to a physician's service (not separately payable), or if supply for implanted prosthetic device or implanted DME. If other, bill DME MAC.

* **A4650** Implantable radiation dosimeter, each

► New ⤾ Revised ✔ Reinstated ~~deleted~~ Deleted ⊘ Not covered or valid by Medicare
Special coverage instructions * Carrier discretion Bill local carrier Bill DME MAC

Supplies for Dialysis

A4653-A4932: Supplies for ESRD - Bill DME MAC (not separately payable).

⊕ **A4651** Calibrated microcapillary tube, each Ⓑ

IOM: 100-04, 3, 40.3

⊕ **A4652** Microcapillary tube sealant Ⓑ

IOM: 100-04, 3, 40.3

* **A4653** Peritoneal dialysis catheter anchoring device, belt, each Ⓑ

⊕ **A4657** Syringe, with or without needle, each Ⓑ

IOM: 100-04, 8, 90.3.2

⊕ **A4660** Sphygmomanometer/blood pressure apparatus with cuff and stethoscope Ⓑ

IOM: 100-04, 8, 90.3.2

⊕ **A4663** Blood pressure cuff only Ⓑ

IOM: 100-04, 8, 90.3.2

⊘ **A4670** Automatic blood pressure monitor Ⓑ

IOM: 100-04, 8, 90.3.2

⊕ **A4671** Disposable cycler set used with cycler dialysis machine, each Ⓑ

IOM: 100-04, 8, 90.3.2

⊕ **A4672** Drainage extension line, sterile, for dialysis, each Ⓑ

IOM: 100-04, 8, 90.3.2

⊕ **A4673** Extension line with easy lock connectors, used with dialysis Ⓑ

IOM: 100-04, 8, 90.3.2

⊕ **A4674** Chemicals/antiseptics solution used to clean/sterilize dialysis equipment, per 8 oz Ⓑ

IOM: 100-04, 8, 90.3.2

⊕ **A4680** Activated carbon filters for hemodialysis, each Ⓑ

IOM: 100-04, 8, 90.3.2

⊕ **A4690** Dialyzers (artificial kidneys), all types, all sizes, for hemodialysis, each Ⓑ

IOM: 100-04, 8, 90.3.2

⊕ **A4706** Bicarbonate concentrate, solution, for hemodialysis, per gallon Ⓑ

IOM: 100-04, 8, 90.3.2

⊕ **A4707** Bicarbonate concentrate, powder, for hemodialysis, per packet Ⓑ

IOM: 100-04, 8, 90.3.2

⊕ **A4708** Acetate concentrate solution, for hemodialysis, per gallon Ⓑ

IOM: 100-04, 8, 90.3.2

⊕ **A4709** Acid concentrate, solution, for hemodialysis, per gallon Ⓑ

IOM: 100-04, 8, 90.3.2

⊕ **A4714** Treated water (deionized, distilled, or reverse osmosis) for peritoneal dialysis, per gallon Ⓑ

IOM: 100-03, 4, 230.7; 100-04, 3, 40.3

⊕ **A4719** "Y set" tubing for peritoneal dialysis Ⓑ

IOM: 100-04, 8, 90.3.2

⊕ **A4720** Dialysate solution, any concentration of dextrose, fluid volume greater than 249 cc, but less than or equal to 999 cc, for peritoneal dialysis Ⓑ

Do not use AX modifier

IOM: 100-04, 8, 90.3.2

⊕ **A4721** Dialysate solution, any concentration of dextrose, fluid volume greater than 999 cc but less than or equal to 1999 cc, for peritoneal dialysis Ⓑ

IOM: 100-04, 8, 90.3.2

⊕ **A4722** Dialysate solution, any concentration of dextrose, fluid volume greater than 1999 cc but less than or equal to 2999 cc, for peritoneal dialysis Ⓑ

IOM: 100-04, 8, 90.3.2

⊕ **A4723** Dialysate solution, any concentration of dextrose, fluid volume greater than 2999 cc but less than or equal to 3999 cc, for peritoneal dialysis Ⓑ

IOM: 100-04, 8, 90.3.2

⊕ **A4724** Dialysate solution, any concentration of dextrose, fluid volume greater than 3999 cc but less than or equal to 4999 cc for peritoneal dialysis Ⓑ

IOM: 100-04, 8, 90.3.2

⊕ **A4725** Dialysate solution, any concentration of dextrose, fluid volume greater than 4999 cc but less than or equal to 5999 cc, for peritoneal dialysis Ⓑ

IOM: 100-04, 8, 90.3.2

⊕ **A4726** Dialysate solution, any concentration of dextrose, fluid volume greater than 5999 cc, for peritoneal dialysis Ⓑ

IOM: 100-04, 8, 90.3.2

* **A4728** Dialysate solution, non-dextrose containing, 500 ml Ⓑ

⊕ **A4730** Fistula cannulation set for hemodialysis, each Ⓑ

IOM: 100-04, 8, 90.3.2

⊕ **A4736** Topical anesthetic, for dialysis, per gram Ⓑ

IOM: 100-04, 8, 90.3.2

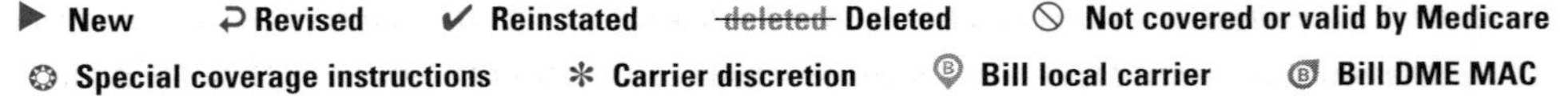

◌ **A4737** Injectable anesthetic, for dialysis, per 10 ml Ⓑ
IOM: 100-04, 8, 90.3.2

◌ **A4740** Shunt accessory, for hemodialysis, any type, each Ⓑ
IOM: 100-04, 8, 90.3.2

◌ **A4750** Blood tubing, arterial or venous, for hemodialysis, each Ⓑ
IOM: 100-04, 8, 90.3.2

◌ **A4755** Blood tubing, arterial and venous combined, for hemodialysis, each Ⓑ
IOM: 100-04, 8, 90.3.2

◌ **A4760** Dialysate solution test kit, for peritoneal dialysis, any type, each Ⓑ
IOM: 100-04, 8, 90.3.2

◌ **A4765** Dialysate concentrate, powder, additive for peritoneal dialysis, per packet Ⓑ
IOM: 100-04, 8, 90.3.2

◌ **A4766** Dialysate concentrate, solution, additive for peritoneal dialysis, per 10 ml Ⓑ
IOM: 100-04, 8, 90.3.2

◌ **A4770** Blood collection tube, vacuum, for dialysis, per 50 Ⓑ
IOM: 100-04, 8, 90.3.2

◌ **A4771** Serum clotting time tube, for dialysis, per 50 Ⓑ
IOM: 100-04, 8, 90.3.2

◌ **A4772** Blood glucose test strips, for dialysis, per 50 Ⓑ
IOM: 100-04, 8, 90.3.2

◌ **A4773** Occult blood test strips, for dialysis, per 50 Ⓑ
IOM: 100-04, 8, 90.3.2

◌ **A4774** Ammonia test strips, for dialysis, per 50 Ⓑ
IOM: 100-04, 8, 90.3.2

◌ **A4802** Protamine sulfate, for hemodialysis, per 50 mg Ⓑ
IOM: 100-04, 8, 90.3.2

◌ **A4860** Disposable catheter tips for peritoneal dialysis, per 10 Ⓑ
IOM: 100-04, 8, 90.3.2

◌ **A4870** Plumbing and/or electrical work for home hemodialysis equipment Ⓑ
IOM: 100-04, 8, 90.3.2

◌ **A4890** Contracts, repair and maintenance, for hemodialysis equipment Ⓑ
IOM: 100-02, 15, 110.2

◌ **A4911** Drain bag/bottle, for dialysis, each Ⓑ

◌ **A4913** Miscellaneous dialysis supplies, not otherwise specified Ⓑ
Items not related to dialysis must not be billed with the miscellaneous codes A4913 or E1699.

◌ **A4918** Venous pressure clamp, for hemodialysis, each Ⓑ

◌ **A4927** Gloves, non-sterile, per 100 Ⓑ

◌ **A4928** Surgical mask, per 20 Ⓑ

◌ **A4929** Tourniquet for dialysis, each Ⓑ

◌ **A4930** Gloves, sterile, per pair Ⓑ

* **A4931** Oral thermometer, reusable, any type, each Ⓑ

* **A4932** Rectal thermometer, reusable, any type, each Ⓑ

Additional Ostomy Supplies

A5051-A5093: If provided in the physician's office for a temporary condition, the item is incident to the physician's service and billed to the Local Carrier. If provided in the physician's office or other place of service for a permanent condition, the item is a prosthetic device and billed to the DME MAC.

◌ **A5051** Ostomy pouch, closed; with barrier attached (1 piece), each Ⓑ Ⓑ
IOM: 100-02, 15, 120

◌ **A5052** Ostomy pouch, closed; without barrier attached (1 piece), each Ⓑ Ⓑ
IOM: 100-02, 15, 120

◌ **A5053** Ostomy pouch, closed; for use on faceplate, each Ⓑ Ⓑ
IOM: 100-02, 15, 120

◌ **A5054** Ostomy pouch, closed; for use on barrier with flange (2 piece), each Ⓑ Ⓑ
IOM: 100-02, 15, 120

◌ **A5055** Stoma cap Ⓑ Ⓑ
IOM: 100-02, 15, 120

◌ **A5056** Ostomy pouch, drainable, with extended wear barrier attached, with filter, (1 piece), each Ⓑ Ⓑ
IOM: 100-02, 15, 120

◌ **A5057** Ostomy pouch, drainable, with extended wear barrier attached, with built in convexity, with filter, (1 piece), each Ⓑ Ⓑ
IOM: 100-02, 15, 120

* **A5061** Ostomy pouch, drainable; with barrier attached, (1 piece), each Ⓑ Ⓑ
IOM: 100-02, 15, 120

▶ New ⤾ Revised ✔ Reinstated ~~deleted~~ Deleted ⊘ Not covered or valid by Medicare
◌ Special coverage instructions * Carrier discretion Ⓑ Bill local carrier Ⓑ Bill DME MAC

⊕ **A5062** Ostomy pouch, drainable; without barrier attached (1 piece), each Ⓑ Ⓑ
IOM: 100-02, 15, 120

⊕ **A5063** Ostomy pouch, drainable; for use on barrier with flange (2 piece system), each Ⓑ Ⓑ
IOM: 100-02, 15, 120

⊕ **A5071** Ostomy pouch, urinary; with barrier attached (1 piece), each Ⓑ Ⓑ
IOM: 100-02, 15, 120

⊕ **A5072** Ostomy pouch, urinary; without barrier attached (1 piece), each Ⓑ Ⓑ
IOM: 100-02, 15, 120

⊕ **A5073** Ostomy pouch, urinary; for use on barrier with flange (2 piece), each Ⓑ Ⓑ
IOM: 100-02, 15, 120

⊕ **A5081** Stoma plug or seal, any type Ⓑ Ⓑ
IOM: 100-02, 15, 120

⊕ **A5082** Continent device; catheter for continent stoma Ⓑ Ⓑ
IOM: 100-02, 15, 120

* **A5083** Continent device, stoma absorptive cover for continent stoma Ⓑ Ⓑ

⊕ **A5093** Ostomy accessory; convex insert Ⓑ Ⓑ
IOM: 100-02, 15, 120

Additional Incontinence and Ostomy Supplies

A5102-A5200: If provided in the physician's office for a temporary condition, the item is incident to the physician's service and billed to the Local Carrier. If provided in the physician's office or other place of service for a permanent condition, the item is a prosthetic device and billed to the DME MAC.

⊕ **A5102** Bedside drainage bottle with or without tubing, rigid or expandable, each Ⓑ Ⓑ
IOM: 100-02, 15, 120

⊕ **A5105** Urinary suspensory, with leg bag, with or without tube, each Ⓑ Ⓑ
IOM: 100-02, 15, 120

⊕ **A5112** Urinary drainage bag, leg bag, leg or abdomen, latex, with or without tube, with straps, each Ⓑ Ⓑ
IOM: 100-02, 15, 120

⊕ **A5113** Leg strap; latex, replacement only, per set Ⓑ Ⓑ
IOM: 100-02, 15, 120

⊕ **A5114** Leg strap; foam or fabric, replacement only, per set Ⓑ Ⓑ
IOM: 100-02, 15, 120

⊕ **A5120** Skin barrier, wipes or swabs, each Ⓑ Ⓑ
IOM: 100-02, 15, 120

⊕ **A5121** Skin barrier; solid, 6 × 6 or equivalent, each Ⓑ Ⓑ
IOM: 100-02, 15, 120

⊕ **A5122** Skin barrier; solid, 8 × 8 or equivalent, each Ⓑ Ⓑ
IOM: 100-02, 15, 120

⊕ **A5126** Adhesive or non-adhesive; disk or foam pad Ⓑ Ⓑ
IOM: 100-02, 15, 120

⊕ **A5131** Appliance cleaner, incontinence and ostomy appliances, per 16 oz Ⓑ Ⓑ
IOM: 100-02, 15, 120

⊕ **A5200** Percutaneous catheter/tube anchoring device, adhesive skin attachment Ⓑ Ⓑ
IOM: 100-02, 15, 120

Diabetic Shoes, Fitting, and Modifications

⊕ **A5500** For diabetics only, fitting (including follow-up), custom preparation and supply of off-the-shelf depth-inlay shoe manufactured to accommodate multi-density insert(s), per shoe Ⓑ
IOM: 100-02, 15, 140

⊕ **A5501** For diabetics only, fitting (including follow-up), custom preparation and supply of shoe molded from cast(s) of patient's foot (custom-molded shoe), per shoe Ⓑ

The diabetic patient must have at least one of the following conditions: peripheral neuropathy with evidence of callus formation, pre-ulcerative calluses, previous ulceration, foot deformity, previous amputation or poor circulation

IOM: 100-02, 15, 140

⊕ **A5503** For diabetics only, modification (including fitting) of off-the-shelf depth-inlay shoe or custom-molded shoe with roller or rigid rocker bottom, per shoe Ⓑ
IOM: 100-02, 15, 140

A5504 For diabetics only, modification (including fitting) of off-the-shelf depth-inlay shoe or custom-molded shoe with wedge(s), per shoe

IOM: 100-02, 15, 140

A5505 For diabetics only, modification (including fitting) of off-the-shelf depth-inlay shoe or custom-molded shoe with metatarsal bar, per shoe

IOM: 100-02, 15, 140

A5506 For diabetics only, modification (including fitting) of off-the-shelf depth-inlay shoe or custom-molded shoe with off-set heel(s), per shoe

IOM: 100-02, 15, 140

A5507 For diabetics only, not otherwise specified modification (including fitting) of off-the-shelf depth-inlay shoe or custom-molded shoe, per shoe

Only used for not otherwise specified therapeutic modifications to shoe or for repairs to a diabetic shoe(s)

IOM: 100-02, 15, 140

A5508 For diabetics only, deluxe feature of off-the-shelf depth-inlay shoe or custom-molded shoe, per shoe

IOM: 100-02, 15, 40

A5510 For diabetics only, direct formed, compression molded to patient's foot without external heat source, multiple-density insert(s) prefabricated, per shoe

IOM: 100-02, 15, 140

* **A5512** For diabetics only, multiple density insert, direct formed, molded to foot after external heat source of 230 degrees Fahrenheit or higher, total contact with patient's foot, including arch, base layer minimum of 1/4 inch material of shore a 35 durometer or 3/16 inch material of shore a 40 durometer (or higher), prefabricated, each

* **A5513** For diabetics only, multiple density insert, custom molded from model of patient's foot, total contact with patient's foot, including arch, base layer minimum of 3/16 inch material of shore a 35 durometer (or higher), includes arch filler and other shaping material, custom fabricated, each

Dressings

A6010-A6512: Bill Local Carrier if incident to a physician's service (not separately payable) or if supply for implanted prosthetic device or implanted DME. If other, bill DME MAC.

A6000 Non-contact wound warming wound cover for use with the non-contact wound warming device and warming card

IOM: 100-02, 16, 20

A6010 Collagen based wound filler, dry form, sterile, per gram of collagen

IOM: 100-02, 15, 100

A6011 Collagen based wound filler, gel/paste, per gram of collagen

IOM: 100-02, 15, 100

A6021 Collagen dressing, sterile, size 16 sq. in. or less, each

IOM: 100-02, 15, 100

A6022 Collagen dressing, sterile, size more than 16 sq. in. but less than or equal to 48 sq. in., each

IOM: 100-02, 15, 100

A6023 Collagen dressing, sterile, size more than 48 sq. in., each

IOM: 100-02, 15, 100

A6024 Collagen dressing wound filler, sterile, per 6 inches

IOM: 100-02, 15, 100

* **A6025** Gel sheet for dermal or epidermal application, (e.g., silicone, hydrogel, other), each

If used for the treatment of keloids or other scars, a silicone gel sheet will not meet the definition of the surgical dressing benefit and will be denied as noncovered.

A6154 Wound pouch, each

Waterproof collection device with drainable port that adheres to skin around wound. Usual dressing change is up to 3 × per week.

IOM: 100-02, 15, 100

A6196 Alginate or other fiber gelling dressing, wound cover, sterile, pad size 16 sq. in. or less, each dressing

IOM: 100-02, 15, 100

A6197 Alginate or other fiber gelling dressing, wound cover, sterile, pad size more than 16 sq. in., but less than or equal to 48 sq. in., each dressing

IOM: 100-02, 15, 100

A6198 Alginate or other fiber gelling dressing, wound cover, sterile, pad size more than 48 sq. in., each dressing

IOM: 100-02, 15, 100

A6199 Alginate or other fiber gelling dressing, wound filler, sterile, per 6 inches

IOM: 100-02, 15, 100

A6203 Composite dressing, sterile, pad size 16 sq. in. or less, with any size adhesive border, each dressing

Usual composite dressing change is up to 3 times per week, one wound cover per dressing change.

IOM: 100-02, 15, 100

A6204 Composite dressing, sterile, pad size more than 16 sq. in. but less than or equal to 48 sq. in., with any size adhesive border, each dressing

Usual composite dressing change is up to 3 times per week, one wound cover per dressing change.

IOM: 100-02, 15, 100

A6205 Composite dressing, sterile, pad size more than 48 sq. in., with any size adhesive border, each dressing

Usual composite dressing change is up to 3 times per week, one wound cover per dressing change.

IOM: 100-02, 15, 100

A6206 Contact layer, sterile, 16 sq. in. or less, each dressing

Contact layers are porous to allow wound fluid to pass through for absorption by separate overlying dressing and are not intended to be changed with each dressing change. Usual dressing change is up to once per week.

IOM: 100-02, 15, 100

A6207 Contact layer, sterile, more than 16 sq. in. but less than or equal to 48 sq. in., each dressing

Contact layer dressings are used to line the entire wound; they are not intended to be changed with each dressing change. Usual dressing change is up to once per week.

IOM: 100-02, 15, 100

A6208 Contact layer, sterile, more than 48 sq. in., each dressing

Contact layer dressings are used to line the entire wound; they are not intended to be changed with each dressing change. Usual dressing change is up to once per week.

IOM: 100-02, 15, 100

A6209 Foam dressing, wound cover, sterile, pad size 16 sq. in. or less, without adhesive border, each dressing

Made of open cell, medical grade expanded polymer; with nonadherent property over wound site

IOM: 100-02, 15, 100

A6210 Foam dressing, wound cover, sterile, pad size more than 16 sq. in. but less than or equal to 48 sq. in., without adhesive border, each dressing

Foam dressings are covered items when used on full thickness wounds (e.g., stage III or IV ulcers) with moderate to heavy exudates. Usual dressing change for a foam wound cover when used as primary dressing is up to 3 times per week. When foam wound cover is used as a secondary dressing for wounds with very heavy exudates, dressing change may be up to 3 times per week. Usual dressing change for foam wound fillers is up to once per day (A6209-A6215).

IOM: 100-02, 15, 100

A6211 Foam dressing, wound cover, sterile, pad size more than 48 sq. in., without adhesive border, each dressing

IOM: 100-02, 15, 100

A6212 Foam dressing, wound cover, sterile, pad size 16 sq. in. or less, with any size adhesive border, each dressing

IOM: 100-02, 15, 100

A6213 Foam dressing, wound cover, sterile, pad size more than 16 sq. in. but less than or equal to 48 sq. in., with any size adhesive border, each dressing

IOM: 100-02, 15, 100

A6214 Foam dressing, wound cover, sterile, pad size more than 48 sq. in., with any size adhesive border, each dressing

IOM: 100-02, 15, 100

A6215 Foam dressing, wound filler, sterile, per gram

IOM: 100-02, 15, 100

A6216 Gauze, non-impregnated, non-sterile, pad size 16 sq. in. or less, without adhesive border, each dressing

IOM: 100-02, 15, 100

A6217 Gauze, non-impregnated, non-sterile, pad size more than 16 sq. in. but less than or equal to 48 sq. in., without adhesive border, each dressing

IOM: 100-02, 15, 100

A6218 Gauze, non-impregnated, non-sterile, pad size more than 48 sq. in., without adhesive border, each dressing

IOM: 100-02, 15, 100

A6219 Gauze, non-impregnated, sterile, pad size 16 sq. in. or less, with any size adhesive border, each dressing

IOM: 100-02, 15, 100

A6220 Gauze, non-impregnated, sterile, pad size more than 16 sq. in. but less than or equal to 48 sq. in., with any size adhesive border, each dressing

IOM: 100-02, 15, 100

A6221 Gauze, non-impregnated, sterile, pad size more than 48 sq. in., with any size adhesive border, each dressing

IOM: 100-02, 15, 100

A6222 Gauze, impregnated with other than water, normal saline, or hydrogel, sterile, pad size 16 sq. in. or less, without adhesive border, each dressing

Substances may have been incorporated into dressing material (i.e., iodinated agents, petrolatum, zinc paste, crystalline sodium chloride, chlorhexadine gluconate [CHG], bismuth tribromophenate [BTP], water, aqueous saline, hydrogel, or agents).

IOM: 100-02, 15, 100

A6223 Gauze, impregnated with other than water, normal saline, or hydrogel, sterile, pad size more than 16 sq. in. but less than or equal to 48 sq. in., without adhesive border, each dressing

IOM: 100-02, 15, 100

A6224 Gauze, impregnated with other than water, normal saline, or hydrogel, sterile, pad size more than 48 square inches, without adhesive border, each dressing

IOM: 100-02, 15, 100

A6228 Gauze, impregnated, water or normal saline, sterile, pad size 16 sq. in. or less, without adhesive border, each dressing

IOM: 100-02, 15, 100

A6229 Gauze, impregnated, water or normal saline, sterile, pad size more than 16 sq. in. but less than or equal to 48 sq. in., without adhesive border, each dressing

IOM: 100-02, 15, 100

A6230 Gauze, impregnated, water or normal saline, sterile, pad size more than 48 sq. in., without adhesive border, each dressing

IOM: 100-02, 15, 100

A6231 Gauze, impregnated, hydrogel, for direct wound contact, sterile, pad size 16 sq. in. or less, each dressing

IOM: 100-02, 15, 100

A6232 Gauze, impregnated, hydrogel, for direct wound contact, sterile, pad size greater than 16 sq. in., but less than or equal to 48 sq. in., each dressing

IOM: 100-02, 15, 100

A6233 Gauze, impregnated, hydrogel, for direct wound contact, sterile, pad size more than 48 sq. in., each dressing

IOM: 100-02, 15, 100

A6234 Hydrocolloid dressing, wound cover, sterile, pad size 16 sq. in. or less, without adhesive border, each dressing

This type of dressing is usually used on wounds with light to moderate exudate with an average of three dressing changes per week.

IOM: 100-02, 15, 100

A6235 Hydrocolloid dressing, wound cover, sterile, pad size more than 16 sq. in. but less than or equal to 48 sq. in., without adhesive border, each dressing

IOM: 100-02, 15, 100

A6236 Hydrocolloid dressing, wound cover, sterile, pad size more than 48 sq. in., without adhesive border, each dressing

IOM: 100-02, 15, 100

A6237 Hydrocolloid dressing, wound cover, sterile, pad size 16 sq. in. or less, with any size adhesive border, each dressing

IOM: 100-02, 15, 100

A6238 Hydrocolloid dressing, wound cover, sterile, pad size more than 16 sq. in. but less than or equal to 48 sq. in., with any size adhesive border, each dressing

IOM: 100-02, 15, 100

A6239 Hydrocolloid dressing, wound cover, sterile, pad size more than 48 sq. in., with any size adhesive border, each dressing

IOM: 100-02, 15, 100

A6240 Hydrocolloid dressing, wound filler, paste, sterile, per ounce

IOM: 100-02, 15, 100

A6241 Hydrocolloid dressing, wound filler, dry form, sterile, per gram

IOM: 100-02, 15, 100

A6242 Hydrogel dressing, wound cover, sterile, pad size 16 sq. in. or less, without adhesive border, each dressing

Considered medically necessary when used on full thickness wounds with minimal or no exudate (e.g., stage III or IV ulcers)

Usually up to one dressing change per day is considered medically necessary, but if well documented and medically necessary, the payer may allow more frequent dressing changes.

IOM: 100-02, 15, 100

A6243 Hydrogel dressing, wound cover, sterile, pad size more than 16 sq. in. but less than or equal to 48 sq. in., without adhesive border, each dressing

IOM: 100-02, 15, 100

A6244 Hydrogel dressing, wound cover, sterile, pad size more than 48 sq. in., without adhesive border, each dressing

IOM: 100-02, 15, 100

A6245 Hydrogel dressing, wound cover, sterile, pad size 16 sq. in. or less, with any size adhesive border, each dressing

Coverage of a non-elastic gradient compression wrap is limited to one per 6 months per leg.

IOM: 100-02, 15, 100

A6246 Hydrogel dressing, wound cover, sterile, pad size more than 16 sq. in. but less than or equal to 48 sq. in., with any size adhesive border, each dressing

IOM: 100-02, 15, 100

A6247 Hydrogel dressing, wound cover, sterile, pad size more than 48 sq. in., with any size adhesive border, each dressing

IOM: 100-02, 15, 100

A6248 Hydrogel dressing, wound filler, gel, per fluid ounce

IOM: 100-02, 15, 100

A6250 Skin sealants, protectants, moisturizers, ointments, any type, any size

IOM: 100-02, 15, 100

A6251 Specialty absorptive dressing, wound cover, sterile, pad size 16 sq. in. or less, without adhesive border, each dressing

IOM: 100-02, 15, 100

A6252 Specialty absorptive dressing, wound cover, sterile, pad size more than 16 sq. in. but less than or equal to 48 sq. in., without adhesive border, each dressing

IOM: 100-02, 15, 100

A6253 Specialty absorptive dressing, wound cover, sterile, pad size more than 48 sq. in., without adhesive border, each dressing

IOM: 100-02, 15, 100

A6254 Specialty absorptive dressing, wound cover, sterile, pad size 16 sq. in. or less, with any size adhesive border, each dressing

IOM: 100-02, 15, 100

A6255 Specialty absorptive dressing, wound cover, sterile, pad size more than 16 sq. in. but less than or equal to 48 sq. in., with any size adhesive border, each dressing

A6256 Specialty absorptive dressing, wound cover, sterile, pad size more than 48 sq. in., with any size adhesive border, each dressing

Considered medically necessary when used for moderately or highly exudative wounds (e.g., stage III or IV ulcers)

IOM: 100-02, 15, 100

A6257 Transparent film, sterile, 16 sq. in. or less, each dressing

Considered medically necessary when used on open partial thickness wounds with minimal exudate or closed wounds

IOM: 100-02, 15, 100

A6258 Transparent film, sterile, more than 16 sq. in. but less than or equal to 48 sq. in., each dressing

IOM: 100-02, 15, 100

▶ New ↻ Revised ✔ Reinstated ~~deleted~~ Deleted ⊘ Not covered or valid by Medicare
Special coverage instructions ✻ Carrier discretion Bill local carrier Bill DME MAC

⚙ **A6259** Transparent film, sterile, more than 48 sq. in., each dressing Ⓑ Ⓑ

IOM: 100-02, 15, 100

⚙ **A6260** Wound cleansers, any type, any size Ⓑ Ⓑ

IOM: 100-02, 15, 100

⚙ **A6261** Wound filler, gel/paste, per fluid ounce, not otherwise specified Ⓑ Ⓑ

Units of service for wound fillers are 1 gram, 1 fluid ounce, 6-inch length, or 1 yard depending on product

IOM: 100-02, 15, 100

⚙ **A6262** Wound filler, dry form, per gram, not otherwise specified Ⓑ Ⓑ

Dry forms (e.g., powder, granules, beads) are used to eliminate dead space in an open wound.

IOM: 100-02, 15, 100

⚙ **A6266** Gauze, impregnated, other than water, normal saline, or zinc paste, sterile, any width, per linear yard Ⓑ Ⓑ

IOM: 100-02, 15, 100

⚙ **A6402** Gauze, non-impregnated, sterile, pad size 16 sq. in. or less, without adhesive border, each dressing Ⓑ Ⓑ

IOM: 100-02, 15, 100

⚙ **A6403** Gauze, non-impregnated, sterile, pad size more than 16 sq. in., less than or equal to 48 sq. in., without adhesive border, each dressing Ⓑ Ⓑ

IOM: 100-02, 15, 100

⚙ **A6404** Gauze, non-impregnated, sterile, pad size more than 48 sq. in., without adhesive border, each dressing Ⓑ Ⓑ

IOM: 100-02, 15, 100

* **A6407** Packing strips, non-impregnated, sterile, up to 2 inches in width, per linear yard Ⓑ Ⓑ

IOM: 100-02, 15, 100

⚙ **A6410** Eye pad, sterile, each Ⓑ Ⓑ

IOM: 100-02, 15, 100

⚙ **A6411** Eye pad, non-sterile, each Ⓑ Ⓑ

IOM: 100-02, 15, 100

* **A6412** Eye patch, occlusive, each Ⓑ Ⓑ

⃠ **A6413** Adhesive bandage, first-aid type, any size, each Ⓑ Ⓑ

First aid type bandage is a wound cover with a pad size of less than 4 square inches. Does not meet the definition of the surgical dressing benefit and will be denied as non-covered.

Medicare Statute 1861(s)(5)

* **A6441** Padding bandage, non-elastic, non-woven/non-knitted, width greater than or equal to three inches and less than five inches, per yard Ⓑ Ⓑ

* **A6442** Conforming bandage, non-elastic, knitted/woven, non-sterile, width less than three inches, per yard Ⓑ Ⓑ

Non-elastic, moderate or high compression that is typically sustained for one week

* **A6443** Conforming bandage, non-elastic, knitted/woven, non-sterile, width greater than or equal to three inches and less than five inches, per yard Ⓑ Ⓑ

* **A6444** Conforming bandage, non-elastic, knitted/woven, non-sterile, width greater than or equal to five inches, per yard Ⓑ Ⓑ

* **A6445** Conforming bandage, non-elastic, knitted/woven, sterile, width less than three inches, per yard Ⓑ Ⓑ

* **A6446** Conforming bandage, non-elastic, knitted/woven, sterile, width greater than or equal to three inches and less than five inches, per yard Ⓑ Ⓑ

* **A6447** Conforming bandage, non-elastic, knitted/woven, sterile, width greater than or equal to five inches, per yard Ⓑ Ⓑ

* **A6448** Light compression bandage, elastic, knitted/woven, width less than three inches, per yard Ⓑ Ⓑ

Used to hold wound cover dressings in place over a wound. Example is an ACE type elastic bandage.

* **A6449** Light compression bandage, elastic, knitted/woven, width greater than or equal to three inches and less than five inches, per yard Ⓑ Ⓑ

* **A6450** Light compression bandage, elastic, knitted/woven, width greater than or equal to five inches, per yard Ⓑ Ⓑ

* **A6451** Moderate compression bandage, elastic, knitted/woven, load resistance of 1.25 to 1.34 foot pounds at 50% maximum stretch, width greater than or equal to three inches and less than five inches, per yard Ⓑ Ⓑ

Elastic bandages that produce moderate compression that is typically sustained for one week

Medicare considers coverage if part of a multi-layer compression bandage system for the treatment of a venous stasis ulcer. Do not assign for strains or sprains.

✻ **A6452** High compression bandage, elastic, knitted/woven, load resistance greater than or equal to 1.35 foot pounds at 50% maximum stretch, width greater than or equal to three inches and less than five inches, per yard

Elastic bandages that produce high compression that is typically sustained for one week

✻ **A6453** Self-adherent bandage, elastic, non-knitted/non-woven, width less than three inches, per yard

✻ **A6454** Self-adherent bandage, elastic, non-knitted/non-woven, width greater than or equal to three inches and less than five inches, per yard

✻ **A6455** Self-adherent bandage, elastic, non-knitted/non-woven, width greater than or equal to five inches, per yard

✻ **A6456** Zinc paste impregnated bandage, non-elastic, knitted/woven, width greater than or equal to three inches and less than five inches, per yard

✻ **A6457** Tubular dressing with or without elastic, any width, per linear yard

❂ **A6501** Compression burn garment, bodysuit (head to foot), custom fabricated

Garments used to reduce hypertrophic scarring and joint contractures following burn injury

IOM: 100-02, 15, 100

❂ **A6502** Compression burn garment, chin strap, custom fabricated

IOM: 100-02, 15, 100

❂ **A6503** Compression burn garment, facial hood, custom fabricated

IOM: 100-02, 15, 100

❂ **A6504** Compression burn garment, glove to wrist, custom fabricated

IOM: 100-02, 15, 100

❂ **A6505** Compression burn garment, glove to elbow, custom fabricated

IOM: 100-02, 15, 100

❂ **A6506** Compression burn garment, glove to axilla, custom fabricated

IOM: 100-02, 15, 100

❂ **A6507** Compression burn garment, foot to knee length, custom fabricated

IOM: 100-02, 15, 100

❂ **A6508** Compression burn garment, foot to thigh length, custom fabricated

IOM: 100-02, 15, 100

❂ **A6509** Compression burn garment, upper trunk to waist including arm openings (vest), custom fabricated

IOM: 100-02, 15, 100

❂ **A6510** Compression burn garment, trunk, including arms down to leg openings (leotard), custom fabricated

IOM: 100-02, 15, 100

❂ **A6511** Compression burn garment, lower trunk including leg openings (panty), custom fabricated

IOM: 100-02, 15, 100

❂ **A6512** Compression burn garment, not otherwise classified

IOM: 100-02, 15, 100

✻ **A6513** Compression burn mask, face and/or neck, plastic or equal, custom fabricated

GRADIENT COMPRESSION STOCKINGS (A6530-A6549)

⊘ **A6530** Gradient compression stocking, below knee, 18–30 mmHg, each

IOM: 100-03, 4, 280.1

❂ **A6531** Gradient compression stocking, below knee, 30–40 mmHg, each

Covered when used in treatment of open venous stasis ulcer. Modifiers A1-A9 are not assigned. Must be billed with AW, RT, or LT

IOM: 100-02, 15, 100

❂ **A6532** Gradient compression stocking, below knee, 40–50 mmHg, each

Covered when used in treatment of open venous stasis ulcer. Modifiers A1-A9 are not assigned. Must be billed with AW, RT, or LT

IOM: 100-02, 15, 100

⊘ **A6533** Gradient compression stocking, thigh length, 18–30 mmHg, each

IOM: 100-02, 15, 130; 100-03, 4, 280.1

⊘ **A6534** Gradient compression stocking, thigh length, 30–40 mmHg, each

IOM: 100-02, 15, 130; 100-03, 4, 280.1

⊘ **A6535** Gradient compression stocking, thigh length, 40–50 mmHg, each

IOM: 100-02, 15, 130; 100-03, 4, 280.1

⊘ **A6536** Gradient compression stocking, full length/chap style, 18–30 mmHg, each

IOM: 100-02, 15, 130; 100-03, 4, 280.1

⊘ **A6537** Gradient compression stocking, full length/chap style, 30–40 mmHg, each Ⓑ

IOM: 100-02, 15, 130; 100-03, 4, 280.1

⊘ **A6538** Gradient compression stocking, full length/chap style, 40–50 mmHg, each Ⓑ

IOM: 100-02, 15, 130; 100-03, 4, 280.1

⊘ **A6539** Gradient compression stocking, waist length, 18–30 mmHg, each Ⓑ

IOM: 100-02, 15, 130; 100-03, 4, 280.1

⊘ **A6540** Gradient compression stocking, waist length, 30–40 mmHg, each Ⓑ

IOM: 100-02, 15, 130; 100-03, 4, 280.1

⊘ **A6541** Gradient compression stocking, waist length, 40–50 mmHg, each Ⓑ

IOM: 100-02, 15, 130; 100-03, 4, 280.1

⊘ **A6544** Gradient compression stocking, garter belt Ⓑ

IOM: 100-02, 15, 130; 100-03, 4, 280.1

✪ **A6545** Gradient compression wrap, non-elastic, below knee, 30-50 mm hg, each Ⓑ

Modifiers RT and/or LT must be appended. When assigned for bilateral items (left/right) on the same date of service, bill both items on the same claim line using RT/LT modifiers and 2 units of service.

IOM: 10-02, 15, 100

⊘ **A6549** Gradient compression stocking/sleeve, not otherwise specified Ⓑ

IOM: 100-02, 15, 130; 100-03, 4, 280.1

WOUND CARE (A6550)

✻ **A6550** Wound care set, for negative pressure wound therapy electrical pump, includes all supplies and accessories Ⓑ

RESPIRATORY DURABLE MEDICAL EQUIPMENT, INEXPENSIVE AND ROUTINELY PURCHASED (A7000-A7509)

✻ **A7000** Canister, disposable, used with suction pump, each Ⓑ

✻ **A7001** Canister, non-disposable, used with suction pump, each Ⓑ

✻ **A7002** Tubing, used with suction pump, each Ⓑ

✻ **A7003** Administration set, with small volume nonfiltered pneumatic nebulizer, disposable Ⓑ

✻ **A7004** Small volume nonfiltered pneumatic nebulizer, disposable Ⓑ

✻ **A7005** Administration set, with small volume nonfiltered pneumatic nebulizer, non-disposable Ⓑ

✻ **A7006** Administration set, with small volume filtered pneumatic nebulizer Ⓑ

✻ **A7007** Large volume nebulizer, disposable, unfilled, used with aerosol compressor Ⓑ

✻ **A7008** Large volume nebulizer, disposable, prefilled, used with aerosol compressor Ⓑ

✻ **A7009** Reservoir bottle, nondisposable, used with large volume ultrasonic nebulizer Ⓑ

✻ **A7010** Corrugated tubing, disposable, used with large volume nebulizer, 100 feet Ⓑ

✻ **A7012** Water collection device, used with large volume nebulizer Ⓑ

✻ **A7013** Filter, disposable, used with aerosol compressor or ultrasonic generator Ⓑ

✻ **A7014** Filter, non-disposable, used with aerosol compressor or ultrasonic generator Ⓑ

✻ **A7015** Aerosol mask, used with DME nebulizer Ⓑ

✻ **A7016** Dome and mouthpiece, used with small volume ultrasonic nebulizer Ⓑ

✪ **A7017** Nebulizer, durable, glass or autoclavable plastic, bottle type, not used with oxygen Ⓑ

IOM: 100-03, 4, 280.1

✻ **A7018** Water, distilled, used with large volume nebulizer, 1000 ml Ⓑ

✻ **A7020** Interface for cough stimulating device, includes all components, replacement only Ⓑ

✻ **A7025** High frequency chest wall oscillation system vest, replacement for use with patient owned equipment, each Ⓑ

✻ **A7026** High frequency chest wall oscillation system hose, replacement for use with patient owned equipment, each Ⓑ

✻ **A7027** Combination oral/nasal mask, used with continuous positive airway pressure device, each Ⓑ

✻ **A7028** Oral cushion for combination oral/nasal mask, replacement only, each Ⓑ

✻ **A7029** Nasal pillows for combination oral/nasal mask, replacement only, pair Ⓑ

* **A7030** Full face mask used with positive airway pressure device, each Ⓑ
* **A7031** Face mask interface, replacement for full face mask, each Ⓑ
* **A7032** Cushion for use on nasal mask interface, replacement only, each Ⓑ
* **A7033** Pillow for use on nasal cannula type interface, replacement only, pair Ⓑ
* **A7034** Nasal interface (mask or cannula type) used with positive airway pressure device, with or without head strap Ⓑ
* **A7035** Headgear used with positive airway pressure device Ⓑ
* **A7036** Chinstrap used with positive airway pressure device Ⓑ
* **A7037** Tubing used with positive airway pressure device Ⓑ
* **A7038** Filter, disposable, used with positive airway pressure device Ⓑ
* **A7039** Filter, non disposable, used with positive airway pressure device Ⓑ
* **A7040** One way chest drain valve Ⓑ
* **A7041** Water seal drainage container and tubing for use with implanted chest tube Ⓑ
* **A7044** Oral interface used with positive airway pressure device, each Ⓑ

⚙ **A7045** Exhalation port with or without swivel used with accessories for positive airway devices, replacement only Ⓑ

IOM: 100-03, 4, 230.17

⚙ **A7046** Water chamber for humidifier, used with positive airway pressure device, replacement, each Ⓑ

IOM: 100-03, 4, 230.17

* **A7047** Oral interface used with respiratory suction pump, each Ⓑ
* **A7048** Vacuum drainage collection unit and tubing kit, including all supplies needed for collection unit change, for use with implanted catheter, each Ⓑ

⚙ **A7501** Tracheostoma valve, including diaphragm, each Ⓑ

IOM: 100-02, 15, 120

⚙ **A7502** Replacement diaphragm/faceplate for tracheostoma valve, each Ⓑ

IOM: 100-02, 15, 120

⚙ **A7503** Filter holder or filter cap, reusable, for use in a tracheostoma heat and moisture exchange system, each Ⓑ

IOM: 100-02, 15, 120

⚙ **A7504** Filter for use in a tracheostoma heat and moisture exchange system, each Ⓑ

IOM: 100-02, 15, 120

⚙ **A7505** Housing, reusable without adhesive, for use in a heat and moisture exchange system and/or with a tracheostoma valve, each Ⓑ

IOM: 100-02, 15, 120

⚙ **A7506** Adhesive disc for use in a heat and moisture exchange system and/or with tracheostoma valve, any type, each Ⓑ

IOM: 100-02, 15, 120

⚙ **A7507** Filter holder and integrated filter without adhesive, for use in a tracheostoma heat and moisture exchange system, each Ⓑ

IOM: 100-02, 15, 120

⚙ **A7508** Housing and integrated adhesive, for use in a tracheostoma heat and moisture exchange system and/or with a tracheostoma valve, each Ⓑ

IOM: 100-02, 15, 120

⚙ **A7509** Filter holder and integrated filter housing, and adhesive, for use as a tracheostoma heat and moisture exchange system, each Ⓑ

IOM: 100-02, 15, 120

* **A7520** Tracheostomy/laryngectomy tube, non-cuffed, polyvinylchloride (PVC), silicone or equal, each Ⓑ

Tracheostomy Supplies

* **A7521** Tracheostomy/laryngectomy tube, cuffed, polyvinylchloride (PVC), silicone or equal, each Ⓑ
* **A7522** Tracheostomy/laryngectomy tube, stainless steel or equal (sterilizable and reusable), each Ⓑ
* **A7523** Tracheostomy shower protector, each Ⓑ
* **A7524** Tracheostoma stent/stud/button, each Ⓑ
* **A7525** Tracheostomy mask, each Ⓑ
* **A7526** Tracheostomy tube collar/holder, each Ⓑ
* **A7527** Tracheostomy/laryngectomy tube plug/stop, each Ⓑ

▶ New ⮌ Revised ✔ Reinstated ~~deleted~~ Deleted ⊘ Not covered or valid by Medicare
⚙ Special coverage instructions * Carrier discretion Ⓑ Bill local carrier Ⓑ Bill DME MAC

HELMETS (A8000-A8004)

✻ **A8000** Helmet, protective, soft, prefabricated, includes all components and accessories Ⓑ

✻ **A8001** Helmet, protective, hard, prefabricated, includes all components and accessories Ⓑ

✻ **A8002** Helmet, protective, soft, custom fabricated, includes all components and accessories Ⓑ

✻ **A8003** Helmet, protective, hard, custom fabricated, includes all components and accessories Ⓑ

✻ **A8004** Soft interface for helmet, replacement only Ⓑ

ADMINISTRATIVE, MISCELLANEOUS, AND INVESTIGATIONAL (A9000-A9999)

Note: The following codes do not imply that codes in other sections are necessarily covered.

✪ **A9150** Non-prescription drugs Ⓑ

IOM: 100-02, 15, 50

⃠ **A9152** Single vitamin/mineral/trace element, oral, per dose, not otherwise specified Ⓑ

⃠ **A9153** Multiple vitamins, with or without minerals and trace elements, oral, per dose, not otherwise specified Ⓑ

✻ **A9155** Artificial saliva, 30 ml Ⓑ

⃠ **A9180** Pediculosis (lice infestation) treatment, topical, for administration by patient/caretaker Ⓑ

⃠ **A9270** Non-covered item or service Ⓑ

IOM: 100-02, 16, 20

⃠ **A9272** Wound suction, disposable, includes dressing, all accessories and components, any type, each Ⓑ

Medicare Statute 1861(n)

⃠ **A9273** Hot water bottle, ice cap or collar, heat and/or cold wrap, any type Ⓑ

⃠ **A9274** External ambulatory insulin delivery system, disposable, each, includes all supplies and accessories Ⓑ

Medicare Statute 1861(n)

⃠ **A9275** Home glucose disposable monitor, includes test strips Ⓑ

⃠ **A9276** Sensor; invasive (e.g., subcutaneous), disposable, for use with interstitial continuous glucose monitoring system, one unit = 1 day supply Ⓑ

Medicare Statute 1861(n)

⃠ **A9277** Transmitter; external, for use with interstitial continuous glucose monitoring system Ⓑ

Medicare Statute 1861(n)

⃠ **A9278** Receiver (monitor); external, for use with interstitial continuous glucose monitoring system Ⓑ

Medicare Statute 1861(n)

⃠ **A9279** Monitoring feature/device, stand-alone or integrated, any type, includes all accessories, components and electronics, not otherwise classified Ⓑ

Medicare Statute 1861(n)

⃠ **A9280** Alert or alarm device, not otherwise classified Ⓑ

Medicare Statute 1861

⃠ **A9281** Reaching/grabbing device, any type, any length, each Ⓑ

Medicare Statute 1862 SSA

⃠ **A9282** Wig, any type, each Ⓑ

Medicare Statute 1862 SSA

⃠ **A9283** Foot pressure off loading/supportive device, any type, each Ⓑ

Medicare Statute 1862A(i)13

✪ **A9284** Spirometer, non-electronic, includes all accessories Ⓑ

▶ ✻ **A9285** Inversion/eversion correction device

▶ ⃠ **A9286** Hygienic item or device, disposable or non-disposable, any type, each

Medicare Statute 1834

⃠ **A9300** Exercise equipment Ⓑ

IOM: 100-02, 15, 110.1; 100-03, 4, 280.1

Supplies for Radiology Procedures (Radiopharmaceuticals)

✻ **A9500** Technetium Tc-99m sestamibi, diagnostic, per study dose Ⓑ

Should be filed on same claim as procedure code reporting radiopharmaceutical. Verify with payer definition of a "study."

✻ **A9501** Technetium Tc-99m teboroxime, diagnostic, per study dose Ⓑ

▶ New ⮌ Revised ✔ Reinstated ~~deleted~~ Deleted ⃠ Not covered or valid by Medicare
✪ Special coverage instructions ✻ Carrier discretion Ⓑ Bill local carrier Ⓑ Bill DME MAC

* **A9502** Technetium Tc-99m tetrofosmin, diagnostic, per study dose
* **A9503** Technetium Tc-99m medronate, diagnostic, per study dose, up to 30 millicuries
* **A9504** Technetium Tc-99m apcitide, diagnostic, per study dose, up to 20 millicuries
* **A9505** Thallium Tl-201 thallous chloride, diagnostic, per millicurie
* **A9507** Indium In-111 capromab pendetide, diagnostic, per study dose, up to 10 millicuries
* **A9508** Iodine I-131 iobenguane sulfate, diagnostic, per 0.5 millicurie
* **A9509** Iodine I-123 sodium iodide, diagnostic, per millicurie
* **A9510** Technetium Tc-99m disofenin, diagnostic, per study dose, up to 15 millicuries
* **A9512** Technetium Tc-99m pertechnetate, diagnostic, per millicurie
* ▶ **A9515** Choline C-11, diagnostic, per study dose up to 20 millicuries
* **A9516** Iodine I-123 sodium iodide, diagnostic, per 100 microcuries, up to 999 microcuries
* **A9517** Iodine I-131 sodium iodide capsule(s), therapeutic, per millicurie
* **A9520** Technetium Tc-99m tilmanocept, diagnostic, up to 0.5 millicuries
* **A9521** Technetium Tc-99m exametazime, diagnostic, per study dose, up to 25 millicuries
* **A9524** Iodine I-131 iodinated serum albumin, diagnostic, per 5 microcuries
* **A9526** Nitrogen N-13 ammonia, diagnostic, per study dose, up to 40 millicuries
* **A9527** Iodine I-125, sodium iodide solution, therapeutic, per millicurie
* **A9528** Iodine I-131 sodium iodide capsule(s), diagnostic, per millicurie
* **A9529** Iodine I-131 sodium iodide solution, diagnostic, per millicurie
* **A9530** Iodine I-131 sodium iodide solution, therapeutic, per millicurie
* **A9531** Iodine I-131 sodium iodide, diagnostic, per microcurie (up to 100 microcuries)
* **A9532** Iodine I-125 serum albumin, diagnostic, per 5 microcuries
* **A9536** Technetium Tc-99m depreotide, diagnostic, per study dose, up to 35 millicuries
* **A9537** Technetium Tc-99m mebrofenin, diagnostic, per study dose, up to 15 millicuries
* **A9538** Technetium Tc-99m pyrophosphate, diagnostic, per study dose, up to 25 millicuries
* **A9539** Technetium Tc-99m pentetate, diagnostic, per study dose, up to 25 millicuries
* **A9540** Technetium Tc-99m macroaggregated albumin, diagnostic, per study dose, up to 10 millicuries
* **A9541** Technetium Tc-99m sulfur colloid, diagnostic, per study dose, up to 20 millicuries
* **A9542** Indium In-111 ibritumomab tiuxetan, diagnostic, per study dose, up to 5 millicuries

  Specifically for diagnostic use.
* **A9543** Yttrium Y-90 ibritumomab tiuxetan, therapeutic, per treatment dose, up to 40 millicuries

  Specifically for therapeutic use.

~~A9544 Iodine I-131 tositumomab, diagnostic, per study dose~~ ✖

~~A9545 Iodine I-131 tositumomab, therapeutic, per treatment dose~~ ✖

* **A9546** Cobalt Co-57/58, cyanocobalamin, diagnostic, per study dose, up to 1 microcurie
* **A9547** Indium In-111 oxyquinoline, diagnostic, per 0.5 millicurie
* **A9548** Indium In-111 pentetate, diagnostic, per 0.5 millicurie
* **A9550** Technetium Tc-99m sodium gluceptate, diagnostic, per study dose, up to 25 millicuries
* **A9551** Technetium Tc-99m succimer, diagnostic, per study dose, up to 10 millicuries
* **A9552** Fluorodeoxyglucose F-18 FDG, diagnostic, per study dose, up to 45 millicuries
* **A9553** Chromium Cr-51 sodium chromate, diagnostic, per study dose, up to 250 microcuries
* **A9554** Iodine I-125 sodium Iothalamate, diagnostic, per study dose, up to 10 microcuries

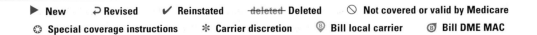

✻ **A9555** Rubidium Rb-82, diagnostic, per study dose, up to 60 millicuries Ⓑ

✻ **A9556** Gallium Ga-67 citrate, diagnostic, per millicurie Ⓑ

✻ **A9557** Technetium Tc-99m bicisate, diagnostic, per study dose, up to 25 millicuries Ⓑ

✻ **A9558** Xenon Xe-133 gas, diagnostic, per 10 millicuries Ⓑ

✻ **A9559** Cobalt Co-57 cyanocobalamin, oral, diagnostic, per study dose, up to 1 microcurie Ⓑ

✻ **A9560** Technetium Tc-99m labeled red blood cells, diagnostic, per study dose, up to 30 millicuries Ⓑ

✻ **A9561** Technetium Tc-99m oxidronate, diagnostic, per study dose, up to 30 millicuries Ⓑ

✻ **A9562** Technetium Tc-99m mertiatide, diagnostic, per study dose, up to 15 millicuries Ⓑ

✻ **A9563** Sodium phosphate P-32, therapeutic, per millicurie Ⓑ

✻ **A9564** Chromic phosphate P-32 suspension, therapeutic, per millicurie Ⓑ

✻ **A9566** Technetium Tc-99m fanolesomab, diagnostic, per study dose, up to 25 millicuries Ⓑ

✻ **A9567** Technetium Tc-99m pentetate, diagnostic, aerosol, per study dose, up to 75 millicuries Ⓑ

✻ **A9568** Technetium TC-99m arcitumomab, diagnostic, per study dose, up to 45 millicuries Ⓑ

✻ **A9569** Technetium Tc-99m exametazime labeled autologous white blood cells, diagnostic, per study dose Ⓑ

✻ **A9570** Indium In-111 labeled autologous white blood cells, diagnostic, per study dose Ⓑ

✻ **A9571** Indium In-111 labeled autologous platelets, diagnostic, per study dose Ⓑ

✻ **A9572** Indium In-111 pentetreotide, diagnostic, per study dose, up to 6 millicuries Ⓑ

✻ **A9575** Injection, gadoterate meglumine, 0.1 ml Ⓑ

NDC: Dotarem

✻ **A9576** Injection, gadoteridol, (ProHance Multipack), per ml Ⓑ

✻ **A9577** Injection, gadobenate dimeglumine (MultiHance), per ml Ⓑ

✻ **A9578** Injection, gadobenate dimeglumine (MultiHance Multipack), per ml Ⓑ

✻ **A9579** Injection, gadolinium-based magnetic resonance contrast agent, not otherwise specified (NOS), per ml Ⓑ

NDC: Magnevist, Omniscan, Optimark, Prohance

✻ **A9580** Sodium fluoride F-18, diagnostic, per study dose, up to 30 millicuries Ⓑ

✻ **A9581** Injection, gadoxetate disodium, 1 ml Ⓑ

Local Medicare contractors may require the use of modifier JW to identify unused product from single-dose vials that are appropriately discarded.

NDC: Eovist

✻ **A9582** Iodine I-123 iobenguane, diagnostic, per study dose, up to 15 millicuries Ⓑ

Molecular imaging agent that assists in the identification of rare neuroendocrine tumors.

✻ **A9583** Injection, gadofosveset trisodium, 1 ml Ⓑ

NDC: Ablavar

✻ **A9584** Iodine 1-123 ioflupane, diagnostic, per study dose, up to 5 millicuries Ⓑ

✻ **A9585** Injection, gadobutrol, 0.1 ml Ⓑ

NDC: Gadavist

⚙ **A9586** Florbetapir F18, diagnostic, per study dose, up to 10 millicuries Ⓑ

▶ ✻ **A9587** Gallium Ga-68, dotatate, diagnostic, 0.1 millicurie

▶ ✻ **A9588** Fluciclovine F-18, diagnostic, 1 millicurie

▶ ✻ **A9597** Positron emission tomography radiopharmaceutical, diagnostic, for tumor identification, not otherwise classified

▶ ✻ **A9598** Positron emission tomography radiopharmaceutical, diagnostic, for non-tumor identification, not otherwise classified

↩ ⚙ **A9599** Radiopharmaceutical, diagnostic, for beta-amyloid positron emission tomography (PET) imaging, per study dose, not otherwise specified Ⓑ

✻ **A9600** Strontium Sr-89 chloride, therapeutic, per millicurie Ⓑ

✻ **A9604** Samarium SM-153 lexidronam, therapeutic, per treatment dose, up to 150 millicuries Ⓑ

✻ **A9606** Radium Ra-223 dichloride, therapeutic, per microcurie

▶ New ↩ Revised ✔ Reinstated ~~deleted~~ Deleted ⊘ Not covered or valid by Medicare
⚙ Special coverage instructions ✻ Carrier discretion Ⓑ Bill local carrier Ⓑ Bill DME MAC

⚙ **A9698** Non-radioactive contrast imaging material, not otherwise classified, per study Ⓑ

IOM: 100-04, 12, 70; 100-04, 13, 20

✻ **A9699** Radiopharmaceutical, therapeutic, not otherwise classified Ⓑ

⚙ **A9700** Supply of injectable contrast material for use in echocardiography, per study Ⓑ

IOM: 100-04, 12, 30.4

Miscellaneous Service Component

✻ **A9900** Miscellaneous DME supply, accessory, and/or service component of another HCPCS code Ⓑ Ⓑ

Bill Local Carrier if used with implanted DME. If other, bill DME MAC.

On DMEPOS fee schedule as a payable replacement for miscellaneous implanted or non-implanted items.

✻ **A9901** DME delivery, set up, and/or dispensing service component of another HCPCS code Ⓑ

✻ **A9999** Miscellaneous DME supply or accessory, not otherwise specified Ⓑ Ⓑ

Bill Local Carrier if used with implanted DME. If other, bill DME MAC.

On DMEPOS fee schedule as a payable replacement for miscellaneous implanted or non-implanted items.

▶ New ↩ Revised ✔ Reinstated ~~deleted~~ Deleted ⊘ Not covered or valid by Medicare
⚙ Special coverage instructions ✻ Carrier discretion Ⓑ Bill local carrier Ⓑ Bill DME MAC

ENTERAL AND PARENTERAL THERAPY (B4000-B9999)

Enteral Formulae and Enteral Medical Supplies

❂ **B4034** Enteral feeding supply kit; syringe fed, per day, includes but not limited to feeding/flushing syringe, administration set tubing, dressings, tape Ⓑ

Dressings used with gastrostomy tubes for enteral nutrition (covered under the prosthetic device benefit) are included in the payment.

IOM: 100-02, 15, 120; 100-03, 3, 180.2; 100-04, 20, 100.2.2

❂ **B4035** Enteral feeding supply kit; pump fed, per day, includes but not limited to feeding/flushing syringe, administration set tubing, dressings, tape Ⓑ

IOM: 100-02, 15, 120; 100-03, 3, 180.2; 100-04, 20, 100.2.2

❂ **B4036** Enteral feeding supply kit; gravity fed, per day, includes but not limited to feeding/flushing syringe, administration set tubing, dressings, tape Ⓑ

IOM: 100-02, 15, 120; 100-03, 3, 180.2; 100-04, 20, 100.2.2

❂ **B4081** Nasogastric tubing with stylet Ⓑ

More than 3 nasogastric tubes (B4081-B4083), or 1 gastrostomy/jejunostomy tube (B4087-B4088) every three months is rarely medically necessary

IOM: 100-02, 15, 120; 100-03, 3, 180.2; 100-04, 20, 100.2.2

❂ **B4082** Nasogastric tubing without stylet Ⓑ

IOM: 100-02, 15, 120; 100-03, 3, 180.2; 100-04, 20, 100.2.2

❂ **B4083** Stomach tube - Levine type Ⓑ

IOM: 100-02, 15, 120; 100-03, 3, 180.2; 100-04, 20, 100.2.2

✻ **B4087** Gastrostomy/jejunostomy tube, standard, any material, any type, each Ⓑ

✻ **B4088** Gastrostomy/jejunostomy tube, low-profile, any material, any type, each Ⓑ

⦸ **B4100** Food thickener, administered orally, per ounce Ⓑ

❂ **B4102** Enteral formula, for adults, used to replace fluids and electrolytes (e.g., clear liquids), 500 ml = 1 unit Ⓑ

IOM: 100-03, 3, 180.2

❂ **B4103** Enteral formula, for pediatrics, used to replace fluids and electrolytes (e.g., clear liquids), 500 ml = 1 unit Ⓑ

IOM: 100-03, 3, 180.2

❂ **B4104** Additive for enteral formula (e.g., fiber) Ⓑ

IOM: 100-03, 3, 180.2

❂ **B4149** Enteral formula, manufactured blenderized natural foods with intact nutrients, includes proteins, fats, carbohydrates, vitamins and minerals, may include fiber, administered through an enteral feeding tube, 100 calories = 1 unit Ⓑ

Produced to meet unique nutrient needs for specific disease conditions; medical record must document specific condition and need for special nutrient

IOM: 100-02, 15, 120; 100-03, 3, 180.2; 100-04, 20, 100.2.2

❂ **B4150** Enteral formulae, nutritionally complete with intact nutrients, includes proteins, fats, carbohydrates, vitamins, and minerals, may include fiber, administered through an enteral feeding tube, 100 calories = 1 unit Ⓑ

IOM: 100-02, 15, 120; 100-03, 3, 180.2; 100-04, 20, 100.2.2

❂ **B4152** Enteral formula, nutritionally complete, calorically dense (equal to or greater than 1.5 kcal/ml) with intact nutrients, includes proteins, fats, carbohydrates, vitamins and minerals, may include fiber, administered through an enteral feeding tube, 100 calories = 1 unit Ⓑ

IOM: 100-02, 15, 120; 100-03, 3, 180.2; 100-04, 20, 100.2.2

❂ **B4153** Enteral formula, nutritionally complete, hydrolyzed proteins (amino acids and peptide chain), includes fats, carbohydrates, vitamins and minerals, may include fiber, administered through an enteral feeding tube, 100 calories = 1 unit Ⓑ

If 2 enteral nutrition products described by same HCPCS code and provided at same time billed on single claim line with units of service reflecting total calories of both nutrients

IOM: 100-02, 15, 120; 100-03, 3, 180.2; 100-04, 20, 100.2.2

Modifier BA is the only modifier specific to enteral feedings.

B4154 Enteral formula, nutritionally complete, for special metabolic needs, excludes inherited disease of metabolism, includes altered composition of proteins, fats, carbohydrates, vitamins and/or minerals, may include fiber, administered through an enteral feeding tube, 100 calories = 1 unit

IOM: 100-02, 15, 120; 100-03, 3, 180.2; 100-04, 20, 100.2.2

B4155 Enteral formula, nutritionally incomplete/modular nutrients, includes specific nutrients, carbohydrates (e.g., glucose polymers), proteins/amino acids (e.g., glutamine, arginine), fat (e.g., medium chain triglycerides) or combination, administered through an enteral feeding tube, 100 calories = 1 unit

IOM: 100-02, 15, 120; 100-03, 3, 180.2; 100-04, 20, 100.2.2

B4157 Enteral formula, nutritionally complete, for special metabolic needs for inherited disease of metabolism, includes proteins, fats, carbohydrates, vitamins and minerals, may include fiber, administered through an enteral feeding tube, 100 calories = 1 unit

IOM: 100-03, 3, 180.2

B4158 Enteral formula, for pediatrics, nutritionally complete with intact nutrients, includes proteins, fats, carbohydrates, vitamins and minerals, may include fiber and/or iron, administered through an enteral feeding tube, 100 calories = 1 unit

IOM: 100-03, 3, 180.2

B4159 Enteral formula, for pediatrics, nutritionally complete soy based with intact nutrients, includes proteins, fats, carbohydrates, vitamins and minerals, may include fiber and/or iron, administered through an enteral feeding tube, 100 calories = 1 unit

IOM: 100-03, 3, 180.2

B4160 Enteral formula, for pediatrics, nutritionally complete calorically dense (equal to or greater than 0.7 kcal/ml) with intact nutrients, includes proteins, fats, carbohydrates, vitamins and minerals, may include fiber, administered through an enteral feeding tube, 100 calories = 1 unit

IOM: 100-03, 3, 180.2

B4161 Enteral formula, for pediatrics, hydrolyzed/amino acids and peptide chain proteins, includes fats, carbohydrates, vitamins and minerals, may include fiber, administered through an enteral feeding tube, 100 calories = 1 unit

IOM: 100-03, 3, 180.2

B4162 Enteral formula, for pediatrics, special metabolic needs for inherited disease of metabolism, includes proteins, fats, carbohydrates, vitamins and minerals, may include fiber, administered through an enteral feeding tube, 100 calories = 1 unit

IOM: 100-03, 3, 180.2

Parenteral Nutritional Solutions and Supplies

B4164 Parenteral nutrition solution: carbohydrates (dextrose), 50% or less (500 ml = 1 unit) - home mix

IOM: 100-02, 15, 120; 100-03, 3, 180.2; 100-04, 20, 100.2.2

B4168 Parenteral nutrition solution; amino acid, 3.5%, (500 ml = 1 unit) - home mix

IOM: 100-02, 15, 120; 100-03, 3, 180.2; 100-04, 20, 100.2.2

B4172 Parenteral nutrition solution; amino acid, 5.5% through 7%, (500 ml = 1 unit) - home mix

IOM: 100-02, 15, 120; 100-03, 3, 180.2; 100-04, 20, 100.2.2

B4176 Parenteral nutrition solution; amino acid, 7% through 8.5%, (500 ml = 1 unit) - home mix

IOM: 100-02, 15, 120; 100-03, 3, 180.2; 100-04, 20, 100.2.2

B4178 Parenteral nutrition solution: amino acid, greater than 8.5% (500 ml = 1 unit) - home mix

IOM: 100-02, 15, 120; 100-03, 3, 180.2; 100-04, 20, 100.2.2

B4180 Parenteral nutrition solution; carbohydrates (dextrose), greater than 50% (500 ml = 1 unit) - home mix

IOM: 100-02, 15, 120; 100-03, 3, 180.2; 100-04, 20, 100.2.2

B4185 Parenteral nutrition solution, per 10 grams lipids

⊛ **B4189** Parenteral nutrition solution; compounded amino acid and carbohydrates with electrolytes, trace elements, and vitamins, including preparation, any strength, 10 to 51 grams of protein - premix Ⓑ

IOM: 100-02, 15, 120; 100-03, 3, 180.2; 100-04, 20, 100.2.2

⊛ **B4193** Parenteral nutrition solution; compounded amino acid and carbohydrates with electrolytes, trace elements, and vitamins, including preparation, any strength, 52 to 73 grams of protein - premix Ⓑ

IOM: 100-02, 15, 120; 100-03, 3, 180.2; 100-04, 20, 100.2.2

⊛ **B4197** Parenteral nutrition solution; compounded amino acid and carbohydrates with electrolytes, trace elements and vitamins, including preparation, any strength, 74 to 100 grams of protein - premix Ⓑ

IOM: 100-02, 15, 120; 100-03, 3, 180.2; 100-04, 20, 100.2.2

⊛ **B4199** Parenteral nutrition solution; compounded amino acid and carbohydrates with electrolytes, trace elements and vitamins, including preparation, any strength, over 100 grams of protein - premix Ⓑ

IOM: 100-02, 15, 120; 100-03, 3, 180.2; 100-04, 20, 100.2.2

⊛ **B4216** Parenteral nutrition; additives (vitamins, trace elements, heparin, electrolytes) home mix per day Ⓑ

IOM: 100-02, 15, 120; 100-03, 3, 180.2; 100-04, 20, 100.2.2

⊛ **B4220** Parenteral nutrition supply kit; premix, per day Ⓑ

IOM: 100-02, 15, 120; 100-03, 3, 180.2; 100-04, 20, 100.2.2

⊛ **B4222** Parenteral nutrition supply kit; home mix, per day Ⓑ

IOM: 100-02, 15, 120; 100-03, 3, 180.2; 100-04, 20, 100.2.2

⊛ **B4224** Parenteral nutrition administration kit, per day Ⓑ

Dressings used with parenteral nutrition (covered under the prosthetic device benefit) are included in the payment. (www.cms.gov/medicare-coverage-database/)

IOM: 100-02, 15, 120; 100-03, 3, 180.2; 100-04, 20, 100.2.2

⊛ **B5000** Parenteral nutrition solution compounded amino acid and carbohydrates with electrolytes, trace elements, and vitamins, including preparation, any strength, renal - Aminosyn-RF, NephrAmine, RenAmine - premix Ⓑ

IOM: 100-02, 15, 120; 100-03, 3, 180.2; 100-04, 20, 100.2.2

⊛ **B5100** Parenteral nutrition solution compounded amino acid and carbohydrates with electrolytes, trace elements, and vitamins, including preparation, any strength, hepatic, HepatAmine - premix Ⓑ

IOM: 100-02, 15, 120; 100-03, 3, 180.2; 100-04, 20, 100.2.2

⊛ **B5200** Parenteral nutrition solution compounded amino acid and carbohydrates with electrolytes, trace elements, and vitamins, including preparation, any strength, stress-branch chain amino acids-FreAmine-HBC - premix Ⓑ

IOM: 100-02, 15, 120; 100-03, 3, 180.2; 100-04, 20, 100.2.2

Enteral and Parenteral Pumps

~~B9000 Enteral nutrition infusion pump - without alarm~~ ✖

↻⊛ **B9002** Enteral nutrition infusion pump, any type Ⓑ

IOM: 100-02, 15, 120; 100-03, 3, 180.2; 100-04, 20, 100.2.2

⊛ **B9004** Parenteral nutrition infusion pump, portable Ⓑ

IOM: 100-02, 15, 120; 100-03, 3, 180.2; 100-04, 20, 100.2.2

⊛ **B9006** Parenteral nutrition infusion pump, stationary Ⓑ

IOM: 100-02, 15, 120; 100-03, 3, 180.2; 100-04, 20, 100.2.2

⊛ **B9998** NOC for enteral supplies Ⓑ

IOM: 100-02, 15, 120; 100-03, 3, 180.2; 100-04, 20, 100.2.2

⊛ **B9999** NOC for parenteral supplies Ⓑ

Determine if an alternative HCPCS Level II or a CPT code better describes the service being reported. This code should be reported only if a more specific code is unavailable.

IOM: 100-02, 15, 120; 100-03, 3, 180.2; 100-04, 20, 100.2.2

CMS HOSPITAL OUTPATIENT PAYMENT SYSTEM (C1000-C9999)

NOTE: C-codes are used on Medicare Ambulatory Surgical Center (ASC) and Hospital Outpatient Prospective Payment System (OPPS) claims, but may also be recognized on claims from other providers or by other payment systems. As of 10/01/2006, the following non-OPPS providers have been able to bill Medicare using the C-codes, or an appropriate CPT code on Types of Bill (TOBs) 12X, 13X, or 85X:

- Critical Access Hospitals (CAHs);
- Indian Health Service Hospitals (IHS);
- Hospitals located in American Samoa, Guam, Saipan or the Virgin Islands; and
- Maryland waiver hospitals.

The billing of C-codes by Method I and Method II Critical Access Hospitals (CAHs) is limited to the billing for facility (technical) services. The C-codes shall not be billed by Method II CAHs for professional services with revenue codes (RCs) 96X, 97X, or 98X.

C codes are updated quarterly by the Centers for Medicare and Medicaid Services (CMS).

C1713 Anchor/Screw for opposing bone-to-bone or soft tissue-to-bone (implantable)
Medicare Statute 1833(t)

C1714 Catheter, transluminal atherectomy, directional
Medicare Statute 1833(t)

C1715 Brachytherapy needle
Medicare Statute 1833(t)

C1716 Brachytherapy source, non-stranded, gold-198, per source
Medicare Statute 1833(t)

C1717 Brachytherapy source, non-stranded, high dose rate iridium 192, per source
Medicare Statute 1833(t)

C1719 Brachytherapy source, non-stranded, non-high dose rate iridium-192, per source
Medicare Statute 1833(t)

C1721 Cardioverter-defibrillator, dual chamber (implantable)
Related CPT codes: 33224, 33240, 33249.
Medicare Statute 1833(t)

C1722 Cardioverter-defibrillator, single chamber (implantable)
Related CPT codes: 33240, 33249.
Medicare Statute 1833(t)

C1724 Catheter, transluminal atherectomy, rotational
Medicare Statute 1833(t)

C1725 Catheter, transluminal angioplasty, non-laser (may include guidance, infusion/perfusion capability)
Medicare Statute 1833(t)

C1726 Catheter, balloon dilatation, non-vascular
Medicare Statute 1833(t)

C1727 Catheter, balloon tissue dissector, non-vascular (insertable)
Medicare Statute 1833(t)

C1728 Catheter, brachytherapy seed administration
Medicare Statute 1833(t)

C1729 Catheter, drainage
Medicare Statute 1833(t)

C1730 Catheter, electrophysiology, diagnostic, other than 3D mapping (19 or fewer electrodes)
Medicare Statute 1833(t)

C1731 Catheter, electrophysiology, diagnostic, other than 3D mapping (20 or more electrodes)
Medicare Statute 1833(t)

C1732 Catheter, electrophysiology, diagnostic/ablation, 3D or vector mapping
Medicare Statute 1833(t)

C1733 Catheter, electrophysiology, diagnostic/ablation, other than 3D or vector mapping, other than cool-tip
Medicare Statute 1833(t)

C1749 Endoscope, retrograde imaging/illumination colonoscope device (implantable)
Medicare Statute 1833(t)

C1750 Catheter, hemodialysis/peritoneal, long-term
Medicare Statute 1833(t)

C1751 Catheter, infusion, inserted peripherally, centrally, or midline (other than hemodialysis)
Medicare Statute 1833(t)

New | Revised | Reinstated | ~~deleted~~ Deleted | Not covered or valid by Medicare
Special coverage instructions | * Carrier discretion | Bill local carrier | Bill DME MAC

 HCPCS C Codes can only be reported by facilities, not physicians

◎ **C1752** Catheter, hemodialysis/peritoneal, short-term
Medicare Statute 1833(t)

◎ **C1753** Catheter, intravascular ultrasound
Medicare Statute 1833(t)

◎ **C1754** Catheter, intradiscal
Medicare Statute 1833(t)

◎ **C1755** Catheter, instraspinal
Medicare Statute 1833(t)

◎ **C1756** Catheter, pacing, transesophageal
Medicare Statute 1833(t)

◎ **C1757** Catheter, thrombectomy/embolectomy
Medicare Statute 1833(t)

◎ **C1758** Catheter, ureteral
Medicare Statute 1833(t)

◎ **C1759** Catheter, intracardiac echocardiography
Medicare Statute 1833(t)

◎ **C1760** Closure device, vascular (implantable/insertable)
Medicare Statute 1833(t)

◎ **C1762** Connective tissue, human (includes fascia lata)
Medicare Statute 1833(t)

◎ **C1763** Connective tissue, non-human (includes synthetic)
Medicare Statute 1833(t)

◎ **C1764** Event recorder, cardiac (implantable)
Medicare Statute 1833(t)

◎ **C1765** Adhesion barrier
Medicare Statute 1833(t)

◎ **C1766** Introducer/sheath, guiding, intracardiac electrophysiological, steerable, other than peel-away
Medicare Statute 1833(t)

◎ **C1767** Generator, neurostimulator (implantable), nonrechargeable
Related CPT codes: 61885, 61886, 63685, 64590.
Medicare Statute 1833(t)

◎ **C1768** Graft, vascular
Medicare Statute 1833(t)

◎ **C1769** Guide wire
Medicare Statute 1833(t)

◎ **C1770** Imaging coil, magnetic reasonance (insertable)
Medicare Statute 1833(t)

◎ **C1771** Repair device, urinary, incontinence, with sling graft
Medicare Statute 1833(t)

◎ **C1772** Infusion pump, programmable (implantable)
Medicare Statute 1833(t)

◎ **C1773** Retrieval device, insertable (used to retrieve fractured medical devices)
Medicare Statute 1833(t)

◎ **C1776** Joint device (implantable)
Medicare Statute 1833(t)

◎ **C1777** Lead, cardioverter-defibrillator, endocardial single coil (implantable)
Related CPT codes: 33216, 33217, 33249.
Medicare Statute 1833(t)

◎ **C1778** Lead, neurostimulator (implantable)
Related CPT codes: 43647, 63650, 63655, 63663, 63664, 64553, 64555, 64560, 64561, 64565, 64573, 64575, 64577, 64580, 64581.
Medicare Statute 1833(t)

◎ **C1779** Lead, pacemaker, trasvenous VDD single pass
Related CPT codes: 33206, 33207, 33208, 33210, 33211, 33214, 33216, 33217, 33249.
Medicare Statute 1833(t)

◎ **C1780** Lens, intraocular (new technology)
Medicare Statute 1833(t)

◎ **C1781** Mesh (implantable)
Medicare Statute 1833(t)

◎ **C1782** Morcellator
Medicare Statute 1833(t)

◎ **C1783** Ocular implant, aqueous drainage assist device
Medicare Statute 1833(t)

◎ **C1784** Ocular device, intraoperative, detached retina
Medicare Statute 1833(t)

◎ **C1785** Pacemaker, dual chamber, rate-responsive (implantable)
Related CPT codes: 33206, 33207, 33208, 33213, 33214, 33224.
Medicare Statute 1833(t)

◎ **C1786** Pacemaker, single chamber, rate-responsive (implantable)
Related CPT codes: 33206, 33207, 33212.
Medicare Statute 1833(t)

⊕ **C1787** Patient programmer, neurostimulator
Medicare Statute 1833(t)

⊕ **C1788** Port, indwelling (implantable)
Medicare Statute 1833(t)

⊕ **C1789** Prosthesis, breast (implantable)
Medicare Statute 1833(t)

⊕ **C1813** Prosthesis, penile, inflatable
Medicare Statute 1833(t)

⊕ **C1814** Retinal tamponade device, silicone oil
Medicare Statute 1833(t)

⊕ **C1815** Prosthesis, urinary sphincter (implantable)
Medicare Statute 1833(t)

⊕ **C1816** Receiver and/or transmitter, neurostimulator (implantable)
Medicare Statute 1833(t)

⊕ **C1817** Septal defect implant system, intracardiac
Medicare Statute 1833(t)

⊕ **C1818** Integrated keratoprosthesic
Medicare Statute 1833(t)

⊕ **C1819** Surgical tissue localization and excision device (implantable)
Medicare Statute 1833(t)

⊕ **C1820** Generator, neurostimulator (implantable), with rechargeable battery and charging system
Related CPT codes: 61885, 61886, 63685, 64590.
Medicare Statute 1833(t)

⊕ **C1821** Interspinous process distraction device (implantable)
Medicare Statute 1833(t)

⊕ **C1822** Generator, neurostimulator (implantable), high frequency, with rechargeable battery and charging system
Medicare Statute 1833(T)

⊕ **C1830** Powered bone marrow biopsy needle
Medicare Statute 1833(t)

⊕ **C1840** Lens, intraocular (telescopic)
Medicare Statute 1833(t)

⊕ **C1841** Retinal prosthesis, includes all internal and external components
Medicare Statute 1833(t)

⊕ **C1874** Stent, coated/covered, with delivery system
Medicare Statute 1833(t)

⊕ **C1875** Stent, coated/covered, without delivery system
Medicare Statute 1833(t)

⊕ **C1876** Stent, non-coated/non-covered, with delivery system
Medicare Statute 1833(t)

⊕ **C1877** Stent, non-coated/non-covered, without delivery system
Medicare Statute 1833(t)

⊕ **C1878** Material for vocal cord medialization, synthetic (implantable)
Medicare Statute 1833(t)

⊕ **C1880** Vena cava filter
Medicare Statute 1833(t)

⊕ **C1881** Dialysis access system (implantable)
Medicare Statute 1833(t)

⊕ **C1882** Cardioverter-defibrillator, other than single or dual chamber (implantable)
Related CPT codes: 33224, 33240, 33249.
Medicare Statute 1833(t)

⊕ **C1883** Adapter/Extension, pacing lead or neurostimulator lead (implantable)
Medicare Statute 1833(t)

⊕ **C1884** Embolization protective system
Medicare Statute 1833(t)

⊕ **C1885** Catheter, transluminal angioplasty, laser
Medicare Statute 1833(t)

⊕ **C1886** Catheter, extravascular tissue ablation, any modality (insertable)
Medicare Statute 1833(t)

⊕ **C1887** Catheter, guiding (may include infusion/perfusion capability)
Medicare Statute 1833(t)

⊕ **C1888** Catheter, ablation, non-cardiac, endovascular (implantable)
Medicare Statute 1833(t)

▶ ⊕ **C1889** Implantable/insertable device for device intensive procedure, not otherwise classified
Medicare Statute 1833(T)

⊕ **C1891** Infusion pump, non-programmable, permanent (implantable)
Medicare Statute 1833(t)

⊕ **C1892** Introducer/sheath, guiding, intracardiac electrophysiological, fixed-curve, peel-away
Medicare Statute 1833(t)

▶ New ⊋ Revised ✔ Reinstated ~~deleted~~ Deleted ⊘ Not covered or valid by Medicare
⊕ Special coverage instructions ✻ Carrier discretion Ⓑ Bill local carrier Ⓑ Bill DME MAC

⊕ **C1893** Introducer/sheath, guiding, intracardiac electrophysiological, fixed-curve, other than peel-away

Medicare Statute 1833(t)

⊕ **C1894** Introducer/sheath, other than guiding, other than intracardiac electrophysiological, non-laser

Medicare Statute 1833(t)

⊕ **C1895** Lead, cardioverter-defibrillator, endocardial dual coil (implantable)

Related CPT codes: 33216, 33217, 33249.

Medicare Statute 1833(t)

⊕ **C1896** Lead, cardioverter-defibrillator, other than endocardial single or dual coil (implantable)

Related CPT codes: 33216, 33217, 33249.

Medicare Statute 1833(t)

⊕ **C1897** Lead, neurostimulator test kit (implantable)

Related CPT codes: 43647, 63650, 63655, 63663, 63664, 64553, 64555, 64560, 64561, 64565, 64575, 64577, 64580, 64581.

Medicare Statute 1833(t)

⊕ **C1898** Lead, pacemaker, other than transvenous VDD single pass

Related CPT codes: 33206, 33207, 33208, 33210, 33211, 33214, 33216, 33217, 33249.

Medicare Statute 1833(t)

⊕ **C1899** Lead, pacemaker/cardioverter-defibrillator combination (implantable)

Related CPT codes: 33216, 33217, 33249.

Medicare Statute 1833(t)

⊕ **C1900** Lead, left ventricular coronary venous system

Related CPT codes: 33224, 33225.

Medicare Statute 1833(t)

⊕ **C2613** Lung biopsy plug with delivery system

Medicare Statute 1833(t)

⊕ **C2614** Probe, percutaneous lumbar discectomy

Medicare Statute 1833(t)

⊕ **C2615** Sealant, pulmonary, liquid

Medicare Statute 1833(t)

⊕ **C2616** Brachytherapy source, non-stranded, yttrium-90, per source

Medicare Statute 1833(t)

⊕ **C2617** Stent, non-coronary, temporary, without delivery system

Medicare Statute 1833(t)

⊕ **C2618** Probe/needle, cryoablation

Medicare Statute 1833(t)

⊕ **C2619** Pacemaker, dual chamber, non rate-responsive (implantable)

Related CPT codes: 33206, 33207, 33208, 33213, 33214, 33224.

Medicare Statute 1833(t)

⊕ **C2620** Pacemaker, single chamber, non rate-responsive (implantable)

Related CPT codes: 33206, 33207, 33212, 33224.

Medicare Statute 1833(t)

⊕ **C2621** Pacemaker, other than single or dual chamber (implantable)

Related CPT codes: 33206, 33207, 33208, 33212, 33213, 33214, 33224.

Medicare Statute 1833(t)

⊕ **C2622** Prosthesis, penile, non-inflatable

Medicare Statute 1833(t)

⊕ **C2623** Catheter, transluminal angioplasty, drug-coated, non-laser

Medicare Statute 1833(t)

⊕ **C2624** Implantable wireless pulmonary artery pressure sensor with delivery catheter, including all system components

Medicare Statute 1833(t)

⊕ **C2625** Stent, non-coronary, temporary, with delivery system

Medicare Statute 1833(t)

⊕ **C2626** Infusion pump, non-programmable, temporary (implantable)

Medicare Statute 1833(t)

⊕ **C2627** Catheter, suprapubic/ cystoscopic

Medicare Statute 1833(t)

⊕ **C2628** Catheter, occlusion

Medicare Statute 1833(t)

⊕ **C2629** Introducer/Sheath, other than guiding, other than intracardiac electrophysiological, laser

Medicare Statute 1833(t)

⊕ **C2630** Catheter, electrophysiology, diagnostic/ ablation, other than 3D or vector mapping, cool-tip

Medicare Statute 1833(t)

⊕ **C2631** Repair device, urinary, incontinence, without sling graft
Medicare Statute 1833(t)

⊕ **C2634** Brachytherapy source, non-stranded, high activity, iodine-125, greater than 1.01 mci (NIST), per source
Medicare Statute 1833(t)

⊕ **C2635** Brachytherapy source, non-stranded, high activity, palladium-103, greater than 2.2 mci (NIST), per source
Medicare Statute 1833(t)

⊕ **C2636** Brachytherapy linear source, non-stranded, palladium-103, per 1 mm

⊕ **C2637** Brachytherapy source, non-stranded, Ytterbium-169, per source
Medicare Statute 1833(t)

⊕ **C2638** Brachytherapy source, stranded, iodine-125, per source
Medicare Statute 1833(t)(2)

⊕ **C2639** Brachytherapy source, non-stranded, iodine-125, per source
Medicare Statute 1833(t)(2)

⊕ **C2640** Brachytherapy source, stranded, palladium-103, per source
Medicare Statute 1833(t)(2)

⊕ **C2641** Brachytherapy source, non-stranded, palladium-103, per source
Medicare Statute 1833(t)(2)

⊕ **C2642** Brachytherapy source, stranded, cesium-131, per source
Medicare Statute 1833(t)(2)

⊕ **C2643** Brachytherapy source, non-stranded, cesium-131, per source
Medicare Statute 1833(t)(2)

⊕ **C2644** Brachytherapy source, Cesium-131 chloride solution, per millicurie
Medicare Statute 1833(t)

⊕ **C2645** Brachytherapy planar source, palladium-103, per square millimeter
Medicare Statute 1833(T)

⊕ **C2698** Brachytherapy source, stranded, not otherwise specified, per source
Medicare Statute 1833(t)(2)

⊕ **C2699** Brachytherapy source, non-stranded, not otherwise specified, per source
Medicare Statute 1833(t)(2)

⊕ **C5271** Application of low cost skin substitute graft to trunk, arms, legs, total wound surface area up to 100 sq cm; first 25 sq cm or less wound surface area
Medicare Statute 1833(t)

⊕ **C5272** Application of low cost skin substitute graft to trunk, arms, legs, total wound surface area up to 100 sq cm; each additional 25 sq cm wound surface area, or part thereof (list separately in addition to code for primary procedure)
Medicare Statute 1833(t)

⊕ **C5273** Application of low cost skin substitute graft to trunk, arms, legs, total wound surface area greater than or equal to 100 sq cm; first 100 sq cm wound surface area, or 1% of body area of infants and children
Medicare Statute 1833(t)

⊕ **C5274** Application of low cost skin substitute graft to trunk, arms, legs, total wound surface area greater than or equal to 100 sq cm; each additional 100 sq cm wound surface area, or part thereof, or each additional 1% of body area of infants and children, or part thereof (list separately in addition to code for primary procedure)
Medicare Statute 1833(t)

⊕ **C5275** Application of low cost skin substitute graft to face, scalp, eyelids, mouth, neck, ears, orbits, genitalia, hands, feet, and/or multiple digits, total wound surface area up to 100 sq cm; first 25 sq cm or less wound surface area
Medicare Statute 1833(t)

⊕ **C5276** Application of low cost skin substitute graft to face, scalp, eyelids, mouth, neck, ears, orbits, genitalia, hands, feet, and/or multiple digits, total wound surface area up to 100 sq cm; each additional 25 sq cm wound surface area, or part thereof (list separately in addition to code for primary procedure)
Medicare Statute 1833(t)

◎ **C5277** Application of low cost skin substitute graft to face, scalp, eyelids, mouth, neck, ears, orbits, genitalia, hands, feet, and/or multiple digits, total wound surface area greater than or equal to 100 sq cm; first 100 sq cm wound surface area, or 1% of body area of infants and children

Medicare Statute 1833(t)

◎ **C5278** Application of low cost skin substitute graft to face, scalp, eyelids, mouth, neck, ears, orbits, genitalia, hands, feet, and/or multiple digits, total wound surface area greater than or equal to 100 sq cm; each additional 100 sq cm wound surface area, or part thereof, or each additional 1% of body area of infants and children, or part thereof (list separately in addition to code for primary procedure)

Medicare Statute 1833(t)

◎ **C8900** Magnetic resonance angiography with contrast, abdomen

Medicare Statute 1833(t)(2)

◎ **C8901** Magnetic resonance angiography without contrast, abdomen

Medicare Statute 1833(t)(2)

◎ **C8902** Magnetic resonance angiography without contrast followed by with contrast, abdomen

Medicare Statute 1833(t)(2)

◎ **C8903** Magnetic resonance imaging with contrast, breast; unilateral

Medicare Statute 1833(t)(2)

◎ **C8904** Magnetic resonance imaging without contrast, breast; unilateral

Medicare Statute 1833(t)(2)

◎ **C8905** Magnetic resonance imaging without contrast followed by with contrast, breast; unilateral

Medicare Statute 1833(t)(2)

◎ **C8906** Magnetic resonance imaging with contrast, breast; bilateral

Medicare Statute 1833(t)(2)

◎ **C8907** Magnetic resonance imaging without contrast, breast; bilateral

Medicare Statute 1833(t)(2)

◎ **C8908** Magnetic resonance imaging without contrast followed by with contrast, breast; bilateral

Medicare Statute 1833(t)(2)

◎ **C8909** Magnetic resonance angiography with contrast, chest (excluding myocardium)

Medicare Statute 1833(t)(2)

◎ **C8910** Magnetic resonance angiography without contrast, chest (excluding myocardium)

Medicare Statute 1833(t)(2)

◎ **C8911** Magnetic resonance angiography without contrast followed by with contrast, chest (excluding myocardium)

Medicare Statute 1833(t)(2)

◎ **C8912** Magnetic resonance angiography with contrast, lower extremity

Medicare Statute 1833(t)(2)

◎ **C8913** Magnetic resonance angiography without contrast, lower extremity

Medicare Statute 1833(t)(2)

◎ **C8914** Magnetic resonance angiography without contrast followed by with contrast, lower extremity

Medicare Statute 1833(t)(2)

◎ **C8918** Magnetic resonance angiography with contrast, pelvis

Medicare Statute 1833(t)(2)

◎ **C8919** Magnetic resonance angiography without contrast, pelvis

Medicare Statute 1833(t)(2)

◎ **C8920** Magnetic resonance angiography without contrast followed by with contrast, pelvis

Medicare Statute 1833(t)(2)

◎ **C8921** Transthoracic echocardiography with contrast, or without contrast followed by with contrast, for congenital cardiac anomalies; complete

Medicare Statute 1833(t)(2)

◎ **C8922** Transthoracic echocardiography with contrast, or without contrast followed by with contrast, for congenital cardiac anomalies; follow-up or limited study

Medicare Statute 1833(t)(2)

◎ **C8923** Transthoracic echocardiography with contrast, or without contrast followed by with contrast, real-time with image documentation (2D), includes M-mode recording, when performed, complete, without spectral or color Doppler echocardiography

Medicare Statute 1833(t)(2)

C8924 Transthoracic echocardiography with contrast, or without contrast followed by with contrast, real-time with image documentation (2D), includes M-mode recording, when performed, follow-up or limited study

Medicare Statute 1833(t)(2)

C8925 Transesophageal echocardiography (TEE) with contrast, or without contrast followed by with contrast, real time with image documentation (2D) (with or without M-mode recording); including probe placement, image acquisition, interpretation and report

Medicare Statute 1833(t)(2)

C8926 Transesophageal echocardiography (TEE) with contrast, or without contrast followed by with contrast, for congenital cardiac anomalies; including probe placement, image acquisition, interpretation and report

Medicare Statute 1833(t)(2)

C8927 Transesophageal echocardiography (TEE) with contrast, or without contrast followed by with contrast, for monitoring purposes, including probe placement, real time 2-dimensional image acquisition and interpretation leading to ongoing (continuous) assessment of (dynamically changing) cardiac pumping function and to therapeutic measures on an immediate time basis

Medicare Statute 1833(t)(2)

C8928 Transthoracic echocardiography with contrast, or without contrast followed by with contrast, real-time with image documentation (2D), includes M-mode recording, when performed, during rest and cardiovascular stress test using treadmill, bicycle exercise and/or pharmacologically induced stress, with interpretation and report

Medicare Statute 1833(t)(2)

C8929 Transthoracic echocardiography with contrast, or without contrast followed by with contrast, real-time with image documentation (2D), includes M-mode recording, when performed, complete, with spectral Doppler echocardiography, and with color flow Doppler echocardiography

Medicare Statute 1833(t)(2)

C8930 Transthoracic echocardiography, with contrast, or without contrast followed by with contrast, real-time with image documentation (2D), includes M-mode recording, when performed, during rest and cardiovascular stress test using treadmill, bicycle exercise and/or pharmacologically induced stress, with interpretation and report; including performance of continuous electrocardiographic monitoring, with physician supervision

Medicare Statute 1833(t)(2)

C8931 Magnetic resonance angiography with contrast, spinal canal and contents

Medicare Statute 1833(t)

C8932 Magnetic resonance angiography without contrast, spinal canal and contents

Medicare Statute 1833(t)

C8933 Magnetic resonance angiography without contrast followed by with contrast, spinal canal and contents

Medicare Statute 1833(t)

C8934 Magnetic resonance angiography with contrast, upper extremity

Medicare Statute 1833(t)

C8935 Magnetic resonance angiography without contrast, upper extremity

Medicare Statute 1833(t)

C8936 Magnetic resonance angiography without contrast followed by with contrast, upper extremity

Medicare Statute 1833(t)

C8957 Intravenous infusion for therapy/diagnosis; initiation of prolonged infusion (more than 8 hours), requiring use of portable or implantable pump

Medicare Statute 1833(t)

C9113 Injection, pantoprazole sodium, per vial

Medicare Statute 1833(t)

~~C9121 Injection, argatroban, per 5 mg~~ ✖

C9132 Prothrombin complex concentrate (human), Kcentra, per i.u. of Factor IX activity

Medicare Statute 1833(t)

~~C9137 Injection, factor viii (antihemophilic factor, recombinant) pegylated, 1 i.u.~~ ✖

Cross Reference J7207

~~C9138 Injection, factor viii (antihemophilic factor, recombinant) (nuwiq), 1 i.u.~~ ✖

Cross Reference J7209

▶ New ↩ Revised ✔ Reinstated ~~deleted~~ Deleted ⃠ Not covered or valid by Medicare
Special coverage instructions * Carrier discretion Bill local carrier Bill DME MAC

~~C9139~~ ~~Injection, factor ix, albumin fusion protein (recombinant), idelvion, 1 i.u.~~ ✖

Cross Reference J7202

▶ ❂ **C9140** Injection, factor VIII (antihemophilic factor, recombinant) (afstyla), 1 i.u.

Medicare Statute 1833(T)

❂ **C9248** Injection, clevidipine butyrate, 1 mg

Medicare Statute 1833(t)

↩ ❂ **C9250** Human plasma fibrin sealant, vapor-heated, solvent-detergent (ARTISS), 2 ml

Example of diagnosis codes to be reported with C9250: T20.00-T25.799.

Medicare Statute 621MMA

❂ **C9254** Injection, lacosamide, 1 mg

Medicare Statute 621MMA

❂ **C9257** injection, bevacizumab, 0.25 mg

Medicare Statute 1833(t)

❂ **C9275** Injection, hexaminolevulinate hydrochloride, 100 mg, per study dose

Medicare Statute 1833(t)

❂ **C9285** Lidocaine 70 mg/tetracaine 70 mg, per patch

Medicare Statute 1833(t)

❂ **C9290** Injection, bupivacine liposome, 1 mg

Medicare Statute 1833(t)

❂ **C9293** Injection, glucarpidase, 10 units

Medicare Statute 1833(t)

~~C9349~~ ~~Puraply, and Puraply Antimicrobial, any type, per square centimeter~~ ✖

❂ **C9352** Microporous collagen implantable tube (NeuraGen Nerve Guide), per centimeter length

Medicare Statute 621MMA

❂ **C9353** Microporous collagen implantable slit tube (NeuraWrap Nerve Protector), per centimeter length

Medicare Statute 621MMA

❂ **C9354** Acellular pericardial tissue matrix of non-human origin (Veritas), per square centimeter

Medicare Statute 621MMA

❂ **C9355** Collagen nerve cuff (NeuroMatrix), per 0.5 centimeter length

Medicare Statute 621MMA

❂ **C9356** Tendon, porous matrix of cross-linked collagen and glycosaminoglycan matrix (TenoGlide Tendon Protector Sheet), per square centimeter

Medicare Statute 621MMA

❂ **C9358** Dermal substitute, native, non-denatured collagen, fetal bovine origin (SurgiMend Collagen Matrix), per 0.5 square centimeters

Medicare Statute 621MMA

❂ **C9359** Porous purified collagen matrix bone void filler (Integra Mozaik Osteoconductive Scaffold Putty, Integra OS Osteoconductive Scaffold Putty), per 0.5 cc

Medicare Statute 1833(t)

❂ **C9360** Dermal substitute, native, non-denatured collagen, neonatal bovine origin (SurgiMend Collagen Matrix), per 0.5 square centimeters

Medicare Statute 621MMA

❂ **C9361** Collagen matrix nerve wrap (NeuroMend Collagen Nerve Wrap), per 0.5 centimeter length

Medicare Statute 621MMA

❂ **C9362** Porous purified collagen matrix bone void filler (Integra Mozaik Osteoconductive Scaffold Strip), per 0.5 cc

Medicare Statute 621MMA

❂ **C9363** Skin substitute, Integra Meshed Bilayer Wound Matrix, per square centimeter

Medicare Statute 621MMA

❂ **C9364** Porcine implant, Permacol, per square centimeter

Medicare Statute 621MMA

❂ **C9399** Unclassified drugs or biologicals

Medicare Statute 621MMA

❂ **C9447** Injection, phenylephrine and ketorolac, 4 ml vial

Medicare Statute 1833(t)

~~C9458~~ ~~Florbetaben f18, diagnostic, per study dose, up to 8.1 millicuries~~ ✖

Cross Reference Q9983

~~C9459~~ ~~Flutemetamol f18, diagnostic, per study dose, up to 5 millicuries~~ ✖

Cross Reference Q9982

❂ **C9460** Injection, cangrelor, 1 mg

Medicare Statute 1833(t)

~~C9461~~ ~~Choline c 11, diagnostic, per study dose~~ ✖

Cross Reference A9515

~~C9470~~ ~~Injection, aripiprazole lauroxil, 1 mg~~ ✖

Cross Reference J1942

▶ New ↩ Revised ✔ Reinstated ~~deleted~~ Deleted ⊘ Not covered or valid by Medicare
❂ Special coverage instructions ✻ Carrier discretion Ⓑ Bill local carrier Ⓓ Bill DME MAC

~~C9471~~ ~~Hyaluronan or derivative, hymovis, for intra-articular injection, 1 mg~~ ✖
Cross Reference J7322

~~C9472~~ ~~Injection, talimogene laherparepvec, 1 million plaque forming units (pfu)~~ ✖
Cross Reference J9325

~~C9473~~ ~~Injection, mepolizumab, 1 mg~~ ✖
Cross Reference J2182

~~C9474~~ ~~Injection, irinotecan liposome, 1 mg~~ ✖
Cross Reference J9205

~~C9475~~ ~~Injection, necitumumab, 1 mg~~ ✖
Cross Reference J9295

~~C9476~~ ~~Injection, daratumumab, 10 mg~~ ✖
Cross Reference J9145

~~C9477~~ ~~Injection, elotuzumab, 1 mg~~ ✖
Cross Reference J9176

~~C9478~~ ~~Injection, sebelipase alfa, 1 mg~~ ✖
Cross Reference J2840

~~C9479~~ ~~Instillation, ciprofloxacin otic suspension, 6 mg~~ ✖
Cross Reference J7342

~~C9480~~ ~~Injection, trabectedin, 0.1 mg~~ ✖
Cross Reference J9352

~~C9481~~ ~~Injection, reslizumab, 1 mg~~ ✖
Cross Reference J2786

▶ **C9482** Injection, sotalol hydrochloride, 1 mg
Medicare Statute 1833(t)

▶ **C9483** Injection, atezolizumab, 10 mg
Medicare Statute 1833(t)

⚙ **C9497** Loxapine, inhalation powder, 10 mg
Medicare Statute 1833(t)

⚙ **C9600** Percutaneous transcatheter placement of drug eluting intracoronary stent(s), with coronary angioplasty when performed; a single major coronary artery or branch
Medicare Statute 1833(t)

⚙ **C9601** Percutaneous transcatheter placement of drug-eluting intracoronary stent(s), with coronary angioplasty when performed; each additional branch of a major coronary artery (list separately in addition to code for primary procedure)
Medicare Statute 1833(t)

⚙ **C9602** Percutaneous transluminal coronary atherectomy, with drug eluting intracoronary stent, with coronary angioplasty when performed; a single major coronary artery or branch
Medicare Statute 1833(t)

⚙ **C9603** Percutaneous transluminal coronary atherectomy, with drug-eluting intracoronary stent, with coronary angioplasty when performed; each additional branch of a major coronary artery (list separately in addition to code for primary procedure)
Medicare Statute 1833(t)

⚙ **C9604** Percutaneous transluminal revascularization of or through coronary artery bypass graft (internal mammary, free arterial, venous), any combination of drug-eluting intracoronary stent, atherectomy and angioplasty, including distal protection when performed; a single vessel

⚙ **C9605** Percutaneous transluminal revascularization of or through coronary artery bypass graft (internal mammary, free arterial, venous), any combination of drug-eluting intracoronary stent, atherectomy and angioplasty, including distal protection when performed; each additional branch subtended by the bypass graft (list separately in addition to code for primary procedure)
Medicare Statute 1833(t)

⚙ **C9606** Percutaneous transluminal revascularization of acute total/subtotal occlusion during acute myocardial infarction, coronary artery or coronary artery bypass graft, any combination of drug-eluting intracoronary stent, atherectomy and angioplasty, including aspiration thrombectomy when performed, single vessel
Medicare Statute 1833(t)

⚙ **C9607** Percutaneous transluminal revascularization of chronic total occlusion, coronary artery, coronary artery branch, or coronary artery bypass graft, any combination of drug-eluting intracoronary stent, atherectomy and angioplasty; single vessel
Medicare Statute 1833(t)

C9608 Percutaneous transluminal revascularization of chronic total occlusion, coronary artery, coronary artery branch, or coronary artery bypass graft, any combination of drug-eluting intracoronary stent, atherectomy and angioplasty; each additional coronary artery, coronary artery branch, or bypass graft (list separately in addition to code for primary procedure)

Medicare Statute 1833(t)

C9725 Placement of endorectal intracavitary applicator for high intensity brachytherapy

Medicare Statute 1833(t)

C9726 Placement and removal (if performed) of applicator into breast for intraoperative radiation therapy, add-on to primary breast procedure

Medicare Statute 1833(t)

C9727 Insertion of implants into the soft palate; minimum of three implants

Medicare Statute 1833(t)

C9728 Placement of interstitial device(s) for radiation therapy/surgery guidance (e.g., fiducial markers, dosimeter), for other than the following sites (any approach): abdomen, pelvis, prostate, retroperitoneum, thorax, single or multiple

Medicare Statute 1833(t)

C9733 Non-ophthalmic fluorescent vascular angiography

Medicare Statute 1833(t)

C9734 Focused ultrasound ablation/therapeutic intervention, other than uterine leiomyomata, with magnetic resonance (MR) guidance

Medicare Statute 1833(t)

C9739 Cystourethroscopy, with insertion of transprostatic implant; 1 to 3 implants

Medicare Statute 1833(t)

C9740 Cystourethroscopy, with insertion of transprostatic implant; 4 or more implants

Medicare Statute 1833(t)

C9741 Right heart catheterization with implantation of wireless pressure sensor in the pulmonary artery, including any type of measurement, angiography, imaging supervision, interpretation, and report

Medicare Statute 1833(t)

~~C9742 Laryngoscopy, flexible fiberoptic, with injection into vocal cord(s), therapeutic, including diagnostic laryngoscopy, if performed~~ ✖

Cross Reference 31573, 31574

~~C9743 Injection/implantation of bulking or spacer material (any type) with or without image guidance (not to be used if a more specific code applies)~~ ✖

Cross Reference 0438T

▶ **C9744** Ultrasound, abdominal, with contrast

Medicare Statute 1833(t)

~~C9800 Dermal injection procedure(s) for facial lipodystrophy syndrome (LDS) and provision of radiesse or sculptra dermal filler, including all items and supplies~~ ✖

Cross Reference G0429

C9898 Radiolabeled product provided during a hospital inpatient stay

C9899 Implanted prosthetic device, payable only for inpatients who do not have inpatient coverage

Medicare Statute 1833(t)

DURABLE MEDICAL EQUIPMENT (E0100-E1841)

Canes

E0100 Cane, includes canes of all materials, adjustable or fixed, with tip

IOM: 100-02, 15, 110.1; 100-03, 4, 280.1; 100-03, 4, 280.2

E0105 Cane, quad or three prong, includes canes of all materials, adjustable or fixed, with tips

IOM: 100-02, 15, 110.1; 100-03, 4, 280.1; 100-03, 4, 280.2

Crutches

E0110 Crutches, forearm, includes crutches of various materials, adjustable or fixed, pair, complete with tips and handgrips

Crutches are covered when prescribed for a patient who is normally ambulatory but suffers from a condition that impairs ambulation. Provides minimal to moderate weight support while ambulating.

IOM: 100-02, 15, 110.1; 100-03, 4, 280.1

E0111 Crutch forearm, includes crutches of various materials, adjustable or fixed, each, with tips and handgrips

IOM: 100-02, 15, 110.1; 100-03, 4, 280.1

E0112 Crutches, underarm, wood, adjustable or fixed, pair, with pads, tips, and handgrips

IOM: 100-02, 15, 110.1; 100-03, 4, 280.1

E0113 Crutch underarm, wood, adjustable or fixed, each, with pad, tip, and handgrip

IOM: 100-02, 15, 110.1; 100-03, 4, 280.1

E0114 Crutches, underarm, other than wood, adjustable or fixed, pair, with pads, tips and handgrips

IOM: 100-02, 15, 110.1; 100-03, 4, 280.1

E0116 Crutch, underarm, other than wood, adjustable or fixed, with pad, tip, handgrip, with or without shock absorber, each

IOM: 100-02, 15, 110.1; 100-03, 4, 280.1

E0117 Crutch, underarm, articulating, spring assisted, each

IOM: 100-02, 15, 110.1

* **E0118** Crutch substitute, lower leg platform, with or without wheels, each

Walkers

E0130 Walker, rigid (pickup), adjustable or fixed height

Standard walker criteria for payment: Individual has a mobility limitation that significantly impairs ability to participate in mobility-related activities of daily living that cannot be adequately or safely addressed by a cane. The patient is able to use the walker safely; the functional mobility deficit can be resolved with use of a standard walker.

IOM: 100-02, 15, 110.1; 100-03, 4, 280.1

E0135 Walker, folding (pickup), adjustable or fixed height

IOM: 100-02, 15, 110.1; 100-03, 4, 280.1

E0140 Walker, with trunk support, adjustable or fixed height, any type

IOM: 100-02, 15, 110.1; 100-03, 4, 280.1

E0141 Walker, rigid, wheeled, adjustable or fixed height

IOM: 100-02, 15, 110.1; 100-03, 4, 280.1

E0143 Walker, folding, wheeled, adjustable or fixed height

IOM: 100-02, 15, 110.1; 100-03, 4, 280.1

E0144 Walker, enclosed, four sided framed, rigid or folding, wheeled, with posterior seat

IOM: 100-02, 15, 110.1; 100-03, 4, 280.1

E0147 Walker, heavy duty, multiple braking system, variable wheel resistance

Heavy-duty walker is labeled as capable of supporting more than 300 pounds

IOM: 100-02, 15, 110.1; 100-03, 4, 280.1

* **E0148** Walker, heavy duty, without wheels, rigid or folding, any type, each

Heavy-duty walker is labeled as capable of supporting more than 300 pounds

* **E0149** Walker, heavy duty, wheeled, rigid or folding, any type

Heavy-duty walker is labeled as capable of supporting more than 300 pounds

* **E0153** Platform attachment, forearm crutch, each

* **E0154** Platform attachment, walker, each

* **E0155** Wheel attachment, rigid pick-up walker, per pair

▶ New ⮌ Revised ✔ Reinstated ~~deleted~~ Deleted ⊘ Not covered or valid by Medicare
Special coverage instructions * Carrier discretion Bill local carrier Bill DME MAC

 DME codes can be reported by ALL providers

Attachments

* ✻ **E0156** Seat attachment, walker Ⓑ
* ✻ **E0157** Crutch attachment, walker, each Ⓑ
* ✻ **E0158** Leg extensions for walker, per set of four (4) Ⓑ

  Leg extensions are considered medically necessary DME for patients 6 feet tall or more
* ✻ **E0159** Brake attachment for wheeled walker, replacement, each Ⓑ

Commodes

* ✪ **E0160** Sitz type bath or equipment, portable, used with or without commode Ⓑ

  IOM: 100-03, 4, 280.1
* ✪ **E0161** Sitz type bath or equipment, portable, used with or without commode, with faucet attachment/s Ⓑ

  IOM: 100-03, 4, 280.1
* ✪ **E0162** Sitz bath chair Ⓑ

  IOM: 100-03, 4, 280.1
* ✪ **E0163** Commode chair, mobile or stationary, with fixed arms Ⓑ

  IOM: 100-02, 15, 110.1; 100-03, 4, 280.1
* ✪ **E0165** Commode chair, mobile or stationary, with detachable arms Ⓑ

  IOM: 100-02, 15, 110.1; 100-03, 4, 280.1
* ✪ **E0167** Pail or pan for use with commode chair, replacement only Ⓑ

  IOM: 100-03, 4, 280.1
* ✻ **E0168** Commode chair, extra wide and/or heavy duty, stationary or mobile, with or without arms, any type, each Ⓑ

  Extra-wide or heavy duty commode chair is labeled as capable of supporting more than 300 pounds
* ✻ **E0170** Commode chair with integrated seat lift mechanism, electric, any type Ⓑ
* ✻ **E0171** Commode chair with integrated seat lift mechanism, non-electric, any type Ⓑ
* ⊘ **E0172** Seat lift mechanism placed over or on top of toilet, any type Ⓑ

  Medicare Statute 1861 SSA
* ✻ **E0175** Foot rest, for use with commode chair, each Ⓑ

Decubitus Care Equipment

* ✪ **E0181** Powered pressure reducing mattress overlay/pad, alternating, with pump, includes heavy duty Ⓑ

  Requires the provider to determine medical necessity compliance. To demonstrate the requirements in the medical policy were met, attach KX.

  IOM: 100-03, 4, 280.1; 100-08, 5, 5.2.3
* ✪ **E0182** Pump for alternating pressure pad, for replacement only Ⓑ

  IOM: 100-03, 4, 280.1; 100-08, 5, 5.2.3
* ✪ **E0184** Dry pressure mattress Ⓑ

  IOM: 100-03, 4, 280.1; 100-08, 5, 5.2.3
* ✪ **E0185** Gel or gel-like pressure pad for mattress, standard mattress length and width Ⓑ

  IOM: 100-03, 4, 280.1; 100-08, 5, 5.2.3
* ✪ **E0186** Air pressure mattress Ⓑ

  IOM: 100-03, 4, 280.1
* ✪ **E0187** Water pressure mattress Ⓑ

  IOM: 100-03, 4, 280.1
* ✪ **E0188** Synthetic sheepskin pad Ⓑ

  IOM: 100-03, 4, 280.1; 100-08, 5, 5.2.3
* ✪ **E0189** Lambswool sheepskin pad, any size Ⓑ

  IOM: 100-03, 4, 280.1; 100-08, 5, 5.2.3
* ✪ **E0190** Positioning cushion/pillow/wedge, any shape or size, includes all components and accessories Ⓑ

  IOM: 100-02, 15, 110.1
* ✻ **E0191** Heel or elbow protector, each Ⓑ
* ✻ **E0193** Powered air flotation bed (low air loss therapy) Ⓑ
* ✪ **E0194** Air fluidized bed Ⓑ

  IOM: 100-03, 4, 280.1
* ✪ **E0196** Gel pressure mattress Ⓑ

  IOM: 100-03, 4, 280.1
* ⮌ ✪ **E0197** Air pressure pad for mattress, standard mattress length and width Ⓑ

  IOM: 100-03, 4, 280.1
* ✪ **E0198** Water pressure pad for mattress, standard mattress length and width Ⓑ

  IOM: 100-03, 4, 280.1
* ✪ **E0199** Dry pressure pad for mattress, standard mattress length and width Ⓑ

  IOM: 100-03, 4, 280.1

▶ New ⮌ Revised ✔ Reinstated ~~deleted~~ Deleted ⊘ Not covered or valid by Medicare
✪ Special coverage instructions ✻ Carrier discretion Ⓑ Bill local carrier Ⓑ Bill DME MAC

Heat/Cold Application

⊕ **E0200** Heat lamp, without stand (table model), includes bulb, or infrared element Ⓑ

Covered when medical review determines patient's medical condition is one for which application of heat by heat lamp is therapeutically effective

IOM: 100-02, 15, 110.1; 100-03, 4, 280.1

* **E0202** Phototherapy (bilirubin) light with photometer Ⓑ

⊘ **E0203** Therapeutic lightbox, minimum 10,000 lux, table top model Ⓑ

IOM: 100-03, 4, 280.1

⊕ **E0205** Heat lamp, with stand, includes bulb, or infrared element Ⓑ

IOM: 100-02, 15, 110.1; 100-03, 4, 280.1

⊕ **E0210** Electric heat pad, standard Ⓑ

Flexible device containing electric resistive elements producing heat; has fabric cover to prevent burns; with or without timing devices for automatic shut-off

IOM: 100-03, 4, 280.1

⊕ **E0215** Electric heat pad, moist Ⓑ

Flexible device containing electric resistive elements producing heat. Must have component that will absorb and retain liquid (water).

IOM: 100-03, 4, 280.1

⊕ **E0217** Water circulating heat pad with pump Ⓑ

Consists of flexible pad containing series of channels through which water is circulated by means of electrical pumping mechanism and heated in external reservoir

IOM: 100-03, 4, 280.1

⊕ **E0218** Water circulating cold pad with pump Ⓑ

IOM: 100-03, 4, 280.1

* **E0221** Infrared heating pad system Ⓑ

⊕ **E0225** Hydrocollator unit, includes pads Ⓑ

IOM: 100-02, 15, 230; 100-03, 4, 280.1

⊘ **E0231** Non-contact wound warming device (temperature control unit, AC adapter and power cord) for use with warming card and wound cover Ⓑ

IOM: 100-02, 16, 20

⊘ **E0232** Warming card for use with the non-contact wound warming device and non-contact wound warming wound cover Ⓑ

IOM: 100-02, 16, 20

⊕ **E0235** Paraffin bath unit, portable (medical supply code A4265 for paraffin) Ⓑ

Ordered by physician and patient's condition expected to be relieved by long-term use of modality

IOM: 100-02, 15, 230; 100-03, 4, 280.1

⊕ **E0236** Pump for water circulating pad Ⓑ

IOM: 100-03, 4, 280.1

⊕ **E0239** Hydrocollator unit, portable Ⓑ

IOM: 100-02, 15, 230; 100-03, 4, 280.1

Bath and Toilet Aids

⊘ **E0240** Bath/shower chair, with or without wheels, any size Ⓑ

IOM: 100-03, 4, 280.1

⊘ **E0241** Bath tub wall rail, each Ⓑ

IOM: 100-02, 15, 110.1; 100-03, 4, 280.1

⊘ **E0242** Bath tub rail, floor base Ⓑ

IOM: 100-02, 15, 110.1; 100-03, 4, 280.1

⊘ **E0243** Toilet rail, each Ⓑ

IOM: 100-02, 15, 110.1; 100-03, 4, 280.1

⊘ **E0244** Raised toilet seat Ⓑ

IOM: 100-03, 4, 280.1

⊘ **E0245** Tub stool or bench Ⓑ

IOM: 100-03, 4, 280.1

* **E0246** Transfer tub rail attachment Ⓑ

⊕ **E0247** Transfer bench for tub or toilet with or without commode opening Ⓑ

IOM: 100-03, 4, 280.1

⊕ **E0248** Transfer bench, heavy duty, for tub or toilet with or without commode opening Ⓑ

Heavy duty transfer bench is labeled as capable of supporting more than 300 pounds

IOM: 100-03, 4, 280.1

Pad for Heating Unit

⊕ **E0249** Pad for water circulating heat unit, for replacement only Ⓑ

Describes durable replacement pad used with water circulating heat pump system

IOM: 100-03, 4, 280.1

Hospital Beds and Accessories

⊕ **E0250** Hospital bed, fixed height, with any type side rails, with mattress Ⓑ

IOM: 100-02, 15, 110.1; 100-03, 4, 280.7

⊕ **E0251** Hospital bed, fixed height, with any type side rails, without mattress Ⓑ

IOM: 100-02, 15, 110.1; 100-03, 4, 280.7

⊕ **E0255** Hospital bed, variable height, hi-lo, with any type side rails, with mattress Ⓑ

IOM: 100-02, 15, 110.1; 100-03, 4, 280.7

⊕ **E0256** Hospital bed, variable height, hi-lo, with any type side rails, without mattress Ⓑ

IOM: 100-02, 15, 110.1; 100-03, 4, 280.7

⊕ **E0260** Hospital bed, semi-electric (head and foot adjustment), with any type side rails, with mattress Ⓑ

IOM: 100-02, 15, 110.1; 100-03, 4, 280.7

⊕ **E0261** Hospital bed, semi-electric (head and foot adjustment), with any type side rails, without mattress Ⓑ

IOM: 100-02, 15, 110.1; 100-03, 4, 280.7

⊕ **E0265** Hospital bed, total electric (head, foot and height adjustments), with any type side rails, with mattress Ⓑ

IOM: 100-02, 15, 110.1; 100-03, 4, 280.7

⊕ **E0266** Hospital bed, total electric (head, foot and height adjustments), with any type side rails, without mattress Ⓑ

IOM: 100-02, 15, 110.1; 100-03, 4, 280.7

⊘ **E0270** Hospital bed, institutional type includes: oscillating, circulating and Stryker frame, with mattress Ⓑ

IOM: 100-03, 4, 280.1

⊕ **E0271** Mattress, innerspring Ⓑ

IOM: 100-03, 4, 280.1; 100-03, 4, 280.7

⊕ **E0272** Mattress, foam rubber Ⓑ

IOM: 100-03, 4, 280.1; 100-03, 4, 280.7

⊘ **E0273** Bed board Ⓑ

IOM: 100-03, 4, 280.1

⊘ **E0274** Over-bed table Ⓑ

IOM: 100-03, 4, 280.1

⊕ **E0275** Bed pan, standard, metal or plastic Ⓑ

IOM: 100-03, 4, 280.1

⊕ **E0276** Bed pan, fracture, metal or plastic Ⓑ

IOM: 100-03, 4, 280.1

⊕ **E0277** Powered pressure-reducing air mattress Ⓑ

IOM: 100-03, 4, 280.1

✻ **E0280** Bed cradle, any type Ⓑ

⊕ **E0290** Hospital bed, fixed height, without side rails, with mattress Ⓑ

IOM: 100-02, 15, 110.1; 100-03, 4, 280.7

⊕ **E0291** Hospital bed, fixed height, without side rails, without mattress Ⓑ

IOM: 100-02, 15, 110.1; 100-03, 4, 280.7

↩ ⊕ **E0292** Hospital bed, variable height, hi-lo, without side rails, with mattress Ⓑ

IOM: 100-02, 15, 110.1; 100-03, 4, 280.7

↩ ⊕ **E0293** Hospital bed, variable height, hi-lo, without side rails, without mattress Ⓑ

IOM: 100-02, 15, 110.1; 100-03, 4, 280.7

⊕ **E0294** Hospital bed, semi-electric (head and foot adjustment), without side rails, with mattress Ⓑ

IOM: 100-02, 15, 110.1; 100-03, 4, 280.7

⊕ **E0295** Hospital bed, semi-electric (head and foot adjustment), without side rails, without mattress Ⓑ

IOM: 100-02, 15, 110.1; 100-03, 4, 280.7

⊕ **E0296** Hospital bed, total electric (head, foot and height adjustments), without side rails, with mattress Ⓑ

IOM: 100-02, 15, 110.1; 100-03, 4, 280.7

⊕ **E0297** Hospital bed, total electric (head, foot and height adjustments), without side rails, without mattress Ⓑ

IOM: 100-02, 15, 110.1; 100-03, 4, 280.7

✻ **E0300** Pediatric crib, hospital grade, fully enclosed, with or without top enclosure Ⓑ

⊕ **E0301** Hospital bed, heavy duty, extra wide, with weight capacity greater than 350 pounds, but less than or equal to 600 pounds, with any type side rails, without mattress Ⓑ

IOM: 100-03, 4, 280.7

⊕ **E0302** Hospital bed, extra heavy duty, extra wide, with weight capacity greater than 600 pounds, with any type side rails, without mattress Ⓑ

IOM: 100-03, 4, 280.7

E0303 Hospital bed, heavy duty, extra wide, with weight capacity greater than 350 pounds, but less than or equal to 600 pounds, with any type side rails, with mattress

IOM: 100-03, 4, 280.7

E0304 Hospital bed, extra heavy duty, extra wide, with weight capacity greater than 600 pounds, with any type side rails, with mattress

IOM: 100-03, 4, 280.7

E0305 Bed side rails, half length

IOM: 100-03, 4, 280.7

E0310 Bed side rails, full length

IOM: 100-03, 4, 280.7

⃠ **E0315** Bed accessory: board, table, or support device, any type

IOM: 100-03, 4, 280.1

* **E0316** Safety enclosure frame/canopy for use with hospital bed, any type

E0325 Urinal; male, jug-type, any material

IOM: 100-03, 4, 280.1

E0326 Urinal; female, jug-type, any aterial

IOM: 100-03, 4, 280.1

* **E0328** Hospital bed, pediatric, manual, 360 degree side enclosures, top of headboard, footboard and side rails up to 24 inches above the spring, includes mattress

* **E0329** Hospital bed, pediatric, electric or semi-electric, 360 degree side enclosures, top of headboard, footboard and side rails up to 24 inches above the spring, includes mattress

* **E0350** Control unit for electronic bowel irrigation/evacuation system

Pulsed Irrigation Enhanced Evacuation (PIEE) is pulsed irrigation of severely impacted fecal material and may be necessary for patients who have not responded to traditional bowel program.

* **E0352** Disposable pack (water reservoir bag, speculum, valving mechanism and collection bag/box) for use with the electronic bowel irrigation/evacuation system

Therapy kit includes 1 B-Valve circuit, 2 containment bags, 1 lubricating jelly, 1 bed pad, 1 tray liner-waste disposable bag, and 2 hose clamps

* **E0370** Air pressure elevator for heel

* **E0371** Non powered advanced pressure reducing overlay for mattress, standard mattress length and width

Patient has at least one large Stage III or Stage IV pressure sore (greater than 2 × 2 cm.) on trunk, with only two turning surfaces on which to lie

* **E0372** Powered air overlay for mattress, standard mattress length and width

* **E0373** Non powered advanced pressure reducing mattress

Oxygen and Related Respiratory Equipment

E0424 Stationary compressed gaseous oxygen system, rental; includes container, contents, regulator, flowmeter, humidifier, nebulizer, cannula or mask, and tubing

IOM: 100-03, 4, 280.1; 100-04, 20, 30.6

E0425 Stationary compressed gas system, purchase; includes regulator, flowmeter, humidifier, nebulizer, cannula or mask, and tubing

IOM: 100-03, 4, 280.1; 100-04, 20, 30.6

E0430 Portable gaseous oxygen system, purchase; includes regulator, flowmeter, humidifier, cannula or mask, and tubing

IOM: 100-03, 4, 280.1; 100-04, 20, 30.6

E0431 Portable gaseous oxygen system, rental; includes portable container, regulator, flowmeter, humidifier, cannula or mask, and tubing

IOM: 100-03, 4, 280.1; 100-04, 20, 30.6

* **E0433** Portable liquid oxygen system, rental; home liquefier used to fill portable liquid oxygen containers, includes portable containers, regulator, flowmeter, humidifier, cannula or mask and tubing, with or without supply reservoir and contents gauge

E0434 Portable liquid oxygen system, rental; includes portable container, supply reservoir, humidifier, flowmeter, refill adaptor, contents gauge, cannula or mask, and tubing

Fee schedule payments for stationary oxygen system rentals are all-inclusive and represent monthly allowance for beneficiary. Non-Medicare payers may rent device to beneficiaries, or arrange for purchase of device.

IOM: 100-03, 4, 280.1; 100-04, 20, 30.6

⚙ **E0435** Portable liquid oxygen system, purchase; includes portable container, supply reservoir, flowmeter, humidifier, contents gauge, cannula or mask, tubing and refill adaptor Ⓑ

IOM: 100-03, 4, 280.1; 100-04, 20, 30.6

⚙ **E0439** Stationary liquid oxygen system, rental; includes container, contents, regulator, flowmeter, humidifier, nebulizer, cannula or mask, & tubing Ⓑ

This allowance includes payment for equipment, contents, and accessories furnished during rental month.

IOM: 100-03, 4, 280.1; 100-04, 20, 30.6

⚙ **E0440** Stationary liquid oxygen system, purchase; includes use of reservoir, contents indicator, regulator, flowmeter, humidifier, nebulizer, cannula or mask, and tubing Ⓑ

IOM: 100-03, 4, 280.1; 100-04, 20, 30.6

⚙ **E0441** Stationary oxygen contents, gaseous, 1 month's supply = 1 unit Ⓑ

IOM: 100-03, 4, 280.1; 100-04, 20, 30.6

⚙ **E0442** Stationary oxygen contents, liquid, 1 month's supply = 1 unit Ⓑ

IOM: 100-03, 4, 280.1; 100-04, 20, 30.6

⚙ **E0443** Portable oxygen contents, gaseous, 1 month's supply = 1 unit Ⓑ

IOM: 100-03, 4, 280.1; 100-04, 20, 30.6

⚙ **E0444** Portable oxygen contents, liquid, 1 month's supply = 1 unit Ⓑ

IOM: 100-03, 4, 280.1; 100-04, 20, 30.6

✻ **E0445** Oximeter device for measuring blood oxygen levels non-invasively Ⓑ

⊘ **E0446** Topical oxygen delivery system, not otherwise specified, includes all supplies and accessories Ⓑ

⚙ **E0455** Oxygen tent, excluding croup or pediatric tents Ⓑ

IOM: 100-03, 4, 280.1; 100-04, 20, 30.6

⊘ **E0457** Chest shell (cuirass) Ⓑ

⊘ **E0459** Chest wrap Ⓑ

✻ **E0462** Rocking bed with or without side rails Ⓑ

⚙ **E0465** Home ventilator, any type, used with invasive interface, (e.g., tracheostomy tube) Ⓑ

IOM: 100-03, 4, 280.1

⚙ **E0466** Home ventilator, any type, used with non-invasive interface, (e.g., mask, chest shell) Ⓑ

IOM: 100-03, 4, 280.1

⚙ **E0470** Respiratory assist device, bi-level pressure capability, without backup rate feature, used with noninvasive interface, e.g., nasal or facial mask (intermittent assist device with continuous positive airway pressure device) Ⓑ

IOM: 100-03, 4, 240.2

⚙ **E0471** Respiratory assist device, bi-level pressure capability, with back-up rate feature, used with noninvasive interface, e.g., nasal or facial mask (intermittent assist device with continuous positive airway pressure device) Ⓑ

IOM: 100-03, 4, 240.2

⚙ **E0472** Respiratory assist device, bi-level pressure capability, with backup rate feature, used with invasive interface, e.g., tracheostomy tube (intermittent assist device with continuous positive airway pressure device) Ⓑ

IOM: 100-03, 4, 240.2

⚙ **E0480** Percussor, electric or pneumatic, home model Ⓑ

IOM: 100-03, 4, 240.2

⊘ **E0481** Intrapulmonary percussive ventilation system and related accessories Ⓑ

IOM: 100-03, 4, 240.2

✻ **E0482** Cough stimulating device, alternating positive and negative airway pressure Ⓑ

✻ **E0483** High frequency chest wall oscillation air-pulse generator system, (includes hoses and vest), each Ⓑ

✻ **E0484** Oscillatory positive expiratory pressure device, non-electric, any type, each Ⓑ

✻ **E0485** Oral device/appliance used to reduce upper airway collapsibility, adjustable or non-adjustable, prefabricated, includes fitting and adjustment Ⓑ

✻ **E0486** Oral device/appliance used to reduce upper airway collapsibility, adjustable or non-adjustable, custom fabricated, includes fitting and adjustment Ⓑ

⚙ **E0487** Spirometer, electronic, includes all accessories Ⓑ

▶ New ⤺ Revised ✔ Reinstated ~~deleted~~ Deleted ⊘ Not covered or valid by Medicare
⚙ Special coverage instructions ✻ Carrier discretion Ⓑ Bill local carrier Ⓑ Bill DME MAC

IPPB Machines

E0500 IPPB machine, all types, with built-in nebulization; manual or automatic valves; internal or external power source
IOM: 100-03, 4, 240.2

Humidifiers/Nebulizers/Compressors for Use with Oxygen IPPB Equipment

E0550 Humidifier, durable for extensive supplemental humidification during IPPB treatments or oxygen delivery
IOM: 100-03, 4, 240.2

E0555 Humidifier, durable, glass or autoclavable plastic bottle type, for use with regulator or flowmeter
IOM: 100-03, 4, 280.1; 100-04, 20, 30.6

E0560 Humidifier, durable for supplemental humidification during IPPB treatment or oxygen delivery
IOM: 100-03, 4, 280.1

* **E0561** Humidifier, non-heated, used with positive airway pressure device

* **E0562** Humidifier, heated, used with positive airway pressure device

* **E0565** Compressor, air power source for equipment which is not self-contained or cylinder driven

E0570 Nebulizer, with compressor
IOM: 100-03, 4, 240.2; 100-03, 4, 280.1

* **E0572** Aerosol compressor, adjustable pressure, light duty for intermittent use

* **E0574** Ultrasonic/electronic aerosol generator with small volume nebulizer

E0575 Nebulizer, ultrasonic, large volume
IOM: 100-03, 4, 240.2

E0580 Nebulizer, durable, glass or autoclavable plastic, bottle type, for use with regulator or flowmeter
IOM: 100-03, 4, 240.2; 100-03, 4, 280.1

E0585 Nebulizer, with compressor and heater
IOM: 100-03, 4, 240.2; 100-03, 4, 280.1

Suction Pump/Room Vaporizers

E0600 Respiratory suction pump, home model, portable or stationary, electric
IOM: 100-03, 4, 240.2

E0601 Continuous positive airway pressure (CPAP) device
IOM: 100-03, 4, 240.4

* **E0602** Breast pump, manual, any type
Bill either manual breast pump or breast pump kit

* **E0603** Breast pump, electric (AC and/or DC), any type

* **E0604** Breast pump, hospital grade, electric (AC and/or DC), any type

E0605 Vaporizer, room type
IOM: 100-03, 4, 240.2

E0606 Postural drainage board
IOM: 100-03, 4, 240.2

Monitoring Equipment

E0607 Home blood glucose monitor
Document recipient or caregiver is competent to monitor equipment and that device is designed for home rather than clinical use
IOM: 100-03, 4, 280.1; 100-03, 1, 40.2

E0610 Pacemaker monitor, self-contained, (checks battery depletion, includes audible and visible check systems)
IOM: 100-03, 1, 20.8

E0615 Pacemaker monitor, self-contained, checks battery depletion and other pacemaker components, includes digital/visible check systems
IOM: 100-03, 1, 20.8

* **E0616** Implantable cardiac event recorder with memory, activator and programmer
Assign when two 30-day pre-symptom external loop recordings fail to establish a definitive diagnosis.

* **E0617** External defibrillator with integrated electrocardiogram analysis

* **E0618** Apnea monitor, without recording feature

* **E0619** Apnea monitor, with recording feature

* **E0620** Skin piercing device for collection of capillary blood, laser, each

Patient Lifts

⊕ **E0621** Sling or seat, patient lift, canvas or nylon Ⓑ

IOM: 100-03, 4, 240.2, 280.4

⊘ **E0625** Patient lift, bathroom or toilet, not otherwise classified Ⓑ

IOM: 100-03, 4, 240.2

↩ ⊕ **E0627** Seat lift mechanism, electric, any type Ⓑ

IOM: 100-03, 4, 280.4; 100-04, 4, 20

Cross Reference Q0080

~~E0628 Separate seat lift mechanism for use with patient owned furniture - electric~~ ✖

Cross Reference Q0078

↩ ⊕ **E0629** Seat lift mechanism, non-electric, any type Ⓑ

IOM: 100-04, 4, 20

Cross Reference Q0079

⊕ **E0630** Patient lift, hydraulic or mechanical, includes any seat, sling, strap(s) or pad(s) Ⓑ

IOM: 100-03, 4, 240.2

⊕ **E0635** Patient lift, electric, with seat or sling Ⓑ

IOM: 100-03, 4, 240.2

✻ **E0636** Multipositional patient support system, with integrated lift, patient accessible controls Ⓑ

⊘ **E0637** Combination sit to stand frame/table system, any size including pediatric, with seat lift feature, with or without wheels Ⓑ

IOM: 100-03, 4, 240.2

⊘ **E0638** Standing frame/table system, one position (e.g., upright, supine or prone stander), any size including pediatric, with or without wheels Ⓑ

IOM: 100-03, 4, 240.2

✻ **E0639** Patient lift, moveable from room to room with disassembly and reassembly, includes all components/accessories Ⓑ

✻ **E0640** Patient lift, fixed system, includes all components/accessories Ⓑ

⊘ **E0641** Standing frame/table system, multi-position (e.g., three-way stander), any size including pediatric, with or without wheels Ⓑ

IOM: 100-03, 4, 240.2

⊘ **E0642** Standing frame/table system, mobile (dynamic stander), any size including pediatric Ⓑ

IOM: 100-03, 4, 240.2

Pneumatic Compressor and Appliances

⊕ **E0650** Pneumatic compressor, non-segmental home model Ⓑ

Lymphedema pumps are classified as segmented or nonsegmented, depending on whether distinct segments of devices can be inflated sequentially.

IOM: 100-03, 4, 280.6

⊕ **E0651** Pneumatic compressor, segmental home model without calibrated gradient pressure Ⓑ

IOM: 100-03, 4, 280.6

⊕ **E0652** Pneumatic compressor, segmental home model with calibrated gradient pressure Ⓑ

IOM: 100-03, 4, 280.6

⊕ **E0655** Non-segmental pneumatic appliance for use with pneumatic compressor, half arm Ⓑ

IOM: 100-03, 4, 280.6

⊕ **E0656** Segmental pneumatic appliance for use with pneumatic compressor, trunk Ⓑ

⊕ **E0657** Segmental pneumatic appliance for use with pneumatic compressor, chest Ⓑ

⊕ **E0660** Non-segmental pneumatic appliance for use with pneumatic compressor, full leg Ⓑ

IOM: 100-03, 4, 280.6

⊕ **E0665** Non-segmental pneumatic appliance for use with pneumatic compressor, full arm Ⓑ

IOM: 100-03, 4, 280.6

⊕ **E0666** Non-segmental pneumatic appliance for use with pneumatic compressor, half leg Ⓑ

IOM: 100-03, 4, 280.6

⊕ **E0667** Segmental pneumatic appliance for use with pneumatic compressor, full leg Ⓑ

IOM: 100-03, 4, 280.6

⊕ **E0668** Segmental pneumatic appliance for use with pneumatic compressor, full arm Ⓑ

IOM: 100-03, 4, 280.6

⊕ **E0669** Segmental pneumatic appliance for use with pneumatic compressor, half leg Ⓑ

IOM: 100-03, 4, 280.6

⊕ **E0670** Segmental pneumatic appliance for use with pneumatic compressor, integrated, 2 full legs and trunk Ⓑ

IOM: 100-03, 4, 280.6

⊕ **E0671** Segmental gradient pressure pneumatic appliance, full leg Ⓑ

IOM: 100-03, 4, 280.6

⊕ **E0672** Segmental gradient pressure pneumatic appliance, full arm Ⓑ

IOM: 100-03, 4, 280.6

⊕ **E0673** Segmental gradient pressure pneumatic appliance, half leg Ⓑ

IOM: 100-03, 4, 280.6

* **E0675** Pneumatic compression device, high pressure, rapid inflation/deflation cycle, for arterial insufficiency (unilateral or bilateral system) Ⓑ

* **E0676** Intermittent limb compression device (includes all accessories), not otherwise specified Ⓑ

Ultraviolet Light Therapy Systems

* **E0691** Ultraviolet light therapy system, includes bulbs/lamps, timer and eye protection; treatment area 2 square feet or less Ⓑ

* **E0692** Ultraviolet light therapy system panel, includes bulbs/lamps, timer and eye protection, 4 foot panel Ⓑ

* **E0693** Ultraviolet light therapy system panel, includes bulbs/lamps, timer and eye protection, 6 foot panel Ⓑ

* **E0694** Ultraviolet multidirectional light therapy system in 6 foot cabinet, includes bulbs/lamps, timer and eye protection Ⓑ

Safety Equipment

* **E0700** Safety equipment, device or accessory, any type Ⓑ

⊕ **E0705** Transfer device, any type, each Ⓑ

Restraints

* **E0710** Restraints, any type (body, chest, wrist or ankle) Ⓑ

Transcutaneous and/or Neuromuscular Electrical Nerve Stimulators (TENS)

⊕ **E0720** Transcutaneous electrical nerve stimulation (TENS) device, two lead, localized stimulation Ⓑ

A Certificate of Medical Necessity (CMN) is not needed for a TENS rental, but is needed purchase.

IOM: 100-03, 2, 160.2; 100-03, 4, 280.1

⊕ **E0730** Transcutaneous electrical nerve stimulation (TENS) device, four or more leads, for multiple nerve stimulation Ⓑ

IOM: 100-03, 2, 160.2; 100-03, 4, 280.1

⊕ **E0731** Form fitting conductive garment for delivery of TENS or NMES (with conductive fibers separated from the patient's skin by layers of fabric) Ⓑ

IOM: 100-03, 2, 160.13

↩⊕ **E0740** Non-implanted pelvic floor electrical stimulator, complete system Ⓑ

IOM: 100-03, 4, 230.8

* **E0744** Neuromuscular stimulator for scoliosis Ⓑ

⊕ **E0745** Neuromuscular stimulator, electronic shock unit Ⓑ

IOM: 100-03, 2, 160.12

⊕ **E0746** Electromyography (EMG), biofeedback device Ⓟ

IOM: 100-03, 1, 30.1

⊕ **E0747** Osteogenesis stimulator, electrical, non-invasive, other than spinal applications Ⓑ

Devices are composed of two basic parts: Coils that wrap around cast and pulse generator that produces electric current.

⊕ **E0748** Osteogenesis stimulator, electrical, non-invasive, spinal applications Ⓑ

Device should be applied within 30 days as adjunct to spinal fusion surgery

⊕ **E0749** Osteogenesis stimulator, electrical, surgically implanted Ⓟ

* **E0755** Electronic salivary reflex stimulator (intra-oral/non-invasive) Ⓑ

▶ New ↩ Revised ✔ Reinstated ~~deleted~~ Deleted ⊘ Not covered or valid by Medicare
⊕ Special coverage instructions * Carrier discretion Ⓟ Bill local carrier Ⓑ Bill DME MAC

✻ **E0760** Osteogenesis stimulator, low intensity ultrasound, non-invasive Ⓑ

Ultrasonic osteogenesis stimulator may not be used concurrently with other noninvasive stimulators

✪ **E0761** Non-thermal pulsed high frequency radiowaves, high peak power electromagnetic energy treatment device Ⓑ

✻ **E0762** Transcutaneous electrical joint stimulation device system, includes all accessories Ⓑ

✪ **E0764** Functional neuromuscular stimulator, transcutaneous stimulation of sequential muscle groups of ambulation with computer control, used for walking by spinal cord injured, entire system, after completion of training program Ⓑ

IOM: 100-03, 2, 160.12

✻ **E0765** FDA approved nerve stimulator, with replaceable batteries, for treatment of nausea and vomiting Ⓑ

✻ **E0766** Electrical stimulation device used for cancer treatment, includes all accessories, any type Ⓑ

✪ **E0769** Electrical stimulation or electromagnetic wound treatment device, not otherwise classified Ⓑ

IOM: 100-04, 32, 11.1

✪ **E0770** Functional electrical stimulator, transcutaneous stimulation of nerve and/or muscle groups, any type, complete system, not otherwise specified Ⓑ

Infusion Supplies

✻ **E0776** IV pole Ⓑ

✻ **E0779** Ambulatory infusion pump, mechanical, reusable, for infusion 8 hours or greater Ⓑ

Requires prior authorization and copy of invoice.

This is a capped rental infusion pump modifier. The correct monthly modifier (KH, KI, KJ) is used to indicate which month the rental is for (i.e., KH, month 1; KI, months 2 and 3; KJ, months 4 through 13).

✻ **E0780** Ambulatory infusion pump, mechanical, reusable, for infusion less than 8 hours Ⓑ

Requires prior authorization and copy of invoice

✪ **E0781** Ambulatory infusion pump, single or multiple channels, electric or battery operated with administrative equipment, worn by patient Ⓑ Ⓑ

Billable to both the Local Carrier and the DME MAC. This item may be billed to the DME MAC whenever the infusion is initiated in the physician's office but the patient does not return during the same business day.

IOM: 100-03, 1, 50.3

✪ **E0782** Infusion pump, implantable, non-programmable (includes all components, e.g., pump, cathether, connectors, etc.) Ⓑ

IOM: 100-03, 1, 50.3

✪ **E0783** Infusion pump system, implantable, programmable (includes all components, e.g., pump, catheter, connectors, etc.) Ⓑ

IOM: 100-03, 1, 50.3

✪ **E0784** External ambulatory infusion pump, insulin Ⓑ

IOM: 100-03, 4, 280.14

✪ **E0785** Implantable intraspinal (epidural/intrathecal) catheter used with implantable infusion pump, replacement Ⓑ

IOM: 100-03, 1, 50.3

✪ **E0786** Implantable programmable infusion pump, replacement (excludes implantable intraspinal catheter) Ⓑ

IOM: 100-03, 1, 50.3

✪ **E0791** Parenteral infusion pump, stationary, single or multi-channel Ⓑ

IOM: 100-02, 15, 120; 100-03, 3, 180.2; 100-04, 20, 100.2.2

Traction Equipment: All Types and Cervical

✪ **E0830** Ambulatory traction device, all types, each Ⓑ

IOM: 100-03, 4, 280.1

✪ **E0840** Traction frame, attached to headboard, cervical traction Ⓑ

IOM: 100-03, 4, 280.1

✻ **E0849** Traction equipment, cervical, free-standing stand/frame, pneumatic, applying traction force to other than mandible Ⓑ

▶ New ↻ Revised ✔ Reinstated ~~deleted~~ Deleted ⊘ Not covered or valid by Medicare
✪ Special coverage instructions ✻ Carrier discretion Ⓑ Bill local carrier Ⓑ Bill DME MAC

⊕ **E0850** Traction stand, free standing, cervical traction Ⓑ
IOM: 100-03, 4, 280.1

✻ **E0855** Cervical traction equipment not requiring additional stand or frame Ⓑ

✻ **E0856** Cervical traction device, with inflatable air bladder(s) Ⓑ

Traction: Overdoor

⊕ **E0860** Traction equipment, overdoor, cervical Ⓑ
IOM: 100-03, 4, 280.1

Traction: Extremity

⊕ **E0870** Traction frame, attached to footboard, extremity traction, (e.g., Buck's) Ⓑ
IOM: 100-03, 4, 280.1

⊕ **E0880** Traction stand, free standing, extremity traction, (e.g., Buck's) Ⓑ
IOM: 100-03, 4, 280.1

Traction: Pelvic

⊕ **E0890** Traction frame, attached to footboard, pelvic traction Ⓑ
IOM: 100-03, 4, 280.1

⊕ **E0900** Traction stand, free standing, pelvic traction, (e.g., Buck's) Ⓑ
IOM: 100-03, 4, 280.1

Trapeze Equipment, Fracture Frame, and Other Orthopedic Devices

⊕ **E0910** Trapeze bars, A/K/A patient helper, attached to bed, with grab bar Ⓑ
IOM: 100-03, 4, 280.1

⊕ **E0911** Trapeze bar, heavy duty, for patient weight capacity greater than 250 pounds, attached to bed, with grab bar Ⓑ
IOM: 100-03, 4, 280.1

⊕ **E0912** Trapeze bar, heavy duty, for patient weight capacity greater than 250 pounds, free standing, complete with grab bar Ⓑ
IOM: 100-03, 4, 280.1

⊕ **E0920** Fracture frame, attached to bed, includes weights Ⓑ
IOM: 100-03, 4, 280.1

⊕ **E0930** Fracture frame, free standing, includes weights Ⓑ
IOM: 100-03, 4, 280.1

⊕ **E0935** Continuous passive motion exercise device for use on knee only Ⓑ
To qualify for coverage, use of device must commence within two days following surgery.
IOM: 100-03, 4, 280.1

⃠ **E0936** Continuous passive motion exercise device for use other than knee Ⓑ

⊕ **E0940** Trapeze bar, free standing, complete with grab bar Ⓑ
IOM: 100-03, 4, 280.1

⊕ **E0941** Gravity assisted traction device, any type Ⓑ
IOM: 100-03, 4, 280.1

✻ **E0942** Cervical head harness/halter Ⓑ

✻ **E0944** Pelvic belt/harness/boot Ⓑ

✻ **E0945** Extremity belt/harness Ⓑ

⊕ **E0946** Fracture, frame, dual with cross bars, attached to bed, (e.g., Balken, 4 poster) Ⓑ
IOM: 100-03, 4, 280.1

⊕ **E0947** Fracture frame, attachments for complex pelvic traction Ⓑ
IOM: 100-03, 4, 280.1

⊕ **E0948** Fracture frame, attachments for complex cervical traction Ⓑ
IOM: 100-03, 4, 280.1

Wheelchair Accessories

⊕ **E0950** Wheelchair accessory, tray, each Ⓑ
IOM: 100-03, 4, 280.1

✻ **E0951** Heel loop/holder, any type, with or without ankle strap, each Ⓑ

⊕ **E0952** Toe loop/holder, any type, each Ⓑ
IOM: 100-03, 4, 280.1

⊋ ✻ **E0955** Wheelchair accessory, headrest, cushioned, any type, including fixed mounting hardware, each Ⓑ

✻ **E0956** Wheelchair accessory, lateral trunk or hip support, any type, including fixed mounting hardware, each Ⓑ

✻ **E0957** Wheelchair accessory, medial thigh support, any type, including fixed mounting hardware, each Ⓑ

✪ **E0958** Manual wheelchair accessory, one-arm drive attachment, each Ⓑ

IOM: 100-03, 4, 280.1

✻ **E0959** Manual wheelchair accessory, adapter for amputee, each Ⓑ

IOM: 100-03, 4, 280.1

✻ **E0960** Wheelchair accessory, shoulder harness/straps or chest strap, including any type mounting hardware Ⓑ

✻ **E0961** Manual wheelchair accessory, wheel lock brake extension (handle), each Ⓑ

IOM: 100-03, 4, 280.1

✻ **E0966** Manual wheelchair accessory, headrest extension, each Ⓑ

IOM: 100-03, 4, 280.1

↩ ✪ **E0967** Manual wheelchair accessory, hand rim with projections, any type, replacement only, each Ⓑ

IOM: 100-03, 4, 280.1

✪ **E0968** Commode seat, wheelchair Ⓑ

IOM: 100-03, 4, 280.1

✪ **E0969** Narrowing device, wheelchair Ⓑ

IOM: 100-03, 4, 280.1

⃠ **E0970** No.2 footplates, except for elevating leg rest Ⓑ

IOM: 100-03, 4, 280.1

Cross Reference K0037, K0042

✻ **E0971** Manual wheelchair accessory, anti-tipping device, each Ⓑ

IOM: 100-03, 4, 280.1

Cross Reference K0021

✪ **E0973** Wheelchair accessory, adjustable height, detachable armrest, complete assembly, each Ⓑ

IOM: 100-03, 4, 280.1

✪ **E0974** Manual wheelchair accessory, anti-rollback device, each Ⓑ

IOM: 100-03, 4, 280.1

✻ **E0978** Wheelchair accessory, positioning belt/safety belt/pelvic strap, each Ⓑ

✻ **E0980** Safety vest, wheelchair Ⓑ

✻ **E0981** Wheelchair accessory, seat upholstery, replacement only, each Ⓑ

✻ **E0982** Wheelchair accessory, back upholstery, replacement only, each Ⓑ

✻ **E0983** Manual wheelchair accessory, power add-on to convert manual wheelchair to motorized wheelchair, joystick control Ⓑ

✻ **E0984** Manual wheelchair accessory, power add-on to convert manual wheelchair to motorized wheelchair, tiller control Ⓑ

↩ ✻ **E0985** Wheelchair accessory, seat lift mechanism Ⓑ

✻ **E0986** Manual wheelchair accessory, push-rim activated power assist system Ⓑ

✻ **E0988** Manual wheelchair accessory, lever-activated, wheel drive, pair Ⓑ

✻ **E0990** Wheelchair accessory, elevating leg rest, complete assembly, each Ⓑ

IOM: 100-03, 4, 280.1

✻ **E0992** Manual wheelchair accessory, solid seat insert Ⓑ

✪ **E0994** Arm rest, each Ⓑ

IOM: 100-03, 4, 280.1

↩ ✻ **E0995** Wheelchair accessory, calf rest/pad, replacement only, each Ⓑ

IOM: 100-03, 4, 280.1

✻ **E1002** Wheelchair accessory, power seating system, tilt only Ⓑ

✻ **E1003** Wheelchair accessory, power seating system, recline only, without shear reduction Ⓑ

✻ **E1004** Wheelchair accessory, power seating system, recline only, with mechanical shear reduction Ⓑ

✻ **E1005** Wheelchair accessory, power seating system, recline only, with power shear reduction Ⓑ

✻ **E1006** Wheelchair accessory, power seating system, combination tilt and recline, without shear reduction Ⓑ

✻ **E1007** Wheelchair accessory, power seating system, combination tilt and recline, with mechanical shear reduction Ⓑ

✻ **E1008** Wheelchair accessory, power seating system, combination tilt and recline, with power shear reduction Ⓑ

✻ **E1009** Wheelchair accessory, addition to power seating system, mechanically linked leg elevation system, including pushrod and leg rest, each Ⓑ

✻ **E1010** Wheelchair accessory, addition to power seating system, power leg elevation system, including leg rest, pair Ⓑ

E1011 Modification to pediatric size wheelchair, width adjustment package (not to be dispensed with initial chair)

IOM: 100-03, 4, 280.1

E1012 Wheelchair accessory, addition to power seating system, center mount power elevating leg rest/platform, complete system, any type, each

E1014 Reclining back, addition to pediatric size wheelchair

IOM: 100-03, 4, 280.1

E1015 Shock absorber for manual wheelchair, each

IOM: 100-03, 4, 280.1

E1016 Shock absorber for power wheelchair, each

IOM: 100-03, 4, 280.1

E1017 Heavy duty shock absorber for heavy duty or extra heavy duty manual wheelchair, each

IOM: 100-03, 4, 280.1

E1018 Heavy duty shock absorber for heavy duty or extra heavy duty power wheelchair, each

IOM: 100-03, 4, 280.1

E1020 Residual limb support system for wheelchair, any type

IOM: 100-03, 3, 280.3

E1028 Wheelchair accessory, manual swing-away, retractable or removable mounting hardware for joystick, other control interface or positioning accessory

E1029 Wheelchair accessory, ventilator tray, fixed

E1030 Wheelchair accessory, ventilator tray, gimbaled

Rollabout Chair and Transfer System

E1031 Rollabout chair, any and all types with casters 5" or greater

IOM: 100-03, 4, 280.1

E1035 Multi-positional patient transfer system, with integrated seat, operated by care giver, patient weight capacity up to and including 300 lbs

IOM: 100-02, 15, 110

E1036 Multi-positional patient transfer system, extra-wide, with integrated seat, operated by caregiver, patient weight capacity greater than 300 lbs

E1037 Transport chair, pediatric size

IOM: 100-03, 4, 280.1

E1038 Transport chair, adult size, patient weight capacity up to and including 300 pounds

IOM: 100-03, 4, 280.1

E1039 Transport chair, adult size, heavy duty, patient weight capacity greater than 300 pounds

Wheelchair: Fully Reclining

E1050 Fully-reclining wheelchair, fixed full length arms, swing away detachable elevating leg rests

IOM: 100-03, 4, 280.1

E1060 Fully-reclining wheelchair, detachable arms, desk or full length, swing away detachable elevating legrests

IOM: 100-03, 4, 280.1

E1070 Fully-reclining wheelchair, detachable arms (desk or full length) swing away detachable footrests

IOM: 100-03, 4, 280.1

E1083 Hemi-wheelchair, fixed full length arms, swing away detachable elevating leg rest

IOM: 100-03, 4, 280.1

E1084 Hemi-wheelchair, detachable arms desk or full length arms, swing away detachable elevating leg rests

IOM: 100-03, 4, 280.1

E1085 Hemi-wheelchair, fixed full length arms, swing away detachable foot rests

IOM: 100-03, 4, 280.1

Cross Reference K0002

E1086 Hemi-wheelchair, detachable arms desk or full length, swing away detachable footrests

IOM: 100-03, 4, 280.1

Cross Reference K0002

E1087 High strength lightweight wheelchair, fixed full length arms, swing away detachable elevating leg rests

IOM: 100-03, 4, 280.1

▶ New ↩ Revised ✔ Reinstated ~~deleted~~ Deleted ⃠ Not covered or valid by Medicare
Special coverage instructions ✻ Carrier discretion Bill local carrier Bill DME MAC

⊕ **E1088** High strength lightweight wheelchair, detachable arms desk or full length, swing away detachable elevating leg rests Ⓑ

IOM: 100-03, 4, 280.1

⊘ **E1089** High strength lightweight wheelchair, fixed length arms, swing away detachable footrest Ⓑ

IOM: 100-03, 4, 280.1

Cross Reference K0004

⊘ **E1090** High strength lightweight wheelchair, detachable arms desk or full length, swing away detachable foot rests Ⓑ

IOM: 100-03, 4, 280.1

Cross Reference K0004

⊕ **E1092** Wide heavy duty wheelchair, detachable arms (desk or full length) swing away detachable elevating leg rests Ⓑ

IOM: 100-03, 4, 280.1

⊕ **E1093** Wide heavy duty wheelchair, detachable arms (desk or full length arms), swing away detachable foot rests Ⓑ

IOM: 100-03, 4, 280.1

Wheelchair: Semi-reclining

⊕ **E1100** Semi-reclining wheelchair, fixed full length arms, swing away detachable elevating leg rests Ⓑ

IOM: 100-03, 4, 280.1

⊕ **E1110** Semi-reclining wheelchair, detachable arms (desk or full length), elevating leg rest Ⓑ

IOM: 100-03, 4, 280.1

Wheelchair: Standard

⊘ **E1130** Standard wheelchair, fixed full length arms, fixed or swing away detachable footrests Ⓑ

IOM: 100-03, 4, 280.1

Cross Reference K0001

⊘ **E1140** Wheelchair, detachable arms, desk or full length, swing away detachable footrests Ⓑ

IOM: 100-03, 4, 280.1

Cross Reference K0001

⊕ **E1150** Wheelchair, detachable arms, desk or full length, swing away detachable elevating legrests Ⓑ

IOM: 100-03, 4, 280.1

⊕ **E1160** Wheelchair, fixed full length arms, swing away detachable elevating legrests Ⓑ

IOM: 100-03, 4, 280.1

* **E1161** Manual adult size wheelchair, includes tilt in space Ⓑ

Wheelchair: Amputee

⊕ **E1170** Amputee wheelchair, fixed full length arms, swing away detachable elevating legrests Ⓑ

IOM: 100-03, 4, 280.1

⊕ **E1171** Amputee wheelchair, fixed full length arms, without footrests or legrest Ⓑ

IOM: 100-03, 4, 280.1

⊕ **E1172** Amputee wheelchair, detachable arms (desk or full length) without footrests or legrest Ⓑ

IOM: 100-03, 4, 280.1

⊕ **E1180** Amputee wheelchair, detachable arms (desk or full length) swing away detachable footrests Ⓑ

IOM: 100-03, 4, 280.1

⊕ **E1190** Amputee wheelchair, detachable arms (desk or full length), swing away detachable elevating legrests Ⓑ

IOM: 100-03, 4, 280.1

⊕ **E1195** Heavy duty wheelchair, fixed full length arms, swing away detachable elevating legrests Ⓑ

IOM: 100-03, 4, 280.1

⊕ **E1200** Amputee wheelchair, fixed full length arms, swing away detachable footrest Ⓑ

IOM: 100-03, 4, 280.1

Wheelchair: Special Size

⊕ **E1220** Wheelchair; specially sized or constructed, (indicate brand name, model number, if any) and justification Ⓑ

IOM: 100-03, 4, 280.3

⊕ **E1221** Wheelchair with fixed arm, footrests Ⓑ

IOM: 100-03, 4, 280.3

⊕ **E1222** Wheelchair with fixed arm, elevating legrests Ⓑ

IOM: 100-03, 4, 280.3

▶ New ↻ Revised ✔ Reinstated ~~deleted~~ Deleted ⊘ Not covered or valid by Medicare
⊕ Special coverage instructions * Carrier discretion Ⓑ Bill local carrier Ⓑ Bill DME MAC

⊕ **E1223** Wheelchair with detachable arms, footrests Ⓑ

IOM: 100-03, 4, 280.3

⊕ **E1224** Wheelchair with detachable arms, elevating legrests Ⓑ

IOM: 100-03, 4, 280.3

⊕ **E1225** Wheelchair accessory, manual semi-reclining back, (recline greater than 15 degrees, but less than 80 degrees), each Ⓑ

IOM: 100-03, 4, 280.3

⊕ **E1226** Wheelchair accessory, manual fully reclining back, (recline greater than 80 degrees), each Ⓑ

IOM: 100-03, 4, 280.1

⊕ **E1227** Special height arms for wheelchair Ⓑ

IOM: 100-03, 4, 280.3

⊕ **E1228** Special back height for wheelchair Ⓑ

IOM: 100-03, 4, 280.3

* **E1229** Wheelchair, pediatric size, not otherwise specified Ⓑ

⊕ **E1230** Power operated vehicle (three or four wheel non-highway), specify brand name and model number Ⓑ

Patient is unable to operate manual wheelchair; patient capable of safely operating controls for scooter; patient can transfer safely in and out of scooter

IOM: 100-08, 5, 5.2.3

⊕ **E1231** Wheelchair, pediatric size, tilt-in-space, rigid, adjustable, with seating system Ⓑ

IOM: 100-03, 4, 280.1

⊕ **E1232** Wheelchair, pediatric size, tilt-in-space, folding, adjustable, with seating system Ⓑ

IOM: 100-03, 4, 280.1

⊕ **E1233** Wheelchair, pediatric size, tilt-in-space, rigid, adjustable, without seating system Ⓑ

IOM: 100-03, 4, 280.1

⊕ **E1234** Wheelchair, pediatric size, tilt-in-space, folding, adjustable, without seating system Ⓑ

IOM: 100-03, 4, 280.1

⊕ **E1235** Wheelchair, pediatric size, rigid, adjustable, with seating system Ⓑ

IOM: 100-03, 4, 280.1

⊕ **E1236** Wheelchair, pediatric size, folding, adjustable, with seating system Ⓑ

IOM: 100-03, 4, 280.1

⊕ **E1237** Wheelchair, pediatric size, rigid, adjustable, without seating system Ⓑ

IOM: 100-03, 4, 280.1

⊕ **E1238** Wheelchair, pediatric size, folding, adjustable, without seating system Ⓑ

IOM: 100-03, 4, 280.1

* **E1239** Power wheelchair, pediatric size, not otherwise specified Ⓑ

Wheelchair: Lightweight

⊕ **E1240** Lightweight wheelchair, detachable arms, (desk or full length) swing away detachable, elevating leg rests Ⓑ

IOM: 100-03, 4, 280.1

⊘ **E1250** Lightweight wheelchair, fixed full length arms, swing away detachable footrest Ⓑ

IOM: 100-03, 4, 280.1

Cross Reference K0003

⊘ **E1260** Lightweight wheelchair, detachable arms (desk or full length) swing away detachable footrest Ⓑ

IOM: 100-03, 4, 280.1

Cross Reference K0003

⊕ **E1270** Lightweight wheelchair, fixed full length arms, swing away detachable elevating legrests Ⓑ

IOM: 100-03, 4, 280.1

Wheelchair: Heavy Duty

⊕ **E1280** Heavy duty wheelchair, detachable arms (desk or full length), elevating legrests Ⓑ

IOM: 100-03, 4, 280.1

⊘ **E1285** Heavy duty wheelchair, fixed full length arms, swing away detachable footrest Ⓑ

IOM: 100-03, 4, 280.1

Cross Reference K0006

⊘ **E1290** Heavy duty wheelchair, detachable arms (desk or full length) swing away detachable footrest Ⓑ

IOM: 100-03, 4, 280.1

Cross Reference K0006

⊕ **E1295** Heavy duty wheelchair, fixed full length arms, elevating legrest Ⓑ

IOM: 100-03, 4, 280.1

⊕ **E1296** Special wheelchair seat height from floor Ⓑ
IOM: 100-03, 4, 280.3

⊕ **E1297** Special wheelchair seat depth, by upholstery Ⓑ
IOM: 100-03, 4, 280.3

⊕ **E1298** Special wheelchair seat depth and/or width, by construction Ⓑ
IOM: 100-03, 4, 280.3

Whirlpool Equipment

⊘ **E1300** Whirlpool, portable (overtub type) Ⓑ
IOM: 100-03, 4, 280.1

⊕ **E1310** Whirlpool, non-portable (built-in type) Ⓑ
IOM: 100-03, 4, 280.1

Additional Oxygen Related Equipment

* **E1352** Oxygen accessory, flow regulator capable of positive inspiratory pressure Ⓑ

⊕ **E1353** Regulator Ⓑ
IOM: 100-03, 4, 240.2

* **E1354** Oxygen accessory, wheeled cart for portable cylinder or portable concentrator, any type, replacement only, each Ⓑ

⊕ **E1355** Stand/rack Ⓑ
IOM: 100-03, 4, 240.2

* **E1356** Oxygen accessory, battery pack/cartridge for portable concentrator, any type, replacement only, each Ⓑ

* **E1357** Oxygen accessory, battery charger for portable concentrator, any type, replacement only, each Ⓑ

⊕ **E1358** Oxygen accessory, DC power adapter for portable concentrator, any type, replacement only, each Ⓑ

⊕ **E1372** Immersion external heater for nebulizer Ⓑ
IOM: 100-03, 4, 240.2

⊕ **E1390** Oxygen concentrator, single delivery port, capable of delivering 85 percent or greater oxygen concentration at the prescribed flow rate Ⓑ
IOM: 100-03, 4, 240.2

⊕ **E1391** Oxygen concentrator, dual delivery port, capable of delivering 85 percent or greater oxygen concentration at the prescribed flow rate, each Ⓑ
IOM: 100-03, 4, 240.2

⊕ **E1392** Portable oxygen concentrator, rental Ⓑ
IOM: 100-03, 4, 240.2

* **E1399** Durable medical equipment, miscellaneous Ⓑ Ⓑ

Bill Local Carrier if implanted DME. If other, bill DME MAC.

Example: Therapeutic exercise putty; rubber exercise tubing; anti-vibration gloves.

On DMEPOS fee schedule as a payable replacement for miscellaneous implanted or non-implanted items.

⊕ **E1405** Oxygen and water vapor enriching system with heated delivery Ⓑ
IOM: 100-03, 4, 240.2

⊕ **E1406** Oxygen and water vapor enriching system without heated delivery Ⓑ
IOM: 100-03, 4, 240.2

Artificial Kidney Machines and Accessories

⊕ **E1500** Centrifuge, for dialysis Ⓑ

⊕ **E1510** Kidney, dialysate delivery syst kidney machine, pump recirculating, air removal syst. flowrate meter, power off, heater and temperature control with alarm, I.V. poles, pressure gauge, concentrate container Ⓑ

⊕ **E1520** Heparin infusion pump for hemodialysis Ⓑ

⊕ **E1530** Air bubble detector for hemodialysis, each, replacement Ⓑ

⊕ **E1540** Pressure alarm for hemodialysis, each, replacement Ⓑ

⊕ **E1550** Bath conductivity meter for hemodialysis, each Ⓑ

⊕ **E1560** Blood leak detector for hemodialysis, each, replacement Ⓑ

⊕ **E1570** Adjustable chair, for ESRD patients Ⓑ

⊕ **E1575** Transducer protectors/fluid barriers for hemodialysis, any size, per 10 Ⓑ

⊕ **E1580** Unipuncture control system for hemodialysis Ⓑ

⊕ **E1590** Hemodialysis machine Ⓑ

⊕ **E1592** Automatic intermittent peritoneal dialysis system Ⓑ

E1594 Cycler dialysis machine for peritoneal dialysis

E1600 Delivery and/or installation charges for hemodialysis equipment

E1610 Reverse osmosis water purification system, for hemodialysis

IOM: 100-03, 4, 230.7

E1615 Deionizer water purification system, for hemodialysis

IOM: 100-03, 4, 230.7

E1620 Blood pump for hemodialysis replacement

E1625 Water softening system, for hemodialysis

IOM: 100-03, 4, 230.7

* **E1630** Reciprocating peritoneal dialysis system

E1632 Wearable artificial kidney, each

E1634 Peritoneal dialysis clamps, each

IOM: 100-04, 8, 60.4.2; 100-04, 8, 90.1; 100-04, 18, 80; 100-04, 18, 90

E1635 Compact (portable) travel hemodialyzer system

E1636 Sorbent cartridges, for hemodialysis, per 10

E1637 Hemostats, each

E1639 Scale, each

E1699 Dialysis equipment, not otherwise specified

Jaw Motion Rehabilitation System and Accessories

* **E1700** Jaw motion rehabilitation system

Must be prescribed by physician

* **E1701** Replacement cushions for jaw motion rehabilitation system, pkg. of 6

* **E1702** Replacement measuring scales for jaw motion rehabilitation system, pkg. of 200

Other Orthopedic Devices

* **E1800** Dynamic adjustable elbow extension/flexion device, includes soft interface material

* **E1801** Static progressive stretch elbow device, extension and/or flexion, with or without range of motion adjustment, includes all components and accessories

* **E1802** Dynamic adjustable forearm pronation/supination device, includes soft interface material

* **E1805** Dynamic adjustable wrist extension/flexion device, includes soft interface material

* **E1806** Static progressive stretch wrist device, flexion and/or extension, with or without range of motion adjustment, includes all components and accessories

* **E1810** Dynamic adjustable knee extension/flexion device, includes soft interface material

* **E1811** Static progressive stretch knee device, extension and/or flexion, with or without range of motion adjustment, includes all components and accessories

* **E1812** Dynamic knee, extension/flexion device with active resistance control

* **E1815** Dynamic adjustable ankle extension/flexion device, includes soft interface material

* **E1816** Static progressive stretch ankle device, flexion and/or extension, with or without range of motion adjustment, includes all components and accessories

* **E1818** Static progressive stretch forearm pronation/supination device with or without range of motion adjustment, includes all components and accessories

* **E1820** Replacement soft interface material, dynamic adjustable extension/flexion device

* **E1821** Replacement soft interface material/cuffs for bi-directional static progressive stretch device

* **E1825** Dynamic adjustable finger extension/flexion device, includes soft interface material

* **E1830** Dynamic adjustable toe extension/flexion device, includes soft interface material

* **E1831** Static progressive stretch toe device, extension and/or flexion, with or without range of motion adjustment, includes all components and accessories

* **E1840** Dynamic adjustable shoulder flexion/abduction/rotation device, includes soft interface material

✻ **E1841** Static progressive stretch shoulder device, with or without range of motion adjustment, includes all components and accessories Ⓑ

MISCELLANEOUS (E1902-E2120)

✻ **E1902** Communication board, non-electronic augmentative or alternative communication device Ⓑ

✻ **E2000** Gastric suction pump, home model, portable or stationary, electric Ⓑ

⚙ **E2100** Blood glucose monitor with integrated voice synthesizer Ⓑ

IOM: 100-03, 4, 230.16

⚙ **E2101** Blood glucose monitor with integrated lancing/blood sample Ⓑ

IOM: 100-03, 4, 230.16

✻ **E2120** Pulse generator system for tympanic treatment of inner ear endolymphatic fluid Ⓑ

Wheelchair Assessories

✻ **E2201** Manual wheelchair accessory, nonstandard seat frame, width greater than or equal to 20 inches and less than 24 inches Ⓑ

✻ **E2202** Manual wheelchair accessory, nonstandard seat frame width, 24-27 inches Ⓑ

✻ **E2203** Manual wheelchair accessory, nonstandard seat frame depth, 20 to less than 22 inches Ⓑ

✻ **E2204** Manual wheelchair accessory, nonstandard seat frame depth, 22 to 25 inches Ⓑ

✻ **E2205** Manual wheelchair accessory, handrim without projections (includes ergonomic or contoured), any type, replacement only, each Ⓑ

⮌ ✻ **E2206** Manual wheelchair accessory, wheel lock assembly, complete, replacement only, each Ⓑ

✻ **E2207** Wheelchair accessory, crutch and cane holder, each Ⓑ

✻ **E2208** Wheelchair accessory, cylinder tank carrier, each Ⓑ

✻ **E2209** Accessory arm trough, with or without hand support, each Ⓑ

✻ **E2210** Wheelchair accessory, bearings, any type, replacement only, each Ⓑ

✻ **E2211** Manual wheelchair accessory, pneumatic propulsion tire, any size, each Ⓑ

✻ **E2212** Manual wheelchair accessory, tube for pneumatic propulsion tire, any size, each Ⓑ

✻ **E2213** Manual wheelchair accessory, insert for pneumatic propulsion tire (removable), any type, any size, each Ⓑ

✻ **E2214** Manual wheelchair accessory, pneumatic caster tire, any size, each Ⓑ

✻ **E2215** Manual wheelchair accessory, tube for pneumatic caster tire, any size, each Ⓑ

✻ **E2216** Manual wheelchair accessory, foam filled propulsion tire, any size, each Ⓑ

✻ **E2217** Manual wheelchair accessory, foam filled caster tire, any size, each Ⓑ

✻ **E2218** Manual wheelchair accessory, foam propulsion tire, any size, each Ⓑ

✻ **E2219** Manual wheelchair accessory, foam caster tire, any size, each Ⓑ

⮌ ✻ **E2220** Manual wheelchair accessory, solid (rubber/plastic) propulsion tire, any size, replacement only, each Ⓑ

⮌ ✻ **E2221** Manual wheelchair accessory, solid (rubber/plastic) caster tire (removable), any size, replacement only, each Ⓑ

⮌ ✻ **E2222** Manual wheelchair accessory, solid (rubber/plastic) caster tire with integrated wheel, any size, replacement only, each Ⓑ

⮌ ✻ **E2224** Manual wheelchair accessory, propulsion wheel excludes tire, any size, replacement only, each Ⓑ

✻ **E2225** Manual wheelchair accessory, caster wheel excludes tire, any size, replacement only, each Ⓑ

✻ **E2226** Manual wheelchair accessory, caster fork, any size, replacement only, each Ⓑ

✻ **E2227** Manual wheelchair accessory, gear reduction drive wheel, each Ⓑ

⮌ ✻ **E2228** Manual wheelchair accessory, wheel braking system and lock, complete, each Ⓑ

✻ **E2230** Manual wheelchair accessory, manual standing system Ⓑ

✻ **E2231** Manual wheelchair accessory, solid seat support base (replaces sling seat), includes any type mounting hardware Ⓑ

✻ **E2291** Back, planar, for pediatric size wheelchair including fixed attaching hardware Ⓑ

✻ **E2292** Seat, planar, for pediatric size wheelchair including fixed attaching hardware Ⓑ

✻ **E2293** Back, contoured, for pediatric size wheelchair including fixed attaching hardware Ⓑ

✻ **E2294** Seat, contoured, for pediatric size wheelchair including fixed attaching hardware Ⓑ

✻ **E2295** Manual wheelchair accessory, for pediatric size wheelchair, dynamic seating frame, allows coordinated movement of multiple positioning features Ⓑ

✻ **E2300** Wheelchair accessory, power seat elevation system, any type Ⓑ

✻ **E2301** Wheelchair accessory, power standing system, any type Ⓑ

✻ **E2310** Power wheelchair accessory, electronic connection between wheelchair controller and one power seating system motor, including all related electronics, indicator feature, mechanical function selection switch, and fixed mounting hardware Ⓑ

✻ **E2311** Power wheelchair accessory, electronic connection between wheelchair controller and two or more power seating system motors, including all related electronics, indicator feature, mechanical function selection switch, and fixed mounting hardware Ⓑ

✻ **E2312** Power wheelchair accessory, hand or chin control interface, mini-proportional remote joystick, proportional, including fixed mounting hardware Ⓑ

✻ **E2313** Power wheelchair accessory, harness for upgrade to expandable controller, including all fasteners, connectors and mounting hardware, each Ⓑ

✻ **E2321** Power wheelchair accessory, hand control interface, remote joystick, nonproportional, including all related electronics, mechanical stop switch, and fixed mounting hardware Ⓑ

✻ **E2322** Power wheelchair accessory, hand control interface, multiple mechanical switches, nonproportional, including all related electronics, mechanical stop switch, and fixed mounting hardware Ⓑ

✻ **E2323** Power wheelchair accessory, specialty joystick handle for hand control interface, prefabricated Ⓑ

✻ **E2324** Power wheelchair accessory, chin cup for chin control interface Ⓑ

✻ **E2325** Power wheelchair accessory, sip and puff interface, nonproportional, including all related electronics, mechanical stop switch, and manual swingaway mounting hardware Ⓑ

✻ **E2326** Power wheelchair accessory, breath tube kit for sip and puff interface Ⓑ

✻ **E2327** Power wheelchair accessory, head control interface, mechanical, proportional, including all related electronics, mechanical direction change switch, and fixed mounting hardware Ⓑ

✻ **E2328** Power wheelchair accessory, head control or extremity control interface, electronic, proportional, including all related electronics and fixed mounting hardware Ⓑ

✻ **E2329** Power wheelchair accessory, head control interface, contact switch mechanism, nonproportional, including all related electronics, mechanical stop switch, mechanical direction change switch, head array, and fixed mounting hardware Ⓑ

✻ **E2330** Power wheelchair accessory, head control interface, proximity switch mechanism, nonproportional, including all related electronics, mechanical stop switch, mechanical direction change switch, head array, and fixed mounting hardware Ⓑ

✻ **E2331** Power wheelchair accessory, attendant control, proportional, including all related electronics and fixed mounting hardware Ⓑ

✻ **E2340** Power wheelchair accessory, nonstandard seat frame width, 20-23 inches

✻ **E2341** Power wheelchair accessory, nonstandard seat frame width, 24-27 inches Ⓑ

✻ **E2342** Power wheelchair accessory, nonstandard seat frame depth, 20 or 21 inches Ⓑ

✻ **E2343** Power wheelchair accessory, nonstandard seat frame depth, 22-25 inches Ⓑ

✻ **E2351** Power wheelchair accessory, electronic interface to operate speech generating device using power wheelchair control interface Ⓑ

✻ **E2358** Power wheelchair accessory, Group 34 non-sealed lead acid battery, each Ⓑ

✻ **E2359** Power wheelchair accessory, Group 34 sealed lead acid battery, each (e.g., gel cell, absorbed glassmat) Ⓑ

✻ **E2360** Power wheelchair accessory, 22 NF non-sealed lead acid battery, each Ⓑ

✻ **E2361** Power wheelchair accessory, 22NF sealed lead acid battery, each, (e.g., gel cell, absorbed glassmat) Ⓑ

✻ **E2362** Power wheelchair accessory, group 24 non-sealed lead acid battery, each Ⓑ

✻ **E2363** Power wheelchair accessory, group 24 sealed lead acid battery, each (e.g., gel cell, absorbed glassmat) Ⓑ

✻ **E2364** Power wheelchair accessory, U-1 non-sealed lead acid battery, each Ⓑ

✻ **E2365** Power wheelchair accessory, U-1 sealed lead acid battery, each (e.g., gel cell, absorbed glassmat) Ⓑ

✻ **E2366** Power wheelchair accessory, battery charger, single mode, for use with only one battery type, sealed or non-sealed, each Ⓑ

✻ **E2367** Power wheelchair accessory, battery charger, dual mode, for use with either battery type, sealed or non-sealed, each Ⓑ

↩ ✻ **E2368** Power wheelchair component, drive wheel motor, replacement only Ⓑ

↩ ✻ **E2369** Power wheelchair component, drive wheel gear box, replacement only Ⓑ

↩ ✻ **E2370** Power wheelchair component, integrated drive wheel motor and gear box combination, replacement only Ⓑ

✻ **E2371** Power wheelchair accessory, group 27 sealed lead acid battery, (e.g., gel cell, absorbed glass mat), each Ⓑ

✻ **E2372** Power wheelchair accessory, group 27 non-sealed lead acid battery, each Ⓑ

✻ **E2373** Power wheelchair accessory, hand or chin control interface, compact remote joystick, proportional, including fixed mounting hardware Ⓑ

⚙ **E2374** Power wheelchair accessory, hand or chin control interface, standard remote joystick (not including controller), proportional, including all related electronics and fixed mounting hardware, replacement only Ⓑ

↩ ⚙ **E2375** Power wheelchair accessory, non-expandable controller, including all related electronics and mounting hardware, replacement only Ⓑ

⚙ **E2376** Power wheelchair accessory, expandable controller, including all related electronics and mounting hardware, replacement only Ⓑ

⚙ **E2377** Power wheelchair accessory, expandable controller, including all related electronics and mounting hardware, upgrade provided at initial issue Ⓑ

✻ **E2378** Power wheelchair component, actuator, replacement only Ⓑ

⚙ **E2381** Power wheelchair accessory, pneumatic drive wheel tire, any size, replacement only, each Ⓑ

⚙ **E2382** Power wheelchair accessory, tube for pneumatic drive wheel tire, any size, replacement only, each Ⓑ

⚙ **E2383** Power wheelchair accessory, insert for pneumatic drive wheel tire (removable), any type, any size, replacement only, each Ⓑ

⚙ **E2384** Power wheelchair accessory, pneumatic caster tire, any size, replacement only, each Ⓑ

⚙ **E2385** Power wheelchair accessory, tube for pneumatic caster tire, any size, replacement only, each Ⓑ

⚙ **E2386** Power wheelchair accessory, foam filled drive wheel tire, any size, replacement only, each Ⓑ

⚙ **E2387** Power wheelchair accessory, foam filled caster tire, any size, replacement only, each Ⓑ

⚙ **E2388** Power wheelchair accessory, foam drive wheel tire, any size, replacement only, each Ⓑ

⚙ **E2389** Power wheelchair accessory, foam caster tire, any size, replacement only, each Ⓑ

⚙ **E2390** Power wheelchair accessory, solid (rubber/plastic) drive wheel tire, any size, replacement only, each Ⓑ

⚙ **E2391** Power wheelchair accessory, solid (rubber/plastic) caster tire (removable), any size, replacement only, each Ⓑ

⚙ **E2392** Power wheelchair accessory, solid (rubber/plastic) caster tire with integrated wheel, any size, replacement only, each Ⓑ

⚙ **E2394** Power wheelchair accessory, drive wheel excludes tire, any size, replacement only, each Ⓑ

⚙ **E2395** Power wheelchair accessory, caster wheel excludes tire, any size, replacement only, each Ⓑ

⊛ **E2396** Power wheelchair accessory, caster fork, any size, replacement only, each Ⓑ

✻ **E2397** Power wheelchair accessory, lithium-based battery, each Ⓑ

Negative Pressure

✻ **E2402** Negative pressure wound therapy electrical pump, stationary or portable Ⓑ

Document at least every 30 calendar days the quantitative wound characteristics, including wound surface area (length, width and depth).

Medicare coverage up to a maximum of 15 dressing kits (A6550) per wound per month unless documentation states that the wound size requires more than one dressing kit for each dressing change.

Speech Device

⊛ **E2500** Speech generating device, digitized speech, using pre-recorded messages, less than or equal to 8 minutes recording time Ⓑ

IOM: 100-03, 1, 50.1

⊛ **E2502** Speech generating device, digitized speech, using pre-recorded messages, greater than 8 minutes but less than or equal to 20 minutes recording time Ⓑ

IOM: 100-03, 1, 50.1

⊛ **E2504** Speech generating device, digitized speech, using pre-recorded messages, greater than 20 minutes but less than or equal to 40 minutes recording time Ⓑ

IOM: 100-03, 1, 50.1

⊛ **E2506** Speech generating device, digitized speech, using pre-recorded messages, greater than 40 minutes recording time Ⓑ

IOM: 100-03, 1, 50.1

⊛ **E2508** Speech generating device, synthesized speech, requiring message formulation by spelling and access by physical contact with the device Ⓑ

IOM: 100-03, 1, 50.1

⊛ **E2510** Speech generating device, synthesized speech, permitting multiple methods of message formulation and multiple methods of device access Ⓑ

IOM: 100-03, 1, 50.1

⊛ **E2511** Speech generating software program, for personal computer or personal digital assistant Ⓑ

IOM: 100-03, 1, 50.1

⊛ **E2512** Accessory for speech generating device, mounting system Ⓑ

IOM: 100-03, 1, 50.1

⊛ **E2599** Accessory for speech generating device, not otherwise classified Ⓑ

IOM: 100-03, 1, 50.1

Wheelchair: Cushion

✻ **E2601** General use wheelchair seat cushion, width less than 22 inches, any depth Ⓑ

✻ **E2602** General use wheelchair seat cushion, width 22 inches or greater, any depth Ⓑ

✻ **E2603** Skin protection wheelchair seat cushion, width less than 22 inches, any depth Ⓑ

✻ **E2604** Skin protection wheelchair seat cushion, width 22 inches or greater, any depth Ⓑ

✻ **E2605** Positioning wheelchair seat cushion, width less than 22 inches, any depth Ⓑ

✻ **E2606** Positioning wheelchair seat cushion, width 22 inches or greater, any depth Ⓑ

✻ **E2607** Skin protection and positioning wheelchair seat cushion, width less than 22 inches, any depth Ⓑ

✻ **E2608** Skin protection and positioning wheelchair seat cushion, width 22 inches or greater, any depth Ⓑ

✻ **E2609** Custom fabricated wheelchair seat cushion, any size Ⓑ

✻ **E2610** Wheelchair seat cushion, powered Ⓑ

✻ **E2611** General use wheelchair back cushion, width less than 22 inches, any height, including any type mounting hardware Ⓑ

✻ **E2612** General use wheelchair back cushion, width 22 inches or greater, any height, including any type mounting hardware Ⓑ

✻ **E2613** Positioning wheelchair back cushion, posterior, width less than 22 inches, any height, including any type mounting hardware Ⓑ

✻ **E2614** Positioning wheelchair back cushion, posterior, width 22 inches or greater, any height, including any type mounting hardware Ⓑ

* **E2615** Positioning wheelchair back cushion, posterior-lateral, width less than 22 inches, any height, including any type mounting hardware Ⓑ
* **E2616** Positioning wheelchair back cushion, posterior-lateral, width 22 inches or greater, any height, including any type mounting hardware Ⓑ
* **E2617** Custom fabricated wheelchair back cushion, any size, including any type mounting hardware Ⓑ
* **E2619** Replacement cover for wheelchair seat cushion or back cushion, each Ⓑ
* **E2620** Positioning wheelchair back cushion, planar back with lateral supports, width less than 22 inches, any height, including any type mounting hardware Ⓑ
* **E2621** Positioning wheelchair back cushion, planar back with lateral supports, width 22 inches or greater, any height, including any type mounting hardware Ⓑ

Wheelchair: Skin Protection

* **E2622** Skin protection wheelchair seat cushion, adjustable, width less than 22 inches, any depth Ⓑ
* **E2623** Skin protection wheelchair seat cushion, adjustable, width 22 inches or greater, any depth Ⓑ
* **E2624** Skin protection and positioning wheelchair seat cushion, adjustable, width less than 22 inches, any depth Ⓑ
* **E2625** Skin protection and positioning wheelchair seat cushion, adjustable, width 22 inches or greater, any depth Ⓑ

Wheelchair: Arm Support

* **E2626** Wheelchair accessory, shoulder elbow, mobile arm support attached to wheelchair, balanced, adjustable Ⓑ
* **E2627** Wheelchair accessory, shoulder elbow, mobile arm support attached to wheelchair, balanced, adjustable rancho type Ⓑ
* **E2628** Wheelchair accessory, shoulder elbow, mobile arm support attached to wheelchair, balanced, reclining Ⓑ
* **E2629** Wheelchair accessory, shoulder elbow, mobile arm support attached to wheelchair, balanced, friction arm support (friction dampening to proximal and distal joints) Ⓑ
* **E2630** Wheelchair accessory, shoulder elbow, mobile arm support, monosuspension arm and hand support, overhead elbow forearm hand sling support, yoke type suspension support Ⓑ
* **E2631** Wheelchair accessory, addition to mobile arm support, elevating proximal arm Ⓑ
* **E2632** Wheelchair accessory, addition to mobile arm support, offset or lateral rocker arm with elastic balance control Ⓑ
* **E2633** Wheelchair accessory, addition to mobile arm support, supinator Ⓑ

GAIT TRAINER (E8000-E8002)

⃠ **E8000** Gait trainer, pediatric size, posterior support, includes all accessories and components Ⓑ

⃠ **E8001** Gait trainer, pediatric size, upright support, includes all accessories and components Ⓑ

⃠ **E8002** Gait trainer, pediatric size, anterior support, includes all accessories and components Ⓑ

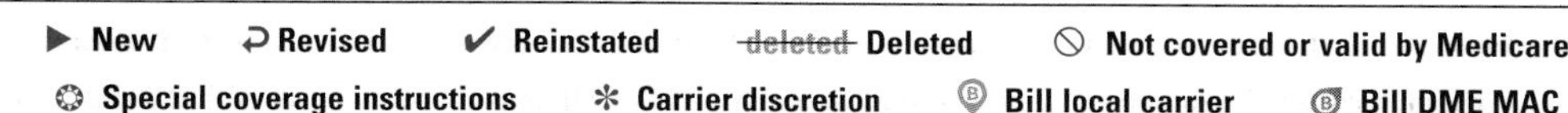

TEMPORARY PROCEDURES/PROFESSIONAL SERVICES (G0000-G9999)

NOTE: Series "G", "K", and "Q" in the Level II coding are reserved for CMS assignment. "G", "K", and "Q" codes are temporary national codes for items or services requiring uniform national coding between one year's update and the next. Sometimes "temporary" codes remain for more than one update. If "G", "K", and "Q" codes are not converted to permanent codes in Level I or Level II series in the following update, they will remain active until converted in following years or until CMS notifies contractors to delete them. All active "G", "K", and "Q" codes at the time of update will be included on the update file for contractors. In addition, deleted codes are retained on the file for informational purposes, with a deleted indicator, for four years.

Administration, Vaccine

* **G0008** Administration of influenza virus vaccine Ⓑ

Coinsurance and deductible do not apply. If provided, report significant, separately identifiable E/M for medically necessary services.

* **G0009** Administration of pneumococcal vaccine Ⓑ

Reported once in a lifetime based on risk; Medicare covers cost of vaccine and administration.

Copayment, coinsurance, and deductible waived. (https://www.cms.gov/MLNProducts/downloads/MPS_QuickReferenceChart_1.pdf)

* **G0010** Administration of hepatitis B vaccine Ⓑ

Report for other than OPPs. Coinsurance and deductible apply; Medicare covers both cost of vaccine and administration.

Copayment/coinsurance and deductible are waived. (https://www.cms.gov/MLNProducts/downloads/MPS_QuickReferenceChart_1.pdf)

Semen Analysis

* **G0027** Semen analysis; presence and/or motility of sperm excluding Huhner Ⓑ

Laboratory Certification: Hematology

Screening, Cervical

G0101 Cervical or vaginal cancer screening; pelvic and clinical breast examination Ⓑ

Covered once every two years and annually if high risk for cervical/vaginal cancer, or if childbearing age patient has had an abnormal Pap smear in preceding three years.

Screening, Prostate

G0102 Prostate cancer screening; digital rectal examination Ⓑ

Covered annually by Medicare. Not separately payable with an E/M code (99201-99499).

IOM: 100-02, 6, 10; 100-04, 4, 240; 100-04, 18, 50.1

G0103 Prostate cancer screening; prostate specific antigen test (PSA) Ⓑ

Covered annually by Medicare

IOM: 100-02, 6, 10; 100-04, 4, 240; 100-04, 18, 50

Laboratory Certification: Routine chemistry

Screening, Colorectal

G0104 Colorectal cancer screening; flexible sigmoidoscopy Ⓑ

Covered once every 48 months for beneficiaries age 50+

Co-insurance waived under Section 4104.

G0105 Colorectal cancer screening; colonoscopy on individual at high risk Ⓑ

Screening colonoscopy covered once every 24 months for high risk for developing colorectal cancer. May use modifier 53 if appropriate (physician fee schedule).

Co-insurance waived under Section 4104.

G0106 Colorectal cancer screening; alternative to G0104, screening sigmoidoscopy, barium enema Ⓑ

Barium enema (not high risk) (alternative to G0104). Covered once every 4 years for beneficiaries age 50+. Use modifier 26 for professional component only.

▶ New ↻ Revised ✔ Reinstated ~~deleted~~ Deleted ⊘ Not covered or valid by Medicare
Special coverage instructions * Carrier discretion Ⓑ Bill local carrier Ⓓ Bill DME MAC

Training Services, Diabetes

✻ **G0108** Diabetes outpatient self-management training services, individual, per 30 minutes Ⓑ

Report for beneficiaries diagnosed with diabetes.

Effective January 2011, DSMT will be included in the list of reimbursable Medicare telehealth services.

✻ **G0109** Diabetes outpatient self-management training services, group session (2 or more) per 30 minutes Ⓑ

Report for beneficiaries diagnosed with diabetes.

Effective January 2011, DSMT will be included in the list of reimbursable Medicare telehealth services.

Screening, Glaucoma

✻ **G0117** Glaucoma screening for high risk patients furnished by an optometrist or ophthalmologist Ⓑ

Covered once per year (full 11 months between screenings). Bundled with all other ophthalmic services provided on same day. Diagnosis code Z13.5

✻ **G0118** Glaucoma screening for high risk patient furnished under the direct supervision of an optometrist or ophthalmologist Ⓑ

Covered once per year (full 11 months between screenings). Diagnosis code Z13.5

Screening, Colorectal, Other

*USE For Digital rectal exam. ie. Prostate exam

✪ **G0120** Colorectal cancer screening; alternative to G0105, screening colonoscopy, barium enema. Ⓑ

Barium enema for patients with a high risk of developing colorectal. Covered once every 2 years. Used as an alternative to G0105. Use modifier 26 for professional component only.

✪ **G0121** Colorectal cancer screening; colonoscopy on individual not meeting criteria for high risk Ⓑ

Screening colonoscopy for patients that are not high risk. Covered once every 10 years, but not within 48 months of a G0104. For non-Medicare patients report 45378.

Co-insurance waived under Section 4104.

⃠ **G0122** Colorectal cancer screening; barium enema Ⓑ

Medicare: this service is denied as noncovered, because it fails to meet the requirements of the benefit. The beneficiary is liable for payment.

Screening, Cytopathology

✪ **G0123** Screening cytopathology, cervical or vaginal (any reporting system), collected in preservative fluid, automated thin layer preparation, screening by cytotechnologist under physician supervision Ⓑ

Use G0123 or G0143 or G0144 or G0145 or G0147 or G0148 or P3000 for Pap smears NOT requiring physician interpretation (technical component).

IOM: 100-03, 3, 190.2; 100-04, 18, 30

Laboratory Certification: Cytology

✪ **G0124** Screening cytopathology, cervical or vaginal (any reporting system), collected in preservative fluid, automated thin layer preparation, requiring interpretation by physician Ⓑ

Report professional component for Pap smears requiring physician interpretation

IOM: 100-03, 3, 190.2; 100-04, 18, 30

Laboratory Certification: Cytology

Trimming, Nail

✪ **G0127** Trimming of dystrophic nails, any number Ⓑ

Must be used with a modifier (Q7, Q8, or Q9) to show that the foot care service is needed because the beneficiary has a systemic disease. Limit 1 unit of service

IOM: 100-02, 15, 290

▶ New ⤾ Revised ✔ Reinstated ~~deleted~~ Deleted ⃠ Not covered or valid by Medicare
✪ Special coverage instructions ✻ Carrier discretion Ⓑ Bill local carrier Ⓓ Bill DME MAC

Service, Nursing and OT

⚙ **G0128** Direct (face-to-face with patient) skilled nursing services of a registered nurse provided in a comprehensive outpatient rehabilitation facility, each 10 minutes beyond the first 5 minutes Ⓑ

A separate nursing service that is clearly identifiable in the Plan of Treatment and not part of other services. Documentation must support this service. Examples include: Insertion of a urinary catheter, intramuscular injections, bowel disimpaction, nursing assessment, and education. Restricted coverage by Medicare.

Medicare Statute 1833(a)

* **G0129** Occupational therapy services requiring the skills of a qualified occupational therapist, furnished as a component of a partial hospitalization treatment program, per session (45 minutes or more) Ⓑ

Study, SEXA

⚙ **G0130** Single energy x-ray absorptiometry (SEXA) bone density study, one or more sites; appendicular skeleton (peripheral) (e.g., radius, wrist, heel) Ⓑ

Covered every 24 months (more frequently if medically necessary). Use modifier 26 for professional component only.

Preventive service; no deductible

IOM: 100-03, 2, 150.3; 100-04, 13, 140.1

Screening, Cytopathology, Other

* **G0141** Screening cytopathology smears, cervical or vaginal, performed by automated system, with manual rescreening, requiring interpretation by physician Ⓑ

Co-insurance, copay, and deductible waived

Report professional component for Pap smears requiring physician interpretation.

Laboratory Certification: Cytology

* **G0143** Screening cytopathology, cervical or vaginal (any reporting system), collected in preservative fluid, automated thin layer preparation, with manual screening and rescreening by cytotechnologist under physician supervision Ⓑ

Co-insurance, copay, and deductible waived

Laboratory Certification: Cytology

* **G0144** Screening cytopathology, cervical or vaginal (any reporting system), collected in preservative fluid, automated thin layer preparation, with screening by automated system, under physician supervision Ⓑ

Co-insurance, copay, and deductible waived

Laboratory Certification: Cytology

* **G0145** Screening cytopathology, cervical or vaginal (any reporting system), collected in preservative fluid, automated thin layer preparation, with screening by automated system and manual rescreening under physician supervision Ⓑ

Co-insurance, copay, and deductible waived

Laboratory Certification: Cytology

* **G0147** Screening cytopathology smears, cervical or vaginal; performed by automated system under physician supervision Ⓑ

Co-insurance, copay, and deductible waived

Laboratory Certification: Cytology

* **G0148** Screening cytopathology smears, cervical or vaginal; performed by automated system with manual rescreening Ⓑ

Co-insurance, copay, and deductible waived

Laboratory Certification: Cytology

Services, Allied Health

* **G0151** Services performed by a qualified physical therapist in the home health or hospice setting, each 15 minutes Ⓑ

* **G0152** Services performed by a qualified occupational therapist in the home health or hospice setting, each 15 minutes Ⓑ

✻ **G0153** Services performed by a qualified speech-language pathologist in the home health or hospice setting, each 15 minutes Ⓑ

~~G0154 Direct skilled nursing services of a licensed nurse (LPN or RN) in the home health or hospice setting, each 15 minutes~~ ✖

✻ **G0155** Services of clinical social worker in home health or hospice settings, each 15 minutes Ⓑ

✻ **G0156** Services of home health/health aide in home health or hospice settings, each 15 minutes Ⓑ

✻ **G0157** Services performed by a qualified physical therapist assistant in the home health or hospice setting, each 15 minutes Ⓑ

✻ **G0158** Services performed by a qualified occupational therapist assistant in the home health or hospice setting, each 15 minutes Ⓑ

✻ **G0159** Services performed by a qualified physical therapist, in the home health setting, in the establishment or delivery of a safe and effective physical therapy maintenance program, each 15 minutes Ⓑ

✻ **G0160** Services performed by a qualified occupational therapist, in the home health setting, in the establishment or delivery of a safe and effective occupational therapy maintenance program, each 15 minutes Ⓑ

✻ **G0161** Services performed by a qualified speech-language pathologist, in the home health setting, in the establishment or delivery of a safe and effective speech-language pathology maintenance program, each 15 minutes Ⓑ

✻ **G0162** Skilled services by a registered nurse (RN) for management and evaluation of the plan of care; each 15 minutes (the patient's underlying condition or complication requires an RN to ensure that essential non-skilled care achieves its purpose in the home health or hospice setting) Ⓑ

Transmittal No. 824 (CR7182)

~~G0163 Skilled services of a licensed nurse (LPN or RN) for the observation and assessment of the patient's condition, each 15 minutes (the of change in the patient's condition requires skilled nursing personnel to identify and evaluate the patient's need for possible modification of treatment in the home health or hospice setting)~~ ✖

~~G0164 Skilled services of a licensed nurse (LPN or RN), in the training and/or education of a patient or family member, in the home health or hospice setting, each 15 minutes~~ ✖

⚙ **G0166** External counterpulsation, per treatment session Ⓑ

IOM: 100-03, 1, 20.20

Wound Closure

✻ **G0168** Wound closure utilizing tissue adhesive(s) only Ⓑ

Report for wound closure with only tissue adhesive. If a practitioner utilizes tissue adhesive in addition to staples or sutures to close a wound, HCPCS code G0168 is not separately reportable, but is included in the tissue repair.

The only closure material used for a simple repair, coverage based on payer

Team Conference

✻ **G0175** Scheduled interdisciplinary team conference (minimum of three exclusive of patient care nursing staff) with patient present Ⓑ

Therapy, Activity

OPPS not separately payable

⚙ **G0176** Activity therapy, such as music, dance, art or play therapies not for recreation, related to the care and treatment of patient's disabling mental health problems, per session (45 minutes or more) Ⓑ

Paid in partial hospitalization

⚙ **G0177** Training and educational services related to the care and treatment of patient's disabling mental health problems per session (45 minutes or more) Ⓑ

Paid in partial hospitalization

▶ New ↩ Revised ✔ Reinstated ~~deleted~~ Deleted ⊘ Not covered or valid by Medicare
⚙ Special coverage instructions ✻ Carrier discretion Ⓑ Bill local carrier Ⓑ Bill DME MAC

Physician Services

✻ **G0179** Physician re-certification for Medicare-covered home health services under a home health plan of care (patient not present), including contacts with home health agency and review of reports of patient status required by physicians to affirm the initial implementation of the plan of care that meets patient's needs, per re-certification period

The recertification code is used after a patient has received services for at least 60 days (or one certification period) when the physician signs the certification after the initial certification period.

✻ **G0180** Physician certification for Medicare-covered home health services under a home health plan of care (patient not present), including contacts with home health agency and review of reports of patient status required by physicians to affirm the initial implementation of the plan of care that meets patient's needs, per certification period

This code can be billed only when the patient has not received Medicare covered home health services for at least 60 days.

✻ **G0181** Physician supervision of a patient receiving Medicare-covered services provided by a participating home health agency (patient not present) requiring complex and multidisciplinary care modalities involving regular physician development and/or revision of care plans, review of subsequent reports of patient status, review of laboratory and other studies, communication (including telephone calls) with other health care professionals involved in the patient's care, integration of new information into the medical treatment plan and/or adjustment of medical therapy, within a calendar month, 30 minutes or more

✻ **G0182** Physician supervision of a patient under a Medicare-approved hospice (patient not present) requiring complex and multidisciplinary care modalities involving regular physician development and/or revision of care plans, review of subsequent reports of patient status, review of laboratory and other studies, communication (including telephone calls) with other health care professionals involved in the patient's care, integration of new information into the medical treatment plan and/or adjustment of medical therapy, within a calendar month, 30 minutes or more

Destruction

✻ **G0186** Destruction of localized lesion of choroid (for example, choroidal neovascularization); photocoagulation, feeder vessel technique (one or more sessions)

Mammography

↻ ✻ **G0202** Screening mammography, bilateral (2-view study of each breast), including computer-aided detection (CAD) when performed

Screening mammogram reported based on technique, such as 76082, 76083, 76092, or G0202. Requires coinsurance, but no deductible. Diagnosis code, Z12.31. Use modifier 26 for professional component only.

↻ ✻ **G0204** Diagnostic mammography, including computer-aided detection (CAD) when performed; bilateral

Use modifier 26 for professional component only.

↻ ✻ **G0206** Diagnostic mammography, including computer-aided detection (CAD) when performed; unilateral

Use modifier 26 for professional component only.

Imaging, PET

⃠ **G0219** PET imaging whole body; melanoma for non-covered indications

Example: Assessing regional lymph nodes in melanoma.

IOM: 100-03, 4, 220.6

▶ New ↻ Revised ✔ Reinstated ~~deleted~~ Deleted ⃠ Not covered or valid by Medicare
Special coverage instructions ✻ Carrier discretion Bill local carrier Bill DME MAC

⃠ **G0235** PET imaging, any site, not otherwise specified Ⓑ

Example: Prostate cancer diagnosis and initial staging.

IOM: 100-03, 4, 220.6

Therapeutic Procedures

* **G0237** Therapeutic procedures to increase strength or endurance of respiratory muscles, face to face, one on one, each 15 minutes (includes monitoring) Ⓑ
* **G0238** Therapeutic procedures to improve respiratory function, other than described by G0237, one on one, face to face, per 15 minutes (includes monitoring) Ⓑ
* **G0239** Therapeutic procedures to improve respiratory function or increase strength or endurance of respiratory muscles, two or more individuals (includes monitoring) Ⓑ

Physician Service, Diabetic

G0245 Initial physician evaluation and management of a diabetic patient with diabetic sensory neuropathy resulting in a loss of protective sensation (LOPS) which must include (1) the diagnosis of LOPS, (2) a patient history, (3) a physical examination that consist of at least the following elements: (A) visual inspection of the forefoot, hindfoot and toe web spaces, (B) evaluation of a protective sensation, (C) evaluation of foot structure and biomechanics, (D) evaluation of vascular status and skin integrity, and (E) evaluation and recommendation of footwear, and (4) patient education Ⓑ

IOM: 100-03, 1, 70.2.1

G0246 Follow-up physician evaluation and management of a diabetic patient with diabetic sensory neuropathy resulting in a loss of protective sensation (LOPS) to include at least the following: (1) a patient history, (2) a physical examination that includes: (A) visual inspection of the forefoot, hindfoot and toe web spaces, (B) evaluation of protective sensation, (C) evaluation of foot structure and biomechanics, (D) evaluation of vascular status and skin integrity, and (E) evaluation and recommendation of footwear, and (3) patient education Ⓑ

IOM: 100-03, 1, 70.2.1; 100-02, 15, 290

Foot Care

G0247 Routine foot care by a physician of a diabetic patient with diabetic sensory neuropathy resulting in a loss of protective sensation (LOPS) to include, the local care of superficial wounds (i.e. superficial to muscle and fascia) and at least the following if present: (1) local care of superficial wounds, (2) debridement of corns and calluses, and (3) trimming and debridement of nails Ⓑ

IOM: 100-03, 1, 70.2.1

Demonstration, INR

G0248 Demonstration, prior to initiation, of home INR monitoring for patient with either mechanical heart valve(s), chronic atrial fibrillation, or venous thromboembolism who meets Medicare coverage criteria, under the direction of a physician; includes: face-to-face demonstration of use and care of the INR monitor, obtaining at least one blood sample, provision of instructions for reporting home INR test results, and documentation of patient's ability to perform testing and report results Ⓑ

G0249 Provision of test materials and equipment for home INR monitoring of patient with either mechanical heart valve(s), chronic atrial fibrillation, or venous thromboembolism who meets Medicare coverage criteria; includes provision of materials for use in the home and reporting of test results to physician; testing not occurring more frequently than once a week; testing materials, billing units of service include 4 tests Ⓑ

G0250 Physician review, interpretation, and patient management of home INR testing for patient with either mechanical heart valve(s), chronic atrial fibrillation, or venous thromboembolism who meets Medicare coverage criteria; testing not occurring more frequently than once a week; billing units of service include 4 tests Ⓑ

Imaging, PET

⊘ **G0252** PET imaging, full and partial-ring PET scanners only, for initial diagnosis of breast cancer and/or surgical planning for breast cancer (e.g., initial staging of axillary lymph nodes) Ⓑ

SNCT

⊘ **G0255** Current perception threshold/sensory nerve conduction test (SNCT), per limb, any nerve Ⓑ

IOM: 100-03, 2, 160.23

Dialysis, Emergency

✪ **G0257** Unscheduled or emergency dialysis treatment for an ESRD patient in a hospital outpatient department that is not certified as an ESRD facility Ⓑ

Injection, Arthrography

✪ **G0259** Injection procedure for sacroiliac joint; arthrography Ⓑ

Replaces 27096 for reporting injections for Medicare beneficiaries

Used by Part A only (facility), not priced by Part B Medicare.

✪ **G0260** Injection procedure for sacroiliac joint; provision of anesthetic, steroid and/or other therapeutic agent, with or without arthrography Ⓑ

ASCs report when a therapeutic sacroiliac joint injection is administered in ASC

Removal, Cerumen

* **G0268** Removal of impacted cerumen (one or both ears) by physician on same date of service as audiologic function testing Ⓑ

Report only when a physician, not an audiologist, performs the procedure.

Use with DX H61.2- when performed by physician.

Placement, Occlusive Device

✪ **G0269** Placement of occlusive device into either a venous or arterial access site, post surgical or interventional procedure (e.g., angioseal plug, vascular plug) Ⓑ

Report for replacement of vasoseal. Hospitals may report the closure device as a supply with C1760. Bundled status on Physician Fee Schedule.

Therapy, Nutrition

* **G0270** Medical nutrition therapy; reassessment and subsequent intervention(s) following second referral in same year for change in diagnosis, medical condition or treatment regimen (including additional hours needed for renal disease), individual, face to face with the patient, each 15 minutes Ⓑ

Requires physician referral for beneficiaries with diabetes or renal disease. Services must be provided by dietitian/nutritionist. Co-insurance and deductible waived.

* **G0271** Medical nutrition therapy, reassessment and subsequent intervention(s) following second referral in same year for change in diagnosis, medical condition, or treatment regimen (including additional hours needed for renal disease), group (2 or more individuals), each 30 minutes Ⓑ

Requires physician referral for beneficiaries with diabetes or renal disease. Services must be provided by dietitian/nutritionist. Co-insurance and deductible waived.

Blinded Procedure

✪ **G0276** Blinded procedure for lumbar stenosis, percutaneous image-guided lumbar decompression (PILD) or placebo-control, performed in an approved coverage with evidence development (CED) clinical trial Ⓑ

Therapy, Hyperbaric Oxygen

✪ **G0277** Hyperbaric oxygen under pressure, full body chamber, per 30 minute interval Ⓑ

IOM: 100-03, 1, 20.29

▶ New ↻ Revised ✔ Reinstated ~~deleted~~ Deleted ⊘ Not covered or valid by Medicare
✪ Special coverage instructions * Carrier discretion Ⓑ Bill local carrier Ⓓ Bill DME MAC

Angiography

✻ **G0278** Iliac and/or femoral artery angiography, non-selective, bilateral or ipsilateral to catheter insertion, performed at the same time as cardiac catheterization and/or coronary angiography, includes positioning or placement of the catheter in the distal aorta or ipsilateral femoral or iliac artery, injection of dye, production of permanent images, and radiologic supervision and interpretation (list separately in addition to primary procedure) Ⓑ

Medicare specific code not reported for iliac injection used as a guiding shot for a closure device

Diagnostic

✻ **G0279** Diagnostic digital breast tomosynthesis, unilateral or bilateral (list separately in addition to G0204 or G0206) Ⓑ

Stimulation, Electrical

✻ **G0281** Electrical stimulation, (unattended), to one or more areas, for chronic stage III and stage IV pressure ulcers, arterial ulcers, diabetic ulcers, and venous stasis ulcers not demonstrating measurable signs of healing after 30 days of conventional care, as part of a therapy plan of care Ⓑ

Reported by encounter/areas and not by site. Therapists report G0281 and G0283 rather than 97014.

⃠ **G0282** Electrical stimulation, (unattended), to one or more areas, for wound care other than described in G0281 Ⓑ

IOM: 100-03, 4, 270.1

✻ **G0283** Electrical stimulation (unattended), to one or more areas for indication(s) other than wound care, as part of a therapy plan of care Ⓑ

Reported by encounter/areas and not by site. Therapists report G0281 and G0283 rather than 97014.

Angiography, Arthroscopy

✻ **G0288** Reconstruction, computed tomographic angiography of aorta for surgical planning for vascular surgery Ⓑ

✻ **G0289** Arthroscopy, knee, surgical, for removal of loose body, foreign body, debridement/shaving of articular cartilage (chondroplasty) at the time of other surgical knee arthroscopy in a different compartment of the same knee Ⓑ

Add-on code reported with knee arthroscopy code for major procedure performed-reported once per extra compartment

"The code may be reported twice (or with a unit of two) if the physician performs these procedures in two compartments, in addition to the compartment where the main procedure was performed." (http://www.ama-assn.org/resources/doc/cpt/orthopaedics.pdf)

Procedure, Non-Covered

✪ **G0293** Noncovered surgical procedure(s) using conscious sedation, regional, general or spinal anesthesia in a Medicare qualifying clinical trial, per day Ⓑ

✪ **G0294** Noncovered procedure(s) using either no anesthesia or local anesthesia only, in a Medicare qualifying clinical trial, per day Ⓑ

Therapy, Electromagnetic

⃠ **G0295** Electromagnetic therapy, to one or more areas, for wound care other than described in G0329 or for other uses Ⓑ

IOM: 100-03, 4, 270.1

Other

✻ **G0296** Counseling visit to discuss need for lung cancer screening (LDCT) using low dose CT scan (service is for eligibility determination and shared decision making) Ⓑ

✻ **G0297** Low dose CT scan (LDCT) for lung cancer screening Ⓑ

✻ **G0299** Direct skilled nursing services of a registered nurse (RN) in the home health or hospice setting, each 15 minutes Ⓑ

✻ **G0300** Direct skilled nursing services of a licensed practical nurse (LPN) in the home health or hospice setting, each 15 minutes Ⓑ

▶ New ↩ Revised ✔ Reinstated ~~deleted~~ Deleted ⃠ Not covered or valid by Medicare
✪ Special coverage instructions ✻ Carrier discretion Ⓑ Bill local carrier Ⓓ Bill DME MAC

Services, Pulmonary Surgery

✻ **G0302** Pre-operative pulmonary surgery services for preparation for LVRS, complete course of services, to include a minimum of 16 days of services Ⓑ

✻ **G0303** Pre-operative pulmonary surgery services for preparation for LVRS, 10 to 15 days of services Ⓑ

✻ **G0304** Pre-operative pulmonary surgery services for preparation for LVRS, 1 to 9 days of services Ⓑ

✻ **G0305** Post-discharge pulmonary surgery services after LVRS, minimum of 6 days of services Ⓑ

Laboratory

✻ **G0306** Complete CBC, automated (HgB, HCT, RBC, WBC, without platelet count) and automated WBC differential count Ⓑ

Laboratory Certification: Hematology

✻ **G0307** Complete CBC, automated (HgB, HCT, RBC, WBC; without platelet count) Ⓑ

Laboratory Certification: Hematology

✪ **G0328** Colorectal cancer screening; fecal occult blood test, immunoassay, 1-3 simultaneous Ⓑ

Co-insurance and deductible waived

Reported for Medicare patients 50+; one FOBT per year, with either G0107 (guaiac-based) or G0328 (immunoassay-based)

Laboratory Certification: Routine chemistry, Hematology

Therapy, Electromagnetic

✻ **G0329** Electromagnetic therapy, to one or more areas for chronic stage III and stage IV pressure ulcers, arterial ulcers, and diabetic ulcers and venous stasis ulcers not demonstrating measurable signs of healing after 30 days of conventional care as part of a therapy plan of care Ⓑ

Fee, Pharmacy

✪ **G0333** Pharmacy dispensing fee for inhalation drug(s); initial 30-day supply as a beneficiary Ⓑ (DME MAC)

Medicare will reimburse an initial dispensing fee to a pharmacy for initial 30-day period of inhalation drugs furnished through DME.

Hospice

✻ **G0337** Hospice evaluation and counseling services, pre-election Ⓑ

Radiosurgery, Robotic

✻ **G0339** Image-guided robotic linear accelerator-based stereotactic radiosurgery, complete course of therapy in one session or first session of fractionated treatment Ⓑ

✻ **G0340** Image-guided robotic linear accelerator-based stereotactic radiosurgery, delivery including collimator changes and custom plugging, fractionated treatment, all lesions, per session, second through fifth sessions, maximum five sessions per course of treatment Ⓑ

Islet Cell

✪ **G0341** Percutaneous islet cell transplant, includes portal vein catheterization and infusion Ⓑ

IOM: 100-03, 4, 260.3; 100-04, 32, 70

✪ **G0342** Laparoscopy for islet cell transplant, includes portal vein catheterization and infusion Ⓑ

IOM: 100-03, 4, 260.3

✪ **G0343** Laparotomy for islet cell transplant, includes portal vein catheterization and infusion Ⓑ

IOM: 100-03, 4, 260.3

▶ New ↻ Revised ✔ Reinstated ~~deleted~~ Deleted ⊘ Not covered or valid by Medicare
✪ Special coverage instructions ✻ Carrier discretion Ⓑ Bill local carrier Ⓑ Bill DME MAC

Aspiration, Bone Marrow

✻ **G0364** Bone marrow aspiration performed with bone marrow biopsy through the same incision on the same date of service Ⓑ

For Medicare patients, reported rather than 38220

Mapping, Vessel

✻ **G0365** Vessel mapping of vessels for hemodialysis access (services for preoperative vessel mapping prior to creation of hemodialysis access using an autogenous hemodialysis conduit, including arterial inflow and venous outflow) Ⓑ

Includes evaluation of the relevant arterial and venous vessels. Use modifier 26 for professional component only.

⚙ **G0372** Physician service required to establish and document the need for a power mobility device Ⓑ

Providers should bill the E/M code and G0372 on the same claim.

Services, Observation and ED

⚙ **G0378** Hospital observation service, per hour Ⓑ

Report all related services in addition to G0378. Report units of hours spent in observation (rounded to the nearest hour). Hospitals report the ED or clinic visit with a CPT code or, if applicable, G0379 (direct admit to observation) and G0378 (hospital observation services, per hour).

⚙ **G0379** Direct admission of patient for hospital observation care Ⓑ

Report all related services in addition to G0379. Report units of hours spent in observation (rounded to the nearest hour). Hospitals report the ED or clinic visit with a CPT code or, if applicable, G0379 (direct admit to observation) and G0378 (hospital observation services, per hour).

✻ **G0380** Level 1 hospital emergency department visit provided in a type B emergency department; (the ED must meet at least one of the following requirements: (1) it is licensed by the state in which it is located under applicable state law as an emergency room or emergency department; (2) it is held out to the public (by name, posted signs, advertising, or other means) as a place that provides care for emergency medical conditions on an urgent basis without requiring a previously scheduled appointment; or (3) during the calendar year immediately preceding the calendar year in which a determination under 42 CFR 489.24 is being made, based on a representative sample of patient visits that occurred during that calendar year, it provides at least one-third of all of its outpatient visits for the treatment of emergency medical conditions on an urgent basis without requiring a previously scheduled appointment) Ⓑ

✻ **G0381** Level 2 hospital emergency department visit provided in a type B emergency department; (the ED must meet at least one of the following requirements: (1) it is licensed by the state in which it is located under applicable state law as an emergency room or emergency department; (2) it is held out to the public (by name, posted signs, advertising, or other means) as a place that provides care for emergency medical conditions on an urgent basis without requiring a previously scheduled appointment; or (3) during the calendar year immediately preceding the calendar year in which a determination under 42 CFR 489.24 is being made, based on a representative sample of patient visits that occurred during that calendar year, it provides at least one-third of all of its outpatient visits for the treatment of emergency medical conditions on an urgent basis without requiring a previously scheduled appointment) Ⓑ

✻ **G0382** Level 3 hospital emergency department visit provided in a type B emergency department; (the ED must meet at least one of the following requirements: (1) it is licensed by the state in which it is located under applicable state law as an emergency room or emergency department; (2) it is held out to the public (by name, posted signs, advertising, or other means) as a place that provides care for emergency medical conditions on an urgent basis without requiring a previously scheduled appointment; or (3) during the calendar year immediately preceding the calendar year in which a determination under 42 CFR 489.24 is being made, based on a representative sample of patient visits that occurred during that calendar year, it provides at least one-third of all of its outpatient visits for the treatment of emergency medical conditions on an urgent basis without requiring a previously scheduled appointment) Ⓑ

✻ **G0383** Level 4 hospital emergency department visit provided in a type B emergency department; (the ED must meet at least one of the following requirements: (1) it is licensed by the state in which it is located under applicable state law as an emergency room or emergency department; (2) it is held out to the public (by name, posted signs, advertising, or other means) as a place that provides care for emergency medical conditions on an urgent basis without requiring a previously scheduled appointment; or (3) during the calendar year immediately preceding the calendar year in which a determination under 42 CFR 489.24 is being made, based on a representative sample of patient visits that occurred during that calendar year, it provides at least one-third of all of its outpatient visits for the treatment of emergency medical conditions on an urgent basis without requiring a previously scheduled appointment) Ⓑ

✻ **G0384** Level 5 hospital emergency department visit provided in a type B emergency department; (the ED must meet at least one of the following requirements: (1) it is licensed by the state in which it is located under applicable state law as an emergency room or emergency department; (2) it is held out to the public (by name, posted signs, advertising, or other means) as a place that provides care for emergency medical conditions on an urgent basis without requiring a previously scheduled appointment; or (3) during the calendar year immediately preceding the calendar year in which a determination under 42 CFR § 489.24 is being made, based on a representative sample of patient visits that occurred during that calendar year, it provides at least one-third of all of its outpatient visits for the treatment of emergency medical conditions on an urgent basis without requiring a previously scheduled appointment) Ⓑ

Ultrasound, AAA

~~G0389 Ultrasound B-scan and/or real time with image documentation; for abdominal aortic aneurysm (AAA) screening~~ ✖

Team, Trauma Response

✪ **G0390** Trauma response team associated with hospital critical care service Ⓑ

Assessment/Intervention

✻ **G0396** Alcohol and/or substance (other than tobacco) abuse structured assessment (e.g., audit, DAST), and brief intervention 15 to 30 minutes Ⓑ

Bill instead of 99408 and 99409

✻ **G0397** Alcohol and/or substance (other than tobacco) abuse structured assessment (e.g., audit, DAST), and intervention, greater than 30 minutes Ⓑ

Bill instead of 99408 and 99409

▶ New ↻ Revised ✔ Reinstated ~~deleted~~ Deleted ⊘ Not covered or valid by Medicare
✪ Special coverage instructions ✻ Carrier discretion Ⓑ Bill local carrier Ⓓ Bill DME MAC

Home Sleep Study Test

✻ **G0398** Home sleep study test (HST) with type II portable monitor, unattended; minimum of 7 channels: EEG, EOG, EMG, ECG/heart rate, airflow, respiratory effort and oxygen saturation Ⓑ

✻ **G0399** Home sleep test (HST) with type III portable monitor, unattended; minimum of 4 channels: 2 respiratory movement/airflow, 1 ECG/heart rate and 1 oxygen saturation Ⓑ

✻ **G0400** Home sleep test (HST) with type IV portable monitor, unattended; minimum of 3 channels Ⓑ

Examination, Initial Medicare

✻ **G0402** Initial preventive physical examination; face-to-face visit, services limited to new beneficiary during the first 12 months of Medicare enrollment Ⓑ

Depending on circumstances, 99201-99215 may be assigned with modifier 25 to report an E/M service as a significant, separately identifiable service in addition to the Initial Preventive Physical Examination (IPPE), G0402.

Copayment and coinsurance waived, deductible waived.

Electrocardiogram

✻ **G0403** Electrocardiogram, routine ECG with 12 leads; performed as a screening for the initial preventive physical examination with interpretation and report Ⓑ

Optional service may be ordered or performed at discretion of physician. Once in a life-time screening, stemming from a referral from Initial Preventive Physical Examination (IPPE). Both deductible and co-payment apply.

✻ **G0404** Electrocardiogram, routine ECG with 12 leads; tracing only, without interpretation and report, performed as a screening for the initial preventive physical examination Ⓑ

✻ **G0405** Electrocardiogram, routine ECG with 12 leads; interpretation and report only, performed as a screening for the initial preventive physical examination Ⓑ

Telehealth

✻ **G0406** Follow-up inpatient consultation, limited, physicians typically spend 15 minutes communicating with the patient via telehealth Ⓑ

These telehealth modifers are required when billing for telehealth services with codes G0406-G0408 and G0425-G0427:

- GT, via interactive audio and video telecommunications system
- GQ, via asynchronous telecommunications system

✻ **G0407** Follow-up inpatient consultation, intermediate, physicians typically spend 25 minutes communicating with the patient via telehealth Ⓑ

✻ **G0408** Follow-up inpatient consultation, complex, physicians typically spend 35 minutes communicating with the patient via telehealth Ⓑ

Services, Social, Psychological

✻ **G0409** Social work and psychological services, directly relating to and/or furthering the patient's rehabilitation goals, each 15 minutes, face-to-face; individual (services provided by a CORF-qualified social worker or psychologist in a CORF) Ⓑ

✻ **G0410** Group psychotherapy other than of a multiple-family group, in a partial hospitalization setting, approximately 45 to 50 minutes Ⓑ

✻ **G0411** Interactive group psychotherapy, in a partial hospitalization setting, approximately 45 to 50 minutes Ⓑ

Treatment, Bone

✻ **G0412** Open treatment of iliac spine(s), tuberosity avulsion, or iliac wing fracture(s), unilateral or bilateral for pelvic bone fracture patterns which do not disrupt the pelvic ring includes internal fixation, when performed Ⓑ

✻ **G0413** Percutaneous skeletal fixation of posterior pelvic bone fracture and/or dislocation, for fracture patterns which disrupt the pelvic ring, unilateral or bilateral, (includes ilium, sacroiliac joint and/or sacrum) Ⓑ

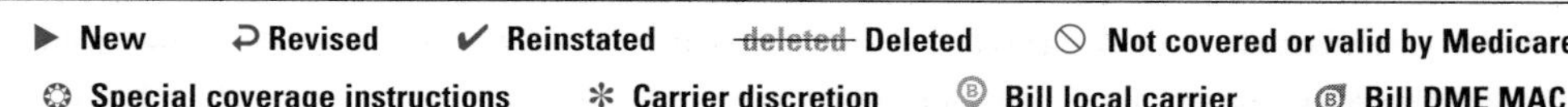

✻ **G0414** Open treatment of anterior pelvic bone fracture and/or dislocation for fracture patterns which disrupt the pelvic ring, unilateral or bilateral, includes internal fixation when performed (includes pubic symphysis and/or superior/inferior rami) Ⓑ

✻ **G0415** Open treatment of posterior pelvic bone fracture and/or dislocation, for fracture patterns which disrupt the pelvic ring, unilateral or bilateral, includes internal fixation, when performed (includes ilium, sacroiliac joint and/or sacrum) Ⓑ

Pathology, Surgical

✻ **G0416** Surgical pathology, gross and microscopic examinations for prostate needle biopsy, any method Ⓑ

This testing requires a facility to have either a CLIA certificate of registration (certificate type code 9), a CLIA certificate of compliance (certificate type code 1), or a CLIA certificate of accreditation (certificate type code 3). A facility without a valid, current, CLIA certificate, with a current CLIA certificate of waiver (certificate type code 2) or with a current CLIA certificate for provider-performed microscopy procedures (certificate type code 4), must not be permitted to be paid for these tests. This code has a TC, 26 (physician), or gobal component.

Laboratory Certification: Histopathology

Educational Services, Rehabilitation, Telehealth, and Miscellaneous

✻ **G0420** Face-to-face educational services related to the care of chronic kidney disease; individual, per session, per one hour Ⓑ

CKD is kidney damage of 3 months or longer, regardless of the cause of kidney damage. Sessions billed in increments of one hour (if session is less than 1 hour, it must last at least 31 minutes to be billable. Sessions less than one hour and longer than 31 minutes is billable as one session. No more than 6 sessions of KDE services in a beneficiary's lifetime

✻ **G0421** Face-to-face educational services related to the care of chronic kidney disease; group, per session, per one hour Ⓑ

Group setting: 2 to 20, report codes G0420 and G0421 with diagnosis code N18.-

✻ **G0422** Intensive cardiac rehabilitation; with or without continuous ECG monitoring with exercise, per session Ⓑ

Includes the same service as 93798 but at a greater frequency; may be reported with as many as six hourly sessions on a single date of service. Includes medical nutrition services to reduce cardiac disease risk factors.

✻ **G0423** Intensive cardiac rehabilitation; with or without continuous ECG monitoring; without exercise, per session Ⓑ

Includes the same service as 93797 but at a greater frequency; may be reported with as many as six hourly sessions on a single date of service. Includes medical nutrition services to reduce cardiac disease risk factors.

✻ **G0424** Pulmonary rehabilitation, including exercise (includes monitoring), one hour, per session, up to two sessions per day Ⓑ

Includes therapeutic services and all related monitoring services to inprove respiratory function. Do not report with G0237, G0238, or G0239.

✻ **G0425** Telehealth consultation, emergency department or initial inpatient, typically 30 minutes communicating with the patient via telehealth Ⓑ

Problem Focused: Problem focused history and examination, with straightforward medical decision making complexity. Typically 30 minutes communicating with patient via telehealth

✻ **G0426** Initial inpatient telehealth consultation, emergency department or initial inpatient, typically 50 minutes communicating with the patient via telehealth Ⓑ

Detailed: Detailed history and examination, with moderate medical decision making complexity. Typically 50 minutes communicating with patient via telehealth.

✻ **G0427** Initial inpatient telehealth consultation, emergency department or initial inpatient, typically 70 minutes or more communicating with the patient via telehealth Ⓑ

Comprehensive: Comprehensive history and examination, with high medical decision making complexity. Typically 70 minutes or more communicating with patient via telehealth.

⃠ **G0428** Collagen meniscus implant procedure for filling meniscal defects (e.g., cmi, collagen scaffold, menaflex) Ⓑ

⮌ ✻ **G0429** Dermal filler injection(s) for the treatment of facial lipodystrophy syndrome (LDS) (e.g., as a result of highly active antiretroviral therapy) Ⓑ

Designated for dermal fillers Sculptra® and Radiesse (Medicare). (https://www.cms.gov/ContractorLearningResources/downloads/JA6953.pdf)

✻ **G0432** Infectious agent antibody detection by enzyme immunoassay (EIA) technique, HIV-1 and/or HIV-2, screening Ⓑ

Laboratory Certification: Virology, General immunology

✻ **G0433** Infectious agent antibody detection by enzyme-linked immunosorbent assay (ELISA) technique, HIV-1 and/or HIV-2, screening Ⓑ

Laboratory Certification: Virology, General immunology

✻ **G0435** Infectious agent antibody detection by rapid antibody test, HIV-1 and/or HIV-2, screening Ⓑ

~~G0436 Smoking and tobacco cessation counseling visit for the asymptomatic patient; intermediate, greater than 3 minutes, up to 10 minutes~~ ✖

Cross Reference 99406, 99407

~~G0437 Smoking and tobacco cessation counseling visit for the asymptomatic patient; intensive, greater than 10 minutes~~ ✖

Cross Reference 99406, 99407

✻ **G0438** Annual wellness visit; includes a personalized prevention plan of service (pps), initial visit Ⓑ

✻ **G0439** Annual wellness visit, includes a personalized prevention plan of service (pps), subsequent visit Ⓑ

✻ **G0442** Annual alcohol misuse screening, 15 minutes Ⓑ

✻ **G0443** Brief face-to-face behavioral counseling for alcohol misuse, 15 minutes Ⓑ

✻ **G0444** Annual depression screening, 15 minutes Ⓑ

✻ **G0445** High intensity behavioral counseling to prevent sexually transmitted infection; face-to-face, individual, includes: education, skills training and guidance on how to change sexual behavior; performed semi-annually, 30 minutes Ⓑ

✻ **G0446** Annual, face-to-face intensive behavioral therapy for cardiovascular disease, individual, 15 minutes Ⓑ

✻ **G0447** Face-to-face behavioral counseling for obesity, 15 minutes Ⓑ

✻ **G0448** Insertion or replacement of a permanent pacing cardioverter-defibrillator system with transvenous lead(s), single or dual chamber with insertion of pacing electrode, cardiac venous system, for left ventricular pacing Ⓑ

✻ **G0451** Development testing, with interpretation and report, per standardized instrument form Ⓑ

✻ **G0452** Molecular pathology procedure; physician interpretation and report Ⓑ

✻ **G0453** Continuous intraoperative neurophysiology monitoring, from outside the operating room (remote or nearby), per patient, (attention directed exclusively to one patient) each 15 minutes (list in addition to primary procedure) Ⓑ

✻ **G0454** Physician documentation of face-to-face visit for durable medical equipment determination performed by nurse practitioner, physician assistant or clinical nurse specialist Ⓑ

✻ **G0455** Preparation with instillation of fecal microbiota by any method, including assessment of donor specimen Ⓑ

✻ **G0458** Low dose rate (LDR) prostate brachytherapy services, composite rate Ⓑ

✻ **G0459** Inpatient telehealth pharmacologic management, including prescription, use, and review of medication with no more than minimal medical psychotherapy Ⓑ

✻ **G0460** Autologous platelet rich plasma for chronic wounds/ulcers, including phlebotomy, centrifugation, and all other preparatory procedures, administration and dressings, per treatment Ⓑ

✻ **G0463** Hospital outpatient clinic visit for assessment and management of a patient Ⓑ

✻ **G0464** Colorectal cancer screening; stool-based DNA and fecal occult hemoglobin (e.g., KRAS, NDRG4 and BMP3) Ⓑ

Laboratory Certification: General immunology, Routine chemistry, Clinical cytogenetics

Cross Reference 81528

✻ **G0466** Federally qualified health center (FQHC) visit, new patient; a medically-necessary, face-to-face encounter (one-on-one) between a new patient and a FQHC practitioner during which time one or more FQHC services are rendered and includes a typical bundle of Medicare-covered services that would be furnished per diem to a patient receiving a FQHC visit Ⓑ

✻ **G0467** Federally qualified health center (FQHC) visit, established patient; a medically-necessary, face-to-face encounter (one-on-one) between an established patient and a FQHC practitioner during which time one or more FQHC services are rendered and includes a typical bundle of Medicare-covered services that would be furnished per diem to a patient receiving a FQHC visit Ⓑ

✻ **G0468** Federally qualified health center (FQHC) visit, IPPE or AWV; a FQHC visit that includes an initial preventive physical examination (IPPE) or annual wellness visit (AWV) and includes a typical bundle of Medicare-covered services that would be furnished per diem to a patient receiving an IPPE or AWV Ⓑ

✻ **G0469** Federally qualified health center (FQHC) visit, mental health, new patient; a medically-necessary, face-to-face mental health encounter (one-on-one) between a new patient and a FQHC practitioner during which time one or more FQHC services are rendered and includes a typical bundle of Medicare-covered services that would be furnished per diem to a patient receiving a mental health visit Ⓑ

✻ **G0470** Federally qualified health center (FQHC) visit, mental health, established patient; a medically-necessary, face-to-face mental health encounter (one-on-one) between an established patient and a FQHC practitioner during which time one or more FQHC services are rendered and includes a typical bundle of Medicare-covered services that would be furnished per diem to a patient receiving a mental health visit Ⓑ

✻ **G0471** Collection of venous blood by venipuncture or urine sample by catheterization from an individual in a skilled nursing facility (SNF) or by a laboratory on behalf of a home health agency (HHA) Ⓑ

✪ **G0472** Hepatitis C antibody screening, for individual at high risk and other covered indication(s) Ⓑ

Medicare Statute 1861SSA

Laboratory Certification: General immunology

✻ **G0473** Face-to-face behavioral counseling for obesity, group (2-10), 30 minutes Ⓑ

✻ **G0475** HIV antigen/antibody, combination assay, screening Ⓑ

✻ **G0476** Infectious agent detection by nucleic acid (DNA or RNA); human papillomavirus (HPV), high-risk types (e.g., 16, 18, 31, 33, 35, 39, 45, 51, 52, 56, 58, 59, 68) for cervical cancer screening, must be performed in addition to pap test Ⓑ

✻ **G0477** Drug test(s), presumptive, any number of drug classes; any number of devices or procedures, (e.g., immunoassay) capable of being read by direct optical observation only (e.g., dipsticks, cups, cards, cartridges), includes sample validation when performed, per date of service Ⓑ

✻ **G0478** Drug test(s), presumptive, any number of drug classes; any number of devices or procedures, (e.g., immunoassay) read by instrument-assisted direct optical observation (e.g., dipsticks, cups, cards, cartridges), includes sample validation when performed, per date of service Ⓑ

✻ **G0479** Drug test(s), presumptive, any number of drug classes; any number of devices or procedures by instrumented chemistry analyzers utilizing immunoassay, enzyme assay, TOF, MALDI, LDTD, DESI, DART, GHPC, GC mass spectrometry), includes sample validation when performed, per date of service Ⓑ

▶ New ↩ Revised ✔ Reinstated ~~deleted~~ Deleted ⊘ Not covered or valid by Medicare
✪ Special coverage instructions ✻ Carrier discretion Ⓑ Bill local carrier Ⓓ Bill DME MAC

* **G0480** Drug test(s), definitive, utilizing drug identification methods able to identify individual drugs and distinguish between structural isomers (but not necessarily stereoisomers), including, but not limited to GC/MS (any type, single or tandem) and LC/MS (any type, single or tandem and excluding immunoassays (e.g., IA, EIA, ELISA, EMIT, FPIA) and enzymatic methods (e.g., alcohol dehydrogenase)); qualitative or quantitative, all sources(s), includes specimen validity testing, per day, 1-7 drug class(es), including metabolite(s) if performed Ⓑ

* **G0481** Drug test(s), definitive, utilizing drug identification methods able to identify individual drugs and distinguish between structural isomers (but not necessarily stereoisomers), including, but not limited to GC/MS (any type, single or tandem) and LC/MS (any type, single or tandem and excluding immunoassays (e.g., IA, EIA, ELISA, EMIT, FPIA) and enzymatic methods (e.g., alcohol dehydrogenase)); qualitative or quantitative, all sources(s), includes specimen validity testing, per day, 8-14 drug class(es), including metabolite(s) if performed Ⓑ

* **G0482** Drug test(s), definitive, utilizing drug identification methods able to identify individual drugs and distinguish between structural isomers (but not necessarily stereoisomers), including, but not limited to GC/MS (any type, single or tandem) and LC/MS (any type, single or tandem and excluding immunoassays (e.g., IA, EIA, ELISA, EMIT, FPIA) and enzymatic methods (e.g., alcohol dehydrogenase)); qualitative or quantitative, all sources(s), includes specimen validity testing, per day, 15-21 drug class(es), including metabolite(s) if performed Ⓑ

* **G0483** Drug test(s), definitive, utilizing drug identification methods able to identify individual drugs and distinguish between structural isomers (but not necessarily stereoisomers), including, but not limited to GC/MS (any type, single or tandem) and LC/MS (any type, single or tandem and excluding immunoassays (e.g., IA, EIA, ELISA, EMIT, FPIA) and enzymatic methods (e.g., alcohol dehydrogenase)); qualitative or quantitative, all sources(s), includes specimen validity testing, per day, 22 or more drug class(es), including metabolite(s) if performed Ⓑ

▶ * **G0490** Face-to-face home health nursing visit by a rural health clinic (RHC) or federally qualified health center (FQHC) in an area with a shortage of home health agencies; (services limited to RN or LPN only) Ⓑ

▶ * **G0491** Dialysis procedure at a Medicare certified ESRD facility for acute kidney injury without ESRD Ⓑ

▶ * **G0492** Dialysis procedure with single evaluation by a physician or other qualified health care professional for acute kidney injury without ESRD Ⓑ

▶ * **G0493** Skilled services of a registered nurse (RN) for the observation and assessment of the patient's condition, each 15 minutes (the change in the patient's condition requires skilled nursing personnel to identify and evaluate the patient's need for possible modification of treatment in the home health or hospice setting) Ⓑ

▶ * **G0494** Skilled services of a licensed practical nurse (LPN) for the observation and assessment of the patient's condition, each 15 minutes (the change in the patient's condition requires skilled nursing personnel to identify and evaluate the patient's need for possible modification of treatment in the home health or hospice setting) Ⓑ

▶ * **G0495** Skilled services of a registered nurse (RN), in the training and/or education of a patient or family member, in the home health or hospice setting, each 15 minutes Ⓑ

▶ * **G0496** Skilled services of a licensed practical nurse (LPN), in the training and/or education of a patient or family member, in the home health or hospice setting, each 15 minutes Ⓑ

* **G0498** Chemotherapy administration, intravenous infusion technique; initiation of infusion in the office/clinic setting using office/clinic pump/ supplies, with continuation of the infusion in the community setting (e.g., home, domiciliary, rest home or assisted living) using a portable pump provided by the office/clinic, includes follow up office/clinic visit at the conclusion of the infusion Ⓑ

▶ * **G0499** Hepatitis B screening in non-pregnant, high risk individual includes hepatitis B surface antigen (HBsAG) followed by a neutralizing confirmatory test for initially reactive results, and antibodies to HBsAG (anti-HBS) and hepatitis B core antigen (anti-HBC) Ⓑ

▶ * **G0500** Moderate sedation services provided by the same physician or other qualified health care professional performing a gastrointestinal endoscopic service that sedation supports, requiring the presence of an independent trained observer to assist in the monitoring of the patient's level of consciousness and physiological status; initial 15 minutes of intra-service time; patient age 5 years or older (additional time may be reported with 99153, as appropriate) Ⓑ

▶ * **G0501** Resource-intensive services for patients for whom the use of specialized mobility-assistive technology (such as adjustable height chairs or tables, patient lift, and adjustable padded leg supports) is medically necessary and used during the provision of an office/outpatient, evaluation and management visit (list separately in addition to primary service) Ⓑ

▶ * **G0502** Initial psychiatric collaborative care management, first 70 minutes in the first calendar month of behavioral health care manager activities, in consultation with a psychiatric consultant, and directed by the treating physician or other qualified health care professional, with the following required elements: outreach to and engagement in treatment of a patient directed by the treating physician or other qualified health care professional; initial assessment of the patient, including administration of validated rating scales, with the development of an individualized treatment plan; review by the psychiatric consultant with modifications of the plan if recommended; entering patient in a registry and tracking patient follow-up and progress using the registry, with appropriate documentation, and participation in weekly caseload consultation with the psychiatric consultant; and provision of brief interventions using evidence-based techniques such as behavioral activation, motivational interviewing, and other focused treatment strategies Ⓑ

▶ * **G0503** Subsequent psychiatric collaborative care management, first 60 minutes in a subsequent month of behavioral health care manager activities, in consultation with a psychiatric consultant, and directed by the treating physician or other qualified health care professional, with the following required elements: tracking patient follow-up and progress using the registry, with appropriate documentation; participation in weekly caseload consultation with the psychiatric consultant; ongoing collaboration with and coordination of the patient's mental health care with the treating physician or other qualified health care professional and any other treating mental health providers; additional review of progress and recommendations for changes in treatment, as indicated, including medications, based on recommendations provided by the psychiatric consultant; provision of brief interventions using evidence-based techniques such as behavioral activation, motivational interviewing, and other focused treatment strategies; monitoring of patient outcomes using validated rating scales; and relapse prevention planning with patients as they achieve remission of symptoms and/or other treatment goals and are prepared for discharge from active treatment Ⓑ

▶ * **G0504** Initial or subsequent psychiatric collaborative care management, each additional 30 minutes in a calendar month of behavioral health care manager activities, in consultation with a psychiatric consultant, and directed by the treating physician or other qualified health care professional (list separately in addition to code for primary procedure); (use G0504 in conjunction with G0502, G0503) Ⓑ

▶ * **G0505** Cognition and functional assessment using standardized instruments with development of recorded care plan for the patient with cognitive impairment, history obtained from patient and/or caregiver, in office or other outpatient setting or home or domiciliary or rest home Ⓑ

▶ * **G0506** Comprehensive assessment of and care planning for patients requiring chronic care management services (list separately in addition to primary monthly care management service) Ⓑ

▶ New ↩ Revised ✔ Reinstated ~~deleted~~ Deleted ⊘ Not covered or valid by Medicare
Special coverage instructions * Carrier discretion Ⓑ Bill local carrier Ⓑ Bill DME MAC

▶ ✻ **G0507** Care management services for behavioral health conditions, at least 20 minutes of clinical staff time, directed by a physician or other qualified health care professional, per calendar month, with the following required elements: initial assessment or follow-up monitoring, including the use of applicable validated rating scales; behavioral health care planning in relation to behavioral/psychiatric health problems, including revision for patients who are not progressing or whose status changes; facilitating and coordinating treatment such as psychotherapy, pharmacotherapy, counseling and/or psychiatric consultation; and continuity of care with a designated member of the care team Ⓑ

▶ ✻ **G0508** Telehealth consultation, critical care, initial, physicians typically spend 60 minutes communicating with the patient and providers via telehealth Ⓑ

▶ ✻ **G0509** Telehealth consultation, critical care, subsequent, physicians typically spend 50 minutes communicating with the patient and providers via telehealth Ⓑ

✻ **G0913** Improvement in visual function achieved within 90 days following cataract surgery Ⓑ

✻ **G0914** Patient care survey was not completed by patient Ⓑ

✻ **G0915** Improvement in visual function not achieved within 90 days following cataract surgery Ⓑ

✻ **G0916** Satisfaction with care achieved within 90 days following cataract surgery Ⓑ

✻ **G0917** Patient satisfaction survey was not completed by patient Ⓑ

✻ **G0918** Satisfaction with care not achieved within 90 days following cataract surgery Ⓑ

Tositumomab

~~G3001 Administration and supply of tositumomab, 450 mg~~ ✖

Guidance

✪ **G6001** Ultrasonic guidance for placement of radiation therapy fields Ⓑ

✻ **G6002** Stereoscopic X-ray guidance for localization of target volume for the delivery of radiation therapy Ⓑ

Treatment, Radiation

✻ **G6003** Radiation treatment delivery, single treatment area, single port or parallel opposed ports, simple blocks or no blocks: up to 5 mev Ⓑ

✻ **G6004** Radiation treatment delivery, single treatment area, single port or parallel opposed ports, simple blocks or no blocks: 6-10 mev Ⓑ

✻ **G6005** Radiation treatment delivery, single treatment area, single port or parallel opposed ports, simple blocks or no blocks: 11-19 mev Ⓑ

✻ **G6006** Radiation treatment delivery, single treatment area, single port or parallel opposed ports, simple blocks or no blocks: 20 mev or greater Ⓑ

✻ **G6007** Radiation treatment delivery, 2 separate treatment areas, 3 or more ports on a single treatment area, use of multiple blocks: up to 5 mev Ⓑ

✻ **G6008** Radiation treatment delivery, 2 separate treatment areas, 3 or more ports on a single treatment area, use of multiple blocks: 6-10 mev Ⓑ

✻ **G6009** Radiation treatment delivery, 2 separate treatment areas, 3 or more ports on a single treatment area, use of multiple blocks: 11-19 mev Ⓑ

✻ **G6010** Radiation treatment delivery, 2 separate treatment areas, 3 or more ports on a single treatment area, use of multiple blocks: 20 mev or greater Ⓑ

✻ **G6011** Radiation treatment delivery, 3 or more separate treatment areas, custom blocking, tangential ports, wedges, rotational beam, compensators, electron beam; up to 5 mev Ⓑ

✻ **G6012** Radiation treatment delivery, 3 or more separate treatment areas, custom blocking, tangential ports, wedges, rotational beam, compensators, electron beam; 6-10 mev Ⓑ

✻ **G6013** Radiation treatment delivery, 3 or more separate treatment areas, custom blocking, tangential ports, wedges, rotational beam, compensators, electron beam; 11-19 mev Ⓑ

✻ **G6014** Radiation treatment delivery, 3 or more separate treatment areas, custom blocking, tangential ports, wedges, rotational beam, compensators, electron beam; 20 mev or greater Ⓑ

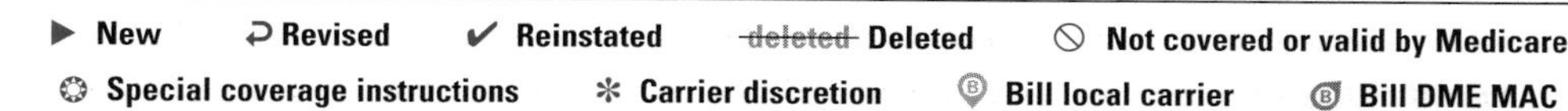

✻ **G6015** Intensity modulated treatment delivery, single or multiple fields/arcs, via narrow spatially and temporally modulated beams, binary, dynamic MLC, per treatment session Ⓑ

✻ **G6016** Compensator-based beam modulation treatment delivery of inverse planned treatment using 3 or more high resolution (milled or cast) compensator, convergent beam modulated fields, per treatment session Ⓑ

✻ **G6017** Intra-fraction localization and tracking of target or patient motion during delivery of radiation therapy (eg, 3D positional tracking, gating, 3D surface tracking), each fraction of treatment Ⓑ

Documentation

✻ **G8395** Left ventricular ejection fraction (LVEF)> = 40% or documentation as normal or mildly depressed left ventricular systolic function Ⓑ

✻ **G8396** Left ventricular ejection fraction (LVEF) not performed or documented Ⓑ

✻ **G8397** Dilated macular or fundus exam performed, including documentation of the presence or absence of macular edema and level of severity of retinopathy Ⓑ

✻ **G8398** Dilated macular or fundus exam not performed Ⓑ

✻ **G8399** Patient with documented results of a central dual-energy x-ray absorptiometry (DXA) ever being performed Ⓑ

✻ **G8400** Patient with central dual-energy x-ray absorptiometry (DXA) results not documented Ⓑ

~~G8401 Clinician documented that patient was not an eligible candidate for screening~~ ✖

✻ **G8404** Lower extremity neurological exam performed and documented Ⓑ

✻ **G8405** Lower extremity neurological exam not performed Ⓑ

✻ **G8410** Footwear evaluation performed and documented Ⓑ

✻ **G8415** Footwear evaluation was not performed Ⓑ

✻ **G8416** Clinician documented that patient was not an eligible candidate for footwear evaluation measure Ⓑ

✻ **G8417** BMI is documented above normal parameters and a follow-up plan is documented Ⓑ

✻ **G8418** BMI is documented below normal parameters and a follow-up plan is documented Ⓑ

✻ **G8419** BMI is documented outside normal parameters, no follow-up plan documented, no reason given Ⓑ

✻ **G8420** BMI is documented within normal parameters and no follow-up plan is required Ⓑ

✻ **G8421** BMI not documented and no reason is given Ⓑ

✻ **G8422** BMI not documented, documentation the patient is not eligible for BMI calculation Ⓑ

⮌ ✻ **G8427** Eligible clinician attests to documenting in the medical record they obtained, updated, or reviewed the patient's current medications Ⓑ

⮌ ✻ **G8428** Current list of medications not documented as obtained, updated, or reviewed by the eligible clinician, reason not given Ⓑ

⮌ ✻ **G8430** Eligible clinician attests to documenting in the medical record the patient is not eligible for a current list of medications being obtained, updated, or reviewed by the eligible clinician Ⓑ

⮌ ✻ **G8431** Screening for depression is documented as being positive and a follow-up plan is documented Ⓑ

⮌ ✻ **G8432** Depression screening not documented, reason not given Ⓑ

⮌ ✻ **G8433** Screening for depression not completed, documented reason Ⓑ

✻ **G8442** Pain assessment not documented as being performed, documentation the patient is not eligible for a pain assessment using a standardized tool Ⓑ

✻ **G8450** Beta-blocker therapy prescribed Ⓑ

✻ **G8451** beta therapy for LVEF < 40% not prescribed for reasons documented by the clinician (e.g., low blood pressure, fluid overload, asthma, patients recently treated with an intravenous positive inotropic agent, allergy, intolerance, other medical reasons, patient declined, other patient reasons or other reasons attributable to the healthcare system) Ⓑ

✻ **G8452** Beta-blocker therapy not prescribed Ⓑ

▶ New ⮌ Revised ✔ Reinstated ~~deleted~~ Deleted ⃠ Not covered or valid by Medicare
Special coverage instructions ✻ Carrier discretion Ⓑ Bill local carrier Ⓑ Bill DME MAC

~~G8458~~ ~~Clinician documented that patient is not an eligible candidate for genotype testing; patient not receiving antiviral treatment for hepatitis C during the measurement period (e.g. genotype test done prior to the reporting period, patient declines, patient not a candidate for antiviral treatment)~~ ✖

~~G8460~~ ~~Clinician documented that patient is not an eligible candidate for quantitative RNA testing at week 12; patient not receiving antiviral treatment for hepatitis C~~ ✖

~~G8461~~ ~~Patient receiving antiviral treatment for hepatitis C during the measurement period~~ ✖

✻ **G8465** High or very high risk of recurrence of prostate cancer Ⓑ

✻ **G8473** Angiotensin converting enzyme (ACE) inhibitor or angiotensin receptor blocker (ARB) therapy prescribed Ⓑ

✻ **G8474** Angiotensin converting enzyme (ACE) inhibitor or angiotensin receptor blocker (ARB) therapy not prescribed for reasons documented by the clinician (e.g., allergy, intolerance, pregnancy, renal failure due to ACE inhibitor, diseases of the aortic or mitral valve, other medical reasons) or (e.g., patient declined, other patient reasons) or (e.g., lack of drug availability, other reasons attributable to the health care system) Ⓑ

✻ **G8475** Angiotensin converting enzyme (ACE) inhibitor or angiotensin receptor blocker (ARB) therapy not prescribed, reason not given Ⓑ

✻ **G8476** Most recent blood pressure has a systolic measurement of < 140 mmHg and a diastolic measurement of < 90 mmHg Ⓑ

✻ **G8477** Most recent blood pressure has a systolic measurement of > = 140 mmHg and/or a diastolic measurement of > = 90 mmHg Ⓑ

✻ **G8478** Blood pressure measurement not performed or documented, reason not given Ⓑ

✻ **G8482** Influenza immunization administered or previously received Ⓑ

✻ **G8483** Influenza immunization was not administered for reasons documented by clinician (e.g., patient allergy or other medical reasons, patient declined or other patient reasons, vacine not available or other system reasons) Ⓑ

✻ **G8484** Influenza immunization was not administered, reason not given Ⓑ

~~G8485~~ ~~I intend to report the diabetes mellitus (DM) measures group~~ ✖

~~G8486~~ ~~I intend to report the preventive care measures group~~ ✖

~~G8487~~ ~~I intend to report the chronic kidney disease (CKD) measures group~~ ✖

~~G8489~~ ~~I intend to report the coronary artery disease (CAD) measures group~~ ✖

~~G8490~~ ~~I intend to report the rheumatoid arthritis (RA) measures group~~ ✖

~~G8491~~ ~~I intend to report the HIV/AIDS measures group~~ ✖

~~G8494~~ ~~All quality actions for the applicable measures in the diabetes mellitus (DM) measures group have been performed for this patient~~ ✖

~~G8495~~ ~~All quality actions for the applicable measures in the chronic kidney disease (CKD) measures group have been performed for this patient~~ ✖

~~G8496~~ ~~All quality actions for the applicable measures in the Preventive Care measures group have been performed for this patient~~ ✖

~~G8497~~ ~~All quality actions for the applicable measures in the Coronary Artery Bypass Graft (CABG) measures group have been performed for this patient~~ ✖

~~G8498~~ ~~All quality actions for the applicable measures in the Coronary Artery Disease (CAD) measures group have been performed for this patient~~ ✖

~~G8499~~ ~~All quality actions for the applicable measures in the Rheumatoid Arthritis (RA) measures group have been performed for this patient~~ ✖

~~G8500~~ ~~All quality actions for the applicable measures in the HIV/AIDS measures group have been performed for this patient~~ ✖

✻ **G8506** Patient receiving angiotensin converting enzyme (ACE) inhibitor or angiotensin receptor blocker (ARB) therapy Ⓑ

✻ **G8509** Pain assessment documented as positive using a standardized tool, follow-up plan not documented, reason not given Ⓑ

⮌ ✻ **G8510** Screening for depression is documented as negative, a follow-up plan is not required Ⓑ

▶ New ⮌ Revised ✔ Reinstated ~~deleted~~ Deleted ⃠ Not covered or valid by Medicare
✪ Special coverage instructions ✻ Carrier discretion Ⓑ Bill local carrier Ⓓ Bill DME MAC

↩ ✻ **G8511** Screening for depression documented as positive, follow up plan not documented, reason not given Ⓑ

✻ **G8535** Elder maltreatment screen not documented; documentation that patient not eligible for the elder maltreatment screen Ⓑ

✻ **G8536** No documentation of an elder maltreatment screen, reason not given Ⓑ

✻ **G8539** Functional outcome assessment documented as positive using a standardized tool and a care plan based on identified deficiencies on the date of functional outcome assessment is documented Ⓑ

✻ **G8540** Functional outcome assessment not documented as being performed, documentation the patient is not eligible for a functional outcome assessment using a standardized tool Ⓑ

✻ **G8541** Functional outcome assessment using a standardized tool not documented, reason not given Ⓑ

✻ **G8542** Functional outcome assessment using a standardized tool is documented; no functional deficiencies identified, care plan not required Ⓑ

✻ **G8543** Documentation of a positive functional outcome assessment using a standardized tool; care plan not documented, reason not given Ⓑ

~~G8544 I intend to report the coronary artery bypass graft (CABG) measures group~~ ✖

~~G8545 I intend to report the Hepatitis C measures group~~ ✖

~~G8548 I intend to report the Heart Failure (HF) measures group~~ ✖

~~G8549 All quality actions for the applicable measures in the Hepatitis C measures group have been performed for this patient~~ ✖

~~G8551 All quality actions for the applicable measures in the Heart Failure (HF) measures group have been performed for this patient~~ ✖

✻ **G8559** Patient referred to a physician (preferably a physician with training in disorders of the ear) for an otologic evaluation Ⓑ

✻ **G8560** Patient has a history of active drainage from the ear within the previous 90 days Ⓑ

✻ **G8561** Patient is not eligible for the referral for otologic evaluation for patients with a history of active drainage measure Ⓑ

✻ **G8562** Patient does not have a history of active drainage from the ear within the previous 90 days Ⓑ

✻ **G8563** Patient not referred to a physician (preferably a physician with training in disorders of the ear) for an otologic evaluation, reason not given Ⓑ

✻ **G8564** Patient was referred to a physician (preferably a physician with training in disorders of the ear) for an otologic evaluation, reason not specified) Ⓑ

✻ **G8565** Verification and documentation of sudden or rapidly progressive hearing loss Ⓑ

✻ **G8566** Patient is not eligible for the "referral for otologic evaluation for sudden or rapidly progressive hearing loss" measure Ⓑ

✻ **G8567** Patient does not have verification and documentation of sudden or rapidly progressive hearing loss Ⓑ

✻ **G8568** Patient was not referred to a physician (preferably a physician with training in disorders of the ear) for an otologic evaluation, reason not given Ⓑ

✻ **G8569** Prolonged postoperative intubation (>24 hrs) required Ⓑ

✻ **G8570** Prolonged postoperative intubation (>24 hrs) not required Ⓑ

✻ **G8571** Development of deep sternal wound infection/mediastinitis within 30 days postoperatively Ⓑ

✻ **G8572** No deep sternal wound infection/ mediastinitis Ⓑ

✻ **G8573** Stroke following isolated CABG surgery Ⓑ

✻ **G8574** No stroke following isolated CABG surgery Ⓑ

✻ **G8575** Developed postoperative renal failure or required dialysis Ⓑ

✻ **G8576** No postoperative renal failure/dialysis not required Ⓑ

✻ **G8577** Re-exploration required due to mediastinal bleeding with or without tamponade, graft occlusion, valve disfunction, or other cardiac reason Ⓑ

✻ **G8578** Re-exploration not required due to mediastinal bleeding with or without tamponade, graft occlusion, valve dysfunction, or other cardiac reason Ⓑ

↺ * **G8598** Aspirin or another antiplatelet therapy used Ⓑ

↺ * **G8599** Aspirin or another antiplatelet therapy not used, reason not given Ⓑ

* **G8600** IV T-PA initiated within three hours (<= 180 minutes) of time last known well Ⓑ

* **G8601** IV T-PA not initiated within three hours (<= 180 minutes) of time last known well for reasons documented by clinician Ⓑ

* **G8602** IV T-PA not initiated within three hours (<= 180 minutes) of time last known well, reason not given Ⓑ

* **G8627** Surgical procedure performed within 30 days following cataract surgery for major complications (e.g., retained nuclear fragments, endophthalmitis, dislocated or wrong power IOL, retinal detachment, or wound dehiscence) Ⓑ

* **G8628** Surgical procedure not performed within 30 days following cataract surgery for major complications (e.g., retained nuclear fragments, endophthalmitis, dislocated or wrong power IOL, retinal detachment, or wound dehiscence) Ⓑ

* **G8633** Pharmacologic therapy (other than minierals/vitamins) for osteoporosis prescribed Ⓑ

~~G8634 Clinician documented patient not an eligible candidate to receive pharmacologic therapy for osteoporosis~~ ✖

* **G8635** Pharmacologic therapy for osteoporosis was not prescribed, reason not given Ⓑ

~~G8645 I intend to report the asthma measures group~~ ✖

~~G8646 All quality actions for the applicable measures in the asthma measures group have been performed for this patient~~ ✖

* **G8647** Risk-adjusted functional status change residual score for the knee successfully calculated and the score was equal to zero (0) or greater than zero (>0) Ⓑ

* **G8648** Risk-adjusted functional status change residual score for the knee successfully calculated and the score was less than zero (< 0) Ⓑ

↺ * **G8649** Risk-adjusted functional status change residual scores for the knee not measured because the patient did not complete FOTO'S status survey near discharge, not appropriate Ⓑ

* **G8650** Risk-adjusted functional status change residual scores for the knee not measured because the patient did not complete FOTO'S functional intake on admission and/or follow up status survey near discharge, reason not given Ⓑ

* **G8651** Risk-adjusted functional status change residual score for the hip successfully calculated and the score was equal to zero (0) or greater than zero (>0) Ⓑ

* **G8652** Risk-adjusted functional status change residual score for the hip successfully calculated and the score was less than zero (< 0) Ⓑ

↺ * **G8653** Risk-adjusted functional status change residual scores for the hip not measured because the patient did not complete follow up status survey near discharge, patient not appropriate Ⓑ

* **G8654** Risk-adjusted functional status change residual scores for the hip not measured because the patient did not complete FOTO'S functional intake on admission and/or follow up status survey near discharge, reason not given Ⓑ

↺ * **G8655** Risk-adjusted functional status change residual score for the foot or ankle successfully calculated and the score was equal to zero (0) or greater than zero (>0) Ⓑ

↺ * **G8656** Risk-adjusted functional status change residual score for the foot or ankle successfully calculated and the score was less than zero (< 0) Ⓑ

↺ * **G8657** Risk-adjusted functional status change residual scores for the foot or ankle not measured because the patient did not complete FOTO'S status survey near discharge, patient not appropriate Ⓑ

↺ * **G8658** Risk-adjusted functional status change residual scores for the foot or ankle not measured because the patient did not complete FOTO'S functional intake on admission and/or follow up status survey near discharge, reason not given Ⓑ

↺ * **G8659** Risk-adjusted functional status change residual score for the lumbar impairment successfully calculated and the score was equal to zero (0) or greater than zero (> 0) Ⓑ

↺ * **G8660** Risk-adjusted functional status change residual score for the lumbar impairment successfully calculated and the score was less than zero (< 0) Ⓑ

▶ New ↺ Revised ✔ Reinstated ~~deleted~~ Deleted ⃠ Not covered or valid by Medicare
✪ Special coverage instructions * Carrier discretion Ⓑ Bill local carrier Ⓓ Bill DME MAC

↩ * **G8661** Risk-adjusted functional status change residual scores for the lumbar impairment not measured because the patient did not complete FOTO'S status survey near discharge, patient not appropriate Ⓑ

↩ * **G8662** Risk-adjusted functional status change residual scores for the lumbar impairment not measured because the patient did not complete FOTO'S functional intake on admission and/or follow up status survey near discharge, reason not given Ⓑ

* **G8663** Risk-adjusted functional status change residual score for the shoulder successfully calculated and the score was equal to zero (0) or greater than zero (>0) Ⓑ

* **G8664** Risk-adjusted functional status change residual score for the shoulder successfully calculated and the score was less than zero (< 0) Ⓑ

↩ * **G8665** Risk-adjusted functional status change residual scores for the shoulder not measured because the patient did not complete FOTO'S functional status survey near discharge, patient not appropriate Ⓑ

* **G8666** Risk-adjusted functional status change residual scores for the shoulder not measured because the patient did not complete FOTO'S functional intake on admission and/or follow up status survey near discharge, reason not given Ⓑ

* **G8667** Risk-adjusted functional status change residual score for the elbow, wrist or hand successfully calculated and the score was equal to zero (0) or greater than zero (>0) Ⓑ

* **G8668** Risk-adjusted functional status change residual score for the elbow, wrist or hand successfully calculated and the score was less than zero (< 0) Ⓑ

↩ * **G8669** Risk-adjusted functional status change residual scores for the elbow, wrist or hand not measured because the patient did not complete FOTO'S functional follow up status survey near discharge, patient not appropriate Ⓑ

* **G8670** Risk-adjusted functional status change residual scores for the elbow, wrist or hand not measured because the patient did not complete FOTO'S functional intake on admission and/or follow up status survey near discharge, reason not given Ⓑ

↩ * **G8671** Risk-adjusted functional status change residual score for the neck, cranium, mandible, thoracic spine, ribs, or other general orthopaedic impairment successfully calculated and the score was equal to zero (0) or greater than zero (> 0) Ⓑ

↩ * **G8672** Risk-adjusted functional status change residual score for the neck, cranium, mandible, thoracic spine, ribs, or other general orthopaedic impairment successfully calculated and the score was less than zero (<0) Ⓑ

↩ * **G8673** Risk-adjusted functional status change residual scores for the neck, cranium, mandible, thoracic spine, ribs, or other general orthopaedic impairment not measured because the patient did not complete FOTO'S functional follow up status survey near discharge, patient not appropriate Ⓑ

↩ * **G8674** Risk-adjusted functional status change residual scores for the neck, cranium, mandible, thoracic spine, ribs, or other general orthopaedic impairment not measured because the patient did not complete FOTO'S functional intake on admission and/or follow up status survey near discharge, reason not given Ⓑ

* **G8694** Left ventriucular ejection fraction (LVEF) < 40% Ⓑ

* **G8696** Antithrombotic therapy prescribed at discharge Ⓑ

↩ * **G8697** Antithrombotic therapy not prescribed for documented reasons (e.g., patient had stroke during hospital stay, patient expired during inpatient stay, other medical reason(s)); (e.g., patient left against medical advice, other patient reason(s)) Ⓑ

* **G8698** Antithrombotic therapy was not prescribed at discharge, reason not given Ⓑ

* **G8708** Patient not prescribed or dispensed antibiotic Ⓑ

▶ New ↩ Revised ✔ Reinstated ~~deleted~~ Deleted ⊘ Not covered or valid by Medicare
Special coverage instructions * Carrier discretion Ⓑ Bill local carrier Ⓓ Bill DME MAC

✻ **G8709** Patient prescribed or dispensed antibiotic for documented medical reason(s) (e.g., intestinal infection, pertussis, bacterial infection, Lyme disease, otitis media, acute sinusitis, acute pharyngitis, acute tonsillitis, chronic sinusitis, infection of the pharynx/larynx/tonsils/adenoids, prostatitis, cellulitis, mastoiditis, or bone infections, acute lymphadenitis, impetigo, skin staph infections, pneumonia/gonococcal infections, venereal disease (syphilis, chlamydia, inflammatory diseases (female reproductive organs), infections of the kidney, cystitis or UTI, and acne) Ⓑ

✻ **G8710** Patient prescribed or dispensed antibiotic Ⓑ

✻ **G8711** Prescribed or dispensed antibiotic Ⓑ

✻ **G8712** Antibiotic not prescribed or dispensed Ⓑ

✻ **G8721** PT category (primary tumor), PN category (regional lymph nodes), and histologic grade were documented in pathology report Ⓑ

✻ **G8722** Documentation of medical reason(s) for not including the PT category, the PN category or the histologic grade in the pathology report (e.g., re-excision without residual tumor; non-carcinomasanal canal) Ⓑ

✻ **G8723** Specimen site is other than anatomic location of primary tumor Ⓑ

✻ **G8724** PT category, PN category and histologic grade were not documented in the pathology report, reason not given Ⓑ

~~G8725 Fasting lipid profile performed (triglycerides, LDL-C, HDL-C and total cholesterol)~~ ✖

~~G8726 Clinician has documented reason for not performing fasting lipid profile (e.g., patient declined, other patient reasons)~~ ✖

~~G8728 Fasting lipid profile not performed, reason not given~~ ✖

✻ **G8730** Pain assessment documented as positive using a standardized tool and a follow-up plan is documented Ⓑ

✻ **G8731** Pain assessment using a standardized tool is documented as negative, no follow-up plan required Ⓑ

✻ **G8732** No documentation of pain assessment, reason not given Ⓑ

✻ **G8733** Elder maltreatment screen documented as positive and a follow-up plan is documented Ⓑ

✻ **G8734** Elder maltreatment screen documented as negative, no follow-up required Ⓑ

✻ **G8735** Elder maltreatment screen documented as positive, follow-up plan not documented, reason not given Ⓑ

✻ **G8749** Absence of signs of melanoma (cough, dyspnea, tenderness, localized neurologic signs such as weakness, jaundice or any other sign suggesting systemic spread) or absence of symptoms of melanoma (pain, paresthesia, or any other symptom suggesting the possibility of systemic spread of melanoma) Ⓑ

✻ **G8752** Most recent systolic blood pressure < 140 mmhg Ⓑ

✻ **G8753** Most recent systolic blood pressure >= 140 mmhg Ⓑ

✻ **G8754** Most recent diastolic blood pressure < 90 mmhg Ⓑ

✻ **G8755** Most recent diastolic blood pressure >= 90 mmhg Ⓑ

✻ **G8756** No documentation of blood pressure measurement, reason not given Ⓑ

~~G8757 All quality actions for the applicable measures in the chronic obstructive pulmonary disease (COPD) measures group have been performed for this patient~~ ✖

~~G8758 All quality actions for the applicable measures in the inflammatory bowel disease (IBD) measures group have been performed for this patient~~ ✖

~~G8759 All quality actions for the applicable measures in the sleep apnea measures group have been performed for this patient~~ ✖

~~G8761 All quality actions for the applicable measures in the dementia measures group have been performed for this patient~~ ✖

~~G8762 All quality actions for the applicable measures in the Parkinson s disease measures group have been performed for this patient~~ ✖

~~G8765 All quality actions for the applicable measures in the cataract measures group have been performed for this patient~~ ✖

✻ **G8783** Normal blood pressure reading documented, follow-up not required Ⓑ

► New ⤾ Revised ✔ Reinstated ~~deleted~~ Deleted ⊘ Not covered or valid by Medicare
✪ Special coverage instructions ✻ Carrier discretion Ⓑ Bill local carrier Ⓓ Bill DME MAC

~~G8784 Patient not eligible (e.g., documentation the patient is not eligible due to active diagnosis of hypertension, patient refuses, urgent or emergent situation)~~ ✖

✻ **G8785** Blood pressure reading not documented, reason not given Ⓑ

✻ **G8797** Specimen site other than anatomic location of esophagus Ⓑ

✻ **G8798** Specimen site other than anatomic location of prostate Ⓑ

✻ **G8806** Performance of trans-abdominal or trans-vaginal ultrasound Ⓑ

✻ **G8807** Trans-abdominal or trans-vaginal ultrasound not performed for reasons documented by clinician (e.g., patient has visited the ED multiple times within 72 hours, patient has a documented intrauterine pregnancy [IUP]) Ⓑ

✻ **G8808** Performance of trans-abdominal or trans-vaginal ultrasound not ordered, reason not given (e.g., patient has visited the ED multiple times with no documentation of a trans-abdominal or trans-vaginal ultrasound within ED or from referring eligible professional) Ⓑ

✻ **G8809** Rh-immunoglobulin (RhoGAM) ordered Ⓑ

✻ **G8810** Rh-immunoglobulin (RhoGAM) not ordered for reasons documented by clinician (e.g., patient had prior documented report of RhoGAM within 12 weeks, patient refusal) Ⓑ

✻ **G8811** Documentation RH-immunoglobulin (RhoGAM) was not ordered, reason not given Ⓑ

⮌ ✻ **G8815** Documented reason in the medical records for why the statin therapy was not prescribed (i.e., lower extremity bypass was for a patient with non-artherosclerotic disease) Ⓑ

✻ **G8816** Statin medication prescribed at discharge Ⓑ

✻ **G8817** Statin therapy not prescribed at discharge, reason not given Ⓑ

✻ **G8818** Patient discharge to home no later than post-operative day #7 Ⓑ

✻ **G8825** Patient not discharged to home by post-operative day #7 Ⓑ

✻ **G8826** Patient discharge to home no later than post-operative day #2 following EVAR Ⓑ

✻ **G8833** Patient not discharged to home by post-operative day #2 following EVAR Ⓑ

✻ **G8834** Patient discharged to home no later than post-operative day #2 following CEA Ⓑ

✻ **G8838** Patient not discharged to home by post-operative day #2 following CEA Ⓑ

✻ **G8839** Sleep apnea symptoms assessed, including presence or absence of snoring and daytime sleepiness Ⓑ

✻ **G8840** Documentation of reason(s) for not documenting an assessment of sleep symptoms (e.g., patient didn't have initial daytime sleepiness, patient visited between initial testing and initiation of therapy) Ⓑ

✻ **G8841** Sleep apnea symptoms not assessed, reason not given Ⓑ

✻ **G8842** Apnea Hypopnea Index (AHI) or Respiratory Disturbance Index (RDI) measured at the time of initial diagnosis Ⓑ

✻ **G8843** Documentation of reason(s) for not measuring an Apnea Hypopnea Index (AHI) or a Respiratory Disturbance Index (RDI) at the time of initial diagnosis (e.g., psychiatric disease, dementia, patient declined, financial, insurance coverage, test ordered but not yet completed) Ⓑ

✻ **G8844** Apnea Hypopnea Index (AHI) or Respiratory Disturbance Index (RDI) not measured at the time of initial diagnosis, reason not given Ⓑ

✻ **G8845** Positive airway pressure therapy prescribed Ⓑ

✻ **G8846** Moderate or severe obstructive sleep apnea (Apnea Hypopnea Index (AHI) or Respiratory Disturbance Index (RDI) of 15 or greater) Ⓑ

~~G8848 Mild obstructive sleep apnea (Apnea Hypopnea Index (AHI) or Respiratory Disturbance Index (RDI) of less than 15)~~ ✖

✻ **G8849** Documentation of reason(s) for not prescribing positive airway pressure therapy (e.g., patient unable to tolerate, alternative therapies use, patient declined, financial, insurance coverage) Ⓑ

✻ **G8850** Positive airway pressure therapy not prescribed, reason not given Ⓑ

✻ **G8851** Objective measurement of adherence to positive airway pressure therapy, documented Ⓑ

▶ New ⮌ Revised ✔ Reinstated ~~deleted~~ Deleted ⊘ Not covered or valid by Medicare
Special coverage instructions ✻ Carrier discretion Ⓑ Bill local carrier Ⓑ Bill DME MAC

✻ **G8852** Positive airway pressure therapy prescribed Ⓑ

~~G8853 Positive airway pressure therapy not prescribed~~ ✖

✻ **G8854** Documentation of reason(s) for not objectively measuring adherence to positive airway pressure therapy (e.g., patient didn't bring data from continuous positive airway pressure [CPAP], therapy was not yet initiated, not available on machine) Ⓑ

✻ **G8855** Objective measurement of adherence to positive airway pressure therapy not performed, reason not given Ⓑ

✻ **G8856** Referral to a physician for an otologic evaluation performed Ⓑ

✻ **G8857** Patient is not eligible for the referral for otologic evaluation measure (e.g., patients who are already under the care of a physician for acute or chronic dizziness) Ⓑ

✻ **G8858** Referral to a physician for an otologic evaluation not performed, reason not given Ⓑ

✻ **G8861** Within the past 2 years, central dual-energy x-ray absorptiometry (DXA) ordered and documented, review of systems and medication history or pharmacologic therapy (other than minerals/vitamins) for osteoporosis prescribed Ⓑ

✻ **G8863** Patients not assessed for risk of bone loss, reason not given Ⓑ

✻ **G8864** Pneumococcal vaccine administered or previously received Ⓑ

✻ **G8865** Documentation of medical reason(s) for not administering or previously receiving pneumococcal vaccine (e.g., patient allergic reaction, potential adverse drug reaction) Ⓑ

✻ **G8866** Documentation of patient reason(s) for not administering or previously receiving pneumococcal vaccine (e.g., patient refusal) Ⓑ

✻ **G8867** Pneumococcal vaccine not administered or previously received, reason not given Ⓑ

~~G8868 Patients receiving a first course of anti-TNF therapy~~

✻ **G8869** Patient has documented immunity to hepatitis B and is receiving a first course of anti-TNF therapy Ⓑ

✻ **G8872** Excised tissue evaluated by imaging intraoperatively to confirm successful inclusion of targeted lesion Ⓑ

✻ **G8873** Patients with needle localization specimens which are not amenable to intraoperative imaging such as MRI needle wire localization, or targets which are tentatively identified on mammogram or ultrasound which do not contain a biopsy marker but which can be verified on intraoperative inspection or pathology (e.g., needle biopsy site where the biopsy marker is remote from the actual biopsy site) Ⓑ

✻ **G8874** Excised tissue not evaluated by imaging intraoperatively to confirm successful inclusion of targeted lesion Ⓑ

✻ **G8875** Clinician diagnosed breast cancer preoperatively by a minimally invasive biopsy method Ⓑ

✻ **G8876** Documentation of reason(s) for not performing minimally invasive biopsy to diagnose breast cancer preoperatively (e.g., lesion too close to skin, implant, chest wall, etc., lesion could not be adequately visualized for needle biopsy, patient condition prevents needle biopsy [weight, breast thickness, etc.], duct excision without imaging abnormality, prophylactic mastectomy, reduction mammoplasty, excisional biopsy performed by another physician) Ⓑ

✻ **G8877** Clinician did not attempt to achieve the diagnosis of breast cancer preoperatively by a minimally invasive biopsy method, reason not given Ⓑ

✻ **G8878** Sentinel lymph node biopsy procedure performed Ⓑ

✻ **G8879** Clinically node negative (T1N0M0 or T2N0M0) invasive breast cancer Ⓑ

✻ **G8880** Documentation of reason(s) sentinel lymph node biopsy not performed (e.g., reasons could include but not limited to; non-invasive cancer, incidental discovery of breast cancer on prophylactic mastectomy, incidental discovery of breast cancer on reduction mammoplasty, pre-operative biopsy proven lymph node (LN) metastases, inflammatory carcinoma, stage 3 locally advanced cancer, recurrent invasive breast cancer, patient refusal after informed consent) Ⓑ

✻ **G8881** Stage of breast cancer is greater than T1N0M0 or T2N0M0 Ⓑ

✻ **G8882** Sentinel lymph node biopsy procedure not performed, reason not given Ⓑ

✻ **G8883** Biopsy results reviewed, communicated, tracked and documented Ⓑ

✻ **G8884** Clinician documented reason that patient's biopsy results were not reviewed Ⓑ

✻ **G8885** Biopsy results not reviewed, communicated, tracked or documented Ⓑ

~~G8898 I intend to report the chronic obstructive pulmonary disease (COPD) measures group~~ ✖

~~G8899 I intend to report the inflammatory bowel disease (IBD) measures group~~ ✖

~~G8900 I intend to report the sleep apnea measures group~~ ✖

~~G8902 I intend to report the dementia measures group~~ ✖

~~G8903 I intend to report the Parkinson's disease measures group~~ ✖

~~G8906 I intend to report the cataract measures group~~ ✖

✻ **G8907** Patient documented not to have experienced any of the following events: a burn prior to discharge; a fall within the facility; wrong site/side/patient/procedure/implant event; or a hospital transfer or hospital admission upon discharge from the facility Ⓑ

✻ **G8908** Patient documented to have received a burn prior to discharge Ⓑ

✻ **G8909** Patient documented not to have received a burn prior to discharge Ⓑ

✻ **G8910** Patient documented to have experienced a fall within ASC Ⓑ

✻ **G8911** Patient documented not to have experienced a fall within ambulatory surgical center Ⓑ

✻ **G8912** Patient documented to have experienced a wrong site, wrong side, wrong patient, wrong procedure or wrong implant event Ⓑ

✻ **G8913** Patient documented not to have experienced a wrong site, wrong side, wrong patient, wrong procedure or wrong implant event Ⓑ

✻ **G8914** Patient documented to have experienced a hospital transfer or hospital admission upon discharge from ASC Ⓑ

✻ **G8915** Patient documented not to have experienced a hospital transfer or hospital admission upon discharge from ASC Ⓑ

✻ **G8916** Patient with preoperative order for IV antibiotic surgical site infection (SSI) prophylaxis, antibiotic initiated on time Ⓑ

✻ **G8917** Patient with preoperative order for IV antibiotic surgical site infection (SSI) prophylaxis, antibiotic not initiated on time Ⓑ

✻ **G8918** Patient without preoperative order for IV antibiotic surgical site infection (SSI) prophylaxis Ⓑ

✻ **G8923** Left ventricular ejection fraction (LVEF) < 40% or documentation of moderately or severely depressed left ventricular systolic function Ⓑ

⮌ ✻ **G8924** Spirometry test results demonstrate FEV1/FVC < 70%, FEV <60% predicted and patient has COPD symptoms (e.g., dyspnea, cough/sputum, wheezing) Ⓑ

⮌ ✻ **G8925** Spirometry test results demonstrate FEV1 > = 60% FEV1/FVC > = 70%, predicted or patient does not have COPD symptoms Ⓑ

✻ **G8926** Spirometry test not performed or documented, reason not given Ⓑ

~~G8927 Adjuvant chemotherapy referred, prescribed or previously received for AJCC stage III, colon cancer~~ ✖

~~G8928 Adjuvant chemotherapy not prescribed or previously received, for documented reasons (e.g., medical co morbidities, diagnosis date more than 5 years prior to the current visit date, patient's diagnosis date is within 120 days of the end of the 12 month reporting period, patient's cancer has metastasized, medical contraindication/allergy, poor performance status, other medical reasons, patient refusal, other patient reasons, patient is currently enrolled in a clinical trial that precludes prescription of chemotherapy, other system reasons)~~ ✖

~~G8929 Adjuvant chemotherapy not prescribed or previously received, reason not given~~ ✖

✻ **G8934** Left ventricular ejection fraction (LVEF) < 40% or documentation of moderately or severely depressed left ventricular systolic function Ⓑ

✻ **G8935** Clinician prescribed angiotensin converting enzyme (ACE) inhibitor or angiotensin receptor blocker (ARB) therapy Ⓑ

✻ **G8936** Clinician documented that patient was not an eligible candidate for angiotensin converting enzyme (ACE) inhibitor or angiotensin receptor blocker (ARB) therapy (eg, allergy, intolerance, pregnancy, renal failure due to ace inhibitor, diseases of the aortic or mitral valve, other medical reasons) or (eg, patient declined, other patient reasons) or (eg, lack of drug availability, other reasons attributable to the health care system) Ⓑ

✻ **G8937** Clinician did not prescribe angiotensin converting enzyme (ACE) inhibitor or angiotensin receptor blocker (ARB) therapy, reason not given Ⓑ

✻ **G8938** BMI is documented as being outside of normal limits, follow-up plan is not documented, documentation the patient is not eligible Ⓑ

✻ **G8939** Pain assessment documented as positive, follow-up plan not documented, documentation the patient is not eligible Ⓑ

~~G8940 Screening for clinical depression documented as positive, a follow up plan not documented, documentation stating the patient is not eligible~~ ✖

✻ **G8941** Elder maltreatment screen documented as positive, follow-up plan not documented, documentation the patient is not eligible Ⓑ

✻ **G8942** Functional outcomes assessment using a standardized tool is documented within the previous 30 days and care plan, based on identified deficiencies on the date of the functional outcome assessment, is documented Ⓑ

✻ **G8944** AJCC melanoma cancer stage 0 through IIC melanoma Ⓑ

✻ **G8946** Minimally invasive biopsy method attempted but not diagnostic of breast cancer (e.g., high risk lesion of breast such as atypical ductal hyperplasia, lobular neoplasia, atypical lobular hyperplasia, lobular carcinoma in situ, atypical columnar hyperplasia, flat epithelial atypia, radial scar, complex sclerosing lesion, papillary lesion, or any lesion with spindle cells) Ⓑ

✻ **G8947** One or more neuropsychiatric symptoms Ⓑ

~~G8948 No neuropsychiatric symptoms~~ ✖

✻ **G8950** Pre-hypertensive or hypertensive blood pressure reading documented, and the indicated follow-up documented Ⓑ

✻ **G8952** Pre-hypertensive or hypertensive blood pressure reading documented, indicated follow-up not documented, reason not given Ⓑ

~~G8953 All quality actions for the applicable measures in the oncology measures group have been performed for this patient~~ ✖

✻ **G8955** Most recent assessment of adequacy of volume management documented Ⓑ

✻ **G8956** Patient receiving maintenance hemodialysis in an outpatient dialysis facility Ⓑ

✻ **G8958** Assessment of adequacy of volume management not documented, reason not given Ⓑ

✻ **G8959** Clinician treating major depressive disorder communicates to clinician treating comorbid condition Ⓑ

✻ **G8960** Clinician treating major depressive disorder did not communicate to clinician treating comorbid condition, reason not given Ⓑ

✻ **G8961** Cardiac stress imaging test primarily performed on low-risk surgery patient for preoperative evaluation within 30 days preceding this surgery Ⓑ

✻ **G8962** Cardiac stress imaging test performed on patient for any reason including those who did not have low risk surgery or test that was performed more than 30 days preceding low risk surgery Ⓑ

✻ **G8963** Cardiac stress imaging performed primarily for monitoring of asymptomatic patient who had PCI within 2 years Ⓑ

✻ **G8964** Cardiac stress imaging test performed primarily for any other reason than monitoring of asymptomatic patient who had PCI within 2 years (e.g., symptomatic patient, patient greater than 2 years since PCI, initial evaluation, etc.) Ⓑ

✻ **G8965** Cardiac stress imaging test primarily performed on low CHD risk patient for initial detection and risk assessment Ⓑ

✻ **G8966** Cardiac stress imaging test performed on symptomatic or higher than low CHD risk patient or for any reason other than initial detection and risk assessment Ⓑ

✻ **G8967** Warfarin or another oral anticoagulant that is FDA approved prescribed Ⓑ

↩ * **G8968** Documentation of medical reason(s) for not prescribing warfarin or another oral anticoagulant that is FDA approved for the prevention of thromboembolism (e.g., allergy, risk of bleeding, other medical reasons) Ⓑ

* **G8969** Documentation of patient reason(s) for not prescribing warfarin or another oral anticoagulant that is FDA approved (e.g., economic, social, and/or religious impediments, noncompliance patient refusal, other patient reasons) Ⓑ

* **G8970** No risk factors or one moderate risk factor for thromboembolism Ⓑ

* **G8971** Warfarin or another oral anticoagulant that is FDA approved not prescribed, reason not given Ⓑ

* **G8972** One or more high risk factors for thromboembolism or more than one moderate risk factor for thromboembolism Ⓑ

* **G8973** Most recent hemoglobin (Hgb) level < 10 g/dl Ⓑ

* **G8974** Hemoglobin level measurement not documented, reason not given Ⓑ

* **G8975** Documentation of medical reason(s) for patient having a hemoglobin level < 10 g/dl (e.g., patients who have non-renal etiologies of anemia [e.g., sickle cell anemia or other hemoglobinopathies, hypersplenism, primary bone marrow disease, anemia related to chemotherapy for diagnosis of malignancy, postoperative bleeding, active bloodstream or peritoneal infection], other medical reasons) Ⓑ

* **G8976** Most recent hemoglobin (Hgb) level >= 10 g/dl Ⓑ

~~G8977 I intend to report the oncology measures group~~ ✖

* **G8978** Mobility: walking & moving around functional limitation, current status, at therapy episode outset and at reporting intervals Ⓑ

* **G8979** Mobility: walking & moving around functional limitation, projected goal status, at therapy episode outset, at reporting intervals, and at discharge or to end reporting Ⓑ

* **G8980** Mobility: walking & moving around functional limitation, discharge status, at discharge from therapy or to end reporting Ⓑ

* **G8981** Changing & maintaining body position functional limitation, current status, at therapy episode outset and at reporting intervals Ⓑ

* **G8982** Changing & maintaining body position functional limitation, projected goal status, at therapy episode outset, at reporting intervals, and at discharge or to end reporting Ⓑ

* **G8983** Changing & maintaining body position functional limitation, discharge status, at discharge from therapy or to end reporting Ⓑ

* **G8984** Carrying, moving & handling objects functional limitation, current status, at therapy episode outset and at reporting intervals Ⓑ

* **G8985** Carrying, moving and handling objects, projected goal status, at therapy episode outset, at reporting intervals, and at discharge or to end reporting Ⓑ

* **G8986** Carrying, moving & handling objects functional limitation, discharge status, at discharge from therapy or to end reporting Ⓑ

* **G8987** Self-care functional limitation, current status, at therapy episode outset and at reporting intervals Ⓑ

* **G8988** Self-care functional limitation, projected goal status, at therapy episode outset, at reporting intervals, and at discharge or to end reporting Ⓑ

* **G8989** Self-care functional limitation, discharge status, at discharge from therapy or to end reporting Ⓑ

* **G8990** Other physical or occupational therapy primary functional limitation, current status, at therapy episode outset and at reporting intervals Ⓑ

* **G8991** Other physical or occupational therapy primary functional limitation, projected goal status, at therapy episode outset, at reporting intervals, and at discharge or to end reporting Ⓑ

* **G8992** Other physical or occupational therapy primary functional limitation, discharge status, at discharge from therapy or to end reporting Ⓑ

* **G8993** Other physical or occupational therapy subsequent functional limitation, current status, at therapy episode outset and at reporting intervals Ⓑ

✻ **G8994** Other physical or occupational therapy subsequent functional limitation, projected goal status, at therapy episode outset, at reporting intervals, and at discharge or to end reporting Ⓑ

✻ **G8995** Other physical or occupational therapy subsequent functional limitation, discharge status, at discharge from therapy or to end reporting Ⓑ

✻ **G8996** Swallowing functional limitation, current status at therapy episode outset and at reporting intervals Ⓑ

✻ **G8997** Swallowing functional limitation, projected goal status, at therapy episode outset, at reporting intervals, and at discharge or to end reporting Ⓑ

✻ **G8998** Swallowing functional limitation, discharge status, at discharge from therapy or to end reporting Ⓑ

✻ **G8999** Motor speech functional limitation, current status at therapy episode outset and at reporting intervals Ⓑ

✪ **G9001** Coordinated care fee, initial rate Ⓑ

✪ **G9002** Coordinated care fee, maintenance rate Ⓑ

✪ **G9003** Coordinated care fee, risk adjusted high, initial Ⓑ

✪ **G9004** Coordinated care fee, risk adjusted low, initial Ⓑ

✪ **G9005** Coordinated care fee, risk adjusted maintenance Ⓑ

✪ **G9006** Coordinated care fee, home monitoring Ⓑ

✪ **G9007** Coordinated care fee, scheduled team conference Ⓑ

✪ **G9008** Coordinated care fee, physician coordinated care oversight services Ⓑ

✪ **G9009** Coordinated care fee, risk adjusted maintenance, level 3 Ⓑ

✪ **G9010** Coordinated care fee, risk adjusted maintenance, level 4 Ⓑ

✪ **G9011** Coordinated care fee, risk adjusted maintenance, level 5 Ⓑ

✪ **G9012** Other specified case management services not elsewhere classified Ⓑ

⊘ **G9013** ESRD demo basic bundle Level I Ⓑ

⊘ **G9014** ESRD demo expanded bundle, including venous access and related services Ⓑ

⊘ **G9016** Smoking cessation counseling, individual, in the absence of or in addition to any other evaluation and management service, per session (6-10 minutes) [demo project code only] Ⓑ

✻ **G9017** Amantadine hydrochloride, oral, per 100 mg (for use in a Medicare-approved demonstration project) Ⓑ

✻ **G9018** Zanamivir, inhalation powder, administered through inhaler, per 10 mg (for use in a Medicare-approved demonstration project) Ⓑ

✻ **G9019** Oseltamivir phosphate, oral, per 75 mg (for use in a Medicare-approved demonstration project) Ⓑ

✻ **G9020** Rimantadine hydrochloride, oral, per 100 mg (for use in a Medicare-approved demonstration project) Ⓑ

✻ **G9033** Amantadine hydrochloride, oral brand, per 100 mg (for use in a Medicare-approved demonstration project) Ⓑ

✻ **G9034** Zanamivir, inhalation powder, administered through inhaler, brand, per 10 mg (for use in a Medicare-approved demonstration project) Ⓑ

✻ **G9035** Oseltamivir phosphate, oral, brand, per 75 mg (for use in a Medicare-approved demonstration project) Ⓑ

✻ **G9036** Rimantadine hydrochloride, oral, brand, per 100 mg (for use in a Medicare-approved demonstration project) Ⓑ

⊘ **G9050** Oncology; primary focus of visit; work-up, evaluation, or staging at the time of cancer diagnosis or recurrence (for use in a Medicare-approved demonstration project) Ⓑ

⊘ **G9051** Oncology; primary focus of visit; treatment decision-making after disease is staged or restaged, discussion of treatment options, supervising/coordinating active cancer directed therapy or managing consequences of cancer directed therapy (for use in a Medicare-approved demonstration project) Ⓑ

⊘ **G9052** Oncology; primary focus of visit; surveillance for disease recurrence for patient who has completed definitive cancer-directed therapy and currently lacks evidence of recurrent disease; cancer directed therapy might be considered in the future (for use in a Medicare-approved demonstration project) Ⓑ

▶ New ⤾ Revised ✔ Reinstated ~~deleted~~ Deleted ⊘ Not covered or valid by Medicare
✪ Special coverage instructions ✻ Carrier discretion Ⓑ Bill local carrier Ⓓ Bill DME MAC

⃠ **G9053** Oncology; primary focus of visit; expectant management of patient with evidence of cancer for whom no cancer directed therapy is being administered or arranged at present; cancer directed therapy might be considered in the future (for use in a Medicare-approved demonstration project) Ⓑ

⃠ **G9054** Oncology; primary focus of visit; supervising, coordinating or managing care of patient with terminal cancer or for whom other medical illness prevents further cancer treatment; includes symptom management, end-of-life care planning, management of palliative therapies (for use in a Medicare-approved demonstration project) Ⓑ

⃠ **G9055** Oncology; primary focus of visit; other, unspecified service not otherwise listed (for use in a Medicare-approved demonstration project) Ⓑ

⃠ **G9056** Oncology; practice guidelines; management adheres to guidelines (for use in a Medicare-approved demonstration project) Ⓑ

⃠ **G9057** Oncology; practice guidelines; management differs from guidelines as a result of patient enrollment in an institutional review board approved clinical trial (for use in a Medicare-approved demonstration project) Ⓑ

⃠ **G9058** Oncology; practice guidelines; management differs from guidelines because the treating physician disagrees with guideline recommendations (for use in a Medicare-approved demonstration project) Ⓑ

⃠ **G9059** Oncology; practice guidelines; management differs from guidelines because the patient, after being offered treatment consistent with guidelines, has opted for alternative treatment or management, including no treatment (for use in a Medicare-approved demonstration project) Ⓑ

⃠ **G9060** Oncology; practice guidelines; management differs from guidelines for reason(s) associated with patient comorbid illness or performance status not factored into guidelines (for use in a Medicare-approved demonstration project) Ⓑ

⃠ **G9061** Oncology; practice guidelines; patient's condition not addressed by available guidelines (for use in a Medicare-approved demonstration project) Ⓑ

⃠ **G9062** Oncology; practice guidelines; management differs from guidelines for other reason(s) not listed (for use in a Medicare-approved demonstration project) Ⓑ

* **G9063** Oncology; disease status; limited to non-small cell lung cancer; extent of disease initially established as stage I (prior to neo-adjuvant therapy, if any) with no evidence of disease progression, recurrence, or metastases (for use in a Medicare-approved demonstration project) Ⓑ

* **G9064** Oncology; disease status; limited to non-small cell lung cancer; extent of disease initially established as stage II (prior to neo-adjuvant therapy, if any) with no evidence of disease progression, recurrence, or metastases (for use in a Medicare-approved demonstration project) Ⓑ

* **G9065** Oncology; disease status; limited to non-small cell lung cancer; extent of disease initially established as stage IIIA (prior to neo-adjuvant therapy, if any) with no evidence of disease progression, recurrence, or metastases (for use in a Medicare-approved demonstration project) Ⓑ

* **G9066** Oncology; disease status; limited to non-small cell lung cancer; stage IIIB-IV at diagnosis, metastatic, locally recurrent, or progressive (for use in a Medicare-approved demonstration project) Ⓑ

* **G9067** Oncology; disease status; limited to non-small cell lung cancer; extent of disease unknown, staging in progress, or not listed (for use in a Medicare-approved demonstration project) Ⓑ

* **G9068** Oncology; disease status; limited to small cell and combined small cell/non-small cell; extent of disease initially established as limited with no evidence of disease progression, recurrence, or metastases (for use in a Medicare-approved demonstration project) Ⓑ

* **G9069** Oncology; disease status; small cell lung cancer, limited to small cell and combined small cell/non-small cell; extensive stage at diagnosis, metastatic, locally recurrent, or progressive (for use in a Medicare-approved demonstration project) Ⓑ

✻ **G9070** Oncology; disease status; small cell lung cancer, limited to small cell and combined small cell/non-small cell; extent of disease unknown, staging in progress, or not listed (for use in a Medicare-approved demonstration project) Ⓑ

✻ **G9071** Oncology; disease status; invasive female breast cancer (does not include ductal carcinoma in situ); adenocarcinoma as predominant cell type; stage I or stage IIA-IIB; or T3, N1, M0; and ER and/or PR positive; with no evidence of disease progression, recurrence, or metastases (for use in a Medicare-approved demonstration project) Ⓑ

✻ **G9072** Oncology; disease status; invasive female breast cancer (does not include ductal carcinoma in situ); adenocarcinoma as predominant cell type; stage I, or stage IIA-IIB; or T3, N1, M0; and ER and PR negative; with no evidence of disease progression, recurrence, or metastases (for use in a Medicare-approved demonstration project) Ⓑ

✻ **G9073** Oncology; disease status; invasive female breast cancer (does not include ductal carcinoma in situ); adenocarcinoma as predominant cell type; stage IIIA-IIIB; and not T3, N1, M0; and ER and/or PR positive; with no evidence of disease progression, recurrence, or metastases (for use in a Medicare-approved demonstration project) Ⓑ

✻ **G9074** Oncology; disease status; invasive female breast cancer (does not include ductal carcinoma in situ); adenocarcinoma as predominant cell type; stage IIIA-IIIB; and not T3, N1, M0; and ER and PR negative; with no evidence of disease progression, recurrence, or metastases (for use in a Medicare-approved demonstration project) Ⓑ

✻ **G9075** Oncology; disease status; invasive female breast cancer (does not include ductal carcinoma in situ); adenocarcinoma as predominant cell type; M1 at diagnosis, metastatic, locally recurrent, or progressive (for use in a Medicare-approved demonstration project) Ⓑ

✻ **G9077** Oncology; disease status; prostate cancer, limited to adenocarcinoma as predominant cell type; T1-T2c and Gleason 2-7 and PSA < or equal to 20 at diagnosis with no evidence of disease progression, recurrence, or metastases (for use in a Medicare-approved demonstration project) Ⓑ

✻ **G9078** Oncology; disease status; prostate cancer, limited to adenocarcinoma as predominant cell type; T2 or T3a Gleason 8-10 or PSA > 20 at diagnosis with no evidence of disease progression, recurrence, or metastases (for use in a Medicare-approved demonstration project) Ⓑ

✻ **G9079** Oncology; disease status; prostate cancer, limited to adenocarcinoma as predominant cell type; T3b-T4, any N; any T, N1 at diagnosis with no evidence of disease progression, recurrence, or metastases (for use in a Medicare-approved demonstration project) Ⓑ

✻ **G9080** Oncology; disease status; prostate cancer, limited to adenocarcinoma; after initial treatment with rising PSA or failure of PSA decline (for use in a Medicare-approved demonstration project) Ⓑ

✻ **G9083** Oncology; disease status; prostate cancer, limited to adenocarcinoma; extent of disease unknown, staging in progress, or not listed (for use in a Medicare-approved demonstration project) Ⓑ

✻ **G9084** Oncology; disease status; colon cancer, limited to invasive cancer, adenocarcinoma as predominant cell type; extent of disease initially established as T1-3, N0, M0 with no evidence of disease progression, recurrence, or metastases (for use in a Medicare-approved demonstration project) Ⓑ

✻ **G9085** Oncology; disease status; colon cancer, limited to invasive cancer, adenocarcinoma as predominant cell type; extent of disease initially established as T4, N0, M0 with no evidence of disease progression, recurrence, or metastases (for use in a Medicare-approved demonstration project) Ⓑ

* **G9086** Oncology; disease status; colon cancer, limited to invasive cancer, adenocarcinoma as predominant cell type; extent of disease initially established as T1-4, N1-2, M0 with no evidence of disease progression, recurrence, or metastases (for use in a Medicare-approved demonstration project) Ⓑ

* **G9087** Oncology; disease status; colon cancer, limited to invasive cancer, adenocarcinoma as predominant cell type; M1 at diagnosis, metastatic, locally recurrent, or progressive with current clinical, radiologic, or biochemical evidence of disease (for use in a Medicare-approved demonstration project) Ⓑ

* **G9088** Oncology; disease status; colon cancer, limited to invasive cancer, adenocarcinoma as predominant cell type; M1 at diagnosis, metastatic, locally recurrent, or progressive without current clinical, radiologic, or biochemical evidence of disease (for use in a Medicare-approved demonstration project) Ⓑ

* **G9089** Oncology; disease status; colon cancer, limited to invasive cancer, adenocarcinoma as predominant cell type; extent of disease unknown, staging in progress, or not listed (for use in a Medicare-approved demonstration project) Ⓑ

* **G9090** Oncology; disease status; rectal cancer, limited to invasive cancer, adenocarcinoma as predominant cell type; extent of disease initially established as T1-2, N0, M0 (prior to neo-adjuvant therapy, if any) with no evidence of disease progression, recurrence, or metastases (for use in a Medicare-approved demonstration project) Ⓑ

* **G9091** Oncology; disease status; rectal cancer, limited to invasive cancer, adenocarcinoma as predominant cell type; extent of disease initially established as T3, N0, M0 (prior to neo-adjuvant therapy, if any) with no evidence of disease progression, recurrence, or metastases (for use in a Medicare-approved demonstration project) Ⓑ

* **G9092** Oncology; disease status; rectal cancer, limited to invasive cancer, adenocarcinoma as predominant cell type; extent of disease initially established as T1-3, N1-2, M0 (prior to neo-adjuvant therapy, if any) with no evidence of disease progression, recurrence or metastases (for use in a Medicare-approved demonstration project) Ⓑ

* **G9093** Oncology; disease status; rectal cancer, limited to invasive cancer, adenocarcinoma as predominant cell type; extent of disease initially established as T4, any N, M0 (prior to neo-adjuvant therapy, if any) with no evidence of disease progression, recurrence, or metastases (for use in a Medicare-approved demonstration project) Ⓑ

* **G9094** Oncology; disease status; rectal cancer, limited to invasive cancer, adenocarcinoma as predominant cell type; M1 at diagnosis, metastatic, locally recurrent, or progressive (for use in a Medicare-approved demonstration project) Ⓑ

* **G9095** Oncology; disease status; rectal cancer, limited to invasive cancer, adenocarcinoma as predominant cell type; extent of disease unknown, staging in progress, or not listed (for use in a Medicare-approved demonstration project) Ⓑ

* **G9096** Oncology; disease status; esophageal cancer, limited to adenocarcinoma or squamous cell carcinoma as predominant cell type; extent of disease initially established as T1-T3, N0-N1 or NX (prior to neo-adjuvant therapy, if any) with no evidence of disease progression, recurrence, or metastases (for use in a Medicare-approved demonstration project) Ⓑ

* **G9097** Oncology; disease status; esophageal cancer, limited to adenocarcinoma or squamous cell carcinoma as predominant cell type; extent of disease initially established as T4, any N, M0 (prior to neo-adjuvant therapy, if any) with no evidence of disease progression, recurrence, or metastases (for use in a Medicare-approved demonstration project) Ⓑ

* **G9098** Oncology; disease status; esophageal cancer, limited to adenocarcinoma or squamous cell carcinoma as predominant cell type; M1 at diagnosis, meta-static, locally recurrent, or progressive (for use in a Medicare-approved demonstration project) Ⓑ

* **G9099** Oncology; disease status; esophageal cancer, limited to adenocarcinoma or squamous cell carcinoma as predominant cell type; extent of disease unknown, staging in progress, or not listed (for use in a Medicare-approved demonstration project) Ⓑ

* **G9100** Oncology; disease status; gastric cancer, limited to adenocarcinoma as predominant cell type; post R0 resection (with or without neoadjuvant therapy) with no evidence of disease recurrence, progression, or metastases (for use in a Medicare-approved demonstration project) Ⓑ

* **G9101** Oncology; disease status; gastric cancer, limited to adenocarcinoma as predominant cell type; post R1 or R2 resection (with or without neoadjuvant therapy) with no evidence of disease progression, or metastases (for use in a Medicare-approved demonstration project) Ⓑ

* **G9102** Oncology; disease status; gastric cancer, limited to adenocarcinoma as predominant cell type; clinical or pathologic M0, unresectable with no evidence of disease progression, or metastases (for use in a Medicare-approved demonstration project Ⓑ

* **G9103** Oncology; disease status; gastric cancer, limited to adenocarcinoma as predominant cell type; clinical or pathologic M1 at diagnosis, metastatic, locally recurrent, or progressive (for use in a Medicare-approved demonstration project) Ⓑ

* **G9104** Oncology; disease status; gastric cancer, limited to adenocarcinoma as predominant cell type; extent of disease unknown, staging in progress, or not listed (for use in a Medicare-approved demonstration project Ⓑ

* **G9105** Oncology; disease status; pancreatic cancer, limited to adenocarcinoma as predominant cell type; post R0 resection without evidence of disease progression, recurrence, or metastases (for use in a Medicare-approved demonstration project) Ⓑ

* **G9106** Oncology; disease status; pancreatic cancer, limited to adenocarcinoma; post R1 or R2 resection with no evidence of disease progression or metastases (for use in a Medicare-approved demonstration project) Ⓑ

* **G9107** Oncology; disease status; pancreatic cancer, limited to adenocarcinoma; unresectable at diagnosis, M1 at diagnosis, metastatic, locally recurrent, or progressive (for use in a Medicare-approved demonstration project) Ⓑ

* **G9108** Oncology; disease status; pancreatic cancer, limited to adenocarcinoma; extent of disease unknown, staging in progress, or not listed (for use in a Medicare-approved demonstration project) Ⓑ

* **G9109** Oncology; disease status; head and neck cancer, limited to cancers of oral cavity, pharynx and larynx with squamous cell as predominant cell type; extent of disease initially established as T1-T2 and N0, M0 (prior to neo-adjuvant therapy, if any) with no evidence of disease progression, recurrence, or metastases (for use in a Medicare-approved demonstration project) Ⓑ

* **G9110** Oncology; disease status; head and neck cancer, limited to cancers of oral cavity, pharynx, and larynx with squamous cell as predominant cell type; extent of disease initially established as T3-4 and/ or N1-3, M0 (prior to neo-adjuvant therapy, if any) with no evidence of disease progression, recurrence, or metastases (for use in a Medicare-approved demonstration project) Ⓑ

* **G9111** Oncology; disease status; head and neck cancer, limited to cancers of oral cavity, pharynx and larynx with squamous cell as predominant cell type; M1 at diagnosis, metastatic, locally recurrent, or progressive (for use in a Medicare-approved demonstration project) Ⓑ

* **G9112** Oncology; disease status; head and neck cancer, limited to cancers of oral cavity, pharynx and larynx with squamous cell as predominant cell type; extent of disease unknown, staging in progress, or not listed (for use in a Medicare-approved demonstration project) Ⓑ

* **G9113** Oncology; disease status; ovarian cancer, limited to epithelial cancer; pathologic stage IA-B (grade 1) without evidence of disease progression, recurrence, or metastases (for use in a Medicare-approved demonstration project) Ⓑ

* **G9114** Oncology; disease status; ovarian cancer, limited to epithelial cancer; pathologic stage IA-B (grade 2-3); or stage IC (all grades); or stage II; without evidence of disease progression, recurrence, or metastases (for use in a Medicare-approved demonstration project) Ⓑ

* **G9115** Oncology; disease status; ovarian cancer, limited to epithelial cancer; pathologic stage III-IV; without evidence of progression, recurrence, or metastases (for use in a Medicare-approved demonstration project) Ⓑ

* **G9116** Oncology; disease status; ovarian cancer, limited to epithelial cancer; evidence of disease progression, or recurrence and/or platinum resistance (for use in a Medicare-approved demonstration project) Ⓑ

* **G9117** Oncology; disease status; ovarian cancer, limited to epithelial cancer; extent of disease unknown, staging in progress, or not listed (for use in a Medicare-approved demonstration project) Ⓑ

* **G9123** Oncology; disease status; chronic myelogenous leukemia, limited to Philadelphia chromosome positive and/or BCR-ABL positive; chronic phase not in hematologic, cytogenetic, or molecular remission (for use in a Medicare-approved demonstration project) Ⓑ

* **G9124** Oncology; disease status; chronic myelogenous leukemia, limited to Philadelphia chromosome positive and/or BCR-ABL positive; accelerated phase not in hematologic cytogenetic, or molecular remission (for use in a Medicare-approved demonstration project) Ⓑ

* **G9125** Oncology; disease status; chronic myelogenous leukemia, limited to Philadelphia chromosome positive and/or BCR-ABL positive; blast phase not in hematologic, cytogenetic, or molecular remission (for use in a Medicare-approved demonstration project) Ⓑ

* **G9126** Oncology; disease status; chronic myelogenous leukemia, limited to Philadelphia chromosome positive and/or BCR-ABL positive; in hematologic, cytogenetic, or molecular remission (for use in a Medicare-approved demonstration project) Ⓑ

* **G9128** Oncology: disease status; limited to multiple myeloma, systemic disease; smouldering, stage I (for use in a Medicare-approved demonstration project) Ⓑ

* **G9129** Oncology; disease status; limited to multiple myeloma, systemic disease; stage II or higher (for use in a Medicare-approved demonstration project) Ⓑ

* **G9130** Oncology; disease status; limited to multiple myeloma, systemic disease; extent of disease unknown, staging in progress, or not listed (for use in a Medicare-approved demonstration project) Ⓑ

* **G9131** Oncology; disease status; invasive female breast cancer (does not include ductal carcinoma in situ); adenocarcinoma as predominant cell type; extent of disease unknown, staging in progress, or not listed (for use in a Medicare-approved demonstration project) Ⓑ

* **G9132** Oncology; disease status; prostate cancer, limited to adenocarcinoma; hormone-refractory/androgen-independent (e.g., rising PSA on anti-androgen therapy or post-orchiectomy); clinical metastases (for use in a Medicare-approved demonstration project) Ⓑ

* **G9133** Oncology; disease status; prostate cancer, limited to adenocarcinoma; hormone-responsive; clinical metastases or M1 at diagnosis (for use in a Medicare-approved demonstration project) Ⓑ

* **G9134** Oncology; disease status; non-Hodgkin's lymphoma, any cellular classification; stage I, II at diagnosis, not relapsed, not refractory (for use in a Medicare-approved demonstration project) Ⓑ

* **G9135** Oncology; disease status; non-Hodgkin's lymphoma, any cellular classification; stage III, IV, not relapsed, not refractory (for use in a Medicare-approved demonstration project) Ⓑ

✻ **G9136** Oncology; disease status; non-Hodgkin's lymphoma, transformed from original cellular diagnosis to a second cellular classification (for use in a Medicare-approved demonstration project) Ⓑ

✻ **G9137** Oncology; disease status; non-Hodgkin's lymphoma, any cellular classification; relapsed/refractory (for use in a Medicare-approved demonstration project) Ⓑ

✻ **G9138** Oncology; disease status; non-Hodgkin's lymphoma, any cellular classification; diagnostic evaluation, stage not determined, evaluation of possible relapse or non-response to therapy, or not listed (for use in a Medicare-approved demonstration project) Ⓑ

✻ **G9139** Oncology; disease status; chronic myelogenous leukemia, limited to Philadelphia chromosome positive and/or BCR-ABL positive; extent of disease unknown, staging in progress, not listed (for use in a Medicare-approved demonstration project) Ⓑ

✻ **G9140** Frontier extended stay clinic demonstration; for a patient stay in a clinic approved for the CMS demonstration project; the following measures should be present: the stay must be equal to or greater than 4 hours; weather or other conditions must prevent transfer or the case falls into a category of monitoring and observation cases that are permitted by the rules of the demonstration; there is a maximum frontier extended stay clinic (FESC) visit of 48 hours, except in the case when weather or other conditions prevent transfer; payment is made on each period up to 4 hours, after the first 4 hours Ⓑ

Influenza A (H1N1) and Warfarin Responsiveness Testing

✻ **G9143** Warfarin responsiveness testing by genetic technique using any method, any number of specimen(s) Ⓑ

This would be a once-in-a-lifetime test unless there is a reason to believe that the patient's personal genetic characteristics would change over time. (https://www.cms.gov/ContractorLearningResources/downloads/JA6715.pdf)

Laboratory Certification: General immunology,Hematology

⃠ **G9147** Outpatient intravenous insulin treatment (OIVIT) either pulsatile or continuous, by any means, guided by the results of measurements for: respiratory quotient; and/or, urine urea nitrogen (UUN); and/or, arterial, venous or capillary glucose; and/or potassium concentration Ⓑ

On December 23, 2009, CMS issued a national non-coverage decision on the use of OIVIT. CR 6775.

Not covered on Physician Fee Schedule

✻ **G9148** National committee for quality assurance - level 1 medical home Ⓑ

✻ **G9149** National committee for quality assurance - level 2 medical home Ⓑ

✻ **G9150** National committee for quality assurance - level 3 medical home Ⓑ

✻ **G9151** MAPCP demonstration - state provided services Ⓑ

✻ **G9152** MAPCP demonstration - community health teams Ⓑ

✻ **G9153** MAPCP demonstration - physician incentive pool Ⓑ

✻ **G9156** Evaluation for wheelchair requiring face to face visit with physician Ⓑ

✻ **G9157** Transesophageal doppler measurement of cardiac output (including probe placement, image acquisition, and interpretation per course of treatment) for monitoring purposes Ⓑ

✻ **G9158** Motor speech functional limitation, discharge status, at discharge from therapy or to end reporting Ⓑ

✻ **G9159** Spoken language comprehension functional limitation, current status at therapy episode outset and at reporting intervals Ⓑ

✻ **G9160** Spoken language comprehension functional limitation, projected goal status at therapy episode outset, at reporting intervals, and at discharge or to end reporting Ⓑ

✻ **G9161** Spoken language comprehension functional limitation, discharge status at discharge from therapy or to end reporting Ⓑ

✻ **G9162** Spoken language expression functional limitation, current status at therapy episode outset and at reporting intervals Ⓑ

✻ **G9163** Spoken language expression functional limitation, projected goal status at therapy episode outset, at reporting intervals, and at discharge or to end reporting Ⓑ

✻ **G9164** Spoken language expression functional limitation, discharge status at discharge from therapy or to end reporting Ⓑ

✻ **G9165** Attention functional limitation, current status at therapy episode outset and at reporting intervals Ⓑ

✻ **G9166** Attention functional limitation, projected goal status at therapy episode outset, at reporting intervals, and at discharge or to end reporting Ⓑ

✻ **G9167** Attention functional limitation, discharge status at discharge from therapy or to end reporting Ⓑ

✻ **G9168** Memory functional limitation, current status at therapy episode outset and at reporting intervals Ⓑ

✻ **G9169** Memory functional limitation, projected goal status at therapy episode outset, at reporting intervals, and at discharge or to end reporting Ⓑ

✻ **G9170** Memory functional limitation, discharge status at discharge from therapy or to end reporting Ⓑ

✻ **G9171** Voice functional limitation, current status at therapy episode outset and at reporting intervals Ⓑ

✻ **G9172** Voice functional limitation, projected goal status at therapy episode outset, at reporting intervals, and at discharge or to end reporting Ⓑ

✻ **G9173** Voice functional limitation, discharge status at discharge from therapy or to end reporting Ⓑ

✻ **G9174** Other speech language pathology functional limitation, current status at therapy episode outset and at reporting intervals Ⓑ

✻ **G9175** Other speech language pathology functional limitation, projected goal status at therapy episode outset, at reporting intervals, and at discharge or to end reporting Ⓑ

✻ **G9176** Other speech language pathology functional limitation, discharge status at discharge from therapy or to end reporting Ⓑ

✻ **G9186** Motor speech functional limitation, projected goal status at therapy episode outset, at reporting intervals, and at discharge or to end reporting Ⓑ

✻ **G9187** Bundled payments for care improvement initiative home visit for patient assessment performed by a qualified health care professional for individuals not considered homebound including, but not limited to, assessment of safety, falls, clinical status, fluid status, medication reconciliation/management, patient compliance with orders/plan of care, performance of activities of daily living, appropriateness of care setting; (for use only in the Medicare-approved bundled payments for care improvement initiative); may not be billed for a 30-day period covered by a transitional care management code Ⓑ

✻ **G9188** Beta-blocker therapy not prescribed, reason not given Ⓑ

✻ **G9189** Beta-blocker therapy prescribed or currently being taken Ⓑ

✻ **G9190** Documentation of medical reason(s) for not prescribing beta-blocker therapy (e.g., allergy, intolerance, other medical reasons) Ⓑ

✻ **G9191** Documentation of patient reason(s) for not prescribing beta-blocker therapy (e.g., patient declined, other patient reasons) Ⓑ

✻ **G9192** Documentation of system reason(s) for not prescribing beta-blocker therapy (e.g., other reasons attributable to the health care system) Ⓑ

✻ **G9196** Documentation of medical reason(s) zfor not ordering a first or second generation cephalosporin for antimicrobial prophylaxis (e.g., patients enrolled in clinical trials, patients with documented infection prior to surgical procedure of interest, patients who were receiving antibiotics more than 24 hours prior to surgery [except colon surgery patients taking oral prophylactic antibiotics], patients who were receiving antibiotics within 24 hours prior to arrival [except colon surgery patients taking oral prophylactic antibiotics], other medical reason(s)) Ⓑ

✻ **G9197** Documentation of order for first or second generation cephalosporin for antimicrobial prophylaxis Ⓑ

✻ **G9198** Order for first or second generation cephalosporin for antimicrobial prophylaxis was not documented, reason not given Ⓑ

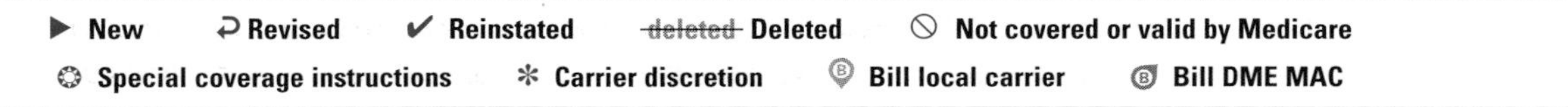

~~G9203 Rna testing for hepatitis C documented as performed within 12 months prior to initiation of antiviral treatment for hepatitis C~~ ✖

~~G9204 Rna testing for hepatitis C was not documented as performed within 12 months prior to initiation of antiviral treatment for hepatitis C, reason not given~~ ✖

~~G9205 Patient starting antiviral treatment for hepatitis C during the measurement period~~ ✖

~~G9206 Patient starting antiviral treatment for hepatitis C during the measurement period~~ ✖

~~G9207 Hepatitis C genotype testing documented as performed within 12 months prior to initiation of antiviral treatment for hepatitis C~~ ✖

~~G9208 Hepatitis C genotype testing was not documented as performed within 12 months prior to initiation of antiviral treatment for hepatitis C, reason not given~~ ✖

~~G9209 Hepatitis C quantitative RNA testing documented as performed between 4-12 weeks after the initiation of antiviral treatment~~ ✖

~~G9210 Hepatitis C quantitative RNA testing not performed between 4-12 weeks after the initiation of antiviral treatment for documented reason(s) (e.g., patients whose treatment was discontinued during the testing period prior to testing, other medical reasons, patient declined, other patient reasons)~~ ✖

~~G9211 Hepatitis C quantitative RNA testing was not documented as performed between 4-12 weeks after the initiation of antiviral treatment, reason not given~~ ✖

* **G9212** DSM-IVTM criteria for major depressive disorder documented at the initial evaluation Ⓑ

* **G9213** DSM-IV-TR criteria for major depressive disorder not documented at the initial evaluation, reason not otherwise specified Ⓑ

~~G9217 PCP prophylaxis was not prescribed within 3 months of low CD4+ cell count below 200 cells/mm3, reason not given~~ ✖

~~G9219 Pneumocystis jiroveci pneumonia prophylaxis not prescribed within 3 months of low CD4+ cell count below 200 cells/mm3 for medical reason (i.e., patient's CD4+ cell count above threshold within 3 months after CD4+ cell count below threshold, indicating that the patient's CD4+ levels are within an acceptable range and the patient does not require PCP prophylaxis)~~ ✖

~~G9222 Pneumocystis jiroveci pneumonia prophylaxis prescribed within 3 months of low CD4+ cell count below 200 cells/mm3~~ ✖

* **G9223** Pneumocystis jiroveci pneumonia prophylaxis prescribed within 3 months of low CD4+ cell count below 500 cells/mm3 or a CD4 percentage below 15% Ⓑ

* **G9225** Foot exam was not performed, reason not given Ⓑ

* **G9226** Foot examination performed (includes examination through visual inspection, sensory exam with 10-g monofilament plus testing any one of the following: vibration using 128-hz tuning fork, pinprick sensation, ankle reflexes, or vibration perception threshold, and pulse exam; report when all of the 3 components are completed) Ⓑ

* **G9227** Functional outcome assessment documented, care plan not documented, documentation the patient is not eligible for a care plan Ⓑ

* **G9228** Chlamydia, gonorrhea and syphilis screening results documented (report when results are present for all of the 3 screenings) Ⓑ

↩ * **G9229** Chlamydia, gonorrhea, and syphilis screening results not documented (patient refusal is the only allowed exception) Ⓑ

* **G9230** Chlamydia, gonorrhea, and syphilis not screened, reason not given Ⓑ

↩ * **G9231** Documentation of end stage renal disease (ESRD), dialysis, renal transplant before or during the measurement period or pregnancy during the measurement period Ⓑ

▶ New ↩ Revised ✔ Reinstated ~~deleted~~ Deleted ⊘ Not covered or valid by Medicare
✪ Special coverage instructions * Carrier discretion Ⓑ Bill local carrier Ⓓ Bill DME MAC

⊋ * **G9232** Clinician treating major depressive disorder did not communicate to clinician treating comorbid condition for specified patient reason (e.g., patient is unable to communicate the diagnosis of a comorbid condition; the patient is unwilling to communicate the diagnosis of a comorbid condition; or the patient is unaware of the comorbid condition, or any other specified patient reason) Ⓑ

~~G9233 All quality actions for the applicable measures in the total knee replacement measures group have been performed for this patient~~ ✖

~~G9234 I intend to report the total knee replacement measures group~~ ✖

~~G9235 All quality actions for the applicable measures in the general surgery measures group have been performed for this patient~~ ✖

~~G9236 All quality actions for the applicable measures in the optimizing patient exposure to ionizing radiation measures group have been performed for this patient~~ ✖

~~G9237 I intend to report the general surgery measures group~~ ✖

~~G9238 I intend to report the optimizing patient exposure to ionizing radiation measures group~~ ✖

⊋ * **G9239** Documentation of reasons for patient initiating maintenance hemodialysis with a catheter as the mode of vascular access (e.g., patient has a maturing AVF/AVG, time-limited trial of hemodialysis, other medical reasons, patient declined AVF/AVG, other patient reasons, patient followed by reporting nephrologist for fewer than 90 days, other system reasons) Ⓑ

* **G9240** Patient whose mode of vascular access is a catheter at the time maintenance hemodialysis is initiated Ⓑ

* **G9241** Patient whose mode of vascular access is not a catheter at the time maintenance hemodialysis is initiated Ⓑ

* **G9242** Documentation of viral load equal to or greater than 200 copies/ml or viral load not performed Ⓑ

* **G9243** Documentation of viral load less than 200 copies/ml Ⓑ

~~G9244 Antiretroviral therapy not prescribed~~ ✖

~~G9245 Antiretroviral therapy prescribed~~ ✖

* **G9246** Patient did not have at least one medical visit in each 6 month period of the 24 month measurement period, with a minimum of 60 days between medical visits Ⓑ

* **G9247** Patient had at least one medical visit in each 6 month period of the 24 month measurement period, with a minimum of 60 days between medical visits Ⓑ

* **G9250** Documentation of patient pain brought to a comfortable level within 48 hours from initial assessment Ⓑ

* **G9251** Documentation of patient with pain not brought to a comfortable level within 48 hours from initial assessment Ⓑ

* **G9254** Documentation of patient discharged to home later than post-operative day 2 following CAS Ⓑ

* **G9255** Documentation of patient discharged to home no later than post operative day 2 following CAS Ⓑ

* **G9256** Documentation of patient death following CAS Ⓑ

* **G9257** Documentation of patient stroke following CAS Ⓑ

* **G9258** Documentation of patient stroke following CEA Ⓑ

* **G9259** Documentation of patient survival and absence of stroke following CAS Ⓑ

* **G9260** Documentation of patient death following CEA Ⓑ

* **G9261** Documentation of patient survival and absence of stroke following CEA Ⓑ

* **G9262** Documentation of patient death in the hospital following endovascular AAA repair Ⓑ

* **G9263** Documentation of patient survival in the hospital following endovascular AAA repair Ⓑ

⊋ * **G9264** Documentation of patient receiving maintenance hemodialysis for greater than or equal to 90 days with a catheter for documented reasons (e.g., other medical reasons, patient declined AVF/AVG, other patient reasons) Ⓑ

* **G9265** Patient receiving maintenance hemodialysis for greater than or equal to 90 days with a catheter as the mode of vascular access Ⓑ

* **G9266** Patient receiving maintenance hemodialysis for greater than or equal to 90 days without a catheter as the mode of vascular access Ⓑ

▶ New ⊋ Revised ✔ Reinstated ~~deleted~~ Deleted ⊘ Not covered or valid by Medicare
⚙ Special coverage instructions * Carrier discretion Ⓑ Bill local carrier Ⓓ Bill DME MAC

* **G9267** Documentation of patient with one or more complications or mortality within 30 days
* **G9268** Documentation of patient with one or more complications within 90 days
* **G9269** Documentation of patient without one or more complications and without mortality within 30 days
* **G9270** Documentation of patient without one or more complications within 90 days
* **G9273** Blood pressure has a systolic value of <140 and a diastolic value of <90
* **G9274** Blood pressure has a systolic value of = 140 and a diastolic value of = 90 or systolic value <140 and diastolic value = 90 or systolic value = 140 and diastolic value < 90
* **G9275** Documentation that patient is a current non-tobacco user
* **G9276** Documentation that patient is a current tobacco user
* **G9277** Documentation that the patient is on daily aspirin or anti-platelet or has documentation of a valid contraindication or exception to aspirin/anti-platelet; contraindications/exceptions include anti-coagulant use, allergy to aspirin or anti-platelets, history of gastrointestinal bleed and bleeding disorder; additionally, the following exceptions documented by the physician as a reason for not taking daily aspirin or anti-platelet are acceptable (use of non-steroidal anti-inflammatory agents, documented risk for drug interaction, uncontrolled hypertension defined as >180 systolic or >110 diastolic or gastroesophageal reflux)
* **G9278** Documentation that the patient is not on daily aspirin or anti-platelet regimen
* **G9279** Pneumococcal screening performed and documentation of vaccination received prior to discharge
* **G9280** Pneumococcal vaccination not administered prior to discharge, reason not specified
* **G9281** Screening performed and documentation that vaccination not indicated/patient refusal
* **G9282** Documentation of medical reason(s) for not reporting the histological type or NSCLC-NOS classification with an explanation (e.g., biopsy taken for other purposes in a patient with a history of non-small cell lung cancer or other documented medical reasons)
* **G9283** Non small cell lung cancer biopsy and cytology specimen report documents classification into specific histologic type or classified as NSCLC-NOS with an explanation
* **G9284** Non small cell lung cancer biopsy and cytology specimen report does not document classification into specific histologic type or classified as NSCLC-NOS with an explanation
* **G9285** Specimen site other than anatomic location of lung or is not classified as non small cell lung cancer
* **G9286** Antibiotic regimen prescribed within 10 days after onset of symptoms
* **G9287** Antibiotic regimen not prescribed within 10 days after onset of symptoms
* **G9288** Documentation of medical reason(s) for not reporting the histological type or NSCLC-NOS classification with an explanation (e.g., a solitary fibrous tumor in a person with a history of non-small cell carcinoma or other documented medical reasons)
* **G9289** Non-small cell lung cancer biopsy and cytology specimen report documents classification into specific histologic type or classified as NSCLC-NOS with an explanation
* **G9290** Non-small cell lung cancer biopsy and cytology specimen report does not document classification into specific histologic type or classified as NSCLC-NOS with an explanation
* **G9291** Specimen site other than anatomic location of lung, is not classified as non small cell lung cancer or classified as NSCLC-NOS
* **G9292** Documentation of medical reason(s) for not reporting PT category and a statement on thickness and ulceration and for PT1, mitotic rate (e.g., negative skin biopsies in a patient with a history of melanoma or other documented medical reasons)
* **G9293** Pathology report does not include the PT category and a statement on thickness and ulceration and for PT1, mitotic rate

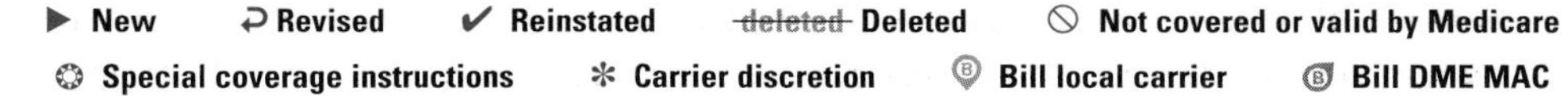

* **G9294** Pathology report includes the PT category and a statement on thickness and ulceration and for PT1, mitotic rate Ⓑ
* **G9295** Specimen site other than anatomic cutaneous location Ⓑ
* **G9296** Patients with documented shared decision-making including discussion of conservative (non-surgical) therapy (e.g., NSAIDs, analgesics, weight loss, exercise, injections) prior to the procedure Ⓑ
* **G9297** Shared decision-making including discussion of conservative (non-surgical) therapy (e.g., NSAIDs, analgesics, weight loss, exercise, injections) prior to the procedure not documented, reason not given Ⓑ
* **G9298** Patients who are evaluated for venous thromboembolic and cardiovascular risk factors within 30 days prior to the procedure (e.g., history of DVT, PE, MI, arrhythmia and stroke) Ⓑ
* **G9299** Patients who are not evaluated for venous thromboembolic and cardiovascular risk factors within 30 days prior to the procedure (e.g., history of DVT, PE, MI, arrhythmia and stroke, reason not given) Ⓑ
* **G9300** Documentation of medical reason(s) for not completely infusing the prophylactic antibiotic prior to the inflation of the proximal tourniquet (e.g., a tourniquet was not used) Ⓑ
* **G9301** Patients who had the prophylactic antibiotic completely infused prior to the inflation of the proximal tourniquet Ⓑ
* **G9302** Prophylactic antibiotic not completely infused prior to the inflation of the proximal tourniquet, reason not given Ⓑ
* **G9303** Operative report does not identify the prosthetic implant specifications including the prosthetic implant manufacturer, the brand name of the prosthetic implant and the size of each prosthetic implant, reason not given Ⓑ
* **G9304** Operative report identifies the prosthetic implant specifications including the prosthetic implant manufacturer, the brand name of the prosthetic implant and the size of each prosthetic implant Ⓑ
* **G9305** Intervention for presence of leak of endoluminal contents through an anastomosis not required Ⓑ
* **G9306** Intervention for presence of leak of endoluminal contents through an anastomosis required Ⓑ
* ⮌ * **G9307** No return to the operating room for a surgical procedure, for complications of the principal operative procedure, within 30 days of the principal operative procedure Ⓑ
* ⮌ * **G9308** Unplanned return to the operating room for a surgical procedure, for complications of the principal operative procedure, within 30 days of the principal operative procedure Ⓑ
* **G9309** No unplanned hospital readmission within 30 days of principal procedure Ⓑ
* **G9310** Unplanned hospital readmission within 30 days of principal procedure Ⓑ
* **G9311** No surgical site infection Ⓑ
* **G9312** Surgical site infection Ⓑ
* **G9313** Amoxicillin, with or without clavulanate, not prescribed as first line antibiotic at the time of diagnosis for documented reason (e.g., cystic fibrosis, immotile cilia disorders, ciliary dyskinesia, immune deficiency, prior history of sinus surgery within the past 12 months, and anatomic abnormalities, such as deviated nasal septum, resistant organisms, allergy to medication, recurrent sinusitis, chronic sinusitis, or other reasons) Ⓑ
* **G9314** Amoxicillin, with or without clavulanate, not prescribed as first line antibiotic at the time of diagnosis, reason not given Ⓑ
* **G9315** Documentation amoxicillin, with or without clavulanate, prescribed as a first line antibiotic at the time of diagnosis Ⓑ
* **G9316** Documentation of patient-specific risk assessment with a risk calculator based on multi-institutional clinical data, the specific risk calculator used, and communication of risk assessment from risk calculator with the patient or family Ⓑ
* **G9317** Documentation of patient-specific risk assessment with a risk calculator based on multi-institutional clinical data, the specific risk calculator used, and communication of risk assessment from risk calculator with the patient or family not completed Ⓑ
* **G9318** Imaging study named according to standardized nomenclature Ⓑ

▶ New ⮌ Revised ✔ Reinstated ~~deleted~~ Deleted ⊘ Not covered or valid by Medicare
Special coverage instructions * Carrier discretion Ⓑ Bill local carrier Ⓓ Bill DME MAC

* **G9319** Imaging study not named according to standardized nomenclature, reason not given Ⓑ

* **G9321** Count of previous CT (any type of CT) and cardiac nuclear medicine (myocardial perfusion) studies documented in the 12-month period prior to the current study Ⓑ

* **G9322** Count of previous CT and cardiac nuclear medicine (myocardial perfusion) studies not documented in the 12-month period prior to the current study, reason not given Ⓑ

~~G9324 All necessary data elements not included, reason not given~~ ✖

⮌ * **G9326** CT studies performed not reported to a radiation dose index registry that is capable of collecting at a minimum all necessary data elements, reason not given Ⓑ

⮌ * **G9327** CT studies performed reported to a radiation dose index registry that is capable of collecting at a minimum all necessary data elements Ⓑ

* **G9329** DICOM format image data available to non-affiliated external healthcare facilities or entities on a secure, media free, reciprocally searchable basis with patient authorization for at least a 12-month period after the study not documented in final report, reason not given Ⓑ

* **G9340** Final report documented that DICOM format image data available to non-affiliated external healthcare facilities or entities on a secure, media free, reciprocally searchable basis with patient authorization for at least a 12-month period after the study Ⓑ

* **G9341** Search conducted for prior patient CT studies completed at non-affiliated external healthcare facilities or entities within the past 12-months and are available through a secure, authorized, media-free, shared archive prior to an imaging study being performed Ⓑ

* **G9342** Search not conducted prior to an imaging study being performed for prior patient CT studies completed at non-affiliated external healthcare facilities or entities within the past 12-months and are available through a secure, authorized, media-free, shared archive, reason not given Ⓑ

* **G9344** Due to system reasons search not conducted for DICOM format images for prior patient CT imaging studies completed at non-affiliated external healthcare facilities or entities within the past 12 months that are available through a secure, authorized, media-free, shared archive (e.g., non-affiliated external healthcare facilities or entities does not have archival abilities through a shared archival system) Ⓑ

* **G9345** Follow-up recommendations documented according to recommended guidelines for incidentally detected pulmonary nodules (e.g., follow-up CT imaging studies needed or that no follow-up is needed) based at a minimum on nodule size and patient risk factors Ⓑ

* **G9347** Follow-up recommendations not documented according to recommended guidelines for incidentally detected pulmonary nodules, reason not given Ⓑ

* **G9348** CT scan of the paranasal sinuses ordered at the time of diagnosis for documented reasons (e.g., persons with sinusitis symptoms lasting at least 7 to 10 days, antibiotic resistance, immunocompromised, recurrent sinusitis, acute frontal sinusitis, acute sphenoid sinusitis, periorbital cellulitis, or other medical) Ⓑ

* **G9349** Documentation of a CT scan of the paranasal sinuses ordered at the time of diagnosis or received within 28 days after date of diagnosis Ⓑ

* **G9350** CT scan of the paranasal sinuses not ordered at the time of diagnosis or received within 28 days after date of diagnosis Ⓑ

* **G9351** More than one CT scan of the paranasal sinuses ordered or received within 90 days after diagnosis Ⓑ

* **G9352** More than one CT scan of the paranasal sinuses ordered or received within 90 days after the date of diagnosis, reason not given Ⓑ

* **G9353** More than one CT scan of the paranasal sinuses ordered or received within 90 days after the date of diagnosis for documented reasons (e.g., patients with complications, second CT obtained prior to surgery, other medical reasons) Ⓑ

* **G9354** One CT scan or no CT scan of the paranasal sinuses ordered within 90 days after the date of diagnosis Ⓑ

* **G9355** Elective delivery or early induction not performed Ⓑ

* **G9356** Elective delivery or early induction performed Ⓑ

* **G9357** Post-partum screenings, evaluations and education performed Ⓑ

* **G9358** Post-partum screenings, evaluations and education not performed Ⓑ

⊋ * **G9359** Documentation of negative or managed positive TB screen with further evidence that TB is not active within one year of patient visit Ⓑ

* **G9360** No documentation of negative or managed positive TB screen Ⓑ

⊋ * **G9361** Medical indication for induction [documentation of reason(s) for elective delivery (c-section) or early induction (e.g., hemorrhage and placental complications, hypertension, preeclampsia and eclampsia, rupture of membranes-premature or prolonged, maternal conditions complicating pregnancy/delivery, fetal conditions complicating pregnancy/delivery, late pregnancy, prior uterine surgery, or participation in clinical trial)] Ⓑ

* **G9364** Sinusitis caused by, or presumed to be caused by, bacterial infection Ⓑ

* **G9365** One high-risk medication ordered Ⓑ

* **G9366** One high-risk medication not ordered Ⓑ

* **G9367** At least two different high-risk medications ordered Ⓑ

* **G9368** At least two different high-risk medications not ordered Ⓑ

* **G9380** Patient offered assistance with end of life issues during the measurement period Ⓑ

⊋ * **G9381** Documentation of medical reason(s) for not offering assistance with end of life issues (e.g., patient in hospice care, patient in terminal phase) during the measurement period Ⓑ

* **G9382** Patient not offered assistance with end of life issues during the measurement period Ⓑ

* **G9383** Patient received screening for HCV infection within the 12 month reporting period Ⓑ

* **G9384** Documentation of medical reason(s) for not receiving annual screening for HCV infection (e.g., decompensated cirrhosis indicating advanced disease [i.e., ascites, esophageal variceal bleeding, hepatic encephalopathy], hepatocellular carcinoma, waitlist for organ transplant, limited life expectancy, other medical reasons) Ⓑ

* **G9385** Documentation of patient reason(s) for not receiving annual screening for HCV infection (e.g., patient declined, other patient reasons) Ⓑ

* **G9386** Screening for HCV infection not received within the 12 month reporting period, reason not given Ⓑ

* **G9389** Unplanned rupture of the posterior capsule requiring vitrectomy during cataract surgery Ⓑ

* **G9390** No unplanned rupture of the posterior capsule requiring vitrectomy during cataract surgery Ⓑ

* **G9393** Patient with an initial PHQ-9 score greater than nine who achieves remission at twelve months as demonstrated by a twelve month (+/- 30 days) PHQ-9 score of less than five Ⓑ

* **G9394** Patient who had a diagnosis of bipolar disorder or personality disorder, death, permanent nursing home resident or receiving hospice or palliative care any time during the measurement or assessment period Ⓑ

* **G9395** Patient with an initial PHQ-9 score greater than nine who did not achieve remission at twelve months as demonstrated by a twelve month (+/- 30 days) PHQ-9 score greater than or equal to five Ⓑ

* **G9396** Patient with an initial PHQ-9 score greater than nine who was not assessed for remission at twelve months (+/- 30 days) Ⓑ

* **G9399** Documentation in the patient record of a discussion between the physician/clinician and the patient that includes all of the following: treatment choices appropriate to genotype, risks and benefits, evidence of effectiveness, and patient preferences toward the outcome of the treatment Ⓑ

✻ **G9400** Documentation of medical or patient reason(s) for not discussing treatment options; medical reasons: patient is not a candidate for treatment due to advanced physical or mental health comorbidity (including active substance use); currently receiving antiviral treatment; successful antiviral treatment (with sustained virologic response) prior to reporting period; other documented medical reasons; patient reasons: patient unable or unwilling to participate in the discussion or other patient reasons Ⓑ

✻ **G9401** No documentation of a discussion in the patient record of a discussion between the physician or other qualified healthcare professional and the patient that includes all of the following: treatment choices appropriate to genotype, risks and benefits, evidence of effectiveness, and patient preferences toward treatment Ⓑ

✻ **G9402** Patient received follow-up on the date of discharge or within 30 days after discharge Ⓑ

✻ **G9403** Clinician documented reason patient was not able to complete 30 day follow-up from acute inpatient setting discharge (e.g., patient death prior to follow-up visit, patient non-compliant for visit follow-up) Ⓑ

✻ **G9404** Patient did not receive follow-up on the date of discharge or within 30 days after discharge Ⓑ

✻ **G9405** Patient received follow-up within 7 days from discharge Ⓑ

✻ **G9406** Clinician documented reason patient was not able to complete 7 day follow-up from acute inpatient setting discharge (i.e patient death prior to follow-up visit, patient non-compliance for visit follow-up) Ⓑ

✻ **G9407** Patient did not receive follow-up on or within 7 days after discharge Ⓑ

✻ **G9408** Patients with cardiac tamponade and/or pericardiocentesis occurring within 30 days Ⓑ

✻ **G9409** Patients without cardiac tamponade and/or pericardiocentesis occurring within 30 days Ⓑ

✻ **G9410** Patient admitted within 180 days, status post CIED implantation, replacement, or revision with an infection requiring device removal or surgical revision Ⓑ

✻ **G9411** Patient not admitted within 180 days, status post CIED implantation, replacement, or revision with an infection requiring device removal or surgical revision Ⓑ

✻ **G9412** Patient admitted within 180 days, status post CIED implantation, replacement, or revision with an infection requiring device removal or surgical revision Ⓑ

✻ **G9413** Patient not admitted within 180 days, status post CIED implantation, replacement, or revision with an infection requiring device removal or surgical revision Ⓑ

✻ **G9414** Patient had one dose of meningococcal vaccine on or between the patient's 11th and 13th birthdays Ⓑ

✻ **G9415** Patient did not have one dose of meningococcal vaccine on or between the patient's 11th and 13th birthdays Ⓑ

⮌ ✻ **G9416** Patient had one tetanus, diphtheria toxoids and acellular pertussis vaccine (Tdap) on or between the patient's 10th and 13th birthdays Ⓑ

⮌ ✻ **G9417** Patient did not have one tetanus, diphtheria toxoids and acellular pertussis vaccine (Tdap) on or between the patient's 10th and 13th birthdays Ⓑ

✻ **G9418** Primary non-small cell lung cancer biopsy and cytology specimen report documents classification into specific histologic type or classified as NSCLC-NOS with an explanation Ⓑ

✻ **G9419** Documentation of medical reason(s) for not including the histological type or NSCLC-NOS classification with an explanation (e.g., biopsy taken for other purposes in a patient with a history of primary non-small cell lung cancer or other documented medical reasons) Ⓑ

✻ **G9420** Specimen site other than anatomic location of lung or is not classified as primary non-small cell lung cancer Ⓑ

✻ **G9421** Primary non-small cell lung cancer biopsy and cytology specimen report does not document classification into specific histologic type or classified as NSCLC-NOS with an explanation Ⓑ

✻ **G9422** Primary lung carcinoma resection report documents pT category, pN category and for non-small cell lung cancer, histologic type (squamous cell carcinoma, adenocarcinoma and not nsclc-nos) Ⓑ

✻ **G9423** Documentation of medical reason for not including pT category, pN category and histologic type [for patient with appropriate exclusion criteria (e.g., metastatic disease, benign tumors, malignant tumors other than carcinomas, inadequate surgical specimens)] Ⓑ

✻ **G9424** Specimen site other than anatomic location of lung, or classified as NSCLC-NOS Ⓑ

✻ **G9425** Primary lung carcinoma resection report does not document pT category, pN category and for non-small cell lung cancer, histologic type (squamous cell carcinoma,adenocarcinoma) Ⓑ

✻ **G9426** Improvement in median time from ED arrival to initial ED oral or parenteral pain medication administration performed for ED admitted patients Ⓑ

✻ **G9427** Improvement in median time from ED arrival to initial ED oral or parenteral pain medication administration not performed for ED admitted patients Ⓑ

✻ **G9428** Pathology report includes the pT category and a statement on thickness and ulceration and for pT1, mitotic rate Ⓑ

✻ **G9429** Documentation of medical reason(s) for not including pT category and a statement on thickness and ulceration and for pT1, mitotic rate (e.g., negative skin biopsies in a patient with a history of melanoma or other documented medical reasons) Ⓑ

✻ **G9430** Specimen site other than anatomic cutaneous location Ⓑ

✻ **G9431** Pathology report does not include the pT category and a statement on thickness and ulceration and for pT1, mitotic rate Ⓑ

✻ **G9432** Asthma well-controlled based on the ACT, C-ACT, ACQ, or ATAQ score and results documented Ⓑ

✻ **G9434** Asthma not well-controlled based on the ACT, C-ACT, ACQ, or ATAQ score, or specified asthma control tool not used, reason not given Ⓑ

~~G9435 Aspirin prescribed at discharge~~ ✖

~~G9436 Aspirin not prescribed for documented reasons (e.g., allergy, medical intolerance, history of bleed)~~ ✖

~~G9437 Aspirin not prescribed at discharge~~ ✖

~~G9438 P2Y inhibitor prescribed at discharge~~ ✖

~~G9439 P2Y inhibitor not prescribed for documented reasons (e.g., allergy, medical intolerance, history of bleed)~~ ✖

~~G9440 P2Y inhibitor not prescribed at discharge~~ ✖

~~G9441 Statin prescribed at discharge~~ ✖

~~G9442 Statin not prescribed for documented reasons (e.g., allergy, medical intolerance)~~ ✖

~~G9443 Statin not prescribed at discharge~~ ✖

✻ **G9448** Patients who were born in the years 1945-1965 Ⓑ

✻ **G9449** History of receiving blood transfusions prior to 1992 Ⓑ

✻ **G9450** History of injection drug use Ⓑ

✻ **G9451** Patient received one-time screening for HCV infection Ⓑ

✻ **G9452** Documentation of medical reason(s) for not receiving one-time screening for HCV infection (e.g., decompensated cirrhosis indicating advanced disease [ie, ascites, esophageal variceal bleeding, hepatic encephalopathy], hepatocellular carcinoma, waitlist for organ transplant, limited life expectancy, other medical reasons) Ⓑ

✻ **G9453** Documentation of patient reason(s) for not receiving one-time screening for HCV infection (e.g., patient declined, other patient reasons) Ⓑ

✻ **G9454** One-time screening for HCV infection not received within 12 month reporting period and no documentation of prior screening for HCV infection, reason not given Ⓑ

✻ **G9455** Patient underwent abdominal imaging with ultrasound, contrast enhanced CT or contrast MRI for HCC Ⓑ

✻ **G9456** Documentation of medical or patient reason(s) for not ordering or performing screening for HCC. medical reason: comorbid medical conditions with expected survival < 5 years, hepatic decompensation and not a candidate for liver transplantation, or other medical reasons; patient reasons: patient declined or other patient reasons (e.g., cost of tests, time related to accessing testing equipment) Ⓑ

✻ **G9457** Patient did not undergo abdominal imaging and did not have a documented reason for not undergoing abdominal imaging in the reporting period Ⓑ

✻ **G9458** Patient documented as tobacco user and received tobacco cessation intervention (must include at least one of the following: advice given to quit smoking or tobacco use, counseling on the benefits of quitting smoking or tobacco use, assistance with or referral to external smoking or tobacco cessation support programs, or current enrollment in smoking or tobacco use cessation program) if identified as a tobacco user Ⓑ

✻ **G9459** Currently a tobacco non-user Ⓑ

✻ **G9460** Tobacco assessment or tobacco cessation intervention not performed, reason not given Ⓑ

~~G9463 I intend to report the sinusitis measures group~~ ✖

~~G9464 All quality actions for the applicable measures in the sinusitis measures group have been performed for this patient~~ ✖

~~G9465 I intend to report the acute otitis externa (AOE) measures group~~ ✖

~~G9466 All quality actions for the applicable measures in the AOE measures group have been performed for this patient~~ ✖

~~G9467 Patient who have received or are receiving corticosteroids greater than or equal to 10 mg/day of prednisone equivalents for 60 or greater consecutive days or a single prescription equating to 600mg prednisone or greater for all fills within the last twelve months~~ ✖

✻ **G9468** Patient not receiving corticosteroids greater than or equal to 10 mg/day of prednisone equivalents for 60 or greater consecutive days or a single prescription equating to 600 mg prednisone or greater for all fills Ⓑ

✻ **G9469** Patients who have received or are receiving corticosteroids greater than or equal to 10 mg/day of prednisone equivalents for 60 or greater consecutive days or a single prescription equating to 600 mg prednisone or greater for all fills Ⓑ

✻ **G9470** Patients not receiving corticosteroids greater than or equal to 10 mg/day of prednisone equivalents for 60 or greater consecutive days or a single prescription equating to 600 mg prednisone or greater for all fills Ⓑ

✻ **G9471** Within the past 2 years, central dual-energy X-ray absorptiometry (DXA) not ordered or documented Ⓑ

✻ **G9472** Within the past 2 years, central dual-energy X-ray absorptiometry (DXA) not ordered and documented, no review of systems and no medication history or pharmacologic therapy (other than minerals/vitamins) for osteoporosis prescribed Ⓑ

✻ **G9473** Services performed by chaplain in the hospice setting, each 15 minutes

✻ **G9474** Services performed by dietary counselor in the hospice setting, each 15 minutes Ⓑ

✻ **G9475** Services performed by other counselor in the hospice setting, each 15 minutes Ⓑ

✻ **G9476** Services performed by volunteer in the hospice setting, each 15 minutes Ⓑ

✻ **G9477** Services performed by care coordinator in the hospice setting, each 15 minutes Ⓑ

✻ **G9478** Services performed by other qualified therapist in the hospice setting, each 15 minutes Ⓑ

✻ **G9479** Services performed by qualified pharmacist in the hospice setting, each 15 minutes Ⓑ

✻ **G9480** Admission to Medicare Care Choice Model program (MCCM) Ⓑ

▶ ✻ **G9481** Remote in-home visit for the evaluation and management of a new patient for use only in the Medicare-approved comprehensive care for joint replacement model, which requires these 3 key components: a problem focused history; a problem focused examination; and straightforward medical decision making, furnished in real time using interactive audio and video technology. Counseling and coordination of care with other physicians, other qualified health care professionals or agencies are provided consistent with the nature of the problem(s) and the needs of the patient or the family or both. Usually, the presenting problem(s) are self limited or minor. Typically, 10 minutes are spent with the patient or family or both via real time, audio and video intercommunications technology Ⓑ

▶ New ⤾ Revised ✔ Reinstated ~~deleted~~ Deleted ⃠ Not covered or valid by Medicare
Special coverage instructions ✻ Carrier discretion Ⓑ Bill local carrier Ⓓ Bill DME MAC

▶ ✻ **G9482** Remote in-home visit for the evaluation and management of a new patient for use only in the Medicare-approved comprehensive care for joint replacement model, which requires these 3 key components: an expanded problem focused history; an expanded problem focused examination; straightforward medical decision making, furnished in real time using interactive audio and video technology. Counseling and coordination of care with other physicians, other qualified health care professionals or agencies are provided consistent with the nature of the problem(s) and the needs of the patient or the family or both. Usually, the presenting problem(s) are of low to moderate severity. Typically, 20 minutes are spent with the patient or family or both via real time, audio and video intercommunications technology Ⓑ

▶ ✻ **G9483** Remote in-home visit for the evaluation and management of a new patient for use only in the Medicare-approved comprehensive care for joint replacement model, which requires these 3 key components: a detailed history; a detailed examination; medical decision making of low complexity, furnished in real time using interactive audio and video technology. Counseling and coordination of care with other physicians, other qualified health care professionals or agencies are provided consistent with the nature of the problem(s) and the needs of the patient or the family or both. Usually, the presenting problem(s) are of moderate severity. Typically, 30 minutes are spent with the patient or family or both via real time, audio and video intercommunications technology Ⓑ

▶ ✻ **G9484** Remote in-home visit for the evaluation and management of a new patient for use only in the Medicare-approved comprehensive care for joint replacement model, which requires these 3 key components: a comprehensive history; a comprehensive examination; medical decision making of moderate complexity, furnished in real time using interactive audio and video technology. Counseling and coordination of care with other physicians, other qualified health care professionals or agencies are provided consistent with the nature of the problem(s) and the needs of the patient or the family or both. Usually, the presenting problem(s) are of moderate to high severity. Typically, 45 minutes are spent with the patient or family or both via real time, audio and video intercommunications technology Ⓑ

▶ ✻ **G9485** Remote in-home visit for the evaluation and management of a new patient for use only in the Medicare-approved comprehensive care for joint replacement model, which requires these 3 key components: a comprehensive history; a comprehensive examination; medical decision making of high complexity, furnished in real time using interactive audio and video technology. Counseling and coordination of care with other physicians, other qualified health care professionals or agencies are provided consistent with the nature of the problem(s) and the needs of the patient or the family or both. Usually, the presenting problem(s) are of moderate to high severity. Typically, 60 minutes are spent with the patient or family or both via real time, audio and video intercommunications technology Ⓑ

▶ ✻ **G9486** Remote in-home visit for the evaluation and management of an established patient for use only in the Medicare-approved comprehensive care for joint replacement model, which requires at least 2 of the following 3 key components: a problem focused history; a problem focused examination; straightforward medical decision making, furnished in real time using interactive audio and video technology. Counseling and coordination of care with other physicians, other qualified health care professionals or agencies are provided consistent with the nature of the problem(s) and the needs of the patient or the family or both. Usually, the presenting problem(s) are self limited or minor. Typically, 10 minutes are spent with the patient or family or both via real time, audio and video intercommunications technology Ⓑ

▶ ✻ **G9487** Remote in-home visit for the evaluation and management of an established patient for use only in the Medicare-approved comprehensive care for joint replacement model, which requires at least 2 of the following 3 key components: an expanded problem focused history; an expanded problem focused examination; medical decision making of low complexity, furnished in real time using interactive audio and video technology. Counseling and coordination of care with other physicians, other qualified health care professionals or agencies are provided consistent with the nature of the problem(s) and the needs of the patient or the family or both. Usually, the presenting problem(s) are of low to moderate severity. Typically, 15 minutes are spent with the patient or family or both via real time, audio and video intercommunications technology Ⓑ

▶ ✻ **G9488** Remote in-home visit for the evaluation and management of an established patient for use only in the Medicare-approved comprehensive care for joint replacement model, which requires at least 2 of the following 3 key components: a detailed history; a detailed examination; medical decision making of moderate complexity, furnished in real time using interactive audio and video technology. Counseling and coordination of care with other physicians, other qualified health care professionals or agencies are provided consistent with the nature of the problem(s) and the needs of the patient or the family or both. Usually, the presenting problem(s) are of moderate to high severity. Typically, 25 minutes are spent with the patient or family or both via real time, audio and video intercommunications technology Ⓑ

▶ ✻ **G9489** Remote in-home visit for the evaluation and management of an established patient for use only in the Medicare-approved comprehensive care for joint replacement model, which requires at least 2 of the following 3 key components: a comprehensive history; a comprehensive examination; medical decision making of high complexity, furnished in real time using interactive audio and video technology. Counseling and coordination of care with other physicians, other qualified health care professionals or agencies are provided consistent with the nature of the problem(s) and the needs of the patient or the family or both. Usually, the presenting problem(s) are of moderate to high severity. Typically, 40 minutes are spent with the patient or family or both via real time, audio and video intercommunications technology Ⓑ

▶ ✻ **G9490** Comprehensive care for joint replacement model, home visit for patient assessment performed by clinical staff for an individual not considered homebound, including, but not necessarily limited to patient assessment of clinical status, safety/ fall prevention, functional status/ ambulation, medication reconciliation/ management, compliance with orders/ plan of care, performance of activities of daily living, and ensuring beneficiary connections to community and other services. (for use only in the Medicare-approved CJR model); may not be billed for a 30 day period covered by a transitional care management code Ⓑ

✻ **G9496** Documentation of reason for not detecting adenoma(s) or other neoplasm. (e.g., neoplasm detected is only diagnosed as traditional serrated adenoma, sessile serrated polyp, or sessile serrated adenoma Ⓑ

⮌ ✻ **G9497** Received instruction from the anesthesiologist or proxy prior to the day of surgery to abstain from smoking on the day of surgery

✻ **G9498** Antibiotic regimen prescribed Ⓑ

~~G9499 Patient did not start or is not receiving antiviral treatment for Hepatitis C during the measurement period~~ ✖

⮌ ✻ **G9500** Radiation exposure indices, or exposure time and number of fluorographic images in final report for procedures using fluoroscopy, documented Ⓑ

⮌ ✻ **G9501** Radiation exposure indices, or exposure time and number of fluorographic images not documented in final report for procedure using fluoroscopy, reason not given Ⓑ

✻ **G9502** Documentation of medical reason for not performing foot exam (i.e., patients who have had either a bilateral amputation above or below the knee, or both a left and right amputation above or below the knee before or during the measurement period) Ⓑ

✻ **G9503** Patient taking tamsulosin hydrochloride Ⓑ

✻ **G9504** Documented reason for not assessing Hepatitis B virus (HBV) status (e.g. patient not receiving a first course of anti-TNF therapy, patient declined) within one year prior to first course of anti-TNF therapy Ⓑ

✻ **G9505** Antibiotic regimen prescribed within 10 days after onset of symptoms for documented medical reason Ⓑ

✻ **G9506** Biologic immune response modifier prescribed Ⓑ

✻ **G9507** Documentation that the patient is on a statin medication or has documentation of a valid contraindication or exception to statin medications; contraindications/exceptions that can be defined by diagnosis codes include pregnancy during the measurement period, active liver disease, rhabdomyolysis, end stage renal disease on dialysis and heart failure; provider documented contraindications/ exceptions include breastfeeding during the measurement period, woman of child-bearing age not actively taking birth control, allergy to statin, drug interaction (HIV protease inhibitors, nefazodone, cyclosporine, gemfibrozil, and danazol) and intolerance (with supporting documentation of trying a statin at least once within the last 5 years or diagnosis codes for myostitis or toxic myopathy related to drugs) Ⓑ

✻ **G9508** Documentation that the patient is not on a statin medication Ⓑ

✻ **G9509** Remission at twelve months as demonstrated by a twelve month (+/- 30 days) PHQ-9 score of less than 5 Ⓑ

✻ **G9510** Remission at twelve months not demonstrated by a twelve month (+/- 30 days) PHQ-9 score of less than five; either PHQ-9 score was not assessed or is greater than or equal to 5 Ⓑ

✻ **G9511** Index date PHQ-9 score greater than 9 documented during the twelve month denominator identification period Ⓑ

✻ **G9512** Individual had a PDC of 0.8 or greater Ⓑ

✻ **G9513** Individual did not have a PDC of 0.8 or greater Ⓑ

✻ **G9514** Patient required a return to the operating room within 90 days of surgery Ⓑ

✻ **G9515** Patient did not require a return to the operating room within 90 days of surgery Ⓑ

✻ **G9516** Patient achieved an improvement in visual acuity, from their preoperative level, within 90 days of surgery Ⓑ

▶ New ⮌ Revised ✔ Reinstated ~~deleted~~ Deleted ⊘ Not covered or valid by Medicare
✪ Special coverage instructions ✻ Carrier discretion Ⓑ Bill local carrier Ⓓ Bill DME MAC

* **G9517** Patient did not achieve an improvement in visual acuity, from their preoperative level, within 90 days of surgery, reason not given Ⓑ

* **G9518** Documentation of active injection drug use Ⓑ

⮌ * **G9519** Patient achieves final refraction (spherical equivalent) +/- 0.5 diopters of their planned refraction within 90 days of surgery Ⓑ

⮌ * **G9520** Patient does not achieve final refraction (spherical equivalent) +/- 0.5 diopters of their planned refraction within 90 days of surgery Ⓑ

* **G9521** Total number of emergency department visits and inpatient hospitalizations less than two in the past 12 months Ⓑ

* **G9522** Total number of emergency department visits and inpatient hospitalizations equal to or greater than two in the past 12 months or patient not screened, reason not given Ⓑ

* **G9523** Patient discontinued from hemodialysis or peritoneal dialysis Ⓑ

* **G9524** Patient was referred to hospice care Ⓑ

* **G9525** Documentation of patient reason(s) for not referring to hospice care (e.g., patient declined, other patient reasons) Ⓑ

* **G9526** Patient was not referred to hospice care, reason not given Ⓑ

* **G9529** Patient with minor blunt head trauma had an appropriate indication(s) for a head CT Ⓑ

* **G9530** Patient presented within 24 hours of a minor blunt head trauma with a GCS score of 15 and had a head CT ordered for trauma by an emergency care provider Ⓑ

⮌ * **G9531** Patient has documentation of ventricular shunt, brain tumor, multisystem trauma, pregnancy, or is currently taking an antiplatelet medication including: asa/dipyridamole, clopidogrel, prasugrel, ticlopidine, ticagrelor or cilstazol) Ⓑ

⮌ * **G9532** Patient's head injury occurred greater than 24 hours before presentation to the emergency department, or has a GCS score less than 15 or does not have a GCS score documented, or had a head CT for trauma ordered by someone other than an emergency care provider, or was ordered for a reason other than trauma Ⓑ

* **G9533** Patient with minor blunt head trauma did not have an appropriate indication(s) for a head CT Ⓑ

* **G9534** Advanced brain imaging (CTA, CT, MRA or MRI) was not ordered Ⓑ

* **G9535** Patients with a normal neurological examination Ⓑ

* **G9536** Documentation of medical reason(s) for ordering an advanced brain imaging study (i.e., patient has an abnormal neurological examination; patient has the coexistence of seizures, or both; recent onset of severe headache; change in the type of headache; signs of increased intracranial pressure (e.g., papilledema, absent venous pulsations on funduscopic examination, altered mental status, focal neurologic deficits, signs of meningeal irritation); HIV-positive patients with a new type of headache; immunocompromised patient with unexplained headache symptoms; patient on coagulopathy/anti-coagulation or anti-platelet therapy; very young patients with unexplained headache symptoms) Ⓑ

* **G9537** Documentation of system reason(s) for ordering an advanced brain imaging study (i.e., needed as part of a clinical trial; other clinician ordered the study) Ⓑ

* **G9538** Advanced brain imaging (CTA, CT, MRA OR MRI) was ordered Ⓑ

* **G9539** Intent for potential removal at time of placement Ⓑ

* **G9540** Patient alive 3 months post procedure Ⓑ

* **G9541** Filter removed within 3 months of placement Ⓑ

* **G9542** Documented re-assessment for the appropriateness of filter removal within 3 months of placement Ⓑ

* **G9543** Documentation of at least two attempts to reach the patient to arrange a clinical re-assessment for the appropriateness of filter removal within 3 months of placement Ⓑ

* **G9544** Patients that do not have the filter removed, documented re-assessment for the appropriateness of filter removal, or documentation of at least two attempts to reach the patient to arrange a clinical re-assessment for the appropriateness of filter removal within 3 months of placement Ⓑ

↩ ✻ **G9547** Incidental finding: liver lesion <= 0.5 cm, cystic kidney lesion < 1.0 cm or adrenal lesion <= 1.0 cm Ⓑ

✻ **G9548** Final reports for abdominal imaging studies with follow-up imaging recommended Ⓑ

↩ ✻ **G9549** Documentation of medical reason(s) that follow-up imaging is not indicated (e.g., patient has a known malignancy that can metastasize, other medical reason(s) such as fever in an immunocompromised patient) Ⓑ

✻ **G9550** Final reports for abdominal imaging studies with follow-up imaging not recommended Ⓑ

↩ ✻ **G9551** Final reports for abdominal imaging studies without an incidentally found lesion noted: liver lesion <= 0.5 cm, cystic kidney lesion < 1.0 cm or adrenal lesion <= 1.0 cm noted or no lesion found Ⓑ

✻ **G9552** Incidental thyroid nodule < 1.0 cm noted in report Ⓑ

✻ **G9553** Prior thyroid disease diagnosis Ⓑ

↩ ✻ **G9554** Final reports for CT CTA, MRI or MRA of the chest or neck or ultrasound of the neck with follow-up imaging recommended Ⓑ

↩ ✻ **G9555** Documentation of medical reason(s) for recommending follow up imaging (e.g., patient has multiple endocrine neoplasia, patient has cervical lymphadenopathy, other medical reason(s)) Ⓑ

↩ ✻ **G9556** Final reports for CT CTA, MRI or MRA of the chest or neck or ultrasound of the neck with follow-up imaging not recommended Ⓑ

↩ ✻ **G9557** Final reports for CT CTA, MRI or MRA studies of the chest or neck or ultrasound of the neck without an incidentally found thyroid nodule < 1.0 cm noted or no nodule found Ⓑ

✻ **G9558** Patient treated with a beta-lactam antibiotic as definitive therapy Ⓑ

✻ **G9559** Documentation of medical reason(s) for not prescribing a beta-lactam antibiotic (e.g., allergy, intolerance to beta-lactam antibiotics) Ⓑ

✻ **G9560** Patient not treated with a beta-lactam antibiotic as definitive therapy, reason not given Ⓑ

✻ **G9561** Patients prescribed opiates for longer than six weeks Ⓑ

✻ **G9562** Patients who had a follow-up evaluation conducted at least every three months during opioid therapy Ⓑ

✻ **G9563** Patients who did not have a follow-up evaluation conducted at least every three months during opioid therapy Ⓑ

~~G9572 Index date PHQ score greater than 9 documented during the twelve month denominator identification period~~ ✖

✻ **G9573** Remission at six months as demonstrated by a six month (+/- 30 days) PHQ-9 score of less than five Ⓑ

✻ **G9574** Remission at six months not demonstrated by a six month (+/- 30 days) PHQ-9 score of less than five either PHQ-9 score was not assessed or is greater than or equal to five Ⓑ

✻ **G9577** Patients prescribed opiates for longer than six weeks Ⓑ

✻ **G9578** Documentation of signed opioid treatment agreement at least once during opioid therapy Ⓑ

✻ **G9579** No documentation of signed an opioid treatment agreement at least once during opioid therapy Ⓑ

✻ **G9580** Door to puncture time of less than 2 hours Ⓑ

~~G9581 Door to puncture time of greater than 2 hours for reasons documented by clinician (e.g., patients who are transferred from one institution to another with a known diagnosis of CVA for endovascular stroke treatment; hospitalized patients with newly diagnosed CVA considered for endovascular stroke treatment)~~ ✖

✻ **G9582** Door to puncture time of greater than 2 hours, no reason given Ⓑ

✻ **G9583** Patients prescribed opiates for longer than six weeks Ⓑ

↩ ✻ **G9584** Patient evaluated for risk of misuse of opiates by using a brief validated instrument (e.g., opioid risk tool, SOAPP-R) or patient interviewed at least once during opioid therapy Ⓑ

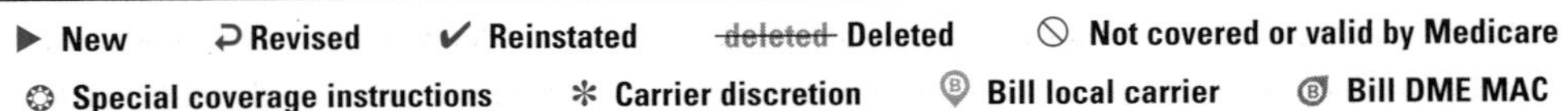

↺ ✻ **G9585** Patient not evaluated for risk of misuse of opiates by using a brief validated instrument (e.g., opioid risk tool, SOAPP-R) or patient not interviewed at least once during opioid therapy Ⓑ

✻ **G9593** Pediatric patient with minor blunt head trauma classified as low risk according to the PECARN Prediction Rules A Ⓑ

✻ **G9594** Patient presented within 24 hours of a minor blunt head trauma with a GCS score of 15 and had a head CT ordered for trauma by an emergency care provider Ⓑ

↺ ✻ **G9595** Patient has documentation of ventricular shunt, brain tumor, coagulopathy, including thrombocytopenia Ⓑ

↺ ✻ **G9596** Pediatric patient's head injury occurred greater than 24 hours before presentation to the emergency department, or has a GCS score less than 15 or does not have a GCS score documented, or had a head CT for trauma ordered by someone other than an emergency care provider, or was ordered for a reason other than trauma A Ⓑ

✻ **G9597** Pediatric patient with minor blunt head trauma not classified as low risk according to the PECARN Prediction Rules A Ⓑ

✻ **G9598** Aortic aneurysm 5.5 - 5.9 cm maximum diameter on centerline formatted CT or minor diameter on axial formatted CT Ⓑ

✻ **G9599** Aortic aneurysm 6.0 cm or greater maximum diameter on centerline formatted CT or minor diameter on axial formatted CT Ⓑ

✻ **G9600** Symptomatic AAAS that required urgent/emergent (non-elective) repair Ⓑ

✻ **G9601** Patient discharge to home no later than post-operative day #7 Ⓑ

✻ **G9602** Patient not discharged to home by post-operative day #7 Ⓑ

✻ **G9603** Patient survey score improved from baseline following treatment Ⓑ

✻ **G9604** Patient survey results not available Ⓑ

✻ **G9605** Patient survey score did not improve from baseline following treatment Ⓑ

✻ **G9606** Intraoperative cystoscopy performed to evaluate for lower tract injury Ⓑ

↺ ✻ **G9607** Documented medical reasons for not performing intraoperative cystoscopy (e.g., urethral pathology precluding cystoscopy, any patient who has a congenital or acquired absence of the urethra) Ⓑ

✻ **G9608** Intraoperative cystoscopy not performed to evaluate for lower tract injury Ⓑ

↺ ✻ **G9609** Documentation of an order for anti-platelet agents Ⓑ

↺ ✻ **G9610** Documentation of medical reason(s) in the patient's record for not ordering anti-platelet agents Ⓑ

↺ ✻ **G9611** Order for anti-platelet agents was not documented in the patient's record, reason not given Ⓑ

✻ **G9612** Photodocumentation of one or more cecal landmarks to establish a complete examination Ⓑ

✻ **G9613** Documentation of post-surgical anatomy (e.g., right hemicolectomy, ileocecal resection, etc.) Ⓑ

✻ **G9614** No photodocumentation of cecal landmarks to establish a complete examination Ⓑ

✻ **G9615** Preoperative assessment documented Ⓑ

✻ **G9616** Documentation of reason(s) for not documenting a preoperative assessment (e.g., patient with a gynecologic or other pelvic malignancy noted at the time of surgery) Ⓑ

✻ **G9617** Preoperative assessment not documented, reason not given Ⓑ

✻ **G9618** Documentation of screening for uterine malignancy or those that had an ultrasound and/or endometrial sampling of any kind Ⓑ

~~G9619 Documentation of reason(s) for not screening for uterine malignancy (e.g., prior hysterectomy)~~ ✖

✻ **G9620** Patient not screened for uterine malignancy, or those that have not had an ultrasound and/or endometrial sampling of any kind, reason not given Ⓑ

✻ **G9621** Patient identified as an unhealthy alcohol user when screened for unhealthy alcohol use using a systematic screening method and received brief counseling Ⓑ

✻ **G9622** Patient not identified as an unhealthy alcohol user when screened for unhealthy alcohol use using a systematic screening method Ⓑ

▶ New ↺ Revised ✔ Reinstated ~~deleted~~ Deleted ⊘ Not covered or valid by Medicare
✪ Special coverage instructions ✻ Carrier discretion Ⓑ Bill local carrier Ⓑ Bill DME MAC

✱ **G9623** Documentation of medical reason(s) for not screening for unhealthy alcohol use (e.g., limited life expectancy, other medical reasons) Ⓑ

✱ **G9624** Patient not screened for unhealthy alcohol screening using a systematic screening method or patient did not receive brief counseling, reason not given Ⓑ

➲ ✱ **G9625** Patient sustained bladder injury at the time of surgery or discovered subsequently up to 1 month post-surgery Ⓑ

➲ ✱ **G9626** Documented medical reason for not reporting bladder injury (e.g., gynecologic or other pelvic malignancy documented, concurrent surgery involving bladder pathology, injury that occurs during urinary incontinence procedure, patient death from non-medical causes not related to surgery, patient died during procedure without evidence of bladder injury) Ⓑ

➲ ✱ **G9627** Patient did not sustain bladder injury at the time of surgery nor discovered subsequently up to 1 month post-surgery Ⓑ

➲ ✱ **G9628** Patient sustained bowel injury at the time of surgery or discovered subsequently up to 1 month post-surgery Ⓑ

➲ ✱ **G9629** Documented medical reasons for not reporting bowel injury (e.g., gynecologic or other pelvic malignancy documented, planned (e.g., not due to an unexpected bowel injury) resection and/or re-anastomosis of bowel, or patient death from non-medical causes not related to surgery, patient died during procedure without evidence of bowel injury) Ⓑ

➲ ✱ **G9630** Patient did not sustain a bowel injury at the time of surgery nor discovered subsequently up to 1 month post-surgery Ⓑ

✱ **G9631** Patient sustained ureter injury at the time of surgery or discovered subsequently up to 1 month post-surgery Ⓑ

➲ ✱ **G9632** Documented medical reasons for not reporting ureter injury (e.g., gynecologic or other pelvic malignancy documented, concurrent surgery involving bladder pathology, injury that occurs during a urinary incontinence procedure, patient death from non-medical causes not related to surgery, patient died during procedure without evidence of ureter injury) Ⓑ

➲ ✱ **G9633** Patient did not sustain ureter injury at the time of surgery nor discovered subsequently up to 1 month post-surgery Ⓑ

✱ **G9634** Health-related quality of life assessed with tool during at least two visits and quality of life score remained the same or improved Ⓑ

✱ **G9635** Health-related quality of life not assessed with tool for documented reason(s) (e.g., patient has a cognitive or neuropsychiatric impairment that impairs his/her ability to complete the HRQOL survey, patient has the inability to read and/or write in order to complete the HRQOL questionnaire) Ⓑ

✱ **G9636** Health-related quality of life not assessed with tool during at least two visits or quality of life score declined Ⓑ

✱ **G9637** Final reports with documentation of one or more dose reduction techniques (e.g., automated exposure control, adjustment of the ma and/or KV according to patient size, use of iterative reconstruction technique) Ⓑ

✱ **G9638** Final reports without documentation of one or more dose reduction techniques (e.g., automated exposure control, adjustment of the ma and/or KV according to patient size, use of iterative reconstruction technique) Ⓑ

✱ **G9639** Major amputation or open surgical bypass not required within 48 hours of the index endovascular lower extremity revascularization procedure Ⓑ

✱ **G9640** Documentation of planned hybrid or staged procedure Ⓑ

✱ **G9641** Major amputation or open surgical bypass required within 48 hours of the index endovascular lower extremity revascularization procedure Ⓑ

↩ ✻ **G9642** Current smokers (e.g., cigarette, cigar, pipe, e-cigarette or marijuana) Ⓑ

✻ **G9643** Elective surgery Ⓑ

✻ **G9644** Patients who abstained from smoking prior to anesthesia on the day of surgery or procedure Ⓑ

✻ **G9645** Patients who did not abstain from smoking prior to anesthesia on the day of surgery or procedure Ⓑ

✻ **G9646** Patients with 90 day MRS score of 0 to 2 Ⓑ

✻ **G9647** Patients in whom MRS score could not be obtained at 90 day follow-up Ⓑ

✻ **G9648** Patients with 90 day MRS score greater than 2 Ⓑ

✻ **G9649** Psoriasis assessment tool documented meeting any one of the specified benchmarks (e.g., (PGA; 6-point scale), body surface area (BSA), psoriasis area and severity index (PASI) and/or dermatology life quality index) (DLQI)) Ⓑ

~~G9650 Documentation that the patient declined therapy change or has documented contraindications (e.g., experienced adverse effects or lack of efficacy with all other therapy options) in order to achieve better disease control as measured by PGA, BSA, PASI, or DLQI~~ ✖

✻ **G9651** Psoriasis assessment tool documented not meeting any one of the specified benchmarks (e.g., (PGA; 6-point scale), body surface area (BSA), psoriasis area and severity index (PASI) and/or dermatology life quality index) (DLQI)) or psoriasis assessment tool not documented Ⓑ

~~G9652 Patient has been treated with a systemic or biologic medication for psoriasis for at least six months~~ ✖

~~G9653 Patient has not been treated with a systemic or biologic medication for psoriasis for at least six months~~ ✖

▶ ✻ **G9654** Monitored anesthesia care (mac) Ⓑ

▶ ✻ **G9655** A transfer of care protocol or handoff tool/checklist that includes the required key handoff elements is used

▶ ✻ **G9656** Patient transferred directly from anesthetizing location to PACU Ⓑ

~~G9657 Transfer of care during an anesthetic or to the intensive care unit~~ ✖

✻ **G9658** A transfer of care protocol or handoff tool/checklist that includes the required key handoff elements is not used Ⓑ

✻ **G9659** Patients greater than 85 years of age who did not have a history of colorectal cancer or valid medical reason for the colonoscopy, including: iron deficiency anemia, lower gastrointestinal bleeding, Crohn's Disease (i.e., regional enteritis), familial adenomatous polyposis, lynch syndrome (i.e., hereditary non-polyposis colorectal cancer), inflammatory bowel disease, ulcerative colitis, abnormal finding of gastrointestinal tract, or changes in bowel habits Ⓑ

✻ **G9660** Documentation of medical reason(s) for a colonoscopy performed on a patient greater than 85 years of age (e.g., last colonoscopy incomplete, last colonoscopy had inadequate prep, iron deficiency anemia, lower gastrointestinal bleeding, Crohn's Disease (i.e., regional enteritis), familial history of adenomatous polyposis, lynch syndrome (i.e., hereditary non-polyposis colorectal cancer), inflammatory bowel disease, ulcerative colitis, abnormal finding of gastrointestinal tract, or changes in bowel habits) Ⓑ

✻ **G9661** Patients greater than 85 years of age who received a routine colonoscopy for a reason other than the following: an assessment of signs/symptoms of GI tract illness, and/or the patient is considered high risk, and/or to follow-up on previously diagnosed advance lesions Ⓑ

✻ **G9662** Previously diagnosed or have an active diagnosis of clinical ASCVD Ⓑ

✻ **G9663** Any fasting or direct LDL-C laboratory test result = 190 mg/dL Ⓑ

✻ **G9664** Patients who are currently statin therapy users or received an order (prescription) for statin therapy Ⓑ

✻ **G9665** Patients who are not currently statin therapy users or did not receive an order (prescription) for statin therapy Ⓑ

✻ **G9666** The highest fasting or direct LDL-C laboratory test result of 70-189 mg/dL in the measurement period or two years prior to the beginning of the measurement period Ⓑ

▶ New ↩ Revised ✔ Reinstated ~~deleted~~ Deleted ⊘ Not covered or valid by Medicare
✪ Special coverage instructions ✻ Carrier discretion Ⓑ Bill local carrier Ⓓ Bill DME MAC

~~G9667 Documentation of medical reason (s) for not currently being a statin therapy user or receive an order (prescription) for statin therapy (e.g., patient with adverse effect, allergy or intolerance to statin medication therapy, patients who have an active diagnosis of pregnancy or who are breastfeeding, patients who are receiving palliative care, patients with active liver disease or hepatic disease or insufficiency, patients with end stage renal disease (ESRD), and patients with diabetes who have a fasting or direct LDL-C laboratory test result < 70 mg/dl and are not taking statin therapy)~~ ✖

~~G9669 I intend to report the multiple chronic conditions measures group~~ ✖

~~G9670 All quality actions for the applicable measures in the multiple chronic conditions measures group have been performed for this patient~~ ✖

~~G9671 I intend to report the diabetic retinopathy measures group~~ ✖

~~G9672 All quality actions for the applicable measures in the diabetic retinopathy measures group have been performed for this patient~~ ✖

~~G9673 I intend to report the cardiovascular prevention measures group~~ ✖

✻ **G9674** Patients with clinical ASCVD diagnosis

✻ **G9675** Patients who have ever had a fasting or direct laboratory result of LDL-C = 190 mg/dL

✻ **G9676** Patients aged 40 to 75 years at the beginning of the measurement period with type 1 or type 2 diabetes and with an LDL-C result of 70-189 mg/dL recorded as the highest fasting or direct laboratory test result in the measurement year or during the two years prior to the beginning of the measurement period

~~G9677 All quality actions for the applicable measures in the cardiovascular prevention measures group have been performed for this patient~~ ✖

▶ ✻ **G9678** Oncology care model (OCM) monthly enhanced oncology services (MEOS) payment for OCM enhanced services. G9678 payments may only be made to OCM practitioners for OCM beneficiaries for the furnishment of enhanced services as defined in the OCM participation agreement

▶ ✻ **G9679** This code is for onsite acute care treatment of a nursing facility resident with pneumonia; may only be billed once per day per beneficiary

▶ ✻ **G9680** This code is for onsite acute care treatment of a nursing facility resident with CHF; may only be billed once per day per beneficiary

▶ ✻ **G9681** This code is for onsite acute care treatment of a resident with COPD or asthma; may only be billed once per day per beneficiary

▶ ✻ **G9682** This code is for the onsite acute care treatment a nursing facility resident with a skin infection; may only be billed once per day per beneficiary

▶ ✻ **G9683** This code is for the onsite acute care treatment of a nursing facility resident with fluid or electrolyte disorder or dehydration (similar pattern); may only be billed once per day per beneficiary

▶ ✻ **G9684** This code is for the onsite acute care treatment of a nursing facility resident for a UTI; may only be billed once per day per beneficiary

▶ ✻ **G9685** This code is for the evaluation and management of a beneficiary's acute change in condition in a nursing facility

▶ ✻ **G9686** Onsite nursing facility conference, that is separate and distinct from an evaluation and management visit, including qualified practitioner and at least one member of the nursing facility interdisciplinary care team

▶ ✻ **G9687** Hospice services provided to patient any time during the measurement period

▶ ✻ **G9688** Patients using hospice services any time during the measurement period

▶ ✻ **G9689** Patient admitted for performance of elective carotid intervention

▶ ✻ **G9690** Patient receiving hospice services any time during the measurement period

▶ ✻ **G9691** Patient had hospice services any time during the measurement period

▶ ✻ **G9692** Hospice services received by patient any time during the measurement period

▶ ✻ **G9693** Patient use of hospice services any time during the measurement period

▶ ✻ **G9694** Hospice services utilized by patient any time during the measurement period

▶ New ⤾ Revised ✔ Reinstated ~~deleted~~ Deleted ⊘ Not covered or valid by Medicare
⚙ Special coverage instructions ✻ Carrier discretion Ⓑ Bill local carrier Ⓔ Bill DME MAC

▶ ✻ **G9695** Long-acting inhaled bronchodilator prescribed

▶ ✻ **G9696** Documentation of medical reason(s) for not prescribing a long-acting inhaled bronchodilator

▶ ✻ **G9697** Documentation of patient reason(s) for not prescribing a long-acting inhaled bronchodilator

▶ ✻ **G9698** Documentation of system reason(s) for not prescribing a long-acting inhaled bronchodilator

▶ ✻ **G9699** Long-acting inhaled bronchodilator not prescribed, reason not otherwise specified

▶ ✻ **G9700** Patients who use hospice services any time during the measurement period

▶ ✻ **G9701** Children who are taking antibiotics in the 30 days prior to the date of the encounter during which the diagnosis was established

▶ ✻ **G9702** Patients who use hospice services any time during the measurement period

▶ ✻ **G9703** Children who are taking antibiotics in the 30 days prior to the diagnosis of pharyngitis

▶ ✻ **G9704** AJCC breast cancer stage I: T1 mic or T1a documented

▶ ✻ **G9705** AJCC breast cancer stage I: T1b (tumor > 0.5 cm but < = 1 cm in greatest dimension) documented

▶ ✻ **G9706** Low (or very low) risk of recurrence, prostate cancer

▶ ✻ **G9707** Patient received hospice services any time during the measurement period

▶ ✻ **G9708** Women who had a bilateral mastectomy or who have a history of a bilateral mastectomy or for whom there is evidence of a right and a left unilateral mastectomy

▶ ✻ **G9709** Hospice services used by patient any time during the measurement period

▶ ✻ **G9710** Patient was provided hospice services any time during the measurement period

▶ ✻ **G9711** Patients with a diagnosis or past history of total colectomy or colorectal cancer

▶ ✻ **G9712** Documentation of medical reason(s) for prescribing or dispensing antibiotic (e.g., intestinal infection, pertussis, bacterial infection, Lyme disease, otitis media, acute sinusitis, acute pharyngitis, acute tonsillitis, chronic sinusitis, infection of the pharynx/larynx/tonsils/adenoids, prostatitis, cellulitis/ mastoiditis/bone infections, acute lymphadenitis, impetigo, skin staph infections, pneumonia, gonococcal infections/venereal disease (syphilis, chlamydia, inflammatory diseases [female reproductive organs]), infections of the kidney, cystitis/UTI, acne, HIV disease/asymptomatic HIV, cystic fibrosis, disorders of the immune system, malignancy neoplasms, chronic bronchitis, emphysema, bronchiectasis, extrinsic allergic alveolitis, chronic airway obstruction, chronic obstructive asthma, pneumoconiosis and other lung disease due to external agents, other diseases of the respiratory system, and tuberculosis)

▶ ✻ **G9713** Patients who use hospice services any time during the measurement period

▶ ✻ **G9714** Patient is using hospice services any time during the measurement period

▶ ✻ **G9715** Patients who use hospice services any time during the measurement period

▶ ✻ **G9716** BMI is documented as being outside of normal limits, follow-up plan is not completed for documented reason

▶ ✻ **G9717** Documentation stating the patient has an active diagnosis of depression or has a diagnosed bipolar disorder, therefore screening or follow-up not required

▶ ✻ **G9718** Hospice services for patient provided any time during the measurement period

▶ ✻ **G9719** Patient is not ambulatory, bed ridden, immobile, confined to chair, wheelchair bound, dependent on helper pushing wheelchair, independent in wheelchair or minimal help in wheelchair

▶ ✻ **G9720** Hospice services for patient occurred any time during the measurement period

▶ ✻ **G9721** Patient not ambulatory, bed ridden, immobile, confined to chair, wheelchair bound, dependent on helper pushing wheelchair, independent in wheelchair or minimal help in wheelchair

▶ ✻ **G9722** Documented history of renal failure or baseline serum creatinine = 4.0 mg/dL; renal transplant recipients are not considered to have preoperative renal failure, unless, since transplantation the CR has been or is 4.0 or higher

▶ ✻ **G9723** Hospice services for patient received any time during the measurement period

▶ ✻ **G9724** Patients who had documentation of use of anticoagulant medications overlapping the measurement year

▶ ✻ **G9725** Patients who use hospice services any time during the measurement period

▶ ✻ **G9726** Patient refused to participate

▶ ✻ **G9727** Patient unable to complete the FOTO knee intake PROM at admission and discharge due to blindness, illiteracy, severe mental incapacity or language incompatibility and an adequate proxy is not available

▶ ✻ **G9728** Patient refused to participate

▶ ✻ **G9729** Patient unable to complete the FOTO hip intake PROM at admission and discharge due to blindness, illiteracy, severe mental incapacity or language incompatibility and an adequate proxy is not available

▶ ✻ **G9730** Patient refused to participate

▶ ✻ **G9731** Patient unable to complete the FOTO foot or ankle intake PROM at admission and discharge due to blindness, illiteracy, severe mental incapacity or language incompatibility and an adequate proxy is not available

▶ ✻ **G9732** Patient refused to participate

▶ ✻ **G9733** Patient unable to complete the FOTO lumbar intake PROM at admission and discharge due to blindness, illiteracy, severe mental incapacity or language incompatibility and an adequate proxy is not available

▶ ✻ **G9734** Patient refused to participate

▶ ✻ **G9735** Patient unable to complete the FOTO shoulder intake PROM at admission and discharge due to blindness, illiteracy, severe mental incapacity or language incompatibility and an adequate proxy is not available

▶ ✻ **G9736** Patient refused to participate

▶ ✻ **G9737** Patient unable to complete the FOTO elbow, wrist or hand intake PROM at admission and discharge due to blindness, illiteracy, severe mental incapacity or language incompatibility and an adequate proxy is not available

▶ ✻ **G9738** Patient refused to participate

▶ ✻ **G9739** Patient unable to complete the FOTO general orthopedic intake PROM at admission and discharge due to blindness, illiteracy, severe mental incapacity or language incompatibility and an adequate proxy is not available

▶ ✻ **G9740** Hospice services given to patient any time during the measurement period

▶ ✻ **G9741** Patients who use hospice services any time during the measurement period

▶ ✻ **G9742** Psychiatric symptoms assessed

▶ ✻ **G9743** Psychiatric symptoms not assessed, reason not otherwise specified

▶ ✻ **G9744** Patient not eligible due to active diagnosis of hypertension

▶ ✻ **G9745** Documented reason for not screening or recommending a follow-up for high blood pressure

▶ ✻ **G9746** Patient has mitral stenosis or prosthetic heart valves or patient has transient or reversible cause of AF (e.g., pneumonia, hyperthyroidism, pregnancy, cardiac surgery)

▶ ✻ **G9747** Patient is undergoing palliative dialysis with a catheter

▶ ✻ **G9748** Patient approved by a qualified transplant program and scheduled to receive a living donor kidney transplant

▶ ✻ **G9749** Patient is undergoing palliative dialysis with a catheter

▶ ✻ **G9750** Patient approved by a qualified transplant program and scheduled to receive a living donor kidney transplant

▶ ✻ **G9751** Patient died at any time during the 24-month measurement period

▶ ✻ **G9752** Emergency surgery

▶ ✻ **G9753** Documentation of medical reason for not conducting a search for DICOM format images for prior patient CT imaging studies completed at non-affiliated external healthcare facilities or entities within the past 12 months that are available through a secure, authorized, media-free, shared archive (e.g., trauma, acute myocardial infarction, stroke, aortic aneurysm where time is of the essence)

▶ ✻ **G9754** A finding of an incidental pulmonary nodule

▶ ✻ **G9755** Documentation of medical reason(s) that follow-up imaging is indicated (e.g., patient has a known malignancy that can metastasize, other medical reason(s))

▶ ✻ **G9756** Surgical procedures that included the use of silicone oil

▶ ✻ **G9757** Surgical procedures that included the use of silicone oil

▶ ✻ **G9758** Patient in hospice and in terminal phase

▶ ✻ **G9759** History of preoperative posterior capsule rupture

▶ ✻ **G9760** Patients who use hospice services any time during the measurement period

▶ ✻ **G9761** Patients who use hospice services any time during the measurement period

▶ ✻ **G9762** Patient had at least three HPV vaccines on or between the patient's 9th and 13th birthdays

▶ ✻ **G9763** Patient did not have at least three HPV vaccines on or between the patient's 9th and 13th birthdays

▶ ✻ **G9764** Patient has been treated with an oral systemic or biologic medication for psoriasis

▶ ✻ **G9765** Documentation that the patient declined therapy change, has documented contraindications, or has not been treated with an oral systemic or biologic for at least six consecutive months (e.g., experienced adverse effects or lack of efficacy with all other therapy options) in order to achieve better disease control as measured by PGA, BSA, PASI, or DLQI

▶ ✻ **G9766** Patients who are transferred from one institution to another with a known diagnosis of CVA for endovascular stroke treatment

▶ ✻ **G9767** Hospitalized patients with newly diagnosed CVA considered for endovascular stroke treatment

▶ ✻ **G9768** Patients who utilize hospice services any time during the measurement period

▶ ✻ **G9769** Patient had a bone mineral density test in the past two years or received osteoporosis medication or therapy in the past 12 months

▶ ✻ **G9770** Peripheral nerve block (PNB)

▶ ✻ **G9771** At least 1 body temperature measurement equal to or greater than 35.5 degrees Celsius (or 95.9 degrees Fahrenheit) achieved within the 30 minutes immediately before or the 15 minutes immediately after anesthesia end time

▶ ✻ **G9772** Documentation of one of the following medical reason(s) for not achieving at least 1 body temperature measurement equal to or greater than 35.5 degrees Celsius (or 95.9 degrees Fahrenheit) achieved within the 30 minutes immediately before or the 15 minutes immediately after anesthesia end time (e.g., emergency cases, intentional hypothermia, etc.)

▶ ✻ **G9773** At least 1 body temperature measurement equal to or greater than 35.5 degrees Celsius (or 95.9 degrees Fahrenheit) not achieved within the 30 minutes immediately before or the 15 minutes immediately after anesthesia end time

▶ ✻ **G9774** Patients who have had a hysterectomy

▶ ✻ **G9775** Patient received at least 2 prophylactic pharmacologic anti-emetic agents of different classes preoperatively and/or intraoperatively

▶ ✻ **G9776** Documentation of medical reason for not receiving at least 2 prophylactic pharmacologic anti-emetic agents of different classes preoperatively and/or intraoperatively (e.g., intolerance or other medical reason)

▶ ✻ **G9777** Patient did not receive at least 2 prophylactic pharmacologic anti-emetic agents of different classes preoperatively and/or intraoperatively

▶ ✻ **G9778** Patients who have a diagnosis of pregnancy

▶ ✻ **G9779** Patients who are breastfeeding

▶ ✻ **G9780** Patients who have a diagnosis of rhabdomyolysis

▶ ✻ **G9781** Documentation of medical reason(s) for not currently being a statin therapy user or receive an order (prescription) for statin therapy (e.g., patient with adverse effect, allergy or intolerance to statin medication therapy, patients who are receiving palliative care, patients with active liver disease or hepatic disease or insufficiency, and patients with end stage renal disease (ESRD))

▶ ✻ **G9782** History of or active diagnosis of familial or pure hypercholesterolemia

▶ ✻ **G9783** Documentation of patients with diabetes who have a most recent fasting or direct LDL-C laboratory test result < 70 mg/dL and are not taking statin therapy

▶ ✻ **G9784** Pathologists/dermatopathologists providing a second opinion on a biopsy

▶ New ⤾ Revised ✔ Reinstated ~~deleted~~ Deleted ⃠ Not covered or valid by Medicare
⚙ Special coverage instructions ✻ Carrier discretion Ⓑ Bill local carrier Ⓓ Bill DME MAC

▶ ✻ **G9785** Pathology report diagnosing cutaneous basal cell carcinoma or squamous cell carcinoma (to include in situ disease) sent from the pathologist/dermatopathologist to the biopsying clinician for review within 7 business days from the time when the tissue specimen was received by the pathologist

▶ ✻ **G9786** Pathology report diagnosing cutaneous basal cell carcinoma or squamous cell carcinoma (to include in situ disease) was not sent from the pathologist/dermatopathologist to the biopsying clinician for review within 7 business days from the time when the tissue specimen was received by the pathologist

▶ ✻ **G9787** Patient alive as of the last day of the measurement year

▶ ✻ **G9788** Most recent BP is less than or equal to 140/90 mm Hg

▶ ✻ **G9789** Blood pressure recorded during inpatient stays, emergency room visits, urgent care visits, and patient self-reported BP's (home and health fair BP results)

▶ ✻ **G9790** Most recent BP is greater than 140/90 mm Hg, or blood pressure not documented

▶ ✻ **G9791** Most recent tobacco status is tobacco free

▶ ✻ **G9792** Most recent tobacco status is not tobacco free

▶ ✻ **G9793** Patient is currently on a daily aspirin or other antiplatelet

▶ ✻ **G9794** Documentation of medical reason(s) for not on a daily aspirin or other antiplatelet (e.g. history of gastrointestinal bleed or intra-cranial bleed or documentation of active anticoagulant use during the measurement period

▶ ✻ **G9795** Patient is not currently on a daily aspirin or other antiplatelet

▶ ✻ **G9796** Patient is currently on a statin therapy

▶ ✻ **G9797** Patient is not on a statin therapy

▶ ✻ **G9798** Discharge(s) for AMI between July 1 of the year prior measurement year to June 30 of the measurement period

▶ ✻ **G9799** Patients with a medication dispensing event indicator of a history of asthma any time during the patient's history through the end of the measure period

▶ ✻ **G9800** Patients who are identified as having an intolerance or allergy to beta-blocker therapy

▶ ✻ **G9801** Hospitalizations in which the patient was transferred directly to a non-acute care facility for any diagnosis

▶ ✻ **G9802** Patients who use hospice services any time during the measurement period

▶ ✻ **G9803** Patient prescribed a 180-day course of treatment with beta-blockers post discharge for AMI

▶ ✻ **G9804** Patient was not prescribed a 180-day course of treatment with beta-blockers post discharge for AMI

▶ ✻ **G9805** Patients who use hospice services any time during the measurement period

▶ ✻ **G9806** Patients who received cervical cytology or an HPV test

▶ ✻ **G9807** Patients who did not receive cervical cytology or an HPV test

▶ ✻ **G9808** Any patients who had no asthma controller medications dispensed during the measurement year

▶ ✻ **G9809** Patients who use hospice services any time during the measurement period

▶ ✻ **G9810** Patient achieved a PDC of at least 75% for their asthma controller medication

▶ ✻ **G9811** Patient did not achieve a PDC of at least 75% for their asthma controller medication

▶ ✻ **G9812** Patient died including all deaths occurring during the hospitalization in which the operation was performed, even if after 30 days, and those deaths occurring after discharge from the hospital, but within 30 days of the procedure

▶ ✻ **G9813** Patient did not die within 30 days of the procedure or during the index hospitalization

▶ ✻ **G9814** Death occurring during hospitalization

▶ ✻ **G9815** Death did not occur during hospitalization

▶ ✻ **G9816** Death occurring 30 days post procedure

▶ ✻ **G9817** Death did not occur 30 days post procedure

▶ ✻ **G9818** Documentation of sexual activity

▶ ✻ **G9819** Patients who use hospice services any time during the measurement period

▶ ✻ **G9820** Documentation of a chlamydia screening test with proper follow-up

▶ ✻ **G9821** No documentation of a chlamydia screening test with proper follow-up

▶ ✻ **G9822** Women who had an endometrial ablation procedure during the year prior to the index date (exclusive of the index date)

▶ ✻ **G9823** Endometrial sampling or hysteroscopy with biopsy and results documented

▶ ✻ **G9824** Endometrial sampling or hysteroscopy with biopsy and results not documented

▶ ✻ **G9825** HER-2/neu negative or undocumented/unknown

▶ ✻ **G9826** Patient transferred to practice after initiation of chemotherapy

▶ ✻ **G9827** HER2-targeted therapies not administered during the initial course of treatment

▶ ✻ **G9828** HER2-targeted therapies administered during the initial course of treatment

▶ ✻ **G9829** Breast adjuvant chemotherapy administered

▶ ✻ **G9830** HER-2/neu positive

▶ ✻ **G9831** AJCC stage at breast cancer diagnosis = II or III

▶ ✻ **G9832** AJCC stage at breast cancer diagnosis = I (Ia or Ib) and T-stage at breast cancer diagnosis does not equal = T1, T1a, T1b

▶ ✻ **G9833** Patient transfer to practice after initiation of chemotherapy

▶ ✻ **G9834** Patient has metastatic disease at diagnosis

▶ ✻ **G9835** Trastuzumab administered within 12 months of diagnosis

▶ ✻ **G9836** Reason for not administering trastuzumab documented (e.g. patient declined, patient died, patient transferred, contraindication or other clinical exclusion, neoadjuvant chemotherapy or radiation not complete)

▶ ✻ **G9837** Trastuzumab not administered within 12 months of diagnosis

▶ ✻ **G9838** Patient has metastatic disease at diagnosis

▶ ✻ **G9839** Anti-EGFR monoclonal antibody therapy

▶ ✻ **G9840** KRAS gene mutation testing performed before initiation of anti-EFGR MoAb

▶ ✻ **G9841** KRAS gene mutation testing not performed before initiation of anti-EFGR MoAb

▶ ✻ **G9842** Patient has metastatic disease at diagnosis

▶ ✻ **G9843** KRAS gene mutation

▶ ✻ **G9844** Patient did not receive anti-EGFR monoclonal antibody therapy

▶ ✻ **G9845** Patient received anti-EGFR monoclonal antibody therapy

▶ ✻ **G9846** Patients who died from cancer

▶ ✻ **G9847** Patient received chemotherapy in the last 14 days of life

▶ ✻ **G9848** Patient did not receive chemotherapy in the last 14 days of life

▶ ✻ **G9849** Patients who died from cancer

▶ ✻ **G9850** Patient had more than one emergency department visit in the last 30 days of life

▶ ✻ **G9851** Patient had one or less emergency department visits in the last 30 days of life

▶ ✻ **G9852** Patients who died from cancer

▶ ✻ **G9853** Patient admitted to the ICU in the last 30 days of life

▶ ✻ **G9854** Patient was not admitted to the ICU in the last 30 days of life

▶ ✻ **G9855** Patients who died from cancer

▶ ✻ **G9856** Patient was not admitted to hospice

▶ ✻ **G9857** Patient admitted to hospice

▶ ✻ **G9858** Patient enrolled in hospice

▶ ✻ **G9859** Patients who died from cancer

▶ ✻ **G9860** Patient spent less than three days in hospice care

▶ ✻ **G9861** Patient spent greater than or equal to three days in hospice care

▶ ✻ **G9862** Documentation of medical reason(s) for not recommending at least a 10 year follow-up interval (e.g., inadequate prep, familial or personal history of colonic polyps, patient had no adenoma and age is = 66 years old, or life expectancy <10 years old, other medical reasons)

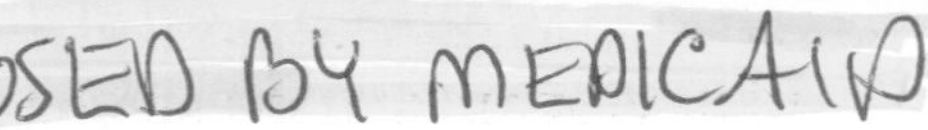

BEHAVIORAL HEALTH AND/OR SUBSTANCE ABUSE TREATMENT SERVICES (H0001-H9999)

NOTE: Used by Medicaid state agencies because no national code exists to meet the reporting needs of these agencies.

⊘ **H0001** Alcohol and/or drug assessment

⊘ **H0002** Behavioral health screening to determine eligibility for admission to treatment program

⊘ **H0003** Alcohol and/or drug screening; laboratory analysis of specimens for presence of alcohol and/or drugs

⊘ **H0004** Behavioral health counseling and therapy, per 15 minutes

⊘ **H0005** Alcohol and/or drug services; group counseling by a clinician

⊘ **H0006** Alcohol and/or drug services; case management

⊘ **H0007** Alcohol and/or drug services; crisis intervention (outpatient)

⊘ **H0008** Alcohol and/or drug services; sub-acute detoxification (hospital inpatient)

⊘ **H0009** Alcohol and/or drug services; acute detoxification (hospital inpatient)

⊘ **H0010** Alcohol and/or drug services; sub-acute detoxification (residential addiction program inpatient)

⊘ **H0011** Alcohol and/or drug services; acute detoxification (residential addiction program inpatient)

⊘ **H0012** Alcohol and/or drug services; sub-acute detoxification (residential addiction program outpatient)

⊘ **H0013** Alcohol and/or drug services; acute detoxification (residential addiction program outpatient)

⊘ **H0014** Alcohol and/or drug services; ambulatory detoxification

⊘ **H0015** Alcohol and/or drug services; intensive outpatient (treatment program that operates at least 3 hours/day and at least 3 days/week and is based on an individualized treatment plan), including assessment, counseling; crisis intervention, and activity therapies or education

⊘ **H0016** Alcohol and/or drug services; medical/somatic (medical intervention in ambulatory setting)

⊘ **H0017** Behavioral health; residential (hospital residential treatment program), without room and board, per diem

⊘ **H0018** Behavioral health; short-term residential (non-hospital residential treatment program), without room and board, per diem

⊘ **H0019** Behavioral health; long-term residential (non-medical, non-acute care in a residential treatment program where stay is typically longer than 30 days), without room and board, per diem

⊘ **H0020** Alcohol and/or drug services; methadone administration and/or service (provision of the drug by a licensed program)

⊘ **H0021** Alcohol and/or drug training service (for staff and personnel not employed by providers)

⊘ **H0022** Alcohol and/or drug intervention service (planned facilitation)

⊘ **H0023** Behavioral health outreach service (planned approach to reach a targeted population)

⊘ **H0024** Behavioral health prevention information dissemination service (one-way direct or non-direct contact with service audiences to affect knowledge and attitude)

⊘ **H0025** Behavioral health prevention education service (delivery of services with target population to affect knowledge, attitude and/or behavior)

⊘ **H0026** Alcohol and/or drug prevention process service, community-based (delivery of services to develop skills of impactors)

⊘ **H0027** Alcohol and/or drug prevention environmental service (broad range of external activities geared toward modifying systems in order to mainstream prevention through policy and law)

⊘ **H0028** Alcohol and/or drug prevention problem identification and referral service (e.g., student assistance and employee assistance programs), does not include assessment

⊘ **H0029** Alcohol and/or drug prevention alternatives service (services for populations that exclude alcohol and other drug use e.g., alcohol-free social events)

⊘ **H0030** Behavioral health hotline service

⊘ **H0031** Mental health assessment, by non-physician

⊘ **H0032** Mental health service plan development by non-physician

⊘ **H0033** Oral medication administration, direct observation

⊘ **H0034** Medication training and support, per 15 minutes

▶ New ⤻ Revised ✔ Reinstated ~~deleted~~ Deleted ⊘ Not covered or valid by Medicare
⚙ Special coverage instructions ✻ Carrier discretion Ⓑ Bill local carrier Ⓑ Bill DME MAC

⊘ **H0035** Mental health partial hospitalization, treatment, less than 24 hours

⊘ **H0036** Community psychiatric supportive treatment, face-to-face, per 15 minutes

⊘ **H0037** Community psychiatric supportive treatment program, per diem

⊘ **H0038** Self-help/peer services, per 15 minutes

⊘ **H0039** Assertive community treatment, face-to-face, per 15 minutes

⊘ **H0040** Assertive community treatment program, per diem

⊘ **H0041** Foster care, child, non-therapeutic, per diem

⊘ **H0042** Foster care, child, non-therapeutic, per month

⊘ **H0043** Supported housing, per diem

⊘ **H0044** Supported housing, per month

⊘ **H0045** Respite care services, not in the home, per diem

⊘ **H0046** Mental health services, not otherwise specified

⊘ **H0047** Alcohol and/or other drug abuse services, not otherwise specified

⊘ **H0048** Alcohol and/or other drug testing: collection and handling only, specimens other than blood

⊘ **H0049** Alcohol and/or drug screening

⊘ **H0050** Alcohol and/or drug services, brief intervention, per 15 minutes

⊘ **H1000** Prenatal care, at-risk assessment

⊘ **H1001** Prenatal care, at-risk enhanced service; antepartum management

⊘ **H1002** Prenatal care, at-risk enhanced service; care coordination

⊘ **H1003** Prenatal care, at-risk enhanced service; education

⊘ **H1004** Prenatal care, at-risk enhanced service; follow-up home visit

⊘ **H1005** Prenatal care, at-risk enhanced service package (includes H1001-H1004)

⊘ **H1010** Non-medical family planning education, per session

⊘ **H1011** Family assessment by licensed behavioral health professional for state defined purposes

⊘ **H2000** Comprehensive multidisciplinary evaluation

⊘ **H2001** Rehabilitation program, per 1/2 day

⊘ **H2010** Comprehensive medication services, per 15 minutes

⊘ **H2011** Crisis intervention service, per 15 minutes

⊘ **H2012** Behavioral health day treatment, per hour

⊘ **H2013** Psychiatric health facility service, per diem

⊘ **H2014** Skills training and development, per 15 minutes

⊘ **H2015** Comprehensive community support services, per 15 minutes

⊘ **H2016** Comprehensive community support services, per diem

⊘ **H2017** Psychosocial rehabilitation services, per 15 minutes

⊘ **H2018** Psychosocial rehabilitation services, per diem

⊘ **H2019** Therapeutic behavioral services, per 15 minutes

⊘ **H2020** Therapeutic behavioral services, per diem

⊘ **H2021** Community-based wrap-around services, per 15 minutes

⊘ **H2022** Community-based wrap-around services, per diem

⊘ **H2023** Supported employment, per 15 minutes

⊘ **H2024** Supported employment, per diem

⊘ **H2025** Ongoing support to maintain employment, per 15 minutes

⊘ **H2026** Ongoing support to maintain employment, per diem

⊘ **H2027** Psychoeducational service, per 15 minutes

⊘ **H2028** Sexual offender treatment service, per 15 minutes

⊘ **H2029** Sexual offender treatment service, per diem

⊘ **H2030** Mental health clubhouse services, per 15 minutes

⊘ **H2031** Mental health clubhouse services, per diem

⊘ **H2032** Activity therapy, per 15 minutes

⊘ **H2033** Multisystemic therapy for juveniles, per 15 minutes

⊘ **H2034** Alcohol and/or drug abuse halfway house services, per diem

⊘ **H2035** Alcohol and/or other drug treatment program, per hour

⊘ **H2036** Alcohol and/or other drug treatment program, per diem

⊘ **H2037** Developmental delay prevention activities, dependent child of client, per 15 minutes

▶ New ⤺ Revised ✔ Reinstated ~~deleted~~ Deleted ⊘ Not covered or valid by Medicare
Special coverage instructions ✻ Carrier discretion Bill local carrier Bill DME MAC

DRUGS OTHER THAN CHEMOTHERAPY DRUGS (J0100-J8999)

J0120-J3570: Bill Local Carrier if incident to a physician's service or used in an implanted infusion pump. If other, bill DME MAC.

J0120 Injection, tetracycline, up to 250 mg

Other: Achromycin

IOM: 100-02, 15, 50

J0129 Injection, abatacept, 10 mg

NDC: Orencia

J0130 Injection, abciximab, 10 (Code may be used for Medicare when drug administered under the direct supervision of a physician; not for use when drug is self-administered)

NDC: ReoPro

IOM: 100-02, 15, 50

J0131 Injection, acetaminophen, 10 mg

J0132 Injection, acetylcysteine, 100 mg

NDC: Acetadote

J0133 Injection, acyclovir, 5 mg

J0135 Injection, adalimumab, 20 mg

NDC: Humira

IOM: 100-02, 15, 50

J0153 Injection, adenosine, 1 mg (not to be used to report any adenosine phosphate compounds)

Other: Adenocard

J0171 Injection, adrenalin, epinephrine, 0.1 mg

IOM: 100-02, 15, 50

J0178 Injection, aflibercept, 1 mg

J0180 Injection, agalsidase beta, 1 mg

NDC: Fabrazyme

IOM: 100-02, 15, 50

J0190 Injection, biperiden lactate, per 5 mg

Other: Akineton

IOM: 100-02, 15, 50

J0200 Injection, alatrofloxacin mesylate, 100 mg

Other: Trovan

IOM: 100-02, 15, 50

J0202 Injection, alemtuzumab, 1 mg

NDC: Lemtrada

J0205 Injection, alglucerase, per 10 units

Other: Ceredase

IOM: 100-02, 15, 50

J0207 Injection, amifostine, 500 mg

Other: Ethyol

IOM: 100-02, 15, 50

J0210 Injection, methyldopate HCL, up to 250 mg

Other: Aldomet

IOM: 100-02, 15, 50

J0215 Injection, alefacept, 0.5 mg

NDC: Amevive

J0220 Injection, alglucosidase alfa, not otherwise specified, 10 mg

J0221 Injection, alglucosidase alfa, (lumizyme), 10 mg

J0256 Injection, alpha 1-proteinase inhibitor (human), not otherwise specified, 10 mg

NDC: Aralast, Aralast NP, Prolastin, Prolastin-C, Zemaira

IOM: 100-02, 15, 50

J0257 Injection, alpha 1 proteinase inhibitor (human), (glassia), 10 mg

IOM: 100-02, 15, 50

J0270 Injection, alprostadil, per 1.25 mcg (Code may be used for Medicare when drug administered under the direct supervision of a physician, not for use when drug is self administered)

Other: Caverject, Prostaglandin E1

IOM: 100-02, 15, 50

J0275 Alprostadil urethral suppository (Code may be used for Medicare when drug administered under the direct supervision of a physician, not for use when drug is self administered)

Other: Muse

IOM: 100-02, 15, 50

J0278 Injection, amikacin sulfate, 100 mg

Other: Amikin

J0280 Injection, aminophylline, up to 250 mg

IOM: 100-02, 15, 50

J0282 Injection, amiodarone hydrochloride, 30 mg

Other: Cordarone

IOM: 100-02, 15, 50

▶ New ⤼ Revised ✔ Reinstated ~~deleted~~ Deleted ⊘ Not covered or valid by Medicare
Special coverage instructions * Carrier discretion Bill local carrier Bill DME MAC

✪ **J0285** Injection, am[illegible]in B, 50 mg
Other: ABLC, A[illegible]ungizone
IOM: 100-02, 15, 50

✪ **J0287** Injection, amphotericin B lipid complex, 10 mg
NDC: Abelcet
IOM: 100-02, 15, 50

✪ **J0288** Injection, amphotericin B cholesteryl sulfate complex, 10 mg
IOM: 100-02, 15, 50

✪ **J0289** Injection, amphotericin B liposome, 10 mg
NDC: AmBisome
IOM: 100-02, 15, 50

✪ **J0290** Injection, ampicillin sodium, 500 mg
Other: Omnipen-N, Polycillin-N, Totacillin-N
IOM: 100-02, 15, 50

✪ **J0295** Injection, ampicillin sodium/sulbactam sodium, per 1.5 gm
NDC: Unasyn
Other: Omnipen-N, Polycillin-N, Totacillin-N
IOM: 100-02, 15, 50

✪ **J0300** Injection, amobarbital, up to 125 mg
Other: Amytal
IOM: 100-02, 15, 50

✪ **J0330** Injection, succinylcholine chloride, up to 20 mg
Other: Anectine, Quelicin
IOM: 100-02, 15, 50

* **J0348** Injection, anidulafungin, 1 mg
NDC: Eraxis

✪ **J0350** Injection, anistreplase, per 30 units
Other: Eminase
IOM: 100-02, 15, 50

✪ **J0360** Injection, hydralazine hydrochloride, up to 20 mg
Other: Apresoline
IOM: 100-02, 15, 50

* **J0364** Injection, apomorphine hydrochloride, 1 mg

✪ **J0365** Injection, aprotinin, 10,000 KIU
NDC: Trasylol
IOM: 100-02, 15, 50

✪ **J0380** Injection, metaraminol bitartrate, per 10 mg
Other: Aramine
IOM: 100-02, 15, 50

✪ **J0390** Injection, chloroquine hydrochloride, up to 250 mg
Benefit only for diagnosed malaria or amebiasis
Other: Aralen
IOM: 100-02, 15, 50

✪ **J0395** Injection, arbutamine HCL, 1 mg
IOM: 100-02, 15, 50

* **J0400** Injection, aripiprazole, intramuscular, 0.25 mg
Other: Abilify

* **J0401** Injection, aripiprazole, extended release, 1 mg
NDC: Abilify

✪ **J0456** Injection, azithromycin, 500 mg
NDC: Zithromax
IOM: 100-02, 15, 50

✪ **J0461** Injection, atropine sulfate, 0.01 mg
IOM: 100-02, 15, 50

✪ **J0470** Injection, dimercaprol, per 100 mg
NDC: BAL In Oil
IOM: 100-02, 15, 50

✪ **J0475** Injection, baclofen, 10 mg
NDC: Gablofen, Lioresal
IOM: 100-02, 15, 50

✪ **J0476** Injection, baclofen 50 mcgfor intrathecal trial
NDC: Gablofen, Lioresal
IOM: 100-02, 15, 50

✪ **J0480** Injection, basiliximab, 20 mg
NDC: Simulect
IOM: 100-02, 15, 50

* **J0485** Injection, belatacept, 1 mg
NDC: Nulojix

* **J0490** Injection, belimumab, 10 mg
NDC: Benlysta

⊛ **J0500** Injection, dicyclomine HCL, up to 20 mg

NDC: Bentyl

Other: Antispas, Dibent, Dicyclocot, Dilomine, Di-Spaz, Neoquess, Or-Tyl, Spasmoject

IOM: 100-02, 15, 50

⊛ **J0515** Injection, benztropine mesylate, per 1 mg

NDC: Cogentin

IOM: 100-02, 15, 50

⊛ **J0520** Injection, bethanechol chloride, myotonachol or urecholine, up to 5 mg

IOM: 100-02, 15, 50

✻ **J0558** Injection, penicillin G benzathine and penicillin G procaine, 100,000 units

NDC: Bicillin C-R

⊛ **J0561** Injection, penicillin G benzathine, 100,000 units

NDC: Bicillin L-A

IOM: 100-02, 15, 50

▶ ✻ **J0570** Buprenorphine implant, 74.2 mg

⊛ **J0571** Buprenorphine, oral, 1 mg

⊛ **J0572** Buprenorphine/naloxone, oral, less than or equal to 3 mg buprenorphine

↩ ⊛ **J0573** Buprenorphine/naloxone, oral, greater than 3 mg, but less than or equal to 6 mg buprenorphine

⊛ **J0574** Buprenorphine/naloxone, oral, greater than 6 mg, but less than or equal to 10 mg buprenorphine

⊛ **J0575** Buprenorphine/naloxone, oral, greater than 10 mg buprenorphine

✻ **J0583** Injection, bivalirudin, 1 mg

NDC: Angiomax

⊛ **J0585** Injection, onabotulinumtoxinaA, 1 unit

NDC: Botox, Botox Cosmetic

Other: Oculinum

IOM: 100-02, 15, 50

✻ **J0586** Injection, abobotulinumtoxinaA, 5 units

NDC: Dysport

⊛ **J0587** Injection, rimabotulinumtoxinB, 100 units

NDC: Myobloc

IOM: 100-02, 15, 50

✻ **J0588** Injection, incobotulinumtoxin A, 1 unit

NDC: Xeomin

⊛ **J0592** Injection, buprenorphine hydrochloride, 0.1 mg

IOM: 100-02, 15, 50

✻ **J0594** Injection, busulfan, 1 mg

✻ **J0595** Injection, butorphanol tartrate, 1 mg

NDC: Stadol

✻ **J0596** Injection, C1 esterase inhibitor (recombinant), ruconest, 10 units

✻ **J0597** Injection, C-1 esterase inhibitor (human), Berinet, 10 units

✻ **J0598** Injection, C1 esterase inhibitor (human), cinryze, 10 units

⊛ **J0600** Injection, edetate calcium disodium, up to 1000 mg

NDC: Calcium Disodium Versenate

IOM: 100-02, 15, 50

⊛ **J0610** Injection, calcium gluconate, per 10 ml

Other: Kaleinate

IOM: 100-02, 15, 50

⊛ **J0620** Injection, calcium glycerophosphate and calcium lactate, per 10 ml

Other: Calphosan

MCM: 2049

IOM: 100-02, 15, 50

⊛ **J0630** Injection, calcitonin (salmon), up to 400 units

NDC: Miacalcin

Other: Calcimar, Calcitonin-salmon

IOM: 100-02, 15, 50

⊛ **J0636** Injection, calcitriol, 0.1 mcg

Non-dialysis use

NDC: Calcijex

IOM: 100-02, 15, 50

✻ **J0637** Injection, caspofungin acetate, 5 mg

NDC: Cancidas

✻ **J0638** Injection, canakinumab, 1 mg

NDC: Ilaris

▶ New ↩ Revised ✔ Reinstated ~~deleted~~ Deleted ⊘ Not covered or valid by Medicare
⊛ Special coverage instructions ✻ Carrier discretion Ⓑ Bill local carrier Ⓑ Bill DME MAC

✪ **J0640** Injection, leucovorin calcium, per 50 mg Ⓑ Ⓑ
NDC: Calcium Folinate (Hungarian import)
Other: Wellcovorin
IOM: 100-02, 15, 50

✪ **J0641** Injection, levoleucovorin calcium, 0.5 mg Ⓑ Ⓑ
Part of treatment regimen for osteosarcoma

✪ **J0670** Injection, mepivacaine HCL, per 10 ml Ⓑ Ⓑ
NDC: Polocaine, Polocaine-MPF
Other: Carbocaine, Isocaine HCl
IOM: 100-02, 15, 50

✪ **J0690** Injection, cefezolin sodium, 500 mg Ⓑ Ⓑ
Other: Ancef, Kefzol
IOM: 100-02, 15, 50

* **J0692** Injection, cefepime HCL, 500 mg Ⓑ Ⓑ
NDC: Maxipime

✪ **J0694** Injection, cefoxitin sodium, 1 gm Ⓑ Ⓑ
Other: Mefoxin
IOM: 100-02, 15, 50,
Cross Reference Q0090

* **J0695** Injection, ceftolozane 50 mg and tazobactam 25 mg Ⓑ Ⓑ

✪ **J0696** Injection, ceftriaxone sodium, per 250 mg Ⓑ Ⓑ
NDC: Rocephin
IOM: 100-02, 15, 50

✪ **J0697** Injection, sterile cefuroxime sodium, per 750 mg Ⓑ Ⓑ
NDC: Zinacef
Other: Kefurox
IOM: 100-02, 15, 50

✪ **J0698** Injection, cefotaxime sodium, per g Ⓑ Ⓑ
NDC: Claforan
IOM: 100-02, 15, 50

✪ **J0702** Injection, betamethasone acetate 3 mg and betamethasone sodium phosphate 3 mg Ⓑ Ⓑ
NDC: Celestone Soluspan
Other: Betameth
IOM: 100-02, 15, 50

* **J0706** Injection, caffeine citrate, 5 mg Ⓑ Ⓑ
Other: Cafcit, Cipro IV, Ciprofloxacin

✪ **J0710** Injection, cephapirin sodium, up to 1 gm Ⓑ Ⓑ
Other: Cefadyl
IOM: 100-02, 15, 50

* **J0712** Injection, ceftaroline fosamil, 10 mg Ⓑ Ⓑ
NDC: Teflaro

✪ **J0713** Injection, ceftazidime, per 500 mg Ⓑ Ⓑ
NDC: Fortaz, Tazicef
IOM: 100-02, 15, 50

* **J0714** Injection, ceftazidime and avibactam, 0.5 g/0.125 g Ⓑ Ⓑ

✪ **J0715** Injection, ceftizoxime sodium, per 500 mg Ⓑ Ⓑ
IOM: 100-02, 15, 50

* **J0716** Injection, centruroides immune F(ab)2, up to 120 milligrams Ⓑ Ⓑ

* **J0717** Injection, certolizumab pegol, 1 mg (code may be used for Medicare when drug administered under the direct supervision of a physician, not for use when drug is self administered) Ⓑ Ⓑ

✪ **J0720** Injection, chloramphenicol sodium succinate, up to 1 gm Ⓑ Ⓑ
IOM: 100-02, 15, 50

✪ **J0725** Injection, chorionic gonadotropin, per 1,000 USP units Ⓑ Ⓑ
NDC: Novarel
Other: A.P.L., Chorex-5, Chorex-10, Chorignon, Choron-10, Corgonject-5, Follutein, Glukor, Gonic, Pregnyl, Profasi HP
IOM: 100-02, 15, 50

✪ **J0735** Injection, clonidine hydrochloride (HCL), 1 mg Ⓑ Ⓑ
NDC: Duraclon
IOM: 100-02, 15, 50

✪ **J0740** Injection, cidofovir, 375 mg Ⓑ Ⓑ
NDC: Vistide
IOM: 100-02, 15, 50

✪ **J0743** Injection, cilastatin sodium; imipenem, per 250 mg Ⓑ Ⓑ
NDC: Primaxin
IOM: 100-02, 15, 50

* **J0744** Injection, ciprofloxacin for intravenous infusion, 200 mg Ⓑ Ⓑ
Other: Cipro IV

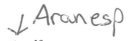

J0745 Injection, codeine phosphate, per 30 mg
IOM: 100-02, 15, 50

~~J0760 Injection, colchicine, per 1 mg~~ ✖

J0770 Injection, colistimethate sodium, up to 150 mg
NDC: Coly-Mycin M Parenteral
IOM: 100-02, 15, 50

* **J0775** Injection, collagenase, clostridium histolyticum, 0.01 mg
NDC: Xiaflex

J0780 Injection, prochlorperazine, up to 10 mg
Other: Compa-Z, Compazine, Cotranzine, Ultrazine-10
IOM: 100-02, 15, 50

J0795 Injection, corticorelin ovine triflutate, 1 microgram
NDC: Acthrel
IOM: 100-02, 15, 50

J0800 Injection, corticotropin, up to 40 units
NDC: Acthar H.P.
Other: Acthar, ACTH
IOM: 100-02, 15, 50

* **J0833** Injection, cosyntropin, not otherwise specified, 0.25 mg

* **J0834** Injection, cosyntropin (Cortrosyn), 0.25 mg

* **J0840** Injection, crotalidae polyvalent immune fab (ovine), up to 1 gram
NDC: Crofab Powder for Solution

J0850 Injection, cytomegalovirus immune globulin intravenous (human), per vial
Prophylaxis to prevent cytomegalovirus disease associated with transplantation of kidney, lung, liver, pancreas, and heart.
NDC: CytoGam
IOM: 100-02, 15, 50

* **J0875** Injection, dalbavancin, 5 mg
NDC: Dalvance

* **J0878** Injection, daptomycin, 1 mg
NDC: Cubicin

J0881 Injection, darbepoetin alfa, 1 microgram (non-ESRD use)
NDC: Aranesp

⤾ **J0882** Injection, darbepoetin alfa, 1 microgram (for ESRD on dialysis)
NDC: Aranesp
IOM: 100-02, 6, 10; 100-04, 4, 240

▶ **J0883** Injection, argatroban, 1 mg (for non-ESRD use)
IOM: 100-02, 15, 50

▶ **J0884** Injection, argatroban, 1 mg (for ESRD on dialysis)
IOM: 100-02, 15, 50

J0885 Injection, epoetin alfa, (for non-ESRD use), 1000 units
NDC: Epogen, Procrit
IOM: 100-02, 15, 50

J0887 Injection, epoetin beta, 1 microgram, (for ESRD on dialysis)
NDC: Mircera

J0888 Injection, epoetin beta, 1 microgram, (for non ESRD use)
NDC: Mircera

* **J0890** Injection, peginesatide, 0.1 mg (for ESRD on dialysis)
NDC: Omontys

* **J0894** Injection, decitabine, 1 mg
Indicated for treatment of myelodysplastic syndromes (MDS)
NDC: Dacogen

J0895 Injection, deferoxamine mesylate, 500 mg
NDC: Desferal
Other: Desferal mesylate
IOM: 100-02, 15, 50,
Cross Reference Q0087

* **J0897** Injection, denosumab, 1 mg
NDC: Prolia, Xgeva

J0945 Injection, brompheniramine maleate, per 10 mg
Other: Codimal-A, Cophene-B, Dehist, Histaject, Nasahist B, ND Stat, Oraminic II, Sinusol-B
IOM: 100-02, 15, 50

J1000 Injection, depo-estradiol cypionate, up to 5 mg
Other: DepGynogen, Depogen, Dura-Estrin, Estra-D, Estro-Cyp, Estroject LA, Estronol-LA
IOM: 100-02, 15, 50

▶ New ⤾ Revised ✔ Reinstated ~~deleted~~ Deleted ⃠ Not covered or valid by Medicare
Special coverage instructions * Carrier discretion Bill local carrier Bill DME MAC

⊕ **J1020** Injection, methylprednisolone acetate, 20 mg Ⓑ Ⓑ

NDC: Depo-Medrol, Methylpred

Other: DepMedalone, Depoject, Depopred, D-Med 80, Duralone, Medralone, M-Prednisol, Rep-Pred

IOM: 100-02, 15, 50

⊕ **J1030** Injection, methylprednisolone acetate, 40 mg Ⓑ Ⓑ

NDC: Depo-Medrol

Other: DepMedalone, Depoject, Depropred, D-Med 80, Duralone, Medralone, M-Prednisol, Rep-Pred

IOM: 100-02, 15, 50

⊕ **J1040** Injection, methylprednisolone acetate, 80 mg Ⓑ Ⓑ

NDC: Depo-Medrol

Other: DepMedalone, Depoject, Depropred, D-Med 80, Duralone, Medralone, M-Prednisol, Rep-Pred

IOM: 100-02, 15, 50

* **J1050** Injection, medroxyprogesterone acetate, 1 mg Ⓑ Ⓑ

Other: Depo-Provera Contraceptive

⊕ **J1071** Injection, testosterone cypionate, 1 mg

⊕ **J1094** Injection, dexamethasone acetate, 1 mg Ⓑ Ⓑ

Other: Dalalone LA, Decadron LA, Decaject LA, Dexacen-LA-8, Dexamethasone Micronized, Dexasone L.A., Dexone-LA

IOM: 100-02, 15, 50

⊕ **J1100** Injection, dexamethasone sodium phosphate, 1 mg Ⓑ Ⓑ

Other: Dalalone, Decadron Phosphate, Decaject, Dexacen-4, Dexone, Hexadrol Phosphate, Solurex

IOM: 100-02, 15, 50

⊕ **J1110** Injection, dihydroergotamine mesylate, per 1 mg Ⓑ Ⓑ

NDC: D.H.E. 45

IOM: 100-02, 15, 50

⊕ **J1120** Injection, acetazolamide sodium, up to 500 mg Ⓑ Ⓑ

Other: Diamox

IOM: 100-02, 15, 50

▶ * **J1130** Injection, diclofenac sodium, 0.5 mg Ⓑ Ⓑ

⊕ **J1160** Injection, digoxin, up to 0.5 mg Ⓑ Ⓑ

NDC: Lanoxin

IOM: 100-02, 15, 50

⊕ **J1162** Injection, digoxin immune Fab (ovine), per vial Ⓑ Ⓑ

NDC: Digibind, DigiFab

IOM: 100-02, 15, 50

⊕ **J1165** Injection, phenytoin sodium, per 50 mg Ⓑ Ⓑ

Other: Dilantin

IOM: 100-02, 15, 50

⊕ **J1170** Injection, hydromorphone, up to 4 mg Ⓑ Ⓑ

Other: Dilaudid

IOM: 100-02, 15, 50

⊕ **J1180** Injection, dyphylline, up to 500 mg Ⓑ Ⓑ

Other: Dilor, Lufyllin

IOM: 100-02, 15, 50

⊕ **J1190** Injection, dexrazoxane hydrochloride, per 250 mg Ⓑ Ⓑ

NDC: Totect, Zinecard

IOM: 100-02, 15, 50

⊕ **J1200** Injection, diphenhydramine HCL, up to 50 mg Ⓑ Ⓑ

NDC: Benadryl

Other: Bena-D, Benahist, Ben-Allergin, Benoject, Truxadryl

⊕ **J1205** Injection, chlorothiazide sodium, per 500 mg Ⓑ Ⓑ

NDC: Diuril

IOM: 100-02, 15, 50

↩ ⊕ **J1212** Injection, DMSO, dimethyl sulfoxide, 50%, 50 ml Ⓑ Ⓑ

NDC: Rimso-50

IOM: 100-02, 15, 50; 100-03, 4, 230.12

⊕ **J1230** Injection, methadone HCL, up to 10 mg Ⓑ Ⓑ

MCM: 2049

IOM: 100-02, 15, 50

⊕ **J1240** Injection, dimenhydrinate, up to 50 mg Ⓑ Ⓑ

Other: Dinate, Dommanate, Dramamine, Dramanate, Dramilin, Dramocen, Dramoject, Dymenate, Hydrate, Marmine, Wehamine

IOM: 100-02, 15, 50

▶ New ↩ Revised ✔ Reinstated ~~deleted~~ Deleted ⊘ Not covered or valid by Medicare
⊕ Special coverage instructions * Carrier discretion Ⓑ Bill local carrier Ⓑ Bill DME MAC

J1245 Injection, dipyridamole, per 10 mg
Other: Persantine
IOM: 100-04, 15, 50; 100-04, 12, 30.6

J1250 Injection, dobutamine HCL, per 250 mg
Other: Dobutrex
IOM: 100-02, 15, 50

J1260 Injection, dolasetron mesylate, 10 mg
NDC: Anzemet
IOM: 100-02, 15, 50

* **J1265** Injection, dopamine HCL, 40 mg

* **J1267** Injection, doripenem, 10 mg
NDC: Doribax

* **J1270** Injection, doxercalciferol, 1 mcg
NDC: Hectorol

* **J1290** Injection, ecallantide, 1 mg
NDC: Kalbitor

* **J1300** Injection, eculizumab, 10 mg
NDC: Soliris

J1320 Injection, amitriptyline HCL, up to 20 mg
Other: Elavil, Enovil
IOM: 100-02, 15, 50

* **J1322** Injection, elosulfase alfa, 1 mg

* **J1324** Injection, enfuvirtide, 1 mg
Other: Fuzeon

J1325 Injection, epoprostenol, 0.5 mg
NDC: Flolan, Veletri
IOM: 100-02, 15, 50

J1327 Injection, eptifibatide, 5 mg
Other: Integrilin
IOM: 100-02, 15, 50

J1330 Injection, ergonovine maleate, up to 0.2 mg
Benefit limited to obstetrical diagnosis
IOM: 100-02, 15, 50

* **J1335** Injection, ertapenem sodium, 500 mg
NDC: Invanz

J1364 Injection, erythromycin lactobionate, per 500 mg
IOM: 100-02, 15, 50

J1380 Injection, estradiol valerate, up to 10 mg
NDC: Delestrogen
Other: Dioval, Duragen, Estra-L, Gynogen L.A., L.A.E. 20, Valergen
IOM: 100-02, 15, 50

J1410 Injection, estrogen conjugated, per 25 mg
NDC: Premarin
IOM: 100-02, 15, 50

J1430 Injection, ethanolamine oleate, 100 mg
Other: Ethamolin
IOM: 100-02, 15, 50

J1435 Injection, estrone, per 1 mg
Other: Estragyn, Estronol, Kestrone 5, Theelin Aqueous
IOM: 100-02, 15, 50

J1436 Injection, etidronate disodium, per 300 mg
Other: Didronel
IOM: 100-02, 15, 50

J1438 Injection, etanercept, 25 mg (Code may be used for Medicare when drug administered under the direct supervision of a physician, not for use when drug is self-administered.)
Other: Enbrel
IOM: 100-02, 15, 50

* **J1439** Injection, ferric carboxymaltose, 1 mg
NDC: Injectafer

J1442 Injection, fi lgrastim (G-CSF), excludes biosimilars, 1 microgram
NDC: Neupogen

* **J1443** Injection, ferric pyrophosphate citrate solution, 0.1 mg of iron

J1447 Injection, TBO-filgrastim, 1 microgram
NDC: GRANIX
IOM: 100-02, 15, 50

J1450 Injection, fluconazole, 200 mg
NDC: Diflucan
IOM: 100-02, 15, 50

J1451 Injection, fomepizole, 15 mg
IOM: 100-02, 15, 50

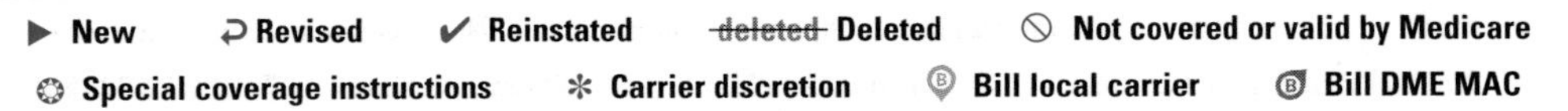

J1452 Injection, fomivirsen sodium, intraocular, 1.65 mg

IOM: 100-02, 15, 50

J1453 Injection, fosaprepitant, 1 mg

Prevents chemotherapy-induced nausea and vomiting

NDC: Emend

J1455 Injection, foscarnet sodium, per 1000 mg

Other: Foscavir

IOM: 100-02, 15, 50

J1457 Injection, gallium nitrate, 1 mg

NDC: Ganite

J1458 Injection, galsulfase, 1 mg

NDC: Naglazyme

J1459 Injection, immune globulin (Privigen), intravenous, non-lyophilized (e.g., liquid), 500 mg

J1460 Injection, gamma globulin, intramuscular, 1 cc

NDC: GamaSTAN

Other: Gammar

IOM: 100-02, 15, 50

J1556 Injection, immune globulin (Bivigam), 500 mg

J1557 Injection, immune globulin, (gammaplex), intravenous, non-lyophilized (e.g., liquid), 500 mg

J1559 Injection, immune globulin, (hizentra), 100 mg

J1560 Injection, gamma globulin, intramuscular, over 10 cc

NDC: GamaSTAN

Other: Gammar

IOM: 100-02, 15, 50

J1561 Injection, immune globulin, (Gamunex-C/Gammaked), non-lyophilized (e.g., liquid), 500 mg

NDC: Gamunex

IOM: 100-02, 15, 50

J1562 Injection, immune globulin (Vivaglobin), 100 mg

J1566 Injection, immune globulin, intravenous, lyophilized (e.g., powder), not otherwise specified, 500 mg

NDC: Carimune, Gammagard S/D

Other: Polygam

IOM: 100-02, 15, 50

J1568 Injection, immune globulin, (Octagam), intravenous, non-lyophilized (e.g., liquid), 500 mg

J1569 Injection, immune globulin, (Gammagard Liquid), non-lyophilized, (e.g., liquid), 500 mg

IOM: 100-02, 15, 50

J1570 Injection, ganciclovir sodium, 500 mg

NDC: Cytovene

IOM: 100-02, 15, 50

J1571 Injection, hepatitis B immune globulin (HepaGam B), intramuscular, 0.5 ml

IOM: 100-02, 15, 50

J1572 Injection, immune globulin, (flebogamma/flebogamma DIF) intravenous, non-lyophilized (e.g., liquid), 500 mg

IOM: 100-02, 15, 50

J1573 Injection, hepatitis B immune globulin (HepaGam B), intravenous, 0.5 ml

J1575 Injection, immune globulin/ hyaluronidase, (HYQVIA), 100 mg immunoglobulin

J1580 Injection, Garamycin, gentamicin, up to 80 mg

NDC: Gentamicin Sulfate

Other: Jenamicin

IOM: 100-02, 15, 50

~~J1590 Injection, gatifloxacin, 10 mg~~

J1595 Injection, glatiramer acetate, 20 mg

Other: Copaxone

IOM: 100-02, 15, 50

J1599 Injection, immune globulin, intravenous, non-lyophilized (e.g., liquid), not otherwise specified, 500 mg

J1600 Injection, gold sodium thiomalate, up to 50 mg

Other: Myochrysine

IOM: 100-02, 15, 50

J1602 Injection, golimumab, 1 mg,for intravenous use

NDC: Simponi Aria

J1610 Injection, glucagon hydrochloride, per 1 mg

Other: GlucaGen, Glucagon Emergency

IOM: 100-02, 15, 50

J1620 Injection, gonadorelin hydrochloride, per 100 mcg
Other: Factrel
IOM: 100-02, 15, 50

J1626 Injection, granisetron hydrochloride, 100 mcg
Other: Kytril
IOM: 100-02, 15, 50

J1630 Injection, haloperidol, up to 5 mg
NDC: Haldol, Haloperidol Lactate
IOM: 100-02, 15, 50

J1631 Injection, haloperidol decanoate, per 50 mg
IOM: 100-02, 15, 50

J1640 Injection, hemin, 1 mg
NDC: Panhematin
IOM: 100-02, 15, 50

J1642 Injection, heparin sodium, (heparin lock flush), per 10 units
NDC: Heparin (Porcine) Lock Flush, Heparin Sodium Flush
Other: Hep-Lock U/P
IOM: 100-02, 15, 50

J1644 Injection, heparin sodium, per 1000 units
NDC: Heparin (Porcine), Heparin Sodium (Porcine)
Other: Liquaemin Sodium
IOM: 100-02, 15, 50

J1645 Injection, dalteparin sodium, per 2500 IU
NDC: Fragmin
IOM: 100-02, 15, 50

* **J1650** Injection, enoxaparin sodium, 10 mg
NDC: Lovenox

J1652 Injection, fondaparinux sodium, 0.5 mg
NDC: Arixtra
IOM: 100-02, 15, 50

* **J1655** Injection, tinzaparin sodium, 1000 IU
Other: Innohep

J1670 Injection, tetanus immune globulin, human, up to 250 units
Indicated for transient protection against tetanus post-exposure to tetanus (Z23).
NDC: Hypertet S/D
Other: Hyper-tet
IOM: 100-02, 15, 50

J1675 Injection, histrelin acetate, 10 micrograms
IOM: 100-02, 15, 50

J1700 Injection, hydrocortisone acetate, up to 25 mg
Other: Hydrocortone Acetate
IOM: 100-02, 15, 50

J1710 Injection, hydrocortisone sodium phosphate, up to 50 mg
Other: A-hydroCort, Hydrocortone phosphate, Solu-Cortef
IOM: 100-02, 15, 50

J1720 Injection, hydrocortisone sodium succinate, up to 100 mg
NDC: Solu-Cortef
Other: A-HydroCort
IOM: 100-02, 15, 50

* **J1725** Injection, hydroxyprogesterone caproate, 1 mg

J1730 Injection, diazoxide, up to 300 mg
Other: Hyperstat
IOM: 100-02, 15, 50

* **J1740** Injection, ibandronate sodium, 1 mg
NDC: Boniva

* **J1741** Injection, ibuprofen, 100 mg

J1742 Injection, ibutilide fumarate, 1 mg
NDC: Corvert
IOM: 100-02, 15, 50

* **J1743** Injection, idursulfase, 1 mg
NDC: Elaprase

* **J1744** Injection, icatibant, 1 mg

J1745 Injection, infliximab, excludes biosimilar, 10 mg
Report total number of 10 mg increments administered
NDC: Remicade
IOM: 100-02, 15, 50

▶ New ⮌ Revised ✔ Reinstated ~~deleted~~ Deleted ⊘ Not covered or valid by Medicare
Special coverage instructions * Carrier discretion Bill local carrier Bill DME MAC

⊛ **J1750** Injection, iron dextran, 50 mg Ⓑ Ⓑ
NDC: Dexferrum, Infed
IOM: 100-02, 15, 50

✻ **J1756** Injection, iron sucrose, 1 mg Ⓑ Ⓑ
NDC: Venofer

⊛ **J1786** Injection, imiglucerase, 10 units Ⓑ Ⓑ
NDC: Cerezyme
IOM: 100-02, 15, 50

⊛ **J1790** Injection, droperidol, up to 5 mg Ⓑ Ⓑ
Other: Inapsine
IOM: 100-02, 15, 50

⊛ **J1800** Injection, propranolol HCL, up to 1 mg Ⓑ Ⓑ
Other: Inderal
IOM: 100-02, 15, 50

⊛ **J1810** Injection, droperidol and fentanyl cit-rate, up to 2 ml ampule Ⓑ Ⓑ
Other: Innovar
IOM: 100-02, 15, 50

⊛ **J1815** Injection, insulin, per 5 units Ⓑ Ⓑ
NDC: Humalog, Humulin, Lantus, Levemir, Novolin, Novolog
IOM: 100-02, 15, 50; 100-30, 4, 280.14

✻ **J1817** Insulin for administration through DME (i.e., insulin pump) per 50 units Ⓑ Ⓑ
NDC: Humalog, Humulin, Novolin, Novolog
Other: Apidra Solostar, Insulin Lispro

↩ ⊘ **J1826** Injection, interferon beta-1a, 30 mcg Ⓑ Ⓑ

⊛ **J1830** Injection, interferon beta-1b, 0.25 mg (Code may be used for Medicare when drug administered under the direct supervision of a physician, not for use when drug is self administered) Ⓑ Ⓑ
Other: Betaseron
IOM: 100-02, 15, 50

✻ **J1833** Injection, isavuconazonium, 1 mg Ⓑ Ⓑ

✻ **J1835** Injection, itraconazole, 50 mg Ⓑ Ⓑ
Other: Sporanox

⊛ **J1840** Injection, kanamycin sulfate, up to 500 mg Ⓑ Ⓑ
Other: Kantrex, Klebcil
IOM: 100-02, 15, 50

⊛ **J1850** Injection, kanamycin sulfate, up to 75 mg Ⓑ Ⓑ
Other: Kantrex, Klebcil
IOM: 100-02, 15, 50

⊛ **J1885** Injection, ketorolac tromethamine, per 15 mg Ⓑ Ⓑ
Other: Toradol
IOM: 100-02, 15, 50

⊛ **J1890** Injection, cephalothin sodium, up to 1 gram Ⓑ Ⓑ
IOM: 100-02, 15, 50

✻ **J1930** Injection, lanreotide, 1 mg Ⓑ Ⓑ
Treats acromegaly and symptoms caused by neuroendocrine tumors
NDC: Somatuline Depot

✻ **J1931** Injection, laronidase, 0.1 mg Ⓑ Ⓑ
NDC: Aldurazyme

⊛ **J1940** Injection, furosemide, up to 20 mg Ⓑ Ⓑ
Other: Lasix
MCM: 2049
IOM: 100-02, 15, 50

▶ ✻ **J1942** Injection, aripiprazole lauroxil, 1 mg Ⓑ Ⓑ

⊛ **J1945** Injection, lepirudin, 50 mg Ⓑ Ⓑ
IOM: 100-02, 15, 50

⊛ **J1950** Injection, leuprolide acetate (for depot suspension), per 3.75 mg Ⓑ Ⓑ
NDC: Lupron Depot, Lupron Depot-Ped
IOM: 100-02, 15, 50

✻ **J1953** Injection, levetiracetam, 10 mg Ⓑ Ⓑ

⊛ **J1955** Injection, levocarnitine, per 1 gm Ⓑ Ⓑ
NDC: Carnitor
IOM: 100-02, 15, 50

⊛ **J1956** Injection, levofloxacin, 250 mg Ⓑ Ⓑ
NDC: Levaquin
IOM: 100-02, 15, 50

⊛ **J1960** Injection, levorphanol tartrate, up to 2 mg Ⓑ Ⓑ
Other: Levo-Dromoran
MCM: 2049
IOM: 100-02, 15, 50

⊛ **J1980** Injection, hyoscyamine sulfate, up to 0.25 mg Ⓑ Ⓑ
NDC: Levsin
IOM: 100-02, 15, 50

J1990 Injection, chlordiazepoxide HCL, up to 100 mg
Other: Librium
IOM: 100-02, 15, 50

J2001 Injection, lidocaine HCL for intravenous infusion, 10 mg
NDC: Lidocaine in D5W
Other: Anestacaine, Caine-1, Dilocaine, L-Caine, Lidoject, Nervocaine, Nulicaine, Xylocaine
IOM: 100-02, 15, 50

J2010 Injection, lincomycin HCL, up to 300 mg
NDC: Lincocin
IOM: 100-02, 15, 50

* **J2020** Injection, linezolid, 200 mg
NDC: Zyvox

J2060 Injection, lorazepam, 2 mg
NDC: Ativan
IOM: 100-02, 15, 50

J2150 Injection, mannitol, 25% in 50 ml
MCM: 2049
IOM: 100-02, 15, 50

* **J2170** Injection, mecasermin, 1 mg
Other: Increlex

J2175 Injection, meperidine hydrochloride, per 100 mg
NDC: Demerol
IOM: 100-02, 15, 50

J2180 Injection, meperidine and promethazine HCL, up to 50 mg
Other: Mepergan
IOM: 100-02, 15, 50

▶ * **J2182** Injection, mepolizumab, 1 mg

* **J2185** Injection, meropenem, 100 mg
NDC: Merrem

J2210 Injection, methylergonovine maleate, up to 0.2 mg
Benefit limited to obstetrical diagnoses for prevention and control of post-partum hemorrhage
NDC: Methergine
IOM: 100-02, 15, 50

* **J2212** Injection, methylnaltrexone, 0.1 mg

* **J2248** Injection, micafungin sodium, 1 mg
Other: Mycamine

J2250 Injection, midazolam hydrochloride, per 1 mg
Other: Versed
IOM: 100-02, 15, 50

J2260 Injection, milrinone lactate, 5 mg
Other: Primacor
IOM: 100-02, 15, 50

* **J2265** Injection, minocycline hydrochloride, 1 mg

J2270 Injection, morphine sulfate, up to 10 mg
Other: Duramorph
IOM: 100-02, 15, 50

J2274 Injection, morphine sulfate, preservative-free for epidural or intrathecal use, 10 mg
NDC: Duramorph, Infumorph
IOM: 100-03, 4, 280.1; 100-02, 15, 50

J2278 Injection, ziconotide, 1 microgram
NDC: Prialt

* **J2280** Injection, moxifloxacin, 100 mg
NDC: Avelox

J2300 Injection, nalbuphine hydrochloride, per 10 mg
Other: Nubain
IOM: 100-02, 15, 50

J2310 Injection, naloxone hydrochloride, per 1 mg
Other: Narcan
IOM: 100-02, 15, 50

* **J2315** Injection, naltrexone, depot form, 1 mg
NDC: Vivitrol

J2320 Injection, nandrolone decanoate, up to 50 mg
Other: Anabolin LA 100, Androlone, Deca-Durabolin, Decolone, Hybolin Decanoate, Nandrobolic LA, Neo-Durabolic
IOM: 100-02, 15, 50

* **J2323** Injection, natalizumab, 1 mg
NDC: Tysabri

J2325 Injection, nesiritide, 0.1 mg
Other: Natrecor
IOM: 100-02, 15, 50

* **J2353** Injection, octreotide, depot form for intramuscular injection, 1 mg
NDC: Sandostatin LAR Depot

▶ New ↩ Revised ✔ Reinstated ~~deleted~~ Deleted ⊘ Not covered or valid by Medicare
Special coverage instructions * Carrier discretion Bill local carrier Bill DME MAC

✻ **J2354** Injection, octreotide, non-depot form for subcutaneous or intravenous injection, 25 mcg
Other: Sandostatin LAR Depot

J2355 Injection, oprelvekin, 5 mg
NDC: Neumega
IOM: 100-02, 15, 50

✻ **J2357** Injection, omalizumab, 5 mg
NDC: Xolair

✻ **J2358** Injection, olanzapine, long-acting, 1 mg
NDC: Zyprexa, Relprevv

J2360 Injection, orphenadrine citrate, up to 60 mg
Other: Antiflex, Banflex, Flexoject, Flexon, K-Flex, Mio-Rel, Neocyten, Norflex, O-Flex, Orfro, Orphenate
IOM: 100-02, 15, 50

J2370 Injection, phenylephrine HCL, up to 1 ml
Other: Neo-Synephrine
IOM: 100-02, 15, 50

J2400 Injection, chloroprocaine hydrochloride, per 30 ml
NDC: Nesacaine, Nesacaine-MPF
IOM: 100-02, 15, 50

J2405 Injection, ondansetron hydrochloride, per 1 mg
NDC: Zofran
IOM: 100-02, 15, 50

J2407 Injection, oritavancin, 10 mg
NDC: Orbactiv
IOM: 100-02, 15, 50

J2410 Injection, oxymorphone HCL, up to 1 mg
NDC: Opana
Other: Numorphan
IOM: 100-02, 15, 50

✻ **J2425** Injection, palifermin, 50 micrograms
NDC: Kepivance

✻ **J2426** Injection, paliperidone palmitate extended release, 1 mg
NDC: Invega Sustenna

J2430 Injection, pamidronate disodium, per 30 mg
Other: Aredia
IOM: 100-02, 15, 50

J2440 Injection, papaverine HCL, up to 60 mg
IOM: 100-02, 15, 50

J2460 Injection, oxytetracycline HCL, up to 50 mg
Other: Terramycin IM
IOM: 100-02, 15, 50

✻ **J2469** Injection, palonosetron HCL, 25 mcg
Example: 0.25 mgm dose = 10 units. Example of use is acute, delayed, nausea and vomiting due to chemotherapy.
NDC: Aloxi

J2501 Injection, paricalcitol, 1 mcg
NDC: Zemplar
IOM: 100-02, 15, 50

✻ **J2502** Injection, pasireotide long acting, 1 mg

✻ **J2503** Injection, pegaptanib sodium, 0.3 mg
NDC: Macugen

J2504 Injection, pegademase bovine, 25 IU
NDC: Adagen
IOM: 100-02, 15, 50

✻ **J2505** Injection, pegfilgrastim, 6 mg
Report 1 unit per 6 mg.
NDC: Neulasta

✻ **J2507** Injection, pegloticase, 1 mg
NDC: Krystexxa

⮌ **J2510** Injection, penicillin G procaine, aqueous, up to 600,000 units
Other: Crysticillin, Duracillin AS, Pfizerpen AS, Wycillin
IOM: 100-02, 15, 50

J2513 Injection, pentastarch, 10% solution, 100 ml
IOM: 100-02, 15, 50

⮌ **J2515** Injection, pentobarbital sodium, per 50 mg
NDC: Nembutal
IOM: 100-02, 15, 50

J2540 Injection, penicillin G potassium, up to 600,000 units
NDC: Pfizerpen-G
IOM: 100-02, 15, 50

▶ New ⮌ Revised ✔ Reinstated ~~deleted~~ Deleted ⦸ Not covered or valid by Medicare
Special coverage instructions ✻ Carrier discretion Bill local carrier Bill DME MAC

J2543 Injection, piperacillin sodium/tazobactam sodium, 1 gram/0.125 grams (1.125 grams)

NDC: Zosyn

IOM: 100-02, 15, 50

J2545 Pentamidine isethionate, inhalation solution, FDA-approved final product, non-compounded, administered through DME, unit dose form, per 300 mg

NDC: Nebupent

* **J2547** Injection, peramivir, 1 mg

J2550 Injection, promethazine HCL, up to 50 mg

Administration of phenergan suppository considered part of E/M encounter

NDC: Phenergan

Other: Anergan, Phenazine, Prorex, Prothazine

IOM: 100-02, 15, 50

J2560 Injection, phenobarbital sodium, up to 120 mg

IOM: 100-02, 15, 50

* **J2562** Injection, plerixafor, 1 mg

FDA approved for non-Hodgkin lymphoma and multiple myeloma in 2008.

NDC: Mozobil

J2590 Injection, oxytocin, up to 10 units

Other: Pitocin, Syntocinon

IOM: 100-02, 15, 50

J2597 Injection, desmopressin acetate, per 1 mcg

NDC: DDAVP

IOM: 100-02, 15, 50

J2650 Injection, prednisolone acetate, up to 1 ml

Other: Cotolone, Key-Pred, Predalone, Predcor, Predicort

IOM: 100-02, 15, 50

J2670 Injection, tolazoline HCL, up to 25 mg

IOM: 100-02, 15, 50

J2675 Injection, progesterone, per 50 mg

Other: Gesterol 50, Progestaject

IOM: 100-02, 15, 50

J2680 Injection, fluphenazine decanoate, up to 25 mg

Other: Prolixin Decanoate

MCM: 2049

IOM: 100-02, 15, 50

J2690 Injection, procainamide HCL, up to 1 gm

Benefit limited to obstetrical diagnoses

Other: Pronestyl, Prostaphlin

IOM: 100-02, 15, 50

J2700 Injection, oxacillin sodium, up to 250 mg

NDC: Bactocill

IOM: 100-02, 15, 50

* **J2704** Injection, propofol, 10 mg

NDC: Diprivan

J2710 Injection, neostigmine methylsulfate, up to 0.5 mg

Other: Prostigmin

IOM: 100-02, 15, 50

J2720 Injection, protamine sulfate, per 10 mg

IOM: 100-02, 15, 50

* **J2724** Injection, protein C concentrate, intravenous, human, 10 IU

NDC: Ceprotin

J2725 Injection, protirelin, per 250 mcg

Other: Relefact TRH, Thypinone

IOM: 100-02, 15, 50

J2730 Injection, pralidoxime chloride, up to 1 gm

Other: Protopam Chloride

IOM: 100-02, 15, 50

J2760 Injection, phentolamine mesylate, up to 5 mg

Other: Regitine

IOM: 100-02, 15, 50

J2765 Injection, metoclopramide HCL, up to 10 mg

Other: Reglan

IOM: 100-02, 15, 50

J2770 Injection, quinupristin/dalfopristin, 500 mg (150/350)

NDC: Synercid

IOM: 100-02, 15, 50

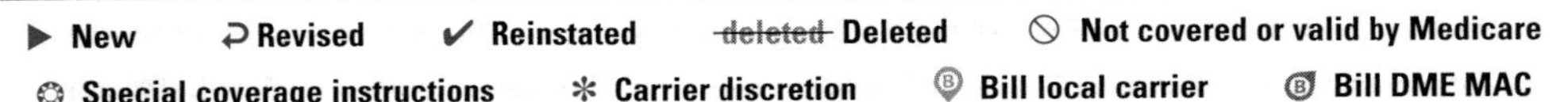

* **J2778** Injection, ranibizumab, 0.1 mg
May be reported for exudative senile macular degeneration (wet AMD) with 67028 (RT or LT)
Other: Lucentis

J2780 Injection, ranitidine hydrochloride, 25 mg
NDC: Zantac
IOM: 100-02, 15, 50

* **J2783** Injection, rasburicase, 0.5 mg
NDC: Elitek

* **J2785** Injection, regadenoson, 0.1 mg
One billing unit equal to 0.1 mg of regadenoson

▶ * **J2786** Injection, reslizumab, 1 mg

J2788 Injection, Rho D immune globulin, human, minidose, 50 mcg (250 IU)
NDC: MicRhoGAM
Other: HypRho-D, RhoGam
IOM: 100-02, 15, 50

J2790 Injection, Rho D immune globulin, human, full dose, 300 mcg (1500 IU)
Administered to pregnant female to prevent hemolistic disease of newborn. Report 90384 to private payer.
NDC: Hyperrho S/D, RhoGAM
Other: Gamulin Rh, HypRho-D, Rhesonativ
IOM: 100-02, 15, 50

J2791 Injection, Rho(D) immune globulin (human), (Rhophylac), intramuscular or intravenous, 100 IU
Agent must be billed per 100 IU in both physician office and hospital outpatient settings
Other: HypRho-D
IOM: 100-02, 15, 50

J2792 Injection, Rho D immune globulin intravenous, human, solvent detergent, 100 IU
NDC: WinRHo-SDF
Other: Gamulin Rh, Hyperrho S/D
IOM: 100-02, 15, 50

J2793 Injection, rilonacept, 1 mg
IOM: 100-02, 15, 50

* **J2794** Injection, risperidone, long acting, 0.5 mg
NDC: Risperdal Costa

* **J2795** Injection, ropivacaine hydrochloride, 1 mg
NDC: Naropin

* **J2796** Injection, romiplostim, 10 micrograms
Stimulates bone marrow megakarocytes to produce platelets (i.e., ITP)
NDC: Nplate

J2800 Injection, methocarbamol, up to 10 ml
NDC: Robaxin
IOM: 100-02, 15, 50

* **J2805** Injection, sincalide, 5 micrograms

J2810 Injection, theophylline, per 40 mg
IOM: 100-02, 15, 50

J2820 Injection, sargramostim (GM-CSF), 50 mcg
NDC: Leukine
Other: Prokine
IOM: 100-02, 15, 50

▶ * **J2840** Injection, sebelipase alfa, 1 mg

J2850 Injection, secretin, synthetic, human, 1 microgram
NDC: Chirhostim
IOM: 100-02, 15, 50

* **J2860** Injection, siltuximab, 10 mg

J2910 Injection, aurothioglucose, up to 50 mg
Other: Solganal
IOM: 100-02, 15, 50

J2916 Injection, sodium ferric gluconate complex in sucrose injection, 12.5 mg
NDC: Ferrlecit
Other: Nulecit
IOM: 100-02, 15, 50

J2920 Injection, methylprednisolone sodium succinate, up to 40 mg
NDC: Solu-Medrol
Other: A-MethaPred
IOM: 100-02, 15, 50

▶ New ↩ Revised ✔ Reinstated ~~deleted~~ Deleted ⊘ Not covered or valid by Medicare
Special coverage instructions * Carrier discretion Bill local carrier Bill DME MAC

J2930 Injection, methylprednisolone sodium succinate, up to 125 mg
NDC: Solu-Medrol
Other: A-MethaPred
IOM: 100-02, 15, 50

J2940 Injection, somatrem, 1 mg
IOM: 100-02, 15, 50,
Medicare Statute 1861s2b

J2941 Injection, somatropin, 1 mg
Other: Genotropin, Humatrope, Nutropin, Omnitrope, Saizen, Serostim, Zorbtive
IOM: 100-02, 15, 50
Medicare Statute 1861s2b

J2950 Injection, promazine HCL, up to 25 mg
Other: Prozine-50, Sparine
IOM: 100-02, 15, 50

J2993 Injection, reteplase, 18.1 mg
Other: Retavase
IOM: 100-02, 15, 50

J2995 Injection, streptokinase, per 250,000 IU
Bill 1 unit for each 250,000 IU
Other: Kabikinase, Streptase
IOM: 100-02, 15, 50

J2997 Injection, alteplase recombinant, 1 mg
Thrombolytic agent, treatment of occluded catheters. Bill units of 1 mg administered.
NDC: Activase, Cathflo Activase
IOM: 100-02, 15, 50

J3000 Injection, streptomycin, up to 1 gm
IOM: 100-02, 15, 50

J3010 Injection, fentanyl citrate, 0.1 mg
NDC: Sublimaze
IOM: 100-02, 15, 50

J3030 Injection, sumatriptan succinate, 6 mg (Code may be used for Medicare when drug administered under the direct supervision of a physician, not for use when drug is self administered)
Other: Imitrex
IOM: 100-02, 15, 150

* **J3060** Injection, taliglucerace alfa, 10 units
NDC: Elelyso

J3070 Injection, pentazocine, 30 mg
Other: Talwin
IOM: 100-02, 15, 50

* **J3090** Injection, tedizolid phosphate, 1 mg
NDC: Sivextro

* **J3095** Injection, televancin, 10 mg
Prescribed for the treatment of adults with complicated skin and skin structure infections (cSSSI) of the following Gram-positive microorganisms: Staphylococcus aureus; Streptococcus pyogenes, Streptococcus agalactiae, Streptococcus anginosusgroup. Separately payable under the ASC payment system.
NDC: Vibativ

* **J3101** Injection, tenecteplase, 1 mg
NDC: TNKase

J3105 Injection, terbutaline sulfate, up to 1 mg
Other: Brethine
IOM: 100-02, 15, 50

J3110 Injection, teriparatide, 10 mcg
Other: Forteo

J3121 Injection, testosterone enanthate, 1 mg

J3145 Injection, testosterone undecanoate, 1 mg

J3230 Injection, chlorpromazine HCL, up to 50 mg
Other: Ormazine, Thorazine
IOM: 100-02, 15, 50

J3240 Injection, thyrotropin alfa, 0.9 mg provided in 1.1 mg vial
NDC: Thyrogen
IOM: 100-02, 15, 50

* **J3243** Injection, tigecycline, 1 mg

* **J3246** Injection, tirofiban HCL, 0.25 mg
Other: Aggrastat

J3250 Injection, trimethobenzamide HCL, up to 200 mg
NDC: Ticon, Tigan
Other: Arrestin, Tiject 20
IOM: 100-02, 15, 50

▶ New ↻ Revised ✔ Reinstated ~~deleted~~ Deleted ⃠ Not covered or valid by Medicare
Special coverage instructions * Carrier discretion Ⓑ Bill local carrier Ⓑ Bill DME MAC

⊕ **J3260** Injection, tobramycin sulfate, up to 80 mg Ⓑ Ⓑ
Other: Nebcin
IOM: 100-02, 15, 50

* **J3262** Injection, tocilizumab, 1 mg Ⓑ Ⓑ
Indicated for the treatment of adult patients with moderately to severely active rheumatoid arthritis (RA) who have had an inadequate response to one or more tumor necrosis factor (TNF) antagonist therapies
NDC: Actemra

⊕ **J3265** Injection, torsemide, 10 mg/ml Ⓑ Ⓑ
Other: Demadex
IOM: 100-02, 15, 50

⊕ **J3280** Injection, thiethylperazine maleate, up to 10 mg Ⓑ Ⓑ
Other: Norzine, Torecan
IOM: 100-02, 15, 50

* **J3285** Injection, treprostinil, 1 mg Ⓑ Ⓑ
NDC: Remodulin

⊕ **J3300** Injection, triamcinolone acetonide, preservative free, 1 mg Ⓑ Ⓑ
Other: Cenacort A-40, Kenaject-40, Triam-A, Triesence, Tri-Kort, Trilog

⊕ **J3301** Injection, triamcinolone acetonide, not otherwise specified, 10 mg Ⓑ Ⓑ
NDC: Kenalog
Other: Cenacort A-40, Kenaject-40, Triam A, Triesence, Tri-Kort, Trilog
IOM: 100-02, 15, 50

⊕ **J3302** Injection, triamcinolone diacetate, per 5 mg Ⓑ Ⓑ
Other: Amcort, Aristocort Forte, Cenacort Forte, Clinacort, Triamcot, Trilone
IOM: 100-02, 15, 50

⊕ **J3303** Injection, triamcinolone hexacetonide, per 5 mg Ⓑ Ⓑ
NDC: Aristospan
IOM: 100-02, 15, 50

⊕ **J3305** Injection, trimetrexate glucuronate, per 25 mg Ⓑ Ⓑ
Other: NeuTrexin
IOM: 100-02, 15, 50

⊕ **J3310** Injection, perphenazine, up to 5 mg Ⓑ Ⓑ
Other: Trilafon
IOM: 100-02, 15, 50

⊕ **J3315** Injection, triptorelin pamoate, 3.75 mg Ⓑ Ⓑ
NDC: Trelstar
IOM: 100-02, 15, 50

⊕ **J3320** Injection, spectinomycin dihydrochloride, up to 2 gm Ⓑ Ⓑ
Other: Trobicin
IOM: 100-02, 15, 50

⊕ **J3350** Injection, urea, up to 40 gm Ⓑ Ⓑ
Other: Ureaphil
IOM: 100-02, 15, 50

⊕ **J3355** Injection, urofollitropin, 75 IU Ⓑ Ⓑ
Other: Bravelle, Metrodin
IOM: 100-02, 15, 50

⮌ * **J3357** Ustekinumab, for subcutaneous injection, 1 mg Ⓑ Ⓑ
Other: Stelara

⊕ **J3360** Injection, diazepam, up to 5 mg Ⓑ Ⓑ
Other: Valium, Zetran
IOM: 100-02, 15, 50

⊕ **J3364** Injection, urokinase, 5000 IU vial Ⓑ Ⓑ
NDC: Abbokinase
IOM: 100-02, 15, 50

⮌ ⊕ **J3365** Injection, IV, urokinase, 250,000 IU vial Ⓑ Ⓑ
Other: Abbokinase
IOM: 100-02, 15, 50,
Cross Reference Q0089

⊕ **J3370** Injection, vancomycin HCL, 500 mg Ⓑ Ⓑ
NDC: Vancocin
Other: Vancoled
IOM: 100-02, 15, 50; 100-03, 4, 280.14

⊕ **J3380** Injection, vedolizumab, 1 mg Ⓑ Ⓑ

* **J3385** Injection, velaglucerase alfa, 100 units Ⓑ Ⓑ
Enzyme replacement therapy in Gaucher Disease that results from a specific enzyme deficiency in the body, caused by a genetic mutation received from both parents. Type 1 is the most prevalent Ashkenazi Jewish genetic disease, occurring in one in every 1,000.
NDC: VPRIV

⊕ **J3396** Injection, verteporfin, 0.1 mg Ⓑ Ⓑ
NDC: Visudyne
IOM: 100-03, 1, 80.2; 100-03, 1, 80.3

▶ New ⮌ Revised ✔ Reinstated ~~deleted~~ Deleted ⊘ Not covered or valid by Medicare
⊕ Special coverage instructions * Carrier discretion Ⓑ Bill local carrier Ⓑ Bill DME MAC

J3400 Injection, triflupromazine HCL, up to 20 mg
Other: Vesprin
IOM: 100-02, 15, 50

J3410 Injection, hydroxyzine HCL, up to 25 mg
Other: Hyzine-50, Vistacot, Vistaject 25
IOM: 100-02, 15, 50

* **J3411** Injection, thiamine HCL, 100 mg

* **J3415** Injection, pyridoxine HCL, 100 mg
Other: Rodex

J3420 Injection, vitamin B-12 cyanocobalamin, up to 1000 mcg
Medicare carriers may have local coverage decisions regarding vitamin B12 injections that provide reimbursement only for patients with certain types of anemia and other conditions.
Other: Cobolin-M, Hydroxocobalamin, Neuroforte-R, Redisol, Rubramin PC, Sytobex, Vita #12
IOM: 100-02, 15, 50; 100-03, 2, 150.6

J3430 Injection, phytonadione (vitamin K), per 1 mg
NDC: Vitamin K1
Other: AquaMephyton, Konakion, Menadione, Synkavite
IOM: 100-02, 15, 50

J3465 Injection, voriconazole, 10 mg
NDC: VFEND
IOM: 100-02, 15, 50

J3470 Injection, hyaluronidase, up to 150 units
Other: Wydase
IOM: 100-02, 15, 50

J3471 Injection, hyaluronidase, ovine, preservative free, per 1 USP unit (up to 999 USP units)
NDC: Vitrase

J3472 Injection, hyaluronidase, ovine, preservative free, per 1000 USP units

J3473 Injection, hyaluronidase, recombinant, 1 USP unit
NDC: Hylenex
IOM: 100-02, 15, 50

J3475 Injection, magnesium sulfate, per 500 mg
IOM: 100-02, 15, 50

J3480 Injection, potassium chloride, per 2 meq
IOM: 100-02, 15, 50

J3485 Injection, zidovudine, 10 mg
NDC: Retrovir
IOM: 100-02, 15, 50

* **J3486** Injection, ziprasidone mesylate, 10 mg
NDC: Geodon

* **J3489** Injection, zoledronic acid, 1 mg
NDC: Reclast, Zometra

J3490 Unclassified drugs
Bill on paper. Bill one unit. Identify drug and total dosage in "Remarks" field.
Other: Acthib, Aminocaproic Acid, Baciim, Bacitracin, Benzocaine, Betamethasone Acetate, Brevital Sodium, Bumetanide, Bupivacaine, Cefotetan, Ciprofloxacin, Cleocin Phosphate, Clindamycin, Definity, Diprivan, Engerix-B, Ethanolamine, Famotidine, Ganirelix, Gonal-F, Hyaluronic Acid, Marcaine, Metronidazole, Nafcillin, Naltrexone, Ovidrel, Pegasys, Peg-Intron, Penicillin G Sodium, Propofol, Protonix, Recombivax, Rifadin, Rifampin, Sensorcaine-MPF, Smz-TMP, Sodium Hyaluronate, Sufentanil Citrate, Treanda, Twinrix, Valcyte, Veritas Collagen Matrix
IOM: 100-02, 15, 50

⃠ **J3520** Edetate disodium, per 150 mg
Other: Chealamide, Disotate, Endrate ethylenediamine-tetra-acetic
IOM: 100-03, 1, 20.21; 100-03, 1, 20.22

J3530 Nasal vaccine inhalation
IOM: 100-02, 15, 50

⃠ **J3535** Drug administered through a metered dose inhaler
Other: Ipratropium bromide
IOM: 100-02, 15, 50

⃠ **J3570** Laetrile, amygdalin, vitamin B-17
IOM: 100-03, 1, 30.7

* **J3590** Unclassified biologics
Bill on paper. Bill one unit. Identify drug and total dosage in "Remarks" field.
Other: Bayhep B, Hyperhep-B, Nabi-HB

▶ New ↩ Revised ✔ Reinstated ~~deleted~~ Deleted ⃠ Not covered or valid by Medicare
Special coverage instructions * Carrier discretion Bill local carrier Bill DME MAC

Miscellaneous Drugs and Solutions

J7030-J7131: Bill Local Carrier if incident to a physician's service or used in an implanted infusion pump. If other, bill DME MAC.

J7030 Infusion, normal saline solution, 1000 cc

NDC: Sodium Chloride

IOM: 100-02, 15, 50

J7040 Infusion, normal saline solution, sterile (500 ml= 1 unit)

NDC: Sodium Chloride

IOM: 100-02, 15, 50

J7042 5% dextrose/normal saline (500 ml = 1 unit)

NDC: Dextrose-Nacl

IOM: 100-02, 15, 50

J7050 Infusion, normal saline solution, 250 cc

NDC: Sodium Chloride

IOM: 100-02, 15, 50

J7060 5% dextrose/water (500 ml = 1 unit)

IOM: 100-02, 15, 50

J7070 Infusion, D 5 W, 1000 cc

NDC: Dextrose

IOM: 100-02, 15, 50

J7100 Infusion, dextran 40, 500 ml

Other: Gentran, LMD, Rheomacrodex

IOM: 100-02, 15, 50

J7110 Infusion, dextran 75, 500 ml

Other: Gentran

IOM: 100-02, 15, 50

J7120 Ringer's lactate infusion, up to 1000 cc

Replacement fluid or electrolytes.

NDC: Lactated Ringers

IOM: 100-02, 15, 50

J7121 5% dextrose in lactated ringers infusion, up to 1000 cc

IOM: 100-02, 15, 50

J7131 Hypertonic saline solution, 1 ml

IOM: 100-02, 15, 50

▶ ✻ **J7175** Injection, Factor X, (human), 1 IU

Fibrinogen

✻ **J7178** Injection, human fibrinogen concentrate, 1 mg

▶ **J7179** Injection, von Willebrand factor (recombinant), (vonvendi), 1 IU VWF:RCo

Antihemophilic Factor

✻ **J7180** Injection, Factor XIII (antihemophilic factor, human), 1 IU

NDC: Corifact

✻ **J7181** Injection, Factor XIII a-subunit, (recombinant), per iu

✻ **J7182** Injection, Factor VIII, (antihemophilic factor, recombinant), (novoeight), per iu

J7183 Injection, von Willebrand factor complex (human), wilate, 1 IU VWF:RCo

IOM: 100-02, 15, 50

✻ **J7185** Injection, Factor VIII (antihemophilic factor, recombinant) (Xyntha), per IU

Reported in place of temporary code Q2023.

J7186 Injection, anti-hemophilic factor VIII/von Willebrand factor complex (human), per Factor VIII IU

NDC: Alphanate

IOM: 100-02, 15, 50

J7187 Injection, von Willebrand factor complex (HUMATE-P), per IU VWF:RCo

NDC: Humate-P Low Dilutent

Other: Wilate

IOM: 100-02, 15, 50

J7188 Injection, factor VIII (antihemophilic factor, recombinant), (obizur), per IU

IOM: 100-02, 15, 50

J7189 Factor VIIa (anti-hemophilic factor, recombinant), per 1 microgram

NDC: NovoSeven

IOM: 100-02, 15, 50

J7190 Factor VIII anti-hemophilic factor, human, per IU

NDC: Alphanate/von Willebrand factor complex, Hemofil M, Koate DVI, Monoclate-P

Other: Koate-HP, Kogenate, Recombinate

IOM: 100-02, 15, 50

J7191 Factor VIII, anti-hemophilic factor (porcine), per IU

Other: Hyate C, Koate-HP, Kogenate, Monoclate-P, Recombinate

IOM: 100-02, 15, 50

J7192 Factor VIII (anti-hemophilic factor, recombinant) per IU, not otherwise specified

NDC: Advate, Helixate FS, Kogenate FS, Recombinate

Other: Koate-HP, Refacto

IOM: 100-02, 15, 50

J7193 Factor IX (anti-hemophilic factor, purified, non-recombinant) per IU

NDC: AlphaNine SD, Mononine, Profiline, Proplex T

IOM: 100-02, 15, 50

J7194 Factor IX, complex, per IU

NDC: Profilnine SD

Other: Bebulin VH, Konyne-80, Profilnine Heat-treated, Proplex SX-T, Proplex T

IOM: 100-02, 15, 50

J7195 Injection, Factor IX (anti-hemophilic factor, recombinant)per IU, not otherwise specified

NDC: Benefix

Other: Konyne 80, Profiline, Proplex T

IOM: 100-02, 15, 50

Antithrombin III

* **J7196** Injection, antithrombin recombinant, 50 IU

Other: ATryn, Feiba VH Immuno

J7197 Anti-thrombin III (human), per IU

NDC: Thrombate III

IOM: 100-02, 15, 50

Anti-inhibitor

J7198 Anti-inhibitor, per IU

Diagnosis examples: D66, D67, D68.-

Other: Autoplex T, Hemophilia clotting factors

Other Hemophilia Clotting Factors

J7199 Hemophilia clotting factor, not otherwise classified

Other: Autoplex T

IOM: 100-02, 15, 50; 100-03, 2, 110.3

J7200 Injection, Factor IX, (antihemophilic factor, recombinant), rixubis, per iu

IOM: 100-02, 15, 50

J7201 Injection, Factor IX, fc fusion protein (recombinant), alprolix, 1 iu

IOM: 100-02, 15, 50

▶ **J7202** Injection, Factor IX, albumin fusion protein, (recombinant), idelvion, 1 IU

J7205 Injection, Factor VIII Fc fusion protein (recombinant), per iu

NDC: Eloctate

▶ **J7207** Injection, Factor VIII, (antihemophilic factor, recombinant), pegylated, 1 IU

▶ * **J7209** Injection, Factor VIII, (antihemophilic factor, recombinant), (nuwiq), 1 IU

Contraceptives

⦸ **J7297** Levonorgestrel-releasing intrauterine contraceptive system (liletta), 52 mg

Medicare Statute 1862(a)(1)

⦸ **J7298** Levonorgestrel-releasing intrauterine contraceptive system (mirena), 52 mg

Medicare Statute 1862(a)(1)

⦸ **J7300** Intrauterine copper contraceptive

Report IVD insertion with 58300. Bill usual and customary charge.

Other: Paragard T 380 A

Medicare Statute 1862a1

⦸ **J7301** Levonorgestrel-releasing intrauterine contraceptive system (skyla), 13.5 mg

Medicare Statute 1862(a)(1)

⦸ **J7303** Contraceptive supply, hormone containing vaginal ring, each

Medicare Statute 1862.1

▶ New ↩ Revised ✔ Reinstated ~~deleted~~ Deleted ⦸ Not covered or valid by Medicare
Special coverage instructions * Carrier discretion Bill local carrier Bill DME MAC

⃠ **J7304** Contraceptive supply, hormone containing patch, each Ⓑ

Only billed by Family Planning Clinics

Medicare Statute 1862.1

⃠ **J7306** Levonorgestrel (contraceptive) implant system, including implants and supplies Ⓑ

⃠ **J7307** Etonogestrel (contraceptive) implant system, including implant and supplies Ⓑ

Aminolevulinic Acid HCL

✻ **J7308** Aminolevulinic acid HCL for topical administration, 20%, single unit dosage form (354 mg) Ⓑ

NDC: Levulan Kerastick

✪ **J7309** Methyl aminolevulinate (MAL) for topical administration, 16.8%, 1 gram Ⓑ

Other: Metvixia

Ganciclovir

✪ **J7310** Ganciclovir, 4.5 mg, Ⓑ

IOM: 100-02, 15, 50

Ophthalmic Drugs

✻ **J7311** Fluocinolone acetonide, intravitreal implant Ⓑ

Treatment of chronic noninfectious posterior segment uveitis

Other: Retisert

✻ **J7312** Injection, dexamethasone, intravitreal implant, 0.1 mg Ⓑ

To bill for Ozurdex services submit the following codes: J7312 and 67028 with the modifier -22 (for the increased work difficulty and increased risk). Indicated for the treatment of macular edema occurring after branch retinal vein occlusion (BRVO) or central retinal vein occlusion (CRVO) and non-infectious uveitis affecting the posterior segment of the eye.

NDC: Ozurdex

✻ **J7313** Injection, fluocinolone acetonide, intravitreal implant, 0.01 mg Ⓑ

NDC: Iluvien

✻ **J7315** Mitomycin, ophthalmic, 0.2 mg Ⓑ

✻ **J7316** Injection, ocriplasmin, 0.125 mg Ⓑ

NDC: Jetrea

► ✻ **J7320** Hyaluronan or derivitive, genvisc 850, for intra-articular injection, 1 mg

Hyaluronan

✻ **J7321** Hyaluronan or derivative, Hyalgan or Supartz, for intra-articular injection, per dose Ⓑ

Therapeutic goal is to restore visco-elasticity of synovial hyaluronan, thereby decreasing pain, improving mobility and restoring natural protective functions of hyaluronan in joint

► ✻ **J7322** Hyaluronan or derivative, hymovis, for intra-articular injection, 1 mg

✻ **J7323** Hyaluronan or derivative, Euflexxa, for intra-articular injection, per dose Ⓑ

✻ **J7324** Hyaluronan or derivative, Orthovisc, for intra-articular injection, per dose Ⓑ

⮌ ✻ **J7325** Hyaluronan or derivative, Synvisc or Synvisc-One, for intra-articular injection, 1 mg Ⓑ

⮌ ✻ **J7326** Hyaluronan or derivative, Gel-One, for intra-articular injection, per dose Ⓑ

✻ **J7327** Hyaluronan or derivative, monovisc, for intra-articular injection, per dose Ⓑ

⮌ ✻ **J7328** Hyaluronan or derivative, gel-syn, for intra-articular injection, 0.1 mg Ⓑ

Autologous Cultured Chondrocytes

✻ **J7330** Autologous cultured chondrocytes, implant Ⓑ

Other: Carticel

Capsaicin

✻ **J7336** Capsaicin 8% patch, per square centimeter Ⓑ

NDC: Qutenza

► New ⮌ Revised ✔ Reinstated ~~deleted~~ Deleted ⃠ Not covered or valid by Medicare
✪ Special coverage instructions ✻ Carrier discretion Ⓑ Bill local carrier Ⓔ Bill DME MAC

Carbidopa/Levodopa

↩ * **J7340** Carbidopa 5 mg/levodopa 20 mg enteral suspension, 100 ml Ⓑ Ⓑ

Bill Local Carrier if incident to a physician's service or used in an implanted infusion pump. If other, bill DME MAC.

▶ * **J7342** Installation, ciprofloxacin otic suspension, 6 mg

Immunosuppressive Drugs (Includes Non-injectibles)

J7500-J7599: Bill Local Carrier if incident to a physician's service or used in an implanted infusion pump. If other, bill DME MAC.

✪ **J7500** Azathioprine, oral, 50 mg Ⓑ Ⓑ

NDC: Azasan

Other: Imuran

IOM: 100-02, 15, 50

✪ **J7501** Azathioprine, parenteral, 100 mg Ⓑ Ⓑ

Other: Imuran

IOM: 100-02, 15, 50

✪ **J7502** Cyclosporine, oral, 100 mg Ⓑ Ⓑ

NDC: Gengraf, Neoral, Sandimmune

IOM: 100-02, 15, 50

↩ ✪ **J7503** Tacrolimus, extended release, (Envarsus XR), oral, 0.25 mg Ⓑ Ⓑ

IOM: 100-02, 15, 50

✪ **J7504** Lymphocyte immune globulin, antithymocyte globulin, equine, parenteral, 250 mg Ⓑ Ⓑ

NDC: Atgam

IOM: 100-02, 15, 50; 100-03, 2, 110.3

↩ ✪ **J7505** Muromonab-CD3, parenteral, 5 mg Ⓑ Ⓑ

Other: Monoclonal antibodies (parenteral)

IOM: 100-02, 15, 50

✪ **J7507** Tacrolimus, immediate release, oral, 1 mg Ⓑ Ⓑ

NDC: Prograf

IOM: 100-02, 15, 50

✪ **J7508** Tacrolimus, extended release, (Astagraf XL), oral, 0.1 mg Ⓑ Ⓑ

NDC: Astagraf XL

IOM: 100-02, 15, 50

✪ **J7509** Methylprednisolone oral, per 4 mg Ⓑ Ⓑ

Other: Medrol

IOM: 100-02, 15, 50

✪ **J7510** Prednisolone oral, per 5 mg Ⓑ Ⓑ

NDC: Flo-Pred

Other: Cotolone, Delta-Cortef, Orapred, Pediapred, Prelone

IOM: 100-02, 15, 50

* **J7511** Lymphocyte immune globulin, antithymocyte globulin, rabbit, parenteral, 25 mg Ⓑ Ⓑ

NDC: Thymoglobulin

✪ **J7512** Prednisone, immediate release or delayed release, oral, 1 mg Ⓑ Ⓑ

NDC: Cyclosporine

IOM: 100-02, 15, 50

✪ **J7513** Daclizumab, parenteral, 25 mg Ⓑ Ⓑ

Other: Zenapax

IOM: 100-02, 15, 50

* **J7515** Cyclosporine, oral, 25 mg Ⓑ Ⓑ

NDC: Gengraf, Neoral, Sandimmune

* **J7516** Cyclosporin, parenteral, 250 mg Ⓑ Ⓑ

NDC: Sandimmune

* **J7517** Mycophenolate mofetil, oral, 250 mg Ⓑ Ⓑ

NDC: CellCept

✪ **J7518** Mycophenolic acid, oral, 180 mg Ⓑ Ⓑ

NDC: Myfortic

IOM: 100-04, 4, 240; 100-4, 17, 80.3.1

✪ **J7520** Sirolimus, oral, 1 mg Ⓑ Ⓑ

NDC: Rapamune

IOM: 100-02, 15, 50

✪ **J7525** Tacrolimus, parenteral, 5 mg Ⓑ Ⓑ

NDC: Prograf

IOM: 100-02, 15, 50

✪ **J7527** Everolimus, oral, 0.25 mg Ⓑ Ⓑ

NDC: Zortress

IOM: 100-02, 15, 50

✪ **J7599** Immunosuppressive drug, not otherwise classified Ⓑ Ⓑ

Bill on paper. Bill one unit. Identify drug and total dosage in "Remarks" field.

IOM: 100-02, 15, 50

▶ New ↩ Revised ✔ Reinstated ~~deleted~~ Deleted ⊘ Not covered or valid by Medicare
✪ Special coverage instructions * Carrier discretion Ⓑ Bill local carrier Ⓑ Bill DME MAC

Inhalation Solutions

J7604-J7699: Bill Local Carrier if incident to a physician's service. If other, bill DME MAC.

✻ J7604 Acetylcysteine, inhalation solution, compounded product, administered through DME, unit dose form, per gram

Other: Mucomyst (unit dose form), Mucosol

✻ J7605 Arformoterol, inhalation solution, FDA approved final product, non-compounded, administered through DME, unit dose form, 15 micrograms

Maintenance treatment of bronchoconstriction in patients with chronic obstructive pulmonary disease (COPD).

Other: Brovana

✻ J7606 Formoterol fumarate, inhalation solution, FDA approved final product, non-compounded, administered through DME, unit dose form, 20 micrograms

NDC: Perforomist

✻ J7607 Levalbuterol, inhalation solution, compounded product, administered through DME, concentrated form, 0.5 mg

J7608 Acetylcysteine, inhalation solution, FDA-approved final product, non-compounded, administered through DME, unit dose form, per gram

Other: Mucomyst, Mucosol

✻ J7609 Albuterol, inhalation solution, compounded product, administered through DME, unit dose, 1 mg

Patient's home, medications—such as a albuterol when administered through a nebulizer—are considered DME and are payable under Part B.

Other: Proventil, Xopenex, Ventolin

✻ J7610 Albuterol, inhalation solution, compounded product, administered through DME, concentrated form, 1 mg

Other: Proventil, Xopenex, Ventolin

J7611 Albuterol, inhalation solution, FDA-approved final product, non-compounded, administered through DME, concentrated form, 1 mg

Report once for each milligram administered. For example, 2 mg of concentrated albuterol (usually diluted with saline), reported with J7611×2.

Other: Proventil, Ventolin, Xopenex

J7612 Levalbuterol, inhalation solution, FDA-approved final product, non-compounded, administered through DME, concentrated form, 0.5 mg

NDC: Xopenex

J7613 Albuterol, inhalation solution, FDA-approved final product, non-compounded, administered through DME, unit dose, 1 mg

NDC: Proventil, Ventolin

Other: Accuneb, Xopenex

J7614 Levalbuterol, inhalation solution, FDA-approved final product, non-compounded, administered through DME, unit dose, 0.5 mg

NDC: Xopenex

✻ J7615 Levalbuterol, inhalation solution, compounded product, administered through DME, unit dose, 0.5 mg

J7620 Albuterol, up to 2.5 mgand ipratropium bromide, up to 0.5 mg,FDA-approved final product, non-compounded, administered through DME

NDC: DuoNeb

✻ J7622 Beclomethasone, inhalation solution, compounded product, administered through DME, unit dose form, per mg

✻ J7624 Betamethasone, inhalation solution, compounded product, administered through DME, unit dose form, per mg

Other: Celestone Soluspan

✻ J7626 Budesonide inhalation solution, FDA-approved final product, non-compounded, administered through DME, unit dose form, up to 0.5 mg

NDC: Pulmicort

✻ J7627 Budesonide, inhalation solution, compounded product, administered through DME, unit dose form, up to 0.5 mg

Other: Pulmicort Respules

▶ New ↩ Revised ✔ Reinstated ~~deleted~~ Deleted ⦸ Not covered or valid by Medicare
Special coverage instructions ✻ Carrier discretion Bill local carrier Bill DME MAC

J7628 Bitolterol mesylate, inhalation solution, compounded product, administered through DME, concentrated form, per milligram

Other: Tornalate

J7629 Bitolterol mesylate, inhalation solution, compounded product, administered through DME, unit dose form, per milligram

Other: Tornalate

J7631 Cromolyn sodium, inhalation solution, FDA-approved final product, non-compounded, administered through DME, unit dose form, per 10 milligrams

Other: Intal

* **J7632** Cromolyn sodium, inhalation solution, compounded product, administered through DME, unit dose form, per 10 milligrams

Other: Intal

* **J7633** Budesonide, inhalation solution, FDA-approved final product, non-compounded, administered through DME, concentrated form, per 0.25 milligram

Other: Pulmicort Respules

* **J7634** Budesonide, inhalation solution, compounded product, administered through DME, concentrated form, per 0.25 milligram

J7635 Atropine, inhalation solution, compounded product, administered through DME, concentrated form, per milligram

J7636 Atropine, inhalation solution, compounded product, administered through DME, unit dose form, per milligram

J7637 Dexamethasone, inhalation solution, compounded product, administered through DME, concentrated form, per milligram

J7638 Dexamethasone, inhalation solution, compounded product, administered through DME, unit dose form, per milligram

J7639 Dornase alfa, inhalation solution, FDA-approved final product, non-compounded, administered through DME, unit dose form, per milligram

NDC: Pulmozyme

* **J7640** Formoterol, inhalation solution, compounded product, administered through DME, unit dose form, 12 micrograms

* **J7641** Flunisolide, inhalation solution, compounded product, administered through DME, unit dose, per milligram

J7642 Glycopyrrolate, inhalation solution, compounded product, administered through DME, concentrated form, per milligram

J7643 Glycopyrrolate, inhalation solution, compounded product, administered through DME, unit dose form, per milligram

Other: Robinul

J7644 Ipratropium bromide, inhalation solution, FDA-approved final product, non-compounded, administered through DME, unit dose form, per milligram

Other: Atrovent

* **J7645** Ipratropium bromide, inhalation solution, compounded product, administered through DME, unit dose form, per milligram

Other: Atrovent

* **J7647** Isoetharine HCL, inhalation solution, compounded product, administered through DME, concentrated form, per milligram

Other: Bronkosol

J7648 Isoetharine HCL, inhalation solution, FDA-approved final product, non-compounded, administered through DME, concentrated form, per milligram

Other: Bronkosol

J7649 Isoetharine HCL, inhalation solution, FDA-approved final product, non-compounded, administered through DME, unit dose form, per milligram

Other: Bronkosol

* **J7650** Isoetharine HCL, inhalation solution, compounded product, administered through DME, unit dose form, per milligram

Other: Bronkosol

* **J7657** Isoproterenol HCL, inhalation solution, compounded product, administered through DME, concentrated form, per milligram

Other: Isuprel

J7658 Isoproterenol HCL inhalation solution, FDA-approved final product, non-compounded, administered through DME, concentrated form, per milligram

Other: Isuprel

J7659 Isoproterenol HCL, inhalation solution, FDA-approved final product, non-compounded, administered through DME, unit dose form, per milligram

Other: Isuprel

* **J7660** Isoproterenol HCL, inhalation solution, compounded product, administered through DME, unit dose form, per milligram

Other: Isuprel

* **J7665** Mannitol, administered through an inhaler, 5 mg

Other: Aridol

* **J7667** Metaproterenol sulfate, inhalation solution, compounded product, concentrated form, per 10 milligrams

Other: Alupent, Metaprel

J7668 Metaproterenol sulfate, inhalation solution, FDA-approved final product, non-compounded, administered through DME, concentrated form, per 10 milligrams

Other: Alupent, Metaprel

J7669 Metaproterenol sulfate, inhalation solution, FDA-approved final product, non-compounded, administered through DME, unit dose form, per 10 milligrams

Other: Alupent, Metaprel

* **J7670** Metaproterenol sulfate, inhalation solution, compounded product, administered through DME, unit dose form, per 10 milligrams

Other: Alupent, Metaprel

* **J7674** Methacholine chloride administered as inhalation solution through a nebulizer, per 1 mg

NDC: Provocholine

* **J7676** Pentamidine isethionate, inhalation solution, compounded product, administered through DME, unit dose form, per 300 mg

Other: NebuPent, Pentam

J7680 Terbutaline sulfate, inhalation solution, compounded product, administered through DME, concentrated form, per milligram

Other: Brethine

J7681 Terbutaline sulfate, inhalation solution, compounded product, administered through DME, unit dose form, per milligram

Other: Brethine

J7682 Tobramycin, inhalation solution, FDA-approved final product, non-compounded unit dose form, administered through DME, per 300 milligrams

NDC: Bethkis, Kitabis PAK, Tobi

Other: Nebcin

J7683 Triamcinolone, inhalation solution, compounded product, administered through DME, concentrated form, per milligram

J7684 Triamcinolone, inhalation solution, compounded product, administered through DME, unit dose form, per milligram

Other: Triamcinolone acetonide

* **J7685** Tobramycin, inhalation solution, compounded product, administered through DME, unit dose form, per 300 milligrams

* **J7686** Treprostinil, inhalation solution, FDA-approved final product, non-compounded, administered through DME, unit dose form, 1.74 mg

NDC: Tyvaso

J7699 NOC drugs, inhalation solution administered through DME

Other: Gentamicin Sulfate, Sodium chloride

NOC Drugs, Other Than Inhalation Drugs

J7799-J7999: Bill Local Carrier if incident to a physician's service or used in an implanted infusion pump. If other, bill DME MAC.

J7799 NOC drugs, other than inhalation drugs, administered through DME

Bill on paper. Bill one unit and identify drug and total dosage in the "Remark" field.

Other: Epinephrine, Mannitol, Osmitrol, Phenylephrine, Resectisol, Sodium chloride

IOM: 100-02, 15, 110.3

▶ New ↻ Revised ✔ Reinstated ~~deleted~~ Deleted ⊘ Not covered or valid by Medicare
Special coverage instructions * Carrier discretion Ⓑ Bill local carrier Ⓑ Bill DME MAC

J7999 Compounded drug, not otherwise classified

Anti-emetic Drug

J8498 Antiemetic drug, rectal/suppository, not otherwise specified

Other: Compazine, Compro, Phenadoz, Phenergan, Prochlorperazine, Promethazine, Promethegan

Medicare Statute 1861(s)2t

Prescription Drug, Oral, Non-Chemotherapeutic

J8499 Prescription drug, oral, non chemotherapeutic, NOS

Bill Local Carrier if incident to a physician's service. If other, bill DME MAC.

Other: Acyclovir, Zovirax

IOM: 100-02, 15, 50

Oral Anti-Cancer Drugs

J8501 Aprepitant, oral, 5 mg

NDC: Emend

J8510 Busulfan; oral, 2 mg

NDC: Myleran

IOM: 100-02, 15, 50; 100-04, 4, 240; 100-04, 17, 80.1.1

J8515 Cabergoline, oral, 0.25 mg

IOM: 100-02, 15, 50; 100-04, 4, 240

J8520 Capecitabine, oral, 150 mg

NDC: Xeloda

IOM: 100-02, 15, 50; 100-04, 4, 240; 100-04, 17, 80.1.1

J8521 Capecitabine, oral, 500 mg

NDC: Xeloda

IOM: 100-02, 15, 50; 100-04, 4, 240; 100-04, 17, 80.1.1

J8530 Cyclophosphamide; oral, 25 mg

Other: Cytoxan

IOM: 100-02, 15, 50; 100-04, 4, 240; 100-04, 17, 80.1.1

J8540 Dexamethasone, oral, 0.25

Other: Decadron, Dexone, Dexpak

Medicare Statute 1861(s)2t

J8560 Etoposide; oral, 50 mg

NDC: VePesid

IOM: 100-02, 15, 50; 100-04, 4, 230.1; 100-04, 4, 240; 100-04, 17, 80.1.1

J8562 Fludarabine phosphate, oral, 10 mg

Other: Oforta

J8565 Gefitinib, oral, 250 mg

J8597 Antiemetic drug, oral, not otherwise specified

Medicare Statute 1861(s)2t

J8600 Melphalan; oral, 2 mg

NDC: Alkeran

IOM: 100-02, 15, 50; 100-04, 4, 240; 100-04, 17, 80.1.1

J8610 Methotrexate; oral, 2.5 mg

NDC: Rheumatrex, Trexall

IOM: 100-02, 15, 50; 100-04, 4, 240; 100-04, 17, 80.1.1

J8650 Nabilone, oral, 1 mg

J8655 Netupitant 300 mg and palonosetron 0.5 mg

NDC: Akynzeo

▶ **J8670** Rolapitant, oral, 1 mg

J8700 Temozolomide, oral, 5 mg

NDC: Temodar

IOM: 100-02, 15, 50; 100-04, 4, 240

J8705 Topotecan, oral, 0.25 mg

Treatment for ovarian and lung cancers, etc. Report J9350 (Topotecan, 4 mg) for intravenous version.

J8999 Prescription drug, oral, chemotherapeutic, NOS

Other: Arimidex, Aromasin, Droxia, Flutamide, Hydrea, Hydroxyurea, Leukeran, Megace, Megestrol Acetate, Mercaptopurine, Nolvadex, Tamoxifen Citrate

IOM: 100-02, 15, 50; 100-04, 4, 250; 100-04, 17, 80.1.1; 100-04, 17, 80.1.2

▶ New ↩ Revised ✔ Reinstated ~~deleted~~ Deleted ⊘ Not covered or valid by Medicare
Special coverage instructions ✻ Carrier discretion Bill local carrier Bill DME MAC

CHEMOTHERAPY DRUGS (J9000-J9999)

Note: These codes cover the cost of the chemotherapy drug only, not to include the administration

J9000-J9999: Bill Local Carrier if incident to a physician's service or used in an implanted infusion pump. If other, bill DME MAC

J9000 Injection, doxorubicin hydrochloride, 10 mg

Other: Rubex

J9015 Injection, aldesleukin, per single use vial

NDC: Proleukin

IOM: 100-02, 15, 50

* **J9017** Injection, arsenic trioxide, 1 mg

NDC: Trisenox

J9019 Injection, asparaginase (Erwinaze), 1,000 iu

IOM: 100-02, 15, 50

J9020 Injection, asparaginase, not otherwise specified 10,000 units

Other: Elspar

IOM: 100-02, 15, 50

* **J9025** Injection, azacitidine, 1 mg

NDC: Vidaza

* **J9027** Injection, clofarabine, 1 mg

NDC: Clolar

J9031 BCG (intravesical), per instillation

NDC: TheraCys, Tice BCG

IOM: 100-02, 15, 50

* **J9032** Injection, belinostat, 10 mg

NDC: Beleodaq

* **J9033** Injection, bendamustine HCL (treanda), 1 mg

Treatment for form of non-Hodgkin's lymphoma; standard administration time is as an intravenous infusion over 30 minutes

NDC: Treanda

▶ * **J9034** Injection, bendamustine HCL (bendeka), 1 mg

* **J9035** Injection, bevacizumab, 10 mg

For malignant neoplasm of breast, considered J9207.

NDC: Avastin

* **J9039** Injection, blinatumomab, 1 microgram

J9040 Injection, bleomycin sulfate, 15 units

Other: Blenoxane

IOM: 100-02, 15, 50

* **J9041** Injection, bortezomib, 0.1 mg

NDC: Velcade

* **J9042** Injection, brentuximab vedotin, 1 mg

NDC: Adcetris

* **J9043** Injection, cabazitaxel, 1 mg

NDC: Jertana

J9045 Injection, carboplatin, 50 mg

Other: Paraplatin

IOM: 100-02, 15, 50

* **J9047** Injection, carfilzomib, 1 mg

NDC: Kyprolis

J9050 Injection, carmustine, 100 mg

NDC: BiCNU

IOM: 100-02, 15, 50

* **J9055** Injection, cetuximab, 10 mg

NDC: Erbitux

J9060 Injection, cisplatin, powder or solution, 10 mg

Other: Plantinol AQ

IOM: 100-02, 15, 50

J9065 Injection, cladribine, per 1 mg

Other: Leustatin

IOM: 100-02, 15, 50

J9070 Cyclophosphamide, 100 mg

Other: Cytoxan, Neosar

IOM: 100-02, 15, 50

* **J9098** Injection, cytarabine liposome, 10 mg

NDC: DepoCyt

J9100 Injection, cytarabine, 100 mg

Other: Cytosar-U

IOM: 100-02, 15, 50

J9120 Injection, dactinomycin, 0.5 mg

NDC: Cosmegen

IOM: 100-02, 15, 50

J9130 Dacarbazine, 100 mg

Other: DTIC-Dome

IOM: 100-02, 15, 50

► ✪ **J9145** Injection, daratumumab, 10 mg
IOM: 100-02, 15, 50

✪ **J9150** Injection, daunorubicin, 10 mg
Other: Cerubidine
IOM: 100-02, 15, 50

✪ **J9151** Injection, daunorubicin citrate, liposomal formulation, 10 mg
Other: Daunoxome
IOM: 100-02, 15, 50

✻ **J9155** Injection, degarelix, 1 mg
Report 1 unit for every 1 mg.
NDC: Firmagon

✻ **J9160** Injection, denileukin diftitox, 300 micrograms

✪ **J9165** Injection, diethylstilbestrol diphosphate, 250 mg
Other: Stilphostrol
IOM: 100-02, 15, 50

✪ **J9171** Injection, docetaxel, 1 mg
Report 1 unit for every 1 mg.
NDC: Docefrez, Taxotere
IOM: 100-02, 15, 50

✪ **J9175** Injection, Elliott's B solution, 1 ml
IOM: 100-02, 15, 50

► ✻ **J9176** Injection, elotuzumab, 1 mg

✻ **J9178** Injection, epirubicin HCL, 2 mg
NDC: Ellence

✻ **J9179** Injection, eribulin mesylate, 0.1 mg
NDC: Halaven

✪ **J9181** Injection, etoposide, 10 mg
NDC: Etopophos, Toposar, VePesid

✪ **J9185** Injection, fludarabine phosphate, 50 mg
Other: Fludara
IOM: 100-02, 15, 50

✪ **J9190** Injection, fluorouracil, 500 mg
NDC: Adrucil
IOM: 100-02, 15, 50

✪ **J9200** Injection, floxuridine, 500 mg
Other: FUDR
IOM: 100-02, 15, 50

✪ **J9201** Injection, gemcitabine hydrochloride, 200 mg
NDC: Gemzar
IOM: 100-02, 15, 50

✪ **J9202** Goserelin acetate implant, per 3.6 mg
NDC: Zoladex
IOM: 100-02, 15, 50

► ✪ **J9205** Injection, irinotecan liposome, 1 mg
IOM: 100-02, 15, 50

✪ **J9206** Injection, irinotecan, 20 mg
NDC: Camptosar
IOM: 100-02, 15, 50

✻ **J9207** Injection, ixabepilone, 1 mg
NDC: Ixempra Kit

✪ **J9208** Injection, ifosfamide, 1 gm
NDC: Ifex
IOM: 100-02, 15, 50

✪ **J9209** Injection, mesna, 200 mg
NDC: Mesnex
IOM: 100-02, 15, 50

✪ **J9211** Injection, idarubicin hydrochloride, 5 mg
NDC: Idamycin PFS
IOM: 100-02, 15, 50

✪ **J9212** Injection, interferon alfacon-1, recombinant, 1 mcg
Other: Infergen
IOM: 100-02, 15, 50

✪ **J9213** Injection, interferon, alfa-2a, recombinant, 3 million units
IOM: 100-02, 15, 50

✪ **J9214** Injection, interferon, alfa-2b, recombinant, 1 million units
NDC: Intron-A
IOM: 100-02, 15, 50

✪ **J9215** Injection, interferon, alfa-n3 (human leukocyte derived), 250,000 IU
Other: Alferon N
IOM: 100-02, 15, 50

✪ **J9216** Injection, interferon, gamma-1B, 3 million units
Other: Actimmune
IOM: 100-02, 15, 50

✪ **J9217** Leuprolide acetate (for depot suspension), 7.5 mg
NDC: Eligard, Lupron Depot
IOM: 100-02, 15, 50

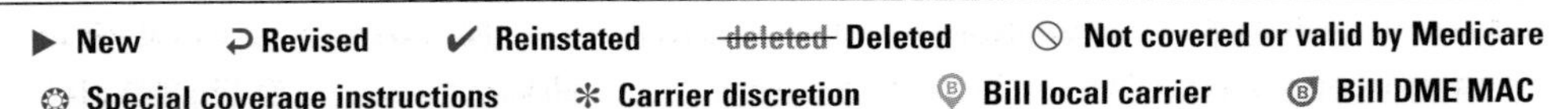

J9218 Leuprolide acetate, per 1 mg
Other: Lupron
IOM: 100-02, 15, 50

J9219 Leuprolide acetate implant, 65 mg
Other: Viadur
IOM: 100-02, 15, 50

J9225 Histrelin implant (Vantas), 50 mg
IOM: 100-02, 15, 50

J9226 Histrelin implant (Supprelin LA), 50 mg
Other: Vantas
IOM: 100-02, 15, 50

* J9228 Injection, ipilimumab, 1 mg
NDC: Yervoy

J9230 Injection, mechlorethamine hydrochloride, (nitrogen mustard), 10 mg
NDC: Mustargen
IOM: 100-02, 15, 50

J9245 Injection, melphalan hydrochloride, 50 mg
NDC: Alkeran, Evomela
IOM: 100-02, 15, 50

J9250 Methotrexate sodium, 5 mg
Other: Folex
IOM: 100-02, 15, 50

J9260 Methotrexate sodium, 50 mg
Other: Folex
IOM: 100-02, 15, 50

* J9261 Injection, nelarabine, 50 mg
NDC: Arranon

* J9262 Injection, omacetaxine mepesuccinate, 0.01 mg

* J9263 Injection, oxaliplatin, 0.5 mg
Eloxatin, platinum-based anticancer drug that destroys cancer cells
NDC: Eloxatin

* J9264 Injection, paclitaxel protein-bound particles, 1 mg
NDC: Abraxane

J9266 Injection, pegaspargase, per single dose vial
NDC: Oncaspar
IOM: 100-02, 15, 50

J9267 Injection, paclitaxel, 1 mg

J9268 Injection, pentostatin, 10 mg
NDC: Nipent
IOM: 100-02, 15, 50

J9270 Injection, plicamycin, 2.5 mg
Other: Mithracin
IOM: 100-02, 15, 50

* J9271 Injection, pembrolizumab, 1 mg
NDC: Keytruda

J9280 Injection, mitomycin, 5 mg
NDC: Mutamycin
IOM: 100-02, 15, 50

J9293 Injection, mitoxantrone hydrochloride, per 5 mg
Other: Novantrone
IOM: 100-02, 15, 50

▶ * J9295 Injection, necitumumab, 1 mg

J9299 Injection, nivolumab, 1 mg
NDC: Opdivo

* J9300 Injection, gemtuzumab ozogamicin, 5 mg
Other: Mylotarg

* J9301 Injection, obinutuzumab, 10 mg
NDC: Gazyva

* J9302 Injection, ofatumumab, 10 mg
NDC: Arzerra

* J9303 Injection, panitumumab, 10 mg
Other: Vectibix

* J9305 Injection, pemetrexed, 10 mg
NDC: Alimta

* J9306 Injection, pertuzumab, 1 mg
NDC: Perjeta

* J9307 Injection, pralatrexate, 1 mg
NDC: Folotyn

* J9308 Injection, ramucirumab, 5 mg
NDC: Cyramza

J9310 Injection, rituximab, 100 mg
NDC: RituXan
IOM: 100-02, 15, 50

* J9315 Injection, romidepsin, 1 mg
NDC: Istodax

J9320 Injection, streptozocin, 1 gram
NDC: Zanosar
IOM: 100-02, 15, 50

▶ * J9325 Injection, talimogene laherparepvec, per 1 million plaque forming units

▶ New ⮐ Revised ✔ Reinstated ~~deleted~~ Deleted ⊘ Not covered or valid by Medicare
Special coverage instructions * Carrier discretion Bill local carrier Bill DME MAC

✻ **J9328** Injection, temozolomide, 1 mg

Intravenous formulation, not for oral administration

NDC: Temodar

✻ **J9330** Injection, temsirolimus, 1 mg

Treatment for advanced renal cell carcinoma; standard administration is intravenous infusion greater than 30-60 minutes

Other: Torisel

❂ **J9340** Injection, thiotepa, 15 mg

Other: Triethylene thio Phosphoramide/T

IOM: 100-02, 15, 50

⮌ ✻ **J9351** Injection, topotecan, 0.1 mg

NDC: Hycamtin

► ✻ **J9352** Injection, trabectedin, 0.1 mg

✻ **J9354** Injection, ado-trastuzumab emtansine, 1 mg

NDC: Kadcyla

✻ **J9355** Injection, trastuzumab, 10 mg

NDC: Herceptin

❂ **J9357** Injection, valrubicin, intravesical, 200 mg

NDC: Valstar

IOM: 100-02, 15, 50

❂ **J9360** Injection, vinblastine sulfate, 1 mg

Other: Alkaban-AQ, Velban, Velsar

IOM: 100-02, 15, 50

❂ **J9370** Vincristine sulfate, 1 mg

Other: Oncovin, Vincasar PFS

IOM: 100-02, 15, 50

✻ **J9371** Injection, vincristine sulfate liposome, 1 mg

❂ **J9390** Injection, vinorelbine tartrate, 10 mg

NDC: Navelbine

IOM: 100-02, 15, 50

✻ **J9395** Injection, fulvestrant, 25 mg

NDC: Faslodex

✻ **J9400** Injection, ziv-aflibercept, 1 mg

NDC: Zaltrap

❂ **J9600** Injection, porfimer sodium, 75 mg

Other: Photofrin

IOM: 100-02, 15, 50

❂ **J9999** Not otherwise classified, antineoplastic drugs

Bill on paper, bill one unit, and identify drug and total dosage in "Remarks" field. Include invoice of cost or NDC number in "Remarks" field.

Other: Ifosfamide/Mesna

IOM: 100-02, 15, 50; 100-03, 2, 110.2

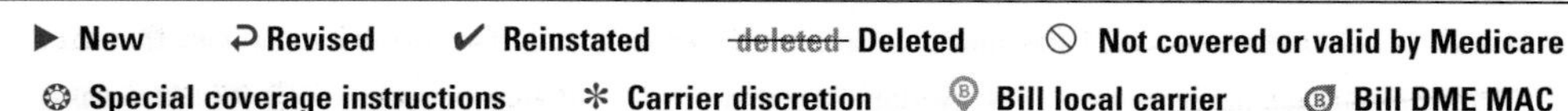

TEMPORARY CODES ASSIGNED TO DME REGIONAL CARRIERS (K0000-K9999)

Wheelchairs and Accessories

NOTE: This section contains national codes assigned by CMS on a temporary basis and for the exclusive use of the durable medical equipment regional carriers (DMERC).

✻ **K0001** Standard wheelchair Ⓑ
Capped rental

✻ **K0002** Standard hemi (low seat) wheelchair Ⓑ
Capped rental

✻ **K0003** Lightweight wheelchair Ⓑ
Capped rental

✻ **K0004** High strength, lightweight wheelchair Ⓑ
Capped rental

✻ **K0005** Ultralightweight wheelchair Ⓑ
Capped rental. Inexpensive and routinely purchased DME

✻ **K0006** Heavy duty wheelchair Ⓑ
Capped rental

✻ **K0007** Extra heavy duty wheelchair Ⓑ
Capped rental

✪ **K0008** Custom manual wheelchair/base Ⓑ

✻ **K0009** Other manual wheelchair/base Ⓑ
Not Otherwise Classified.

✻ **K0010** Standard - weight frame motorized/power wheelchair Ⓑ
Capped rental. Codes K0010-K0014 are not for manual wheelchairs with add-on power packs. Use the appropriate code for the manual wheelchair base provided (K0001-K0009) and code K0460.

✻ **K0011** Standard - weight frame motorized/power wheelchair with programmable control parameters for speed adjustment, tremor dampening, acceleration control and braking Ⓑ
Capped rental. A patient who requires a power wheelchair usually is totally nonambulatory and has severe weakness of the upper extremities due to a neurologic or muscular disease/condition.

✻ **K0012** Lightweight portable motorized/power wheelchair Ⓑ
Capped rental

✪ **K0013** Custom motorized/power wheelchair base Ⓑ

✻ **K0014** Other motorized/power wheelchair base Ⓑ
Capped rental

⮌ ✻ **K0015** Detachable, non-adjustable height armrest, replacement only, each Ⓑ
Inexpensive and routinely purchased DME

✻ **K0017** Detachable, adjustable height armrest, base, replacement only, each Ⓑ
Inexpensive and routinely purchased DME

✻ **K0018** Detachable, adjustable height armrest, upper portion, replacement only, each Ⓑ
Inexpensive and routinely purchased DME

⮌ ✻ **K0019** Arm pad, replacement only, each Ⓑ
Inexpensive and routinely purchased DME

✻ **K0020** Fixed, adjustable height armrest, pair Ⓑ
Inexpensive and routinely purchased DME

⮌ ✻ **K0037** High mount flip-up footrest, replacement only, each Ⓑ
Inexpensive and routinely purchased DME

✻ **K0038** Leg strap, each Ⓑ
Inexpensive and routinely purchased DME

✻ **K0039** Leg strap, H style, each Ⓑ
Inexpensive and routinely purchased DME

✻ **K0040** Adjustable angle footplate, each Ⓑ
Inexpensive and routinely purchased DME

✻ **K0041** Large size footplate, each Ⓑ
Inexpensive and routinely purchased DME

⮌ ✻ **K0042** Standard size footplate, replacement only, each Ⓑ
Inexpensive and routinely purchased DME

⮌ ✻ **K0043** Footrest, lower extension tube, replacement only, each Ⓑ
Inexpensive and routinely purchased DME

↩ ✻ **K0044** Footrest, upper hanger bracket, replacement only, each Ⓑ

Inexpensive and routinely purchased DME

↩ ✻ **K0045** Footrest, complete assembly, replacement only, each Ⓑ

Inexpensive and routinely purchased DME

↩ ✻ **K0046** Elevating legrest, lower extension tube, replacement only, each Ⓑ

Inexpensive and routinely purchased DME

↩ ✻ **K0047** Elevating legrest, upper hanger bracket, replacement only, each Ⓑ

Inexpensive and routinely purchased DME

↩ ✻ **K0050** Ratchet assembly, replacement only Ⓑ

Inexpensive and routinely purchased DME

↩ ✻ **K0051** Cam release assembly, footrest or legrests, replacement only, each Ⓑ

Inexpensive and routinely purchased DME

↩ ✻ **K0052** Swing-away, detachable footrests, replacement only, each Ⓑ

Inexpensive and routinely purchased DME

✻ **K0053** Elevating footrests, articulating (telescoping), each Ⓑ

Inexpensive and routinely purchased DME

✻ **K0056** Seat height less than 17″ or equal to or greater than 21″ for a high strength, lightweight, or ultralightweight wheelchair Ⓑ

Inexpensive and routinely purchased DME

✻ **K0065** Spoke protectors, each Ⓑ

Inexpensive and routinely purchased DME

↩ ✻ **K0069** Rear wheel assembly, complete, with solid tire, spokes or molded, replacement only, each Ⓑ

Inexpensive and routinely purchased DME

↩ ✻ **K0070** Rear wheel assembly, complete, with pneumatic tire, spokes or molded, replacement only, each Ⓑ

Inexpensive and routinely purchased DME

↩ ✻ **K0071** Front caster assembly, complete, with pneumatic tire, replacement only, each Ⓑ

Caster assembly includes a caster fork (E2396), wheel rim, and tire. Inexpensive and routinely purchased DME

↩ ✻ **K0072** Front caster assembly, complete, with semi-pneumatic tire, replacement only, each Ⓑ

Inexpensive and routinely purchased DME

✻ **K0073** Caster pin lock, each Ⓑ

Inexpensive and routinely purchased DME

↩ ✻ **K0077** Front caster assembly, complete, with solid tire, replacement only, each Ⓑ

↩ ✻ **K0098** Drive belt for power wheelchair, replacement only Ⓑ

Inexpensive and routinely purchased DME

✻ **K0105** IV hanger, each Ⓑ

Inexpensive and routinely purchased DME

✻ **K0108** Wheelchair component or accessory, not otherwise specified Ⓑ

✪ **K0195** Elevating leg rests, pair (for use with capped rental wheelchair base) Ⓑ

Medically necessary replacement items are covered if rollabout chair or transport chair covered

IOM: 100-03, 4, 280.1

✪ **K0455** Infusion pump used for uninterrupted parenteral administration of medication (e.g., epoprostenol or treprostinol) Ⓑ

An EIP may also be referred to as an external insulin pump, ambulatory pump, or mini-infuser. CMN/DIF required. Frequent and substantial service DME.

IOM: 100-03, 1, 50.3

✪ **K0462** Temporary replacement for patient owned equipment being repaired, any type Ⓑ

Only report for maintenance and service for an item for which initial claim was paid. The term power mobility device (PMD) includes power operated vehicles (POVs) and power wheelchairs (PWCs). Not Otherwise Classified.

IOM: 100-04, 20, 40.1

▶ New ↩ Revised ✔ Reinstated ~~deleted~~ Deleted ⊘ Not covered or valid by Medicare
✪ Special coverage instructions ✻ Carrier discretion Ⓑ Bill local carrier Ⓑ Bill DME MAC

K0552 Supplies for external non-insulin drug infusion pump, syringe type cartridge, sterile, each
Supplies.
IOM: 100-03, 1, 50.3

K0601 Replacement battery for external infusion pump owned by patient, silver oxide, 1.5 volt, each
Inexpensive and routinely purchased DME

K0602 Replacement battery for external infusion pump owned by patient, silver oxide, 3 volt, each
Inexpensive and routinely purchased DME

K0603 Replacement battery for external infusion pump owned by patient, alkaline, 1.5 volt, each
Inexpensive and routinely purchased DME

K0604 Replacement battery for external infusion pump owned by patient, lithium, 3.6 volt, each
Inexpensive and routinely purchased DME

K0605 Replacement battery for external infusion pump owned by patient, lithium, 4.5 volt, each
Inexpensive and routinely purchased DME

K0606 Automatic external defibrillator, with integrated electrocardiogram analysis, garment type
Capped rental

K0607 Replacement battery for automated external defibrillator, garment type only, each
Inexpensive and routinely purchased DME

K0608 Replacement garment for use with automated external defibrillator, each
Inexpensive and routinely purchased DME

K0609 Replacement electrodes for use with automated external defibrillator, garment type only, each
Supplies.

K0669 Wheelchair accessory, wheelchair seat or back cushion, does not meet specific code criteria or no written coding verification from DME PDAC
Inexpensive and routinely purchased DME

K0672 Addition to lower extremity orthosis, removable soft interface, all components, replacement only, each
Prosthetics/Orthotics

K0730 Controlled dose inhalation drug delivery system
Inexpensive and routinely purchased DME

K0733 Power wheelchair accessory, 12 to 24 amp hour sealed lead acid battery, each (e.g., gel cell, absorbed glassmat)
Inexpensive and routinely purchased DME

K0738 Portable gaseous oxygen system, rental; home compressor used to fill portable oxygen cylinders; includes portable containers, regulator, flowmeter, humidifier, cannula or mask, and tubing
Oxygen and oxygen equipment

K0739 Repair or nonroutine service for durable medical equipment other than oxygen equipment requiring the skill of a technician, labor component, per 15 minutes
Bill Local Carrier if implanted DME. If other, bill DME MAC.

K0740 Repair or nonroutine service for oxygen equipment requiring the skill of a technician, labor component, per 15 minutes

K0743 Suction pump, home model, portable, for use on wounds

K0744 Absorptive wound dressing for use with suction pump, home model, portable, pad size 16 square inches or less

K0745 Absorptive wound dressing for use with suction pump, home model, portable, pad size more than 16 square inches but less than or equal to 48 square inches

K0746 Absorptive wound dressing for use with suction pump, home model, portable, pad size greater than 48 square inches

K0800 Power operated vehicle, group 1 standard, patient weight capacity up to and including 300 pounds
Power mobility device (PMD) includes power operated vehicles (POVs) and power wheelchairs (PWCs). Inexpensive and routinely purchased DME.

New | Revised | Reinstated | ~~deleted~~ Deleted | Not covered or valid by Medicare
Special coverage instructions | Carrier discretion | Bill local carrier | Bill DME MAC

* **K0801** Power operated vehicle, group 1 heavy duty, patient weight capacity 301 to 450 pounds Ⓑ

Inexpensive and routinely purchased DME

* **K0802** Power operated vehicle, group 1 very heavy duty, patient weight capacity 451 to 600 pounds Ⓑ

Inexpensive and routinely purchased DME

* **K0806** Power operated vehicle, group 2 standard, patient weight capacity up to and including 300 pounds Ⓑ

Inexpensive and routinely purchased DME

* **K0807** Power operated vehicle, group 2 heavy duty, patient weight capacity 301 to 450 pounds Ⓑ

Inexpensive and routinely purchased DME

* **K0808** Power operated vehicle, group 2 very heavy duty, patient weight capacity 451 to 600 pounds Ⓑ

Inexpensive and routinely purchased DME

* **K0812** Power operated vehicle, not otherwise classified Ⓑ

Not Otherwise Classified.

* **K0813** Power wheelchair, group 1 standard, portable, sling/solid seat and back, patient weight capacity up to and including 300 pounds Ⓑ

Capped rental

* **K0814** Power wheelchair, group 1 standard, portable, captains chair, patient weight capacity up to and including 300 pounds Ⓑ

Capped rental

* **K0815** Power wheelchair, group 1 standard, sling/solid seat and back, patient weight capacity up to and including 300 pounds Ⓑ

Capped rental

* **K0816** Power wheelchair, group 1 standard, captains chair, patient weight capacity up to and including 300 pounds Ⓑ

Capped rental

* **K0820** Power wheelchair, group 2 standard, portable, sling/solid seat/back, patient weight capacity up to and including 300 pounds Ⓑ

Capped rental

* **K0821** Power wheelchair, group 2 standard, portable, captains chair, patient weight capacity up to and including 300 pounds Ⓑ

Capped rental

* **K0822** Power wheelchair, group 2 standard, sling/solid seat/back, patient weight capacity up to and including 300 pounds Ⓑ

Capped rental

* **K0823** Power wheelchair, group 2 standard, captains chair, patient weight capacity up to and including 300 pounds Ⓑ

Capped rental

* **K0824** Power wheelchair, group 2 heavy duty, sling/solid seat/back, patient weight capacity 301 to 450 pounds Ⓑ

Capped rental

* **K0825** Power wheelchair, group 2 heavy duty, captains chair, patient weight capacity 301 to 450 pounds Ⓑ

Capped rental

* **K0826** Power wheelchair, group 2 very heavy duty, sling/solid seat/back, patient weight capacity 451 to 600 pounds Ⓑ

Capped rental

* **K0827** Power wheelchair, group 2 very heavy duty, captains chair, patient weight capacity 451 to 600 pounds Ⓑ

Capped rental

* **K0828** Power wheelchair, group 2 extra heavy duty, sling/solid seat/back, patient weight capacity 601 pounds or more Ⓑ

Capped rental

* **K0829** Power wheelchair, group 2 extra heavy duty, captains chair, patient weight 601 pounds or more Ⓑ

Capped rental

* **K0830** Power wheelchair, group 2 standard, seat elevator, sling/solid seat/back, patient weight capacity up to and including 300 pounds Ⓑ

Capped rental

* **K0831** Power wheelchair, group 2 standard, seat elevator, captains chair, patient weight capacity up to and including 300 pounds Ⓑ

* **K0835** Power wheelchair, group 2 standard, single power option, sling/solid seat/back, patient weight capacity up to and including 300 pounds Ⓑ

Capped rental

✻ K0836 Power wheelchair, group 2 standard, single power option, captains chair, patient weight capacity up to and including 300 pounds Ⓑ
Capped rental

✻ K0837 Power wheelchair, group 2 heavy duty, single power option, sling/solid seat/back, patient weight capacity 301 to 450 pounds Ⓑ
Capped rental

✻ K0838 Power wheelchair, group 2 heavy duty, single power option, captains chair, patient weight capacity 301 to 450 pounds Ⓑ
Capped rental

✻ K0839 Power wheelchair, group 2 very heavy duty, single power option, sling/solid seat/back, patient weight capacity 451 to 600 pounds Ⓑ
Capped rental

✻ K0840 Power wheelchair, group 2 extra heavy duty, single power option, sling/solid seat/back, patient weight capacity 601 pounds or more Ⓑ
Capped rental

✻ K0841 Power wheelchair, group 2 standard, multiple power option, sling/solid seat/back, patient weight capacity up to and including 300 pounds Ⓑ
Capped rental

✻ K0842 Power wheelchair, group 2 standard, multiple power option, captains chair, patient weight capacity up to and including 300 pounds Ⓑ
Capped rental

✻ K0843 Power wheelchair, group 2 heavy duty, multiple power option, sling/solid seat/back, patient weight capacity 301 to 450 pounds Ⓑ
Capped rental

✻ K0848 Power wheelchair, group 3 standard, sling/solid seat/back, patient weight capacity up to and including 300 pounds Ⓑ
Capped rental

✻ K0849 Power wheelchair, group 3 standard, captains chair, patient weight capacity up to and including 300 pounds Ⓑ
Capped rental

✻ K0850 Power wheelchair, group 3 heavy duty, sling/solid seat/back, patient weight capacity 301 to 450 pounds Ⓑ
Capped rental

✻ K0851 Power wheelchair, group 3 heavy duty, captains chair, patient weight capacity 301 to 450 pounds Ⓑ
Capped rental

✻ K0852 Power wheelchair, group 3 very heavy duty, sling/solid seat/back, patient weight capacity 451 to 600 pounds Ⓑ
Capped rental

✻ K0853 Power wheelchair, group 3 very heavy duty, captains chair, patient weight capacity 451 to 600 pounds Ⓑ
Capped rental

✻ K0854 Power wheelchair, group 3 extra heavy duty, sling/solid seat/back, patient weight capacity 601 pounds or more Ⓑ
Capped rental

✻ K0855 Power wheelchair, group 3 extra heavy duty, captains chair, patient weight capacity 601 pounds or more Ⓑ
Capped rental

✻ K0856 Power wheelchair, group 3 standard, single power option, sling/solid seat/back, patient weight capacity up to and including 300 pounds Ⓑ
Capped rental

✻ K0857 Power wheelchair, group 3 standard, single power option, captains chair, patient weight capacity up to and including 300 pounds Ⓑ
Capped rental

✻ K0858 Power wheelchair, group 3 heavy duty, single power option, sling/solid seat/back, patient weight 301 to 450 pounds Ⓑ
Capped rental

✻ K0859 Power wheelchair, group 3 heavy duty, single power option, captains chair, patient weight capacity 301 to 450 pounds Ⓑ
Capped rental

✻ K0860 Power wheelchair, group 3 very heavy duty, single power option, sling/solid seat/back, patient weight capacity 451 to 600 pounds Ⓑ
Capped rental

✻ K0861 Power wheelchair, group 3 standard, multiple power option, sling/solid seat/back, patient weight capacity up to and including 300 pounds Ⓑ
Capped rental

▶ New ↩ Revised ✔ Reinstated ~~deleted~~ Deleted ⃠ Not covered or valid by Medicare
Special coverage instructions ✻ Carrier discretion Ⓑ Bill local carrier Ⓑ Bill DME MAC

✻ **K0862** Power wheelchair, group 3 heavy duty, multiple power option, sling/solid seat/back, patient weight capacity 301 to 450 pounds Ⓑ

Capped rental

✻ **K0863** Power wheelchair, group 3 very heavy duty, multiple power option, sling/solid seat/back, patient weight capacity 451 to 600 pounds Ⓑ

Capped rental

✻ **K0864** Power wheelchair, group 3 extra heavy duty, multiple power option, sling/solid seat/back, patient weight capacity 601 pounds or more Ⓑ

Capped rental

✻ **K0868** Power wheelchair, group 4 standard, sling/solid seat/back, patient weight capacity up to and including 300 pounds Ⓑ

Capped rental

✻ **K0869** Power wheelchair, group 4 standard, captains chair, patient weight capacity up to and including 300 pounds Ⓑ

Capped rental

✻ **K0870** Power wheelchair, group 4 heavy duty, sling/solid seat/back, patient weight capacity 301 to 450 pounds Ⓑ

Capped rental

✻ **K0871** Power wheelchair, group 4 very heavy duty, sling/solid seat/back, patient weight capacity 451 to 600 pounds Ⓑ

Capped rental

✻ **K0877** Power wheelchair, group 4 standard, single power option, sling/solid seat/back, patient weight capacity up to and including 300 pounds Ⓑ

Capped rental

✻ **K0878** Power wheelchair, group 4 standard, single power option, captains chair, patient weight capacity up to and including 300 pounds Ⓑ

Capped rental

✻ **K0879** Power wheelchair, group 4 heavy duty, single power option, sling/solid seat/back, patient weight capacity 301 to 450 pounds Ⓑ

Capped rental

✻ **K0880** Power wheelchair, group 4 very heavy duty, single power option, sling/solid seat/back, patient weight 451 to 600 pounds Ⓑ

Capped rental

✻ **K0884** Power wheelchair, group 4 standard, multiple power option, sling/solid seat/back, patient weight capacity up to and including 300 pounds Ⓑ

Capped rental

✻ **K0885** Power wheelchair, group 4 standard, multiple power option, captains chair, patient weight capacity up to and including 300 pounds Ⓑ

Capped rental

✻ **K0886** Power wheelchair, group 4 heavy duty, multiple power option, sling/solid seat/back, patient weight capacity 301 to 450 pounds Ⓑ

Capped rental

✻ **K0890** Power wheelchair, group 5 pediatric, single power option, sling/solid seat/back, patient weight capacity up to and including 125 pounds Ⓑ

Capped rental

✻ **K0891** Power wheelchair, group 5 pediatric, multiple power option, sling/solid seat/back, patient weight capacity up to and including 125 pounds Ⓑ

Capped rental

✻ **K0898** Power wheelchair, not otherwise classified Ⓑ

✻ **K0899** Power mobility device, not coded by DME PDAC or does not meet criteria Ⓑ

✪ **K0900** Customized durable medical equipment, other than wheelchair Ⓑ

~~K0901 Knee orthosis (KO), single upright, thigh and calf, with adjustable flexion and extension joint (unicentric or polycentric), medial-lateral and rotation control, with or without varus/valgus adjustment, prefabricated, off-the-shelf~~ ✖

Cross Reference L1851

~~K0902 Knee orthosis (KO), double upright, thigh and calf, with adjustable flexion and extension joint (unicentric or polycentric), medial-lateral and rotation control, with or without varus/valgus adjustment, prefabricated, off-the-shelf~~ ✖

Cross Reference L1852

▶ **New** ↻ **Revised** ✔ **Reinstated** ~~deleted~~ **Deleted** ⊘ **Not covered or valid by Medicare**
✪ **Special coverage instructions** ✻ **Carrier discretion** Ⓑ **Bill local carrier** Ⓑ **Bill DME MAC**

use modifiers LT, RT when orthotic or prosthetic is for certain side. Also a Functional modifier (K0 – K4) to define patient's functional state.

ORTHOTICS (L0100-L4999)

DMEPOS fee schedule:

www.cms.gov/DMEPOSFeeSched/LSDMEPOSFEE/list.asp#TopOfPage

Orthotic Devices: Spinal

✻ **L0112** Cranial cervical orthosis, congenital torticollis type, with or without soft interface material, adjustable range of motion joint, custom fabricated Ⓑ

✻ **L0113** Cranial cervical orthosis, torticollis type, with or without joint, with or without soft interface material, prefabricated, includes fitting and adjustment Ⓑ

✻ **L0120** Cervical, flexible, non-adjustable, prefabricated, off-the-shelf (foam collar) Ⓑ

Cervical orthoses, including soft and rigid devices, may be used as nonoperative management for cervical trauma.

✻ **L0130** Cervical, flexible, thermoplastic collar, molded to patient Ⓑ

✻ **L0140** Cervical, semi-rigid, adjustable (plastic collar) Ⓑ

✻ **L0150** Cervical, semi-rigid, adjustable molded chin cup (plastic collar with mandibular/occipital piece) Ⓑ

✻ **L0160** Cervical, semi-rigid, wire frame occipital/mandibular support, prefabricated, off-the-shelf Ⓑ

✻ **L0170** Cervical, collar, molded to patient model Ⓑ

✻ **L0172** Cervical, collar, semi-rigid thermoplastic foam, two-piece, prefabricated, off-the-shelf Ⓑ

✻ **L0174** Cervical, collar, semi-rigid, thermoplastic foam, two piece with thoracic extension, prefabricated, off-the-shelf Ⓑ

✻ **L0180** Cervical, multiple post collar, occipital/mandibular supports, adjustable Ⓑ

✻ **L0190** Cervical, multiple post collar, occipital/mandibular supports, adjustable cervical bars (SOMI, Guilford, Taylor types) Ⓑ

✻ **L0200** Cervical, multiple post collar, occipital/mandibular supports, adjustable cervical bars, and thoracic extension Ⓑ

✻ **L0220** Thoracic, rib belt, custom fabricated Ⓑ

Thoracic-Lumbar-Sacral

✻ **L0450** TLSO, flexible, provides trunk support, upper thoracic region, produces intracavitary pressure to reduce load on the intervertebral disks with rigid stays or panel(s), includes shoulder straps and closures, prefabricated, off-the-shelf Ⓑ

Used to immobilize specified area of spine, and is generally worn under clothing.

✻ **L0452** TLSO, flexible, provides trunk support, upper thoracic region, produces intracavitary pressure to reduce load on the intervertebral disks with rigid stays or panel(s), includes shoulder straps and closures, custom fabricated Ⓑ

✻ **L0454** TLSO flexible, provides trunk support, extends from sacrococcygeal junction to above T-9 vertebra, restricts gross trunk motion in the sagittal plane, produces intracavitary pressure to reduce load on the intervertebral disks with rigid stays or panel(s), includes shoulder straps and closures, prefabricated item that has been trimmed, bent, molded, assembled, or otherwise customized to fit a specific patient by an individual with expertise Ⓑ

Used to immobilize specified areas of spine; and is generally designed to be worn under clothing; not specifically designed for patients in wheelchairs.

✻ **L0455** TLSO, flexible, provides trunk support, extends from sacrococcygeal junction to above T-9 vertebra, restricts gross trunk motion in the sagittal plane, produces intracavitary pressure to reduce load on the intervertebral disks with rigid stays or panel(s), includes shoulder straps and closures, prefabricated, off-the-shelf Ⓑ

✻ **L0456** TLSO, flexible, provides trunk support, thoracic region, rigid posterior panel and soft anterior apron, extends from the sacrococcygeal junction and terminates just inferior to the scapular spine, restricts gross trunk motion in the sagittal plane, produces intracavitary pressure to reduce load on the intervertebral disks, includes straps and closures, prefabricated item that has been trimmed, bent, molded, assembled, or otherwise customized to fit a specific patient by an individual with expertise Ⓑ

* **L0457** TLSO, flexible, provides trunk support, thoracic region, rigid posterior panel and soft anterior apron, extends from the sacrococcygeal junction and terminates just inferior to the scapular spine, restricts gross trunk motion in the sagittal plane, produces intracavitary pressure to reduce load on the intervertebral disks, includes straps and closures, prefabricated, off-the-shelf Ⓑ

* **L0458** TLSO, triplanar control, modular segmented spinal system, two rigid plastic shells, posterior extends from the sacrococcygeal junction and terminates just inferior to the scapular spine, anterior extends from the symphysis pubis to the xiphoid, soft liner, restricts gross trunk motion in the sagittal, coronal, and transverse planes, lateral strength is provided by overlapping plastic and stabilizing closures, includes straps and closures, prefabricated, includes fitting and adjustment Ⓑ

  To meet Medicare's definition of body jacket, orthosis has to have rigid plastic shell that circles trunk with overlapping edges and stabilizing closures, and entire circumference of shell must be made of same rigid material.

* **L0460** TLSO, triplanar control, modular segmented spinal system, two rigid plastic shells, posterior extends from the sacrococcygeal junction and terminates just inferior to the scapular spine, anterior extends from the symphysis pubis to the sternal notch, soft liner, restricts gross trunk motion in the sagittal, coronal, and transverse planes, lateral strength is provided by overlapping plastic and stabilizing closures, includes straps and closures, prefabricated item that has been trimmed, bent, molded, assembled, or otherwise customized to fit a specific patient by an individual with expertise Ⓑ

* **L0462** TLSO, triplanar control, modular segmented spinal system, three rigid plastic shells, posterior extends from the sacrococcygeal junction and terminates just inferior to the scapular spine, anterior extends from the symphysis pubis to the sternal notch, soft liner, restricts gross trunk motion in the sagittal, coronal, and transverse planes, lateral strength is provided by overlapping plastic and stabilizing closures, includes straps and closures, prefabricated, includes fitting and adjustment Ⓑ

* **L0464** TLSO, triplanar control, modular segmented spinal system, four rigid plastic shells, posterior extends from sacrococcygeal junction and terminates just inferior to scapular spine, anterior extends from symphysis pubis to the sternal notch, soft liner, restricts gross trunk motion in sagittal, coronal, and transverse planes, lateral strength is provided by overlapping plastic and stabilizing closures, includes straps and closures, prefabricated, includes fitting and adjustment Ⓑ

* **L0466** TLSO, sagittal control, rigid posterior frame and flexible soft anterior apron with straps, closures and padding, restricts gross trunk motion in sagittal plane, produces intracavitary pressure to reduce load on intervertebral disks, prefabricated item that has been trimmed, bent, molded, assembled, or otherwise customized to fit a specific patient by an individual with expertise Ⓑ

* **L0467** TLSO, sagittal control, rigid posterior frame and flexible soft anterior apron with straps, closures and padding, restricts gross trunk motion in sagittal plane, produces intracavitary pressure to reduce load on intervertebral disks, prefabricated, off-the-shelf Ⓑ

* **L0468** TLSO, sagittal-coronal control, rigid posterior frame and flexible soft anterior apron with straps, closures and padding, extends from sacrococcygeal junction over scapulae, lateral strength provided by pelvic, thoracic, and lateral frame pieces, restricts gross trunk motion in sagittal, and coronal planes, produces intracavitary pressure to reduce load on intervertebral disks, prefabricated item that has been trimmed, bent, molded, assembled, or otherwise customized to fit a specific patient by an individual with expertise Ⓑ

✻ **L0469** TLSO, sagittal-coronal control, rigid posterior frame and flexible soft anterior apron with straps, closures and padding, extends from sacrococcygeal junction over scapulae, lateral strength provided by pelvic, thoracic, and lateral frame pieces, restricts gross trunk motion in sagittal and coronal planes, produces intracavitary pressure to reduce load on intervertebral disks, prefabricated, off-the-shelf Ⓑ

✻ **L0470** TLSO, triplanar control, rigid posterior frame and flexible soft anterior apron with straps, closures and padding, extends from sacrococcygeal junction to scapula, lateral strength provided by pelvic, thoracic, and lateral frame pieces, rotational strength provided by subclavicular extensions, restricts gross trunk motion in sagittal, coronal, and transverse planes, provides intracavitary pressure to reduce load on the intervertebral disks, includes fitting and shaping the frame, prefabricated, includes fitting and adjustment Ⓑ

✻ **L0472** TLSO, triplanar control, hyperextension, rigid anterior and lateral frame extends from symphysis pubis to sternal notch with two anterior components (one pubic and one sternal), posterior and lateral pads with straps and closures, limits spinal flexion, restricts gross trunk motion in sagittal, coronal, and transverse planes, includes fitting and shaping the frame, prefabricated, includes fitting and adjustment Ⓑ

✻ **L0480** TLSO, triplanar control, one piece rigid plastic shell without interface liner, with multiple straps and closures, posterior extends from sacrococcygeal junction and terminates just inferior to scapular spine, anterior extends from symphysis pubis to sternal notch, anterior or posterior opening, restricts gross trunk motion in sagittal, coronal, and transverse planes, includes a carved plaster or CAD-CAM model, custom fabricated Ⓑ

✻ **L0482** TLSO, triplanar control, one piece rigid plastic shell with interface liner, multiple straps and closures, posterior extends from sacrococcygeal junction and terminates just inferior to scapular spine, anterior extends from symphysis pubis to sternal notch, anterior or posterior opening, restricts gross trunk motion in sagittal, coronal, and transverse planes, includes a carved plaster or CAD-CAM model, custom fabricated Ⓑ

✻ **L0484** TLSO, triplanar control, two piece rigid plastic shell without interface liner, with multiple straps and closures, posterior extends from sacrococcygeal junction and terminates just inferior to scapular spine, anterior extends from symphysis pubis to sternal notch, lateral strength is enhanced by overlapping plastic, restricts gross trunk motion in the sagittal, coronal, and transverse planes, includes a carved plaster or CAD-CAM model, custom fabricated Ⓑ

✻ **L0486** TLSO, triplanar control, two piece rigid plastic shell with interface liner, multiple straps and closures, posterior extends from sacrococcygeal junction and terminates just inferior to scapular spine, anterior extends from symphysis pubis to sternal notch, lateral strength is enhanced by overlapping plastic, restricts gross trunk motion in the sagittal, coronal, and transverse planes, includes a carved plaster or CAD-CAM model, custom fabricated Ⓑ

✻ **L0488** TLSO, triplanar control, one piece rigid plastic shell with interface liner, multiple straps and closures, posterior extends from sacrococcygeal junction and terminates just inferior to scapular spine, anterior extends from symphysis pubis to sternal notch, anterior or posterior opening, restricts gross trunk motion in sagittal, coronal, and transverse planes, prefabricated, includes fitting and adjustment Ⓑ

✻ **L0490** TLSO, sagittal-coronal control, one piece rigid plastic shell, with overlapping reinforced anterior, with multiple straps and closures, posterior extends from sacrococcygeal junction and terminates at or before the T-9 vertebra, anterior extends from symphysis pubis to xiphoid, anterior opening, restricts gross trunk motion in sagittal and coronal planes, prefabricated, includes fitting and adjustment Ⓑ

▶ **New** ⤾ **Revised** ✔ **Reinstated** ~~deleted~~ **Deleted** ⃠ **Not covered or valid by Medicare**
Special coverage instructions ✻ **Carrier discretion** **Bill local carrier** Ⓑ **Bill DME MAC**

* **L0491** TLSO, sagittal-coronal control, modular segmented spinal system, two rigid plastic shells, posterior extends from the sacrococcygeal junction and terminates just inferior to the scapular spine, anterior extends from the symphysis pubis to the xiphoid, soft liner, restricts gross trunk motion in the sagittal and coronal planes, lateral strength is provided by overlapping plastic and stabilizing closures, includes straps and closures, prefabricated, includes fitting and adjustment Ⓑ

* **L0492** TLSO, sagittal-coronal control, modular segmented spinal system, three rigid plastic shells, posterior extends from the sacrococcygeal junction and terminates just inferior to the scapular spine, anterior extends from the symphysis pubis to the xiphoid, soft liner, restricts gross trunk motion in the sagittal and coronal planes, lateral strength is provided by overlapping plastic and stabilizing closures, includes straps and closures, prefabricated, includes fitting and adjustment Ⓑ

Sacroilliac, Lumbar, Sacral Orthosis

* **L0621** Sacroiliac orthosis, flexible, provides pelvic-sacral support, reduces motion about the sacroiliac joint, includes straps, closures, may include pendulous abdomen design, prefabricated, off-the-shelf Ⓑ

* **L0622** Sacroiliac orthosis, flexible, provides pelvic-sacral support, reduces motion about the sacroiliac joint, includes straps, closures, may include pendulous abdomen design, custom fabricated Ⓑ

  Type of custom-fabricated device for which impression of specific body part is made (e.g., by means of plaster cast, or CAD-CAM [computer-aided design] technology); impression then used to make specific patient model

* **L0623** Sacroiliac orthosis, provides pelvic-sacral support, with rigid or semi-rigid panels over the sacrum and abdomen, reduces motion about the sacroiliac joint, includes straps, closures, may include pendulous abdomen design, prefabricated, off-the-shelf Ⓑ

* **L0624** Sacroiliac orthosis, provides pelvic-sacral support, with rigid or semi-rigid panels placed over the sacrum and abdomen, reduces motion about the sacroiliac joint, includes straps, closures, may include pendulous abdomen design, custom fabricated Ⓑ

  Custom fitted

* **L0625** Lumbar orthosis, flexible, provides lumbar support, posterior extends from L-1 to below L-5 vertebra, produces intracavitary pressure to reduce load on the intervertebral discs, includes straps, closures, may include pendulous abdomen design, shoulder straps, stays, prefabricated, off-the- shelf Ⓑ

* **L0626** Lumbar orthosis, sagittal control, with rigid posterior panel(s), posterior extends from L-1 to below L-5 vertebra, produces intracavitary pressure to reduce load on the intervertebral discs, includes straps, closures, may include padding, stays, shoulder straps, pendulous abdomen design, prefabricated item that has been trimmed, bent, molded, assembled, or otherwise customized to fit a specific patient by an individual with expertise Ⓑ

* **L0627** Lumbar orthosis, sagittal control, with rigid anterior and posterior panels, posterior extends from L-1 to below L-5 vertebra, produces intracavitary pressure to reduce load on the intervertebral discs, includes straps, closures, may include padding, shoulder straps, pendulous abdomen design, prefabricated item that has been trimmed, bent, molded, assembled, or otherwise customized to fit a specific patient by an individual with expertise Ⓑ

* **L0628** Lumbar-sacral orthosis, flexible, provides lumbo-sacral support, posterior extends from sacrococcygeal junction to T-9 vertebra, produces intracavitary pressure to reduce load on the intervertebral discs, includes straps, closures, may include stays, shoulder straps, pendulous abdomen design, prefabricated, off-the-shelf Ⓑ

* **L0629** Lumbar-sacral orthosis, flexible, provides lumbo-sacral support, posterior extends from sacrococcygeal junction to T-9 vertebra, produces intracavitary pressure to reduce load on the intervertebral discs, includes straps, closures, may include stays, shoulder straps, pendulous abdomen design, custom fabricated Ⓑ

  Custom fitted

▶ New ↩ Revised ✔ Reinstated ~~deleted~~ Deleted ⊘ Not covered or valid by Medicare
✪ Special coverage instructions * Carrier discretion Ⓑ Bill local carrier Ⓑ Bill DME MAC

✻ **L0630** Lumbar-sacral orthosis, sagittal control, with rigid posterior panel(s), posterior extends from sacrococcygeal junction to T-9 vertebra, produces intracavitary pressure to reduce load on the intervertebral discs, includes straps, closures, may include padding, stays, shoulder straps, pendulous abdomen design, prefabricated item that has been trimmed, bent, molded, assembled, or otherwise customized to fit a specific patient by an individual with expertise Ⓑ

✻ **L0631** Lumbar-sacral orthosis, sagittal control, with rigid anterior and posterior panels, posterior extends from sacrococcygeal junction to T-9 vertebra, produces intracavitary pressure to reduce load on the intervertebral discs, includes straps, closures, may include padding, shoulder straps, pendulous abdomen design, prefabricated item that has been trimmed, bent, molded, assembled, or otherwise customized to fit a specific patient by an individual with expertise Ⓑ

✻ **L0632** Lumbar-sacral orthosis, sagittal control, with rigid anterior and posterior panels, posterior extends from sacrococcygeal junction to T-9 vertebra, produces intracavitary pressure to reduce load on the intervertebral discs, includes straps, closures, may include padding, shoulder straps, pendulous abdomen design, custom fabricated Ⓑ

Custom fitted

✻ **L0633** Lumbar-sacral orthosis, sagittal-coronal control, with rigid posterior frame/panel(s), posterior extends from sacrococcygeal junction to T-9 vertebra, lateral strength provided by rigid lateral frame/panels, produces intracavitary pressure to reduce load on intervertebral discs, includes straps, closures, may include padding, stays, shoulder straps, pendulous abdomen design, prefabricated item that has been trimmed, bent, molded, assembled, or otherwise customized to fit a specific patient by an individual with expertise Ⓑ

✻ **L0634** Lumbar-sacral orthosis, sagittal-coronal control, with rigid posterior frame/panel(s), posterior extends from sacrococcygeal junction to T-9 vertebra, lateral strength provided by rigid lateral frame/panel(s), produces intracavitary pressure to reduce load on intervertebral discs, includes straps, closures, may include padding, stays, shoulder straps, pendulous abdomen design, custom fabricated Ⓑ

Custom fitted

✻ **L0635** Lumbar-sacral orthosis, sagittal-coronal control, lumbar flexion, rigid posterior frame/panel(s), lateral articulating design to flex the lumbar spine, posterior extends from sacrococcygeal junction to T-9 vertebra, lateral strength provided by rigid lateral frame/panel(s), produces intracavitary pressure to reduce load on intervertebral discs, includes straps, closures, may include padding, anterior panel, pendulous abdomen design, prefabricated, includes fitting and adjustment Ⓑ

✻ **L0636** Lumbar sacral orthosis, sagittal-coronal control, lumbar flexion, rigid posterior frame/panels, lateral articulating design to flex the lumbar spine, posterior extends from sacrococcygeal junction to T-9 vertebra, lateral strength provided by rigid lateral frame/panels, produces intracavitary pressure to reduce load on intervertebral discs, includes straps, closures, may include padding, anterior panel, pendulous abdomen design, custom fabricated Ⓑ

Custom fitted

✻ **L0637** Lumbar-sacral orthosis, sagittal-coronal control, with rigid anterior and posterior frame/panels, posterior extends from sacrococcygeal junction to T-9 vertebra, lateral strength provided by rigid lateral frame/panels, produces intracavitary pressure to reduce load on intervertebral discs, includes straps, closures, may include padding, shoulder straps, pendulous abdomen design, prefabricated item that has been trimmed, bent, molded, assembled, or otherwise customized to fit a specific patient by an individual with expertise Ⓑ

* **L0638** Lumbar-sacral orthosis, sagittal-coronal control, with rigid anterior and posterior frame/panels, posterior extends from sacrococcygeal junction to T-9 vertebra, lateral strength provided by rigid lateral frame/panels, produces intracavitary pressure to reduce load on intervertebral discs, includes straps, closures, may include padding, shoulder straps, pendulous abdomen design, custom fabricated Ⓑ

* **L0639** Lumbar-sacral orthosis, sagittal-coronal control, rigid shell(s)/panel(s), posterior extends from sacrococcygeal junction to T-9 vertebra, anterior extends from symphysis pubis to xyphoid, produces intracavitary pressure to reduce load on the intervertebral discs, overall strength is provided by overlapping rigid material and stabilizing closures, includes straps, closures, may include soft interface, pendulous abdomen design, prefabricated item that has been trimmed, bent, molded, assembled, or otherwise customized to fit a specific patient by an individual with expertise Ⓑ

  Characterized by rigid plastic shell that encircles trunk with overlapping edges and stabilizing closures and provides high degree of immobility

* **L0640** Lumbar-sacral orthosis, sagittal-coronal control, rigid shell(s)/panel(s), posterior extends from sacrococcygeal junction to T-9 vertebra, anterior extends from symphysis pubis to xyphoid, produces intracavitary pressure to reduce load on the intervertebral discs, overall strength is provided by overlapping rigid material and stabilizing closures, includes straps, closures, may include soft interface, pendulous abdomen design, custom fabricated Ⓑ

  Custom fitted

* **L0641** Lumbar orthosis, sagittal control, with rigid posterior panel(s), posterior extends from L-1 to below L-5 vertebra, produces intracavitary pressure to reduce load on the intervertebral discs, includes straps, closures, may include padding, stays, shoulder straps, pendulous abdomen design, prefabricated, off-the-shelf Ⓑ

* **L0642** Lumbar orthosis, sagittal control, with rigid anterior and posterior panels, posterior extends from L-1 to below L-5 vertebra, produces intracavitary pressure to reduce load on the intervertebral discs, includes straps, closures, may include padding, shoulder straps, pendulous abdomen design, prefabricated, off-the-shelf Ⓑ

* **L0643** Lumbar-sacral orthosis, sagittal control, with rigid posterior panel(s), posterior extends from sacrococcygeal junction to T-9 vertebra, produces intracavitary pressure to reduce load on the intervertebral discs, includes straps, closures, may include padding, stays, shoulder straps, pendulous abdomen design, prefabricated, off-the-shelf Ⓑ

* **L0648** Lumbar-sacral orthosis, sagittal control, with rigid anterior and posterior panels, posterior extends from sacrococcygeal junction to T-9 vertebra, produces intracavitary pressure to reduce load on the intervertebral discs, includes straps, closures, may include padding, shoulder straps, pendulous abdomen design, prefabricated, off-the-shelf Ⓑ

* **L0649** Lumbar-sacral orthosis, sagittal-coronal control, with rigid posterior frame/panel(s), posterior extends from sacrococcygeal junction to T-9 vertebra, lateral strength provided by rigid lateral frame/panels, produces intracavitary pressure to reduce load on intervertebral discs, includes straps, closures, may include padding, stays, shoulder straps, pendulous abdomen design, prefabricated, off-the-shelf Ⓑ

* **L0650** Lumbar-sacral orthosis, sagittal-coronal control, with rigid anterior and posterior frame/panel(s), posterior extends from sacrococcygeal junction to T-9 vertebra, lateral strength provided by rigid lateral frame/panel(s), produces intracavitary pressure to reduce load on intervertebral discs, includes straps, closures, may include padding, shoulder straps, pendulous abdomen design, prefabricated, off-the-shelf Ⓑ

∗ **L0651** Lumbar-sacral orthosis, sagittal-coronal control, rigid shell(s)/panel(s), posterior extends from sacrococcygeal junction to T-9 vertebra, anterior extends from symphysis pubis to xyphoid, produces intracavitary pressure to reduce load on the intervertebral discs, overall strength is provided by overlapping rigid material and stabilizing closures, includes straps, closures, may include soft interface, pendulous abdomen design, prefabricated, off-the-shelf Ⓑ

Cervical-Thoracic-Lumbar-Sacral

∗ **L0700** Cervical-thoracic-lumbar-sacral-orthoses (CTLSO), anterior-posterior-lateral control, molded to patient model, (Minerva type) Ⓑ

∗ **L0710** CTLSO, anterior-posterior-lateral-control, molded to patient model, with interface material, (Minerva type) Ⓑ

HALO Procedure

∗ **L0810** HALO procedure, cervical halo incorporated into jacket vest Ⓑ

∗ **L0820** HALO procedure, cervical halo incorporated into plaster body jacket Ⓑ

∗ **L0830** HALO procedure, cervical halo incorporated into Milwaukee type orthosis Ⓑ

∗ **L0859** Addition to HALO procedure, magnetic resonance image compatible systems, rings and pins, any material Ⓑ

∗ **L0861** Addition to HALO procedure, replacement liner/interface material Ⓑ

Additions to Spinal Orthoses

TLSO - Thoraci-lumbar-sacral orthoses

Spinal orthoses may be prefabricated, prefitted, or custom fabricated. Conservative treatment for back pain may include the use of spinal orthoses.

∗ **L0970** TLSO, corset front Ⓑ

∗ **L0972** LSO, corset front Ⓑ

∗ **L0974** TLSO, full corset Ⓑ

∗ **L0976** LSO, full corset Ⓑ

∗ **L0978** Axillary crutch extension Ⓑ

∗ **L0980** Peroneal straps, prefabricated, off-the-shelf, pair Ⓑ

∗ **L0982** Stocking supporter grips, prefabricated, off-the-shelf, set of four (4) Ⓑ

Convenience item

∗ **L0984** Protective body sock, prefabricated, off-the-shelf, each Ⓑ

Convenience item

Garment made of cloth or similar material that is worn under spinal orthosis and is not primarily medical in nature

∗ **L0999** Addition to spinal orthosis, not otherwise specified Ⓑ

Orthotic Devices: Scoliosis Procedures (L1000-L1520)

Note: Orthotic care of scoliosis differs from other orthotic care in that the treatment is more dynamic in nature and uses ongoing continual modification of the orthosis to the patient's changing condition. This coding structure uses the proper names, or eponyms, of the procedures because they have historic and universal acceptance in the profession. It should be recognized that variations to the basic procedures described by the founders/developers are accepted in various medical and orthotic practices throughout the country. All procedures include a model of patient when indicated.

Scoliosis: Cervical-Thoracic-Lumbar-Sacral (CTLSO) (Milwaukee)

∗ **L1000** Cervical-thoracic-lumbar-sacral orthosis (CTLSO) (Milwaukee), inclusive of furnishing initial orthosis, including model Ⓑ

∗ **L1001** Cervical thoracic lumbar sacral orthosis, immobilizer, infant size, prefabricated, includes fitting and adjustment Ⓑ

∗ **L1005** Tension based scoliosis orthosis and accessory pads, includes fitting and adjustment Ⓑ

∗ **L1010** Addition to cervical-thoracic-lumbar-sacral orthosis (CTLSO) or scoliosis orthosis, axilla sling Ⓑ

Correction Pads

∗ **L1020** Addition to CTLSO or scoliosis orthosis, kyphosis pad Ⓑ

▶ New ↩ Revised ✔ Reinstated ~~deleted~~ Deleted ⦸ Not covered or valid by Medicare
⊛ Special coverage instructions ∗ Carrier discretion Ⓑ Bill local carrier Ⓑ Bill DME MAC

* **L1025** Addition to CTLSO or scoliosis orthosis, kyphosis pad, floating Ⓑ

* **L1030** Addition to CTLSO or scoliosis orthosis, lumbar bolster pad Ⓑ

* **L1040** Addition to CTLSO or scoliosis orthosis, lumbar or lumbar rib pad Ⓑ

* **L1050** Addition to CTLSO or scoliosis orthosis, sternal pad Ⓑ

* **L1060** Addition to CTLSO or scoliosis orthosis, thoracic pad Ⓑ

* **L1070** Addition to CTLSO or scoliosis orthosis, trapezius sling Ⓑ

* **L1080** Addition to CTLSO or scoliosis orthosis, outrigger Ⓑ

* **L1085** Addition to CTLSO or scoliosis orthosis, outrigger, bilateral with vertical extensions Ⓑ

* **L1090** Addition to CTLSO or scoliosis orthosis, lumbar sling Ⓑ

* **L1100** Addition to CTLSO or scoliosis orthosis, ring flange, plastic or leather Ⓑ

* **L1110** Addition to CTLSO or scoliosis orthosis, ring flange, plastic or leather, molded to patient model Ⓑ

* **L1120** Addition to CTLSO, scoliosis orthosis, cover for upright, each Ⓑ

Scoliosis: Thoracic-Lumbar-Sacral (Low Profile)

* **L1200** Thoracic-lumbar-sacral-orthosis (TLSO), inclusive of furnishing initial orthosis only Ⓑ

* **L1210** Addition to TLSO, (low profile), lateral thoracic extension Ⓑ

* **L1220** Addition to TLSO, (low profile), anterior thoracic extension Ⓑ

* **L1230** Addition to TLSO, (low profile), Milwaukee type superstructure Ⓑ

* **L1240** Addition to TLSO, (low profile), lumbar derotation pad Ⓑ

* **L1250** Addition to TLSO, (low profile), anterior ASIS pad Ⓑ

* **L1260** Addition to TLSO, (low profile), anterior thoracic derotation pad Ⓑ

* **L1270** Addition to TLSO, (low profile), abdominal pad Ⓑ

* **L1280** Addition to TLSO, (low profile), rib gusset (elastic), each Ⓑ

* **L1290** Addition to TLSO, (low profile), lateral trochanteric pad Ⓑ

Other Scoliosis Procedures

* **L1300** Other scoliosis procedure, body jacket molded to patient model Ⓑ

* **L1310** Other scoliosis procedure, postoperative body jacket Ⓑ

* **L1499** Spinal orthosis, not otherwise specified Ⓑ

Orthotic Devices: Lower Limb (L1600-L3649)

Note: the procedures in L1600-L2999 are considered as base or basic procedures and may be modified by listing procedure from the Additions Sections and adding them to the base procedure.

Hip: Flexible

* **L1600** Hip orthosis, abduction control of hip joints, flexible, Frejka type with cover, prefabricated item that has been trimmed, bent, molded, assembled, or otherwise customized to fit a specific patient by an individual with expertise Ⓑ

* **L1610** Hip orthosis, abduction control of hip joints, flexible, (Frejka cover only), prefabricated item that has been trimmed, bent, molded, assembled, or otherwise customized to fit a specific patient by an individual with expertise Ⓑ

* **L1620** Hip orthosis, abduction control of hip joints, flexible, (Pavlik harness), prefabricated item that has been trimmed, bent, molded, assembled, or otherwise customized to fit a specific patient by an individual with expertise Ⓑ

* **L1630** Hip orthosis, abduction control of hip joints, semi-flexible (Von Rosen type), custom-fabricated Ⓑ

* **L1640** Hip orthosis, abduction control of hip joints, static, pelvic band or spreader bar, thigh cuffs, custom-fabricated Ⓑ

* **L1650** Hip orthosis, abduction control of hip joints, static, adjustable, (Ilfled type), prefabricated, includes fitting and adjustment Ⓑ

* **L1652** Hip orthosis, bilateral thigh cuffs with adjustable abductor spreader bar, adult size, prefabricated, includes fitting and adjustment, any type Ⓑ

* **L1660** Hip orthosis, abduction control of hip joints, static, plastic, prefabricated, includes fitting and adjustment Ⓑ

* **L1680** Hip orthosis, abduction control of hip joints, dynamic, pelvic control, adjustable hip motion control, thigh cuffs (Rancho hip action type), custom fabrication Ⓑ

* **L1685** Hip orthosis, abduction control of hip joint, postoperative hip abduction type, custom fabricated Ⓑ

* **L1686** Hip orthosis, abduction control of hip joint, postoperative hip abduction type, prefabricated, includes fitting and adjustment Ⓑ

* **L1690** Combination, bilateral, lumbo-sacral, hip, femur orthosis providing adduction and internal rotation control, prefabricated, includes fitting and adjustment Ⓑ

Legg Perthes

* **L1700** Legg-Perthes orthosis, (Toronto type), custom-fabricated Ⓑ

* **L1710** Legg-Perthes orthosis, (Newington type), custom-fabricated Ⓑ

* **L1720** Legg-Perthes orthosis, trilateral, (Tachdjian type), custom-fabricated Ⓑ

* **L1730** Legg-Perthes orthosis, (Scottish Rite type), custom-fabricated Ⓑ

* **L1755** Legg-Perthes orthosis, (Patten bottom type), custom-fabricated Ⓑ

Knee (KO)

* **L1810** Knee orthosis, elastic with joints, prefabricated item that has been trimmed, bent, molded, assembled, or otherwise customized to fit a specific patient by an individual with expertise Ⓑ

* **L1812** Knee orthosis, elastic with joints, prefabricated, off-the-shelf Ⓑ

* **L1820** Knee orthosis, elastic with condylar pads and joints, with or without patellar control, prefabricated, includes fitting and adjustment Ⓑ

* **L1830** Knee orthosis, immobilizer, canvas longitudinal, prefabricated, off-the-shelf Ⓑ

* **L1831** Knee orthosis, locking knee joint(s), positional orthosis, prefabricated, includes fitting and adjustment Ⓑ

* **L1832** Knee orthosis, adjustable knee joints (unicentric or polycentric), positional orthosis, rigid support, prefabricated item that has been trimmed, bent, molded, assembled, or otherwise customized to fit a specific patient by an individual with expertise Ⓑ

* **L1833** Knee orthosis, adjustable knee joints (unicentric or polycentric), positional orthosis, rigid support, prefabricated, off-the-shelf Ⓑ

* **L1834** Knee orthosis, without knee joint, rigid, custom-fabricated Ⓑ

* **L1836** Knee orthosis, rigid, without joint(s), includes soft interface material, prefabricated, off-the-shelf Ⓑ

* **L1840** Knee orthosis, derotation, medial-lateral, anterior cruciate ligament, custom fabricated Ⓑ

* **L1843** Knee orthosis, single upright, thigh and calf, with adjustable flexion and extension joint (unicentric or polycentric), medial-lateral and rotation control, with or without varus/valgus adjustment, prefabricated item that has been trimmed, bent, molded, assembled, or otherwise customized to fit a specific patient by an individual with expertise Ⓑ

* **L1844** Knee orthosis, single upright, thigh and calf, with adjustable flexion and extension joint (unicentric or polycentric), medial-lateral and rotation control, with or without varus/valgus adjustment, custom fabricated Ⓑ

* **L1845** Knee orthosis, double upright, thigh and calf, with adjustable flexion and extension joint (unicentric or polycentric), medial-lateral and rotation control, with or without varus/valgus adjustment, prefabricated item that has been trimmed, bent, molded, assembled, or otherwise customized to fit a specific patient by an individual with expertise Ⓑ

* **L1846** Knee orthrosis, double upright, thigh and calf, with adjustable flexion and extension joint (unicentric or polycentric), medial-lateral and rotation control, with or without varus/valgus adjustment, custom fabricated Ⓑ

▶ New ↻ Revised ✔ Reinstated ~~deleted~~ Deleted ⊘ Not covered or valid by Medicare
Special coverage instructions * Carrier discretion Bill local carrier Ⓑ Bill DME MAC

* **L1847** Knee orthosis, double upright with adjustable joint, with inflatable air support chamber(s), prefabricated item that has been trimmed, bent, molded, assembled, or otherwise customized to fit a specific patient by an individual with expertise Ⓑ
* **L1848** Knee orthosis, double upright with adjustable joint, with inflatable air support chamber(s), prefabricated, off-the-shelf Ⓑ
* **L1850** Knee orthosis, Swedish type, prefabricated, off-the- shelf Ⓑ
▶ * **L1851** Knee orthosis (KO), single upright, thigh and calf, with adjustable flexion and extension joint (unicentric or polycentric), medial-lateral and rotation control, with or without varus/valgus adjustment, prefabricated, off-the-shelf Ⓑ
▶ * **L1852** Knee orthosis (KO), double upright, thigh and calf, with adjustable flexion and extension joint (unicentric or polycentric), medial-lateral and rotation control, with or without varus/valgus adjustment, prefabricated, off-the-shelf Ⓑ
* **L1860** Knee orthosis, modification of supracondylar prosthetic socket, custom fabricated (SK) Ⓑ

Ankle-Foot (AFO)

* **L1900** Ankle foot orthosis (AFO), spring wire, dorsiflexion assist calf band, custom-fabricated Ⓑ
* **L1902** Ankle orthosis, ankle gauntlet or similiar, with or without joints, prefabricated, off-the-shelf Ⓑ
* **L1904** Ankle orthosis, ankle gauntlet or similiar, with or without joints, custom fabricated Ⓑ
⮐ * **L1906** Ankle foot orthosis, multiligamentous ankle support, prefabricated, off-the-shelf Ⓑ
* **L1907** Ankle orthosis, supramalleolar with straps, with or without interface/pads, custom fabricated Ⓑ
* **L1910** Ankle foot orthosis, posterior, single bar, clasp attachment to shoe counter, prefabricated, includes fitting and adjustment Ⓑ
* **L1920** Ankle foot orthosis, single upright with static or adjustable stop (Phelps or Perlstein type), custom fabricated Ⓑ
* **L1930** Ankle-foot orthosis, plastic or other material, prefabricated, includes fitting and adjustment Ⓑ
* **L1932** AFO, rigid anterior tibial section, total carbon fiber or equal material, prefabricated, includes fitting and adjustment Ⓑ
* **L1940** Ankle foot orthosis, plastic or other material, custom fabricated Ⓑ
* **L1945** Ankle foot orthosis, plastic, rigid anterior tibial section (floor reaction), custom fabricated Ⓑ
* **L1950** Ankle foot orthosis, spiral, (Institute of Rehabilitation Medicine type), plastic, custom fabricated Ⓑ
* **L1951** Ankle foot orthosis, spiral, (Institute of Rehabilitative Medicine type), plastic or other material, prefabricated, includes fitting and adjustment Ⓑ
* **L1960** Ankle foot orthosis, posterior solid ankle, plastic, custom fabricated Ⓑ
* **L1970** Ankle foot orthosis, plastic, with ankle joint, custom fabricated Ⓑ
* **L1971** Ankle foot orthosis, plastic or other material with ankle joint, prefabricated, includes fitting and adjustment Ⓑ
* **L1980** Ankle foot orthosis, single upright free plantar dorsiflexion, solid stirrup, calf band/cuff (single bar 'BK' orthosis), custom fabricated Ⓑ
* **L1990** Ankle foot orthosis, double upright free plantar dorsiflexion, solid stirrup, calf band/cuff (double bar 'BK' orthosis), custom fabricated Ⓑ

Hip-Knee-Ankle-Foot (or Any Combination)

NOTE: L2000, L2020, and L2036 are base procedures to be used with any knee joint. L2010 and L2030 are to be used only with no knee joint.

* **L2000** Knee ankle foot orthosis, single upright, free knee, free ankle, solid stirrup, thigh and calf bands/cuffs (single bar 'AK' orthosis), custom-fabricated Ⓑ
* **L2005** Knee ankle foot orthosis, any material, single or double upright, stance control, automatic lock and swing phase release, any type activation; includes ankle joint, any type, custom fabricated Ⓑ
* **L2010** Knee ankle foot orthosis, single upright, free ankle, solid stirrup, thigh and calf bands/cuffs (single bar 'AK' orthosis), without knee joint, custom-fabricated Ⓑ

▶ New ⮐ Revised ✔ Reinstated ~~deleted~~ Deleted ⃠ Not covered or valid by Medicare
Special coverage instructions * Carrier discretion Ⓑ Bill local carrier Ⓑ Bill DME MAC

* **L2020** Knee ankle foot orthosis, double upright, free knee, free ankle, solid stirrup, thigh and calf bands/cuffs (double bar 'AK' orthosis), custom fabricated Ⓑ

* **L2030** Knee ankle foot orthosis, double upright, free ankle, solid stirrup, thigh and calf bands/cuffs (double bar 'AK' orthosis), without knee joint, custom fabricated Ⓑ

* **L2034** Knee ankle foot orthosis, full plastic, single upright, with or without free motion knee, medial lateral rotation control, with or without free motion ankle, custom fabricated Ⓑ

* **L2035** Knee ankle foot orthosis, full plastic, static (pediatric size), without free motion ankle, prefabricated, includes fitting and adjustment Ⓑ

* **L2036** Knee ankle foot orthosis, full plastic, double upright, with or without free motion knee, with or without free motion ankle, custom fabricated Ⓑ

* **L2037** Knee ankle foot orthosis, full plastic, single upright, with or without free motion knee, with or without free motion ankle, custom fabricated Ⓑ

* **L2038** Knee ankle foot orthosis, full plastic, with or without free motion knee, multi-axis ankle, custom fabricated Ⓑ

Torsion Control

* **L2040** Hip knee ankle foot orthosis, torsion control, bilateral rotation straps, pelvic band/belt, custom fabricated Ⓑ

* **L2050** Hip knee ankle foot orthosis, torsion control, bilateral torsion cables, hip joint, pelvic band/belt, custom fabricated Ⓑ

* **L2060** Hip knee ankle foot orthosis, torsion control, bilateral torsion cables, ball bearing hip joint, pelvic band/belt, custom fabricated Ⓑ

* **L2070** Hip knee ankle foot orthosis, torsion control, unilateral rotation straps, pelvic band/belt, custom fabricated Ⓑ

* **L2080** Hip knee ankle foot orthosis, torsion control, unilateral torsion cable, hip joint, pelvic band/belt, custom fabricated Ⓑ

* **L2090** Hip knee ankle foot orthosis, torsion control, unilateral torsion cable, ball bearing hip joint, pelvic band/belt, custom fabricated Ⓑ

Fracture Orthoses

* **L2106** Ankle foot orthosis, fracture orthosis, tibial fracture cast orthosis, thermoplastic type casting material, custom fabricated Ⓑ

* **L2108** Ankle foot orthosis, fracture orthosis, tibial fracture cast orthosis, custom fabricated Ⓑ

* **L2112** Ankle foot orthosis, fracture orthosis, tibial fracture orthosis, soft, prefabricated, includes fitting and adjustment Ⓑ

* **L2114** Ankle foot orthosis, fracture orthosis, tibial fracture orthosis, semi-rigid, prefabricated, includes fitting and adjustment Ⓑ

* **L2116** Ankle foot orthosis, fracture orthosis, tibial fracture orthosis, rigid, prefabricated, includes fitting and adjustment Ⓑ

* **L2126** Knee ankle foot orthosis, fracture orthosis, femoral fracture cast orthosis, thermoplastic type casting material, custom fabricated Ⓑ

* **L2128** Knee ankle foot orthosis, fracture orthosis, femoral fracture cast orthosis, custom fabricated Ⓑ

* **L2132** KAFO, femoral fracture cast orthosis, soft, prefabricated, includes fitting and adjustment Ⓑ

* **L2134** KAFO, femoral fracture cast orthosis, semi-rigid, prefabricated, includes fitting and adjustment Ⓑ

* **L2136** KAFO, fracture orthosis, femoral fracture cast orthosis, rigid, prefabricated, includes fitting and adjustment Ⓑ

Additions to Fracture Orthosis

* **L2180** Addition to lower extremity fracture orthosis, plastic shoe insert with ankle joints Ⓑ

* **L2182** Addition to lower extremity fracture orthosis, drop lock knee joint Ⓑ

* **L2184** Addition to lower extremity fracture orthosis, limited motion knee joint Ⓑ

* **L2186** Addition to lower extremity fracture orthosis, adjustable motion knee joint, Lerman type Ⓑ

* **L2188** Addition to lower extremity fracture orthosis, quadrilateral brim Ⓑ

* **L2190** Addition to lower extremity fracture orthosis, waist belt Ⓑ

* **L2192** Addition to lower extremity fracture orthosis, hip joint, pelvic band, thigh flange, and pelvic belt Ⓑ

Additions to Lower Extremity Orthosis

Shoe-Ankle-Shin-Knee

* **L2200** Addition to lower extremity, limited ankle motion, each joint Ⓑ
* **L2210** Addition to lower extremity, dorsiflexion assist (plantar flexion resist), each joint Ⓑ
* **L2220** Addition to lower extremity, dorsiflexion and plantar flexion assist/resist, each joint Ⓑ
* **L2230** Addition to lower extremity, split flat caliper stirrups and plate attachment Ⓑ
* **L2232** Addition to lower extremity orthosis, rocker bottom for total contact ankle foot orthosis, for custom fabricated orthosis only Ⓑ
* **L2240** Addition to lower extremity, round caliper and plate attachment Ⓑ
* **L2250** Addition to lower extremity, foot plate, molded to patient model, stirrup attachment Ⓑ
* **L2260** Addition to lower extremity, reinforced solid stirrup (Scott-Craig type) Ⓑ
* **L2265** Addition to lower extremity, long tongue stirrup Ⓑ
* **L2270** Addition to lower extremity, varus/valgus correction ('T') strap, padded/lined or malleolus pad Ⓑ
* **L2275** Addition to lower extremity, varus/valgus correction, plastic modification, padded/lined Ⓑ
* **L2280** Addition to lower extremity, molded inner boot Ⓑ
* **L2300** Addition to lower extremity, abduction bar (bilateral hip involvement), jointed, adjustable Ⓑ
* **L2310** Addition to lower extremity, abduction bar-straight Ⓑ
* **L2320** Addition to lower extremity, non-molded lacer, for custom fabricated orthosis only Ⓑ
* **L2330** Addition to lower extremity, lacer molded to patient model, for custom fabricated orthosis only Ⓑ

  Used whether closure is lacer or Velcro
* **L2335** Addition to lower extremity, anterior swing band Ⓑ
* **L2340** Addition to lower extremity, pre-tibial shell, molded to patient model Ⓑ
* **L2350** Addition to lower extremity, prosthetic type, (BK) socket, molded to patient model, (used for 'PTB' and 'AFO' orthoses) Ⓑ
* **L2360** Addition to lower extremity, extended steel shank Ⓑ
* **L2370** Addition to lower extremity, Patten bottom Ⓑ
* **L2375** Addition to lower extremity, torsion control, ankle joint and half solid stirrup Ⓑ
* **L2380** Addition to lower extremity, torsion control, straight knee joint, each joint Ⓑ
* **L2385** Addition to lower extremity, straight knee joint, heavy duty, each joint Ⓑ
* **L2387** Addition to lower extremity, polycentric knee joint, for custom fabricated knee ankle foot orthosis, each joint Ⓑ
* **L2390** Addition to lower extremity, offset knee joint, each joint Ⓑ
* **L2395** Addition to lower extremity, offset knee joint, heavy duty, each joint Ⓑ
* **L2397** Addition to lower extremity orthosis, suspension sleeve Ⓑ

Additions to Straight Knee or Offset Knee Joints

* **L2405** Addition to knee joint, drop lock, each Ⓑ
* **L2415** Addition to knee lock with integrated release mechanism (bail, cable, or equal), any material, each joint Ⓑ
* **L2425** Addition to knee joint, disc or dial lock for adjustable knee flexion, each joint Ⓑ
* **L2430** Addition to knee joint, ratchet lock for active and progressive knee extension, each joint Ⓑ
* **L2492** Addition to knee joint, lift loop for drop lock ring Ⓑ

Additions to Thigh/Weight Bearing Gluteal/Ischial Weight Bearing

* **L2500** Addition to lower extremity, thigh/weight bearing, gluteal/ischial weight bearing, ring Ⓑ
* **L2510** Addition to lower extremity, thigh/weight bearing, quadri-lateral brim, molded to patient model Ⓑ

▶ New ⊋ Revised ✔ Reinstated ~~deleted~~ Deleted ⊘ Not covered or valid by Medicare
⊛ Special coverage instructions * Carrier discretion Ⓑ Bill local carrier Ⓑ Bill DME MAC

✻ **L2520** Addition to lower extremity, thigh/weight bearing, quadri-lateral brim, custom fitted Ⓑ

✻ **L2525** Addition to lower extremity, thigh/weight bearing, ischial containment/narrow M-L brim molded to patient model Ⓑ

✻ **L2526** Addition to lower extremity, thigh/weight bearing, ischial containment/narrow M-L brim, custom fitted Ⓑ

✻ **L2530** Addition to lower extremity, thigh-weight bearing, lacer, non-molded Ⓑ

✻ **L2540** Addition to lower extremity, thigh/weight bearing, lacer, molded to patient model Ⓑ

✻ **L2550** Addition to lower extremity, thigh/weight bearing, high roll cuff Ⓑ

Additions to Pelvic and Thoracic Control

✻ **L2570** Addition to lower extremity, pelvic control, hip joint, Clevis type two position joint, each Ⓑ

✻ **L2580** Addition to lower extremity, pelvic control, pelvic sling Ⓑ

✻ **L2600** Addition to lower extremity, pelvic control, hip joint, Clevis type, or thrust bearing, free, each Ⓑ

✻ **L2610** Addition to lower extremity, pelvic control, hip joint, Clevis or thrust bearing, lock, each Ⓑ

✻ **L2620** Addition to lower extremity, pelvic control, hip joint, heavy duty, each Ⓑ

✻ **L2622** Addition to lower extremity, pelvic control, hip joint, adjustable flexion, each Ⓑ

✻ **L2624** Addition to lower extremity, pelvic control, hip joint, adjustable flexion, extension, abduction control, each Ⓑ

✻ **L2627** Addition to lower extremity, pelvic control, plastic, molded to patient model, reciprocating hip joint and cables Ⓑ

✻ **L2628** Addition to lower extremity, pelvic control, metal frame, reciprocating hip joint and cables Ⓑ

✻ **L2630** Addition to lower extremity, pelvic control, band and belt, unilateral Ⓑ

✻ **L2640** Addition to lower extremity, pelvic control, band and belt, bilateral Ⓑ

✻ **L2650** Addition to lower extremity, pelvic and thoracic control, gluteal pad, each Ⓑ

✻ **L2660** Addition to lower extremity, thoracic control, thoracic band Ⓑ

✻ **L2670** Addition to lower extremity, thoracic control, paraspinal uprights Ⓑ

✻ **L2680** Addition to lower extremity, thoracic control, lateral support uprights Ⓑ

General Additions

✻ **L2750** Addition to lower extremity orthosis, plating chrome or nickel, per bar Ⓑ

✻ **L2755** Addition to lower extremity orthosis, high strength, lightweight material, all hybrid lamination/prepreg composite, per segment, for custom fabricated orthosis only Ⓑ

✻ **L2760** Addition to lower extremity orthosis, extension, per extension, per bar (for lineal adjustment for growth) Ⓑ

✻ **L2768** Orthotic side bar disconnect device, per bar Ⓑ

✻ **L2780** Addition to lower extremity orthosis, non-corrosive finish, per bar Ⓑ

✻ **L2785** Addition to lower extremity orthosis, drop lock retainer, each Ⓑ

✻ **L2795** Addition to lower extremity orthosis, knee control, full kneecap Ⓑ

✻ **L2800** Addition to lower extremity orthosis, knee control, knee cap, medial or lateral pull, for use with custom fabricated orthosis only Ⓑ

✻ **L2810** Addition to lower extremity orthosis, knee control, condylar pad Ⓑ

✻ **L2820** Addition to lower extremity orthosis, soft interface for molded plastic, below knee section Ⓑ

Only report if soft interface provided, either leather or other material

✻ **L2830** Addition to lower extremity orthosis, soft interface for molded plastic, above knee section Ⓑ

✻ **L2840** Addition to lower extremity orthosis, tibial length sock, fracture or equal, each Ⓑ

✻ **L2850** Addition to lower extremity orthosis, femoral length sock, fracture or equal, each Ⓑ

⦸ **L2861** Addition to lower extremity joint, knee or ankle, concentric adjustable torsion style mechanism for custom fabricated orthotics only, each Ⓑ

✻ **L2999** Lower extremity orthoses, not otherwise specified Ⓑ

▶ New ⤼ Revised ✔ Reinstated ~~deleted~~ Deleted ⦸ Not covered or valid by Medicare
✪ Special coverage instructions ✻ Carrier discretion Ⓑ Bill local carrier Ⓑ Bill DME MAC

Foot (Orthopedic Shoes) (L3000-L3649)

Insert, Removable, Molded to Patient Model

⊙ **L3000** Foot, insert, removable, molded to patient model, 'UCB' type, Berkeley shell, each Ⓑ

If both feet casted and supplied with an orthosis, bill L3000-LT and L3000-RT

IOM: 100-02, 15, 290

⊙ **L3001** Foot, insert, removable, molded to patient model, Spenco, each Ⓑ

IOM: 100-02, 15, 290

⊙ **L3002** Foot, insert, removable, molded to patient model, Plastazote or equal, each Ⓑ

IOM: 100-02, 15, 290

⊙ **L3003** Foot, insert, removable, molded to patient model, silicone gel, each Ⓑ

IOM: 100-02, 15, 290

⊙ **L3010** Foot, insert, removable, molded to patient model, longitudinal arch support, each Ⓑ

IOM: 100-02, 15, 290

⊙ **L3020** Foot, insert, removable, molded to patient model, longitudinal/metatarsal support, each Ⓑ

IOM: 100-02, 15, 290

⊙ **L3030** Foot, insert, removable, formed to patient foot, each Ⓑ

IOM: 100-02, 15, 290

* **L3031** Foot, insert/plate, removable, addition to lower extremity orthosis, high strength, lightweight material, all hybrid lamination/prepreg composite, each Ⓑ

Arch Support, Removable, Premolded

⊙ **L3040** Foot, arch support, removable, premolded, longitudinal, each Ⓑ

IOM: 100-02, 15, 290

⊙ **L3050** Foot, arch support, removable, premolded, metatarsal, each Ⓑ

IOM: 100-02, 15, 290

⊙ **L3060** Foot, arch support, removable, premolded, longitudinal/metatarsal, each Ⓑ

IOM: 100-02, 15, 290

Arch Support, Non-removable, Attached to Shoe

⊙ **L3070** Foot, arch support, non-removable attached to shoe, longitudinal, each Ⓑ

IOM: 100-02, 15, 290

⊙ **L3080** Foot, arch support, non-removable attached to shoe, metatarsal, each Ⓑ

IOM: 100-02, 15, 290

⊙ **L3090** Foot, arch support, non-removable attached to shoe, longitudinal/metatarsal, each Ⓑ

IOM: 100-02, 15, 290

⊙ **L3100** Hallus-valgus night dynamic splint, prefabricated, off-the-shelf Ⓑ

IOM: 100-02, 15, 290

Abduction and Rotation Bars

⊙ **L3140** Foot, abduction rotation bar, including shoes Ⓑ

IOM: 100-02, 15, 290

⊙ **L3150** Foot, abduction rotation bar, without shoes Ⓑ

IOM: 100-02, 15, 290

* **L3160** Foot, adjustable shoe-styled positioning device Ⓑ

⊙ **L3170** Foot, plastic, silicone or equal, heel stabilizer, prefabricated, off-the-shelf, each Ⓑ

IOM: 100-02, 15, 290

Orthopedic Footwear

⊙ **L3201** Orthopedic shoe, oxford with supinator or pronator, infant Ⓑ

IOM: 100-02, 15, 290

⊙ **L3202** Orthopedic shoe, oxford with supinator or pronator, child Ⓑ

IOM: 100-02, 15, 290

⊙ **L3203** Orthopedic shoe, oxford with supinator or pronator, junior Ⓑ

IOM: 100-02, 15, 290

⊙ **L3204** Orthopedic shoe, hightop with supinator or pronator, infant Ⓑ

IOM: 100-02, 15, 290

⊙ **L3206** Orthopedic shoe, hightop with supinator or pronator, child Ⓑ

IOM: 100-02, 15, 290

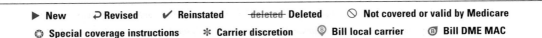

⊕ **L3207** Orthopedic shoe, hightop with supinator or pronator, junior Ⓑ
IOM: 100-02, 15, 290

⊕ **L3208** Surgical boot, infant, each Ⓑ
IOM: 100-02, 15, 100

⊕ **L3209** Surgical boot, each, child Ⓑ
IOM: 100-02, 15, 100

⊕ **L3211** Surgical boot, each, junior Ⓑ
IOM: 100-02, 15, 100

⊕ **L3212** Benesch boot, pair, infant Ⓑ
IOM: 100-02, 15, 100

⊕ **L3213** Benesch boot, pair, child Ⓑ
IOM: 100-02, 15, 100

⊕ **L3214** Benesch boot, pair, junior Ⓑ
IOM: 100-02, 15, 100

⊘ **L3215** Orthopedic footwear, ladies shoe, oxford, each Ⓑ
Medicare Statute 1862a8

⊘ **L3216** Orthopedic footwear, ladies shoe, depth inlay, each Ⓑ
Medicare Statute 1862a8

⊘ **L3217** Orthopedic footwear, ladies shoe, hightop, depth inlay, each Ⓑ
Medicare Statute 1862a8

⊘ **L3219** Orthopedic footwear, mens shoe, oxford, each Ⓑ
Medicare Statute 1862a8

⊘ **L3221** Orthopedic footwear, mens shoe, depth inlay, each Ⓑ
Medicare Statute 1862a8

⊘ **L3222** Orthopedic footwear, mens shoe, hightop, depth inlay, each Ⓑ
Medicare Statute 1862a8

⊕ **L3224** Orthopedic footwear, ladies shoe, oxford, used as an integral part of a brace (orthosis) Ⓑ
IOM: 100-02, 15, 290

⊕ **L3225** Orthopedic footwear, mens shoe, oxford, used as an integral part of a brace (orthosis) Ⓑ
IOM: 100-02, 15, 290

⊕ **L3230** Orthopedic footwear, custom shoe, depth inlay, each Ⓑ
IOM: 100-02, 15, 290

⊕ **L3250** Orthopedic footwear, custom molded shoe, removable inner mold, prosthetic shoe, each Ⓑ
IOM: 100-02, 15, 290

⊕ **L3251** Foot, shoe molded to patient model, silicone shoe, each Ⓑ
IOM: 100-02, 15, 290

⊕ **L3252** Foot, shoe molded to patient model, Plastazote (or similar), custom fabricated, each Ⓑ
IOM: 100-02, 15, 290

⊕ **L3253** Foot, molded shoe Plastazote (or similar), custom fitted, each Ⓑ
IOM: 100-02, 15, 290

⊕ **L3254** Non-standard size or width Ⓑ
IOM: 100-02, 15, 290

⊕ **L3255** Non-standard size or length Ⓑ
IOM: 100-02, 15, 290

⊕ **L3257** Orthopedic footwear, additional charge for split size Ⓑ
IOM: 100-02, 15, 290

⊕ **L3260** Surgical boot/shoe, each Ⓑ
IOM: 100-02, 15, 100

* **L3265** Plastazote sandal, each Ⓑ

Shoe Modifications

Lifts

⊕ **L3300** Lift, elevation, heel, tapered to metatarsals, per inch Ⓑ
IOM: 100-02, 15, 290

⊕ **L3310** Lift, elevation, heel and sole, Neoprene, per inch Ⓑ
IOM: 100-02, 15, 290

⊕ **L3320** Lift, elevation, heel and sole, cork, per inch Ⓑ
IOM: 100-02, 15, 290

⊕ **L3330** Lift, elevation, metal extension (skate) Ⓑ
IOM: 100-02, 15, 290

⊕ **L3332** Lift, elevation, inside shoe, tapered, up to one-half inch Ⓑ
IOM: 100-02, 15, 290

⊕ **L3334** Lift, elevation, heel, per inch Ⓑ
IOM: 100-02, 15, 290

Wedges

⊕ **L3340** Heel wedge, SACH Ⓑ
IOM: 100-02, 15, 290

⊕ **L3350** Heel wedge Ⓑ
IOM: 100-02, 15, 290

▶ New ⤾ Revised ✔ Reinstated ~~deleted~~ Deleted ⊘ Not covered or valid by Medicare
⊕ Special coverage instructions * Carrier discretion Ⓑ Bill local carrier Ⓑ Bill DME MAC

L3360 Sole wedge, outside sole
IOM: 100-02, 15, 290

L3370 Sole wedge, between sole
IOM: 100-02, 15, 290

L3380 Clubfoot wedge
IOM: 100-02, 15, 290

L3390 Outflare wedge
IOM: 100-02, 15, 290

L3400 Metatarsal bar wedge, rocker
IOM: 100-02, 15, 290

L3410 Metatarsal bar wedge, between sole
IOM: 100-02, 15, 290

L3420 Full sole and heel wedge, between sole
IOM: 100-02, 15, 290

Heels

L3430 Heel, counter, plastic reinforced
IOM: 100-02, 15, 290

L3440 Heel, counter, leather reinforced
IOM: 100-02, 15, 290

L3450 Heel, SACH cushion type
IOM: 100-02, 15, 290

L3455 Heel, new leather, standard
IOM: 100-02, 15, 290

L3460 Heel, new rubber, standard
IOM: 100-02, 15, 290

L3465 Heel, Thomas with wedge
IOM: 100-02, 15, 290

L3470 Heel, Thomas extended to ball
IOM: 100-02, 15, 290

L3480 Heel, pad and depression for spur
IOM: 100-02, 15, 290

L3485 Heel, pad, removable for spur
IOM: 100-02, 15, 290

Additions to Orthopedic Shoes

L3500 Orthopedic shoe addition, insole, leather
IOM: 100-02, 15, 290

L3510 Orthopedic shoe addition, insole, rubber
IOM: 100-02, 15, 290

L3520 Orthopedic shoe addition, insole, felt covered with leather
IOM: 100-02, 15, 290

L3530 Orthopedic shoe addition, sole, half
IOM: 100-02, 15, 290

L3540 Orthopedic shoe addition, sole, full
IOM: 100-02, 15, 290

L3550 Orthopedic shoe addition, toe tap standard
IOM: 100-02, 15, 290

L3560 Orthopedic shoe addition, toe tap, horseshoe
IOM: 100-02, 15, 290

L3570 Orthopedic shoe addition, special extension to instep (leather with eyelets)
IOM: 100-02, 15, 290

L3580 Orthopedic shoe addition, convert instep to Velcro closure
IOM: 100-02, 15, 290

L3590 Orthopedic shoe addition, convert firm shoe counter to soft counter
IOM: 100-02, 15, 290

L3595 Orthopedic shoe addition, March bar
IOM: 100-02, 15, 290

Transfer or Replacement

L3600 Transfer of an orthosis from one shoe to another, caliper plate, existing
IOM: 100-02, 15, 290

L3610 Transfer of an orthosis from one shoe to another, caliper plate, new
IOM: 100-02, 15, 290

L3620 Transfer of an orthosis from one shoe to another, solid stirrup, existing
IOM: 100-02, 15, 290

L3630 Transfer of an orthosis from one shoe to another, solid stirrup, new
IOM: 100-02, 15, 290

L3640 Transfer of an orthosis from one shoe to another, Dennis Browne splint (Riveton), both shoes
IOM: 100-02, 15, 290

L3649 Orthopedic shoe, modification, addition or transfer, not otherwise specified
IOM: 100-02, 15, 290

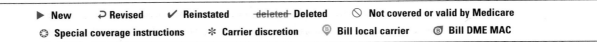

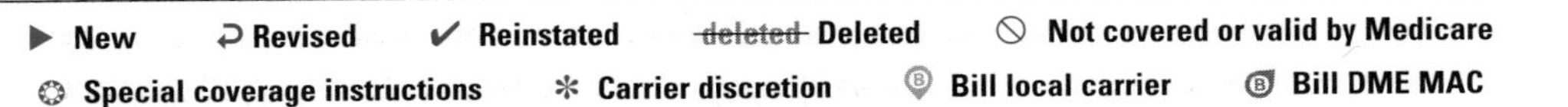

Orthotic Devices: Upper Limb

NOTE: The procedures in this section are considered as base or basic procedures and may be modified by listing procedures from the Additions section and adding them to the base procedure.

Shoulder

✻ **L3650** Shoulder orthosis, figure of eight design abduction restrainer, prefabricated, off-the-shelf Ⓑ

✻ **L3660** Shoulder orthosis, figure of eight design abduction restrainer, canvas and webbing, prefabricated, off-the-shelf Ⓑ

✻ **L3670** Shoulder orthosis, acromio/clavicular (canvas and webbing type), prefabricated, off-the-shelf Ⓑ

✻ **L3671** Shoulder orthosis, shoulder joint design, without joints, may include soft interface, straps, custom fabricated, includes fitting and adjustment Ⓑ

✻ **L3674** Shoulder orthosis, abduction positioning (airplane design), thoracic component and support bar, with or without nontorsion joint/turnbuckle, may include soft interface, straps, custom fabricated, includes fitting and adjustment Ⓑ

✻ **L3675** Shoulder orthosis, vest type abduction restrainer, canvas webbing type or equal, prefabricated, off-the-shelf Ⓑ

✪ **L3677** Shoulder orthosis, shoulder joint design, without joints, may include soft interface, straps, prefabricated item that has been trimmed, bent, molded, assembled, or otherwise customized to fit a specific patient by an individual with expertise Ⓑ

✻ **L3678** Shoulder orthosis, shoulder joint design, without joints, may include soft interface, straps, prefabricated, off-the-shelf Ⓑ

Elbow

✻ **L3702** Elbow orthosis, without joints, may include soft interface, straps, custom fabricated, includes fitting and adjustment Ⓑ

✻ **L3710** Elbow orthosis, elastic with metal joints, prefabricated, off-the-shelf Ⓑ

✻ **L3720** Elbow orthosis, double upright with forearm/arm cuffs, free motion, custom fabricated Ⓑ

✻ **L3730** Elbow orthosis, double upright with forearm/arm cuffs, extension/flexion assist, custom fabricated Ⓑ

✻ **L3740** Elbow orthosis, double upright with forearm/arm cuffs, adjustable position lock with active control, custom fabricated Ⓑ

✻ **L3760** Elbow orthosis, with adjustable position locking joint(s), prefabricated, includes fitting and adjustments, any type Ⓑ

✻ **L3762** Elbow orthosis, rigid, without joints, includes soft interface material, prefabricated, off-the-shelf Ⓑ

✻ **L3763** Elbow wrist hand orthosis, rigid, without joints, may include soft interface, straps, custom fabricated, includes fitting and adjustment Ⓑ

✻ **L3764** Elbow wrist hand orthosis, includes one or more nontorsion joints, elastic bands, turnbuckles, may include soft interface, straps, custom fabricated, includes fitting and adjustment Ⓑ

✻ **L3765** Elbow wrist hand finger orthosis, rigid, without joints, may include soft interface, straps, custom fabricated, includes fitting and adjustment Ⓑ

✻ **L3766** Elbow wrist hand finger orthosis, includes one or more nontorsion joints, elastic bands, turnbuckles, may include soft interface, straps, custom fabricated, includes fitting and adjustment Ⓑ

Wrist-Hand-Finger Orthosis (WHFO)

✻ **L3806** Wrist hand finger orthosis, includes one or more nontorsion joint(s), turnbuckles, elastic bands/springs, may include soft interface material, straps, custom fabricated, includes fitting and adjustment Ⓑ

✻ **L3807** Wrist hand finger orthosis, without joint(s), prefabricated item that has been trimmed, bent, molded, assembled, or otherwise customized to fit a specific patient by an individual with expertise Ⓑ

✻ **L3808** Wrist hand finger orthosis, rigid without joints, may include soft interface material; straps, custom fabricated, includes fitting and adjustment Ⓑ

✻ **L3809** Wrist hand finger orthosis, without joint(s), prefabricated, off-the-shelf, any type Ⓑ

▶ New ↩ Revised ✔ Reinstated ~~deleted~~ Deleted ⃠ Not covered or valid by Medicare
✪ Special coverage instructions ✻ Carrier discretion Ⓑ Bill local carrier Ⓑ Bill DME MAC

Additions and Extensions

⊘ **L3891** Addition to upper extremity joint, wrist or elbow, concentric adjustable torsion style mechanism for custom fabricated orthotics only, each Ⓑ

* **L3900** Wrist hand finger orthosis, dynamic flexor hinge, reciprocal wrist extension/flexion, finger flexion/extension, wrist or finger driven, custom fabricated Ⓑ

* **L3901** Wrist hand finger orthosis, dynamic flexor hinge, reciprocal wrist extension/flexion, finger flexion/extension, cable driven, custom fabricated Ⓑ

External Power

* **L3904** Wrist hand finger orthosis, external powered, electric, custom fabricated Ⓑ

* **L3905** Wrist hand orthosis, includes one or more nontorsion joints, elastic bands, turnbuckles, may include soft interface, straps, custom fabricated, includes fitting and adjustment Ⓑ

Other Wrist-Hand-Finger Orthoses: Custom Fitted

* **L3906** Wrist hand orthosis, without joints, may include soft interface, straps, custom fabricated, includes fitting and adjustment Ⓑ

* **L3908** Wrist hand orthosis, wrist extension control cock-up, non-molded, prefabricated, off-the-shelf Ⓑ

* **L3912** Hand finger orthosis (HFO), flexion glove with elastic finger control, prefabricated, off-the-shelf Ⓑ

* **L3913** Hand finger orthosis, without joints, may include soft interface, straps, custom fabricated, includes fitting and adjustment Ⓑ

* **L3915** Wrist hand orthosis, includes one or more nontorsion joint(s), elastic bands, turnbuckles, may include soft interface, straps, prefabricated item that has been trimmed, bent, molded, assembled, or otherwise customized to fit a specific patient by an individual with expertise Ⓑ

* **L3916** Wrist hand orthosis, includes one or more nontorsion joint(s), elastic bands, turnbuckles, may include soft interface, straps, prefabricated, off-the-shelf Ⓑ

* **L3917** Hand orthosis, metacarpal fracture orthosis, prefabricated item that has been trimmed, bent, molded, assembled, or otherwise customized to fit a specific patient by an individual with expertise Ⓑ

* **L3918** Hand orthosis, metacarpal fracture orthosis, prefabricated, off-the-shelf Ⓑ

* **L3919** Hand orthosis, without joints, may include soft interface, straps, custom fabricated, includes fitting and adjustment Ⓑ

* **L3921** Hand finger orthosis, includes one or more nontorsion joints, elastic bands, turnbuckles, may include soft interface, straps, custom fabricated, includes fitting and adjustment Ⓑ

* **L3923** Hand finger orthosis, without joints, may include soft interface, straps, prefabricated item that has been trimmed, bent, molded, assembled, or otherwise customized to fit a specific patient by an individual with expertise Ⓑ

* **L3924** Hand finger orthosis, without joints, may include soft interface, straps, prefabricated, off-the-shelf Ⓑ

* **L3925** Finger orthosis, proximal interphalangeal (PIP)/distal interphalangeal (DIP), non torsion joint/spring, extension/flexion, may include soft interface material, prefabricated, off-the-shelf Ⓑ

* **L3927** Finger orthosis, proximal interphalangeal (PIP)/distal interphalangeal (DIP), without joint/spring, extension/fl exion (e.g., static or ring type), may include soft interface material, prefabricated, off-the-shelf Ⓑ

* **L3929** Hand finger orthosis, includes one or more nontorsion joint(s), turnbuckles, elastic bands/springs, may include soft interface material, straps, prefabricated item that has been trimmed, bent, molded, assembled, or otherwise customized to fit a specific patient by an individual with expertise Ⓑ

* **L3930** Hand finger orthosis, includes one or more nontorsion joint(s), turnbuckles, elastic bands/springs, may include soft interface material, straps, prefabricated, off-the-shelf Ⓑ

* **L3931** Wrist hand finger orthosis, includes one or more nontorsion joint(s), turnbuckles, elastic bands/springs, may include soft interface material, straps, prefabricated, includes fitting and adjustment Ⓑ

▶ New ⤾ Revised ✔ Reinstated ~~deleted~~ Deleted ⊘ Not covered or valid by Medicare
⚙ Special coverage instructions * Carrier discretion Ⓑ Bill local carrier Ⓑ Bill DME MAC

* **L3933** Finger orthosis, without joints, may include soft interface, custom fabricated, includes fitting and adjustment Ⓑ

* **L3935** Finger orthosis, nontorsion joint, may include soft interface, custom fabricated, includes fitting and adjustment Ⓑ

* **L3956** Addition of joint to upper extremity orthosis, any material, per joint Ⓑ

Shoulder-Elbow-Wrist-Hand Orthosis (SEWHO)

Abduction Positioning: Custom Fitted

* **L3960** Shoulder elbow wrist hand orthosis, abduction positioning, airplane design, prefabricated, includes fitting and adjustment Ⓑ

* **L3961** Shoulder elbow wrist hand orthosis, shoulder cap design, without joints, may include soft interface, straps, custom fabricated, includes fitting and adjustment Ⓑ

* **L3962** Shoulder elbow wrist hand orthosis, abduction positioning, Erb's palsy design, prefabricated, includes fitting and adjustment Ⓑ

* **L3967** Shoulder elbow wrist hand orthosis, abduction positioning (airplane design), thoracic component and support bar, without joints, may include soft interface, straps, custom fabricated, includes fitting and adjustment Ⓑ

Additions to Mobile Arm Supports and SEWHO

* **L3971** Shoulder elbow wrist hand orthosis, shoulder cap design, includes one or more nontorsion joints, elastic bands, turnbuckles, may include soft interface, straps, custom fabricated, includes fitting and adjustment Ⓑ

* **L3973** Shoulder elbow wrist hand orthosis, abduction positioning (airplane design), thoracic component and support bar, includes one or more nontorsion joints, elastic bands, turnbuckles, may include soft interface, straps, custom fabricated, includes fitting and adjustment Ⓑ

* **L3975** Shoulder elbow wrist hand finger orthosis, shoulder cap design, without joints, may include soft interface, straps, custom fabricated, includes fitting and adjustment Ⓑ

* **L3976** Shoulder elbow wrist hand finger orthosis, abduction positioning (airplane design), thoracic component and support bar, without joints, may include soft interface, straps, custom fabricated, includes fitting and adjustment Ⓑ

* **L3977** Shoulder elbow wrist hand finger orthosis, shoulder cap design, includes one or more nontorsion joints, elastic bands, turnbuckles, may include soft interface, straps, custom fabricated, includes fitting and adjustment Ⓑ

* **L3978** Shoulder elbow wrist hand finger orthosis, abduction positioning (airplane design), thoracic component and support bar, includes one or more nontorsion joints, elastic bands, turnbuckles, may include soft interface, straps, custom fabricated, includes fitting and adjustment Ⓑ

Fracture Orthoses

* **L3980** Upper extremity fracture orthosis, humeral, prefabricated, includes fitting and adjustment Ⓑ

* **L3981** Upper extremity fracture orthosis, humeral, prefabricated, includes shoulder cap design, with or without joints, forearm section, may include soft interface, straps, includes fitting and adjustments Ⓑ

* **L3982** Upper extremity fracture orthosis, radius/ulnar, prefabricated, includes fitting and adjustment Ⓑ

* **L3984** Upper extremity fracture orthosis, wrist, prefabricated, includes fitting and adjustment Ⓑ

* **L3995** Addition to upper extremity orthosis, sock, fracture or equal, each Ⓑ

* **L3999** Upper limb orthosis, not otherwise specified Ⓑ

Specific Repair

* **L4000** Replace girdle for spinal orthosis (CTLSO or SO) Ⓑ

* **L4002** Replacement strap, any orthosis, includes all components, any length, any type Ⓑ

* **L4010** Replace trilateral socket brim Ⓑ

* **L4020** Replace quadrilateral socket brim, molded to patient model Ⓑ

* **L4030** Replace quadrilateral socket brim, custom fitted Ⓑ

* L4040 Replace molded thigh lacer, for custom fabricated orthosis only Ⓑ
* L4045 Replace non-molded thigh lacer, for custom fabricated orthosis only Ⓑ
* L4050 Replace molded calf lacer, for custom fabricated orthosis only Ⓑ
* L4055 Replace non-molded calf lacer, for custom fabricated orthosis only Ⓑ
* L4060 Replace high roll cuff Ⓑ
* L4070 Replace proximal and distal upright for KAFO Ⓑ
* L4080 Replace metal bands KAFO, proximal thigh Ⓑ
* L4090 Replace metal bands KAFO-AFO, calf or distal thigh Ⓑ
* L4100 Replace leather cuff KAFO, proximal thigh Ⓑ
* L4110 Replace leather cuff KAFO-AFO, calf or distal thigh Ⓑ
* L4130 Replace pretibial shell Ⓑ

Repairs

⚙ L4205 Repair of orthotic device, labor component, per 15 minutes Ⓑ

IOM: 100-02, 15, 110.2

⚙ L4210 Repair of orthotic device, repair or replace minor parts Ⓑ

IOM: 100-02, 15, 110.2; 100-02, 15, 120

Ancillary Orthotic Services

* L4350 Ankle control orthosis, stirrup style, rigid, includes any type interface (e.g., pneumatic, gel), prefabricated, off-the-shelf Ⓑ
* L4360 Walking boot, pneumatic and/or vacuum, with or without joints, with or without interface material, prefabricated item that has been trimmed, bent, molded, assembled, or otherwise customized to fit a specific patient by an individual with expertise Ⓑ

  Noncovered when walking boots used primarily to relieve pressure, especially on sole of foot, or are used for patients with foot ulcers
* L4361 Walking boot, pneumatic and/or vacuum, with or without joints, with or without interface material, prefabricated, off-the-shelf Ⓑ
* L4370 Pneumatic full leg splint, prefabricated, off-the-shelf Ⓑ
* L4386 Walking boot, non-pneumatic, with or without joints, with or without interface material, prefabricated item that has been trimmed, bent, molded, assembled, or otherwise customized to fit a specific patient by an individual with expertise Ⓑ
* L4387 Walking boot, non-pneumatic, with or without joints, with or without interface material, prefabricated, off-the-shelf Ⓑ
* L4392 Replacement, soft interface material, static AFO Ⓑ
* L4394 Replace soft interface material, foot drop splint Ⓑ
* L4396 Static or dynamic ankle foot orthosis, including soft interface material, adjustable for fit, for positioning, may be used for minimal ambulation, prefabricated item that has been trimmed, bent, molded, assembled, or otherwise customized to fit a specific patient by an individual with expertise Ⓑ
* L4397 Static or dynamic ankle foot orthosis, including soft interface material, adjustable for fit, for positioning, may be used for minimal ambulation, prefabricated, off-the-shelf Ⓑ
* L4398 Foot drop splint, recumbent positioning device, prefabricated, off-the-shelf Ⓑ
* L4631 Ankle foot orthosis, walking boot type, varus/valgus correction, rocker bottom, anterior tibial shell, soft interface, custom arch support, plastic or other material, includes straps and closures, custom fabricated Ⓑ

PROSTHETICS (L5000-L9999)

Lower Limb (L5000-L5999)

NOTE: The procedures in this section are considered as base or basic procedures and may be modified by listing items/procedures or special materials from the Additions section and adding them to the base procedure.

Partial Foot

⚙ L5000 Partial foot, shoe insert with longitudinal arch, toe filler Ⓑ

IOM: 100-02, 15, 290

⚙ L5010 Partial foot, molded socket, ankle height, with toe filler Ⓑ

IOM: 100-02, 15, 290

▶ New ⮌ Revised ✔ Reinstated ~~deleted~~ Deleted ⊘ Not covered or valid by Medicare
⚙ Special coverage instructions * Carrier discretion Ⓑ Bill local carrier Ⓑ Bill DME MAC

✪ **L5020** Partial foot, molded socket, tibial tubercle height, with toe filler Ⓑ

IOM: 100-02, 15, 290

Ankle

* **L5050** Ankle, Symes, molded socket, SACH foot Ⓑ

* **L5060** Ankle, Symes, metal frame, molded leather socket, articulated ankle/foot Ⓑ

Below Knee

* **L5100** Below knee, molded socket, shin, SACH foot Ⓑ

* **L5105** Below knee, plastic socket, joints and thigh lacer, SACH foot Ⓑ

Knee Disarticulation

* **L5150** Knee disarticulation (or through knee), molded socket, external knee joints, shin, SACH foot Ⓑ

* **L5160** Knee disarticulation (or through knee), molded socket, bent knee configuration, external knee joints, shin, SACH foot Ⓑ

Above Knee

* **L5200** Above knee, molded socket, single axis constant friction knee, shin, SACH foot Ⓑ

* **L5210** Above knee, short prosthesis, no knee joint ('stubbies'), with foot blocks, no ankle joints, each Ⓑ

* **L5220** Above knee, short prosthesis, no knee joint ('stubbies'), with articulated ankle/foot, dynamically aligned, each Ⓑ

* **L5230** Above knee, for proximal femoral focal deficiency, constant friction knee, shin, SACH foot Ⓑ

Hip Disarticulation

* **L5250** Hip disarticulation, Canadian type; molded socket, hip joint, single axis constant friction knee, shin, SACH foot Ⓑ

* **L5270** Hip disarticulation, tilt table type; molded socket, locking hip joint, single axis constant friction knee, shin, SACH foot Ⓑ

Hemipelvectomy

* **L5280** Hemipelvectomy, Canadian type; molded socket, hip joint, single axis constant friction knee, shin, SACH foot Ⓑ

Endoskeleton: Below Knee

* **L5301** Below knee, molded socket, shin, SACH foot, endoskeletal system Ⓑ

* **L5312** Knee disarticulation (or through knee), molded socket, single axis knee, pylon, sach foot, endoskeletal system Ⓑ

Endoskeletal: Above Knee

* **L5321** Above knee, molded socket, open end, SACH foot, endoskeletal system, single axis knee Ⓑ

Endoskeletal: Hip Disarticulation

* **L5331** Hip disarticulation, Canadian type, molded socket, endoskeletal system, hip joint, single axis knee, SACH foot Ⓑ

Endoskeletal: Hemipelvectomy

* **L5341** Hemipelvectomy, Canadian type, molded socket, endoskeletal system, hip joint, single axis knee, SACH foot Ⓑ

Immediate Postsurgical or Early Fitting Procedures

* **L5400** Immediate post surgical or early fitting, application of initial rigid dressing, including fitting, alignment, suspension, and one cast change, below knee Ⓑ

* **L5410** Immediate post surgical or early fitting, application of initial rigid dressing, including fitting, alignment and suspension, below knee, each additional cast change and realignment Ⓑ

* **L5420** Immediate post surgical or early fitting, application of initial rigid dressing, including fitting, alignment and suspension and one cast change 'AK' or knee disarticulation Ⓑ

* **L5430** Immediate postsurgical or early fitting, application of initial rigid dressing, including fitting, alignment, and suspension, 'AK' or knee disarticulation, each additional cast change and realignment Ⓑ

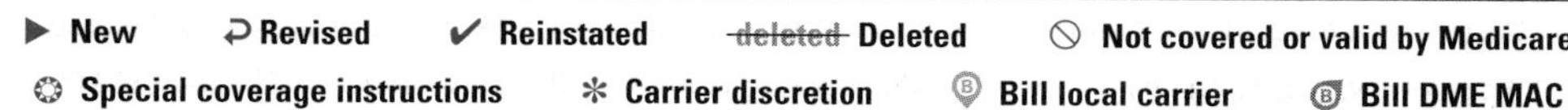

* **L5450** Immediate post surgical or early fitting, application of non-weight bearing rigid dressing, below knee Ⓑ

* **L5460** Immediate post surgical or early fitting, application of non-weight bearing rigid dressing, above knee Ⓑ

Initial Prosthesis

* **L5500** Initial, below knee 'PTB' type socket, non-alignable system, pylon, no cover, SACH foot, plaster socket, direct formed Ⓑ

* **L5505** Initial, above knee-knee disarticulation, ischial level socket, non-alignable system, pylon, no cover, SACH foot, plaster socket, direct formed Ⓑ

Preparatory Prosthesis

* **L5510** Preparatory, below knee 'PTB' type socket, non-alignable system, pylon, no cover, SACH foot, plaster socket, molded to model Ⓑ

* **L5520** Preparatory, below knee 'PTB' type socket, non-alignable system, pylon, no cover, SACH foot, thermoplastic or equal, direct formed Ⓑ

* **L5530** Preparatory, below knee 'PTB' type socket, non-alignable system, pylon, no cover, SACH foot, thermoplastic or equal, molded to model Ⓑ

* **L5535** Preparatory, below knee 'PTB' type socket, non-alignable system, no cover, SACH foot, prefabricated, adjustable open end socket Ⓑ

* **L5540** Preparatory, below knee 'PTB' type socket, non-alignable system, pylon, no cover, SACH foot, laminated socket, molded to model Ⓑ

* **L5560** Preparatory, above knee - knee disarticulation, ischial level socket, non-alignable system, pylon, no cover, SACH foot, plaster socket, molded to model Ⓑ

* **L5570** Preparatory, above knee - knee disarticulation, ischial level socket, non-alignable system, pylon, no cover, SACH foot, thermoplastic or equal, direct formed Ⓑ

* **L5580** Preparatory, above knee - knee disarticulation, ischial level socket, non-alignable system, pylon, no cover, SACH foot, thermoplastic or equal, molded to model Ⓑ

* **L5585** Preparatory, above knee - knee disarticulation, ischial level socket, non-alignable system, pylon, no cover, SACH foot, prefabricated adjustable open end socket Ⓑ

* **L5590** Preparatory, above knee - knee disarticulation, ischial level socket, non-alignable system, pylon, no cover, SACH foot, laminated socket, molded to model Ⓑ

* **L5595** Preparatory, hip disarticulation-hemipelvectomy, pylon, no cover, SACH foot, thermoplastic or equal, molded to patient model Ⓑ

* **L5600** Preparatory, hip disarticulation-hemipelvectomy, pylon, no cover, SACH foot, laminated socket, molded to patient model Ⓑ

Additions to Lower Extremity

* **L5610** Addition to lower extremity, endoskeletal system, above knee, hydracadence system Ⓑ

* **L5611** Addition to lower extremity, endoskeletal system, above knee-knee disarticulation, 4 bar linkage, with friction swing phase control Ⓑ

* **L5613** Addition to lower extremity, endoskeletal system, above knee-knee disarticulation, 4 bar linkage, with hydraulic swing phase control Ⓑ

* **L5614** Addition to lower extremity, exoskeletal system, above knee-knee disarticulation, 4 bar linkage, with pneumatic swing phase control Ⓑ

* **L5616** Addition to lower extremity, endoskeletal system, above knee, universal multiplex system, friction swing phase control Ⓑ

* **L5617** Addition to lower extremity, quick change self-aligning unit, above knee or below knee, each Ⓑ

Additions to Test Sockets

* **L5618** Addition to lower extremity, test socket, Symes Ⓑ

* **L5620** Addition to lower extremity, test socket, below knee Ⓑ

* **L5622** Addition to lower extremity, test socket, knee disarticulation Ⓑ

* **L5624** Addition to lower extremity, test socket, above knee Ⓑ

* **L5626** Addition to lower extremity, test socket, hip disarticulation Ⓑ

✻ **L5628** Addition to lower extremity, test socket, hemipelvectomy Ⓑ

✻ **L5629** Addition to lower extremity, below knee, acrylic socket Ⓑ

Additions to Socket Variations

✻ **L5630** Addition to lower extremity, Symes type, expandable wall socket Ⓑ

✻ **L5631** Addition to lower extremity, above knee or knee disarticulation, acrylic socket Ⓑ

✻ **L5632** Addition to lower extremity, Symes type, 'PTB' brim design socket Ⓑ

✻ **L5634** Addition to lower extremity, Symes type, posterior opening (Canadian) socket Ⓑ

✻ **L5636** Addition to lower extremity, Symes type, medial opening socket Ⓑ

✻ **L5637** Addition to lower extremity, below knee, total contact Ⓑ

✻ **L5638** Addition to lower extremity, below knee, leather socket Ⓑ

✻ **L5639** Addition to lower extremity, below knee, wood socket Ⓑ

✻ **L5640** Addition to lower extremity, knee disarticulation, leather socket Ⓑ

✻ **L5642** Addition to lower extremity, above knee, leather socket Ⓑ

✻ **L5643** Addition to lower extremity, hip disarticulation, flexible inner socket, external frame Ⓑ

✻ **L5644** Addition to lower extremity, above knee, wood socket Ⓑ

✻ **L5645** Addition to lower extremity, below knee, flexible inner socket, external frame Ⓑ

✻ **L5646** Addition to lower extremity, below knee, air, fluid, gel or equal, cushion socket Ⓑ

✻ **L5647** Addition to lower extremity, below knee, suction socket Ⓑ

✻ **L5648** Addition to lower extremity, above knee, air, fluid, gel or equal, cushion socket Ⓑ

✻ **L5649** Addition to lower extremity, ischial containment/narrow M-L socket Ⓑ

✻ **L5650** Additions to lower extremity, total contact, above knee or knee disarticulation socket Ⓑ

✻ **L5651** Addition to lower extremity, above knee, flexible inner socket, external frame Ⓑ

✻ **L5652** Addition to lower extremity, suction suspension, above knee or knee disarticulation socket Ⓑ

✻ **L5653** Addition to lower extremity, knee disarticulation, expandable wall socket Ⓑ

Additions to Socket Insert and Suspension

✻ **L5654** Addition to lower extremity, socket insert, Symes, (Kemblo, Pelite, Aliplast, Plastazote or equal) Ⓑ

✻ **L5655** Addition to lower extremity, socket insert, below knee (Kemblo, Pelite, Aliplast, Plastazote or equal) Ⓑ

✻ **L5656** Addition to lower extremity, socket insert, knee disarticulation (Kemblo, Pelite, Aliplast, Plastazote or equal) Ⓑ

✻ **L5658** Addition to lower extremity, socket insert, above knee (Kemblo, Pelite, Aliplast, Plastazote or equal) Ⓑ

✻ **L5661** Addition to lower extremity, socket insert, multi-durometer Symes Ⓑ

✻ **L5665** Addition to lower extremity, socket insert, multi-durometer, below knee Ⓑ

✻ **L5666** Addition to lower extremity, below knee, cuff suspension Ⓑ

✻ **L5668** Addition to lower extremity, below knee, molded distal cushion Ⓑ

✻ **L5670** Addition to lower extremity, below knee, molded supracondylar suspension ('PTS' or similar) Ⓑ

✻ **L5671** Addition to lower extremity, below knee/above knee suspension locking mechanism (shuttle, lanyard or equal), excludes socket insert Ⓑ

✻ **L5672** Addition to lower extremity, below knee, removable medial brim suspension Ⓑ

✻ **L5673** Addition to lower extremity, below knee/above knee, custom fabricated from existing mold or prefabricated, socket insert, silicone gel, elastomeric or equal, for use with locking mechanism Ⓑ

✻ **L5676** Additions to lower extremity, below knee, knee joints, single axis, pair Ⓑ

✻ **L5677** Additions to lower extremity, below knee, knee joints, polycentric, pair Ⓑ

✻ **L5678** Additions to lower extremity, below knee, joint covers, pair Ⓑ

* **L5679** Addition to lower extremity, below knee/above knee, custom fabricated from existing mold or prefabricated, socket insert, silicone gel, elastomeric or equal, not for use with locking mechanism Ⓑ
* **L5680** Addition to lower extremity, below knee, thigh lacer, non-molded Ⓑ
* **L5681** Addition to lower extremity, below knee/above knee, custom fabricated socket insert for congenital or atypical traumatic amputee, silicone gel, elastomeric or equal, for use with or without locking mechanism, initial only (for other than initial, use code L5673 or L5679) Ⓑ
* **L5682** Addition to lower extremity, below knee, thigh lacer, gluteal/ischial, molded Ⓑ
* **L5683** Addition to lower extremity, below knee/above knee, custom fabricated socket insert for other than congenital or atypical traumatic amputee, silicone gel, elastomeric, or equal, for use with or without locking mechanism, initial only (for other than initial, use code L5673 or L5679) Ⓑ
* **L5684** Addition to lower extremity, below knee, fork strap Ⓑ
* **L5685** Addition to lower extremity prosthesis, below knee, suspension/sealing sleeve, with or without valve, any material, each Ⓑ
* **L5686** Addition to lower extremity, below knee, back check (extension control) Ⓑ
* **L5688** Addition to lower extremity, below knee, waist belt, webbing Ⓑ
* **L5690** Addition to lower extremity, below knee, waist belt, padded and lined Ⓑ
* **L5692** Addition to lower extremity, above knee, pelvic control belt, light Ⓑ
* **L5694** Addition to lower extremity, above knee, pelvic control belt, padded and lined Ⓑ
* **L5695** Addition to lower extremity, above knee, pelvic control, sleeve suspension, neoprene or equal, each Ⓑ
* **L5696** Addition to lower extremity, above knee or knee disarticulation, pelvic joint Ⓑ
* **L5697** Addition to lower extremity, above knee or knee disarticulation, pelvic band Ⓑ
* **L5698** Addition to lower extremity, above knee or knee disarticulation, Silesian bandage Ⓑ
* **L5699** All lower extremity prostheses, shoulder harness Ⓑ

Additions/Replacements to Feet-Ankle Units

* **L5700** Replacement, socket, below knee, molded to patient model Ⓑ
* **L5701** Replacement, socket, above knee/knee disarticulation, including attachment plate, molded to patient model Ⓑ
* **L5702** Replacement, socket, hip disarticulation, including hip joint, molded to patient model Ⓑ
* **L5703** Ankle, Symes, molded to patient model, socket without solid ankle cushion heel (SACH) foot, replacement only Ⓑ
* **L5704** Custom shaped protective cover, below knee Ⓑ
* **L5705** Custom shaped protective cover, above knee Ⓑ
* **L5706** Custom shaped protective cover, knee disarticulation Ⓑ
* **L5707** Custom shaped protective cover, hip disarticulation Ⓑ

Additions to Exoskeletal–Knee-Shin System

* **L5710** Addition, exoskeletal knee-shin system, single axis, manual lock Ⓑ
* **L5711** Additions exoskeletal knee-shin system, single axis, manual lock, ultra-light material Ⓑ
* **L5712** Addition, exoskeletal knee-shin system, single axis, friction swing and stance phase control (safety knee) Ⓑ
* **L5714** Addition, exoskeletal knee-shin system, single axis, variable friction swing phase control Ⓑ
* **L5716** Addition, exoskeletal knee-shin system, polycentric, mechanical stance phase lock Ⓑ
* **L5718** Addition, exoskeletal knee-shin system, polycentric, friction swing and stance phase control Ⓑ
* **L5722** Addition, exoskeletal knee-shin system, single axis, pneumatic swing, friction stance phase control Ⓑ
* **L5724** Addition, exoskeletal knee-shin system, single axis, fluid swing phase control Ⓑ
* **L5726** Addition, exoskeletal knee-shin system, single axis, external joints, fluid swing phase control Ⓑ
* **L5728** Addition, exoskeletal knee-shin system, single axis, fluid swing and stance phase control Ⓑ
* **L5780** Addition, exoskeletal knee-shin system, single axis, pneumatic/hydra pneumatic swing phase control Ⓑ

✻ **L5781** Addition to lower limb prosthesis, vacuum pump, residual limb volume management and moisture evacuation system Ⓑ

✻ **L5782** Addition to lower limb prosthesis, vacuum pump, residual limb volume management and moisture evacuation system, heavy duty Ⓑ

Component Modification

✻ **L5785** Addition, exoskeletal system, below knee, ultra-light material (titanium, carbon fiber, or equal) Ⓑ

✻ **L5790** Addition, exoskeletal system, above knee, ultra-light material (titanium, carbon fiber, or equal) Ⓑ

✻ **L5795** Addition, exoskeletal system, hip disarticulation, ultra-light material (titanium, carbon fiber, or equal) Ⓑ

Endoskeletal

✻ **L5810** Addition, endoskeletal knee-shin system, single axis, manual lock Ⓑ

✻ **L5811** Addition, endoskeletal knee-shin system, single axis, manual lock, ultralight material Ⓑ

✻ **L5812** Addition, endoskeletal knee-shin system, single axis, friction swing and stance phase control (safety knee) Ⓑ

✻ **L5814** Addition, endoskeletal knee-shin system, polycentric, hydraulic swing phase control, mechanical stance phase lock Ⓑ

✻ **L5816** Addition, endoskeletal knee-shin system, polycentric, mechanical stance phase lock Ⓑ

✻ **L5818** Addition, endoskeletal knee-shin system, polycentric, friction swing, and stance phase control Ⓑ

✻ **L5822** Addition, endoskeletal knee-shin system, single axis, pneumatic swing, friction stance phase control Ⓑ

✻ **L5824** Addition, endoskeletal knee-shin system, single axis, fluid swing phase control Ⓑ

✻ **L5826** Addition, endoskeletal knee-shin system, single axis, hydraulic swing phase control, with miniature high activity frame Ⓑ

✻ **L5828** Addition, endoskeletal knee-shin system, single axis, fluid swing and stance phase control Ⓑ

✻ **L5830** Addition, endoskeletal knee-shin system, single axis, pneumatic/swing phase control Ⓑ

✻ **L5840** Addition, endoskeletal knee/shin system, 4-bar linkage or multiaxial, pneumatic swing phase control Ⓑ

✻ **L5845** Addition, endoskeletal, knee-shin system, stance flexion feature, adjustable Ⓑ

✻ **L5848** Addition to endoskeletal, knee-shin system, fluid stance extension, dampening feature, with or without adjustability Ⓑ

✻ **L5850** Addition, endoskeletal system, above knee or hip disarticulation, knee extension assist Ⓑ

✻ **L5855** Addition, endoskeletal system, hip disarticulation, mechanical hip extension assist Ⓑ

✻ **L5856** Addition to lower extremity prosthesis, endoskeletal knee-shin system, microprocessor control feature, swing and stance phase; includes electronic sensor(s), any type Ⓑ

✻ **L5857** Addition to lower extremity prosthesis, endoskeletal knee-shin system, microprocessor control feature, swing phase only; includes electronic sensor(s), any type Ⓑ

✻ **L5858** Addition to lower extremity prosthesis, endoskeletal knee shin system, microprocessor control feature, stance phase only, includes electronic sensor(s), any type Ⓑ

✻ **L5859** Addition to lower extremity prosthesis, endoskeletal knee-shin system, powered and programmable flexion/extension assist control, includes any type motor(s) Ⓑ

✻ **L5910** Addition, endoskeletal system, below knee, alignable system Ⓑ

✻ **L5920** Addition, endoskeletal system, above knee or hip disarticulation, alignable system Ⓑ

✻ **L5925** Addition, endoskeletal system, above knee, knee disarticulation or hip disarticulation, manual lock Ⓑ

✻ **L5930** Addition, endoskeletal system, high activity knee control frame Ⓑ

✻ **L5940** Addition, endoskeletal system, below knee, ultra-light material (titanium, carbon fiber or equal) Ⓑ

✻ **L5950** Addition, endoskeletal system, above knee, ultra-light material (titanium, carbon fiber or equal) Ⓑ

▶ New ⊋ Revised ✔ Reinstated ~~deleted~~ Deleted ⊘ Not covered or valid by Medicare
⚙ Special coverage instructions ✻ Carrier discretion Ⓑ Bill local carrier Ⓑ Bill DME MAC

✻ **L5960** Addition, endoskeletal system, hip disarticulation, ultra-light material (titanium, carbon fiber, or equal)

✻ **L5961** Addition, endoskeletal system, polycentric hip joint, pneumatic or hydraulic control, rotation control, with or without flexion, and/or extension control

✻ **L5962** Addition, endoskeletal system, below knee, flexible protective outer surface covering system

✻ **L5964** Addition, endoskeletal system, above knee, flexible protective outer surface covering system

✻ **L5966** Addition, endoskeletal system, hip disarticulation, flexible protective outer surface covering system

✻ **L5968** Addition to lower limb prosthesis, multiaxial ankle with swing phase active dorsiflexion feature

✻ **L5969** Addition, endoskeletal ankle-foot or ankle system, power assist, includes any type motor(s)

✻ **L5970** All lower extremity prostheses, foot, external keel, SACH foot

✻ **L5971** All lower extremity prosthesis, solid ankle cushion keel (SACH) foot, replacement only

✻ **L5972** All lower extremity prostheses (foot, flexible keel)

✻ **L5973** Endoskeletal ankle foot system, microprocessor controlled feature, dorsiflexion and/or plantar flexion control, includes power source

✻ **L5974** All lower extremity prostheses, foot, single axis ankle/foot

✻ **L5975** All lower extremity prostheses, combination single axis ankle and flexible keel foot

✻ **L5976** All lower extremity prostheses, energy storing foot (Seattle Carbon Copy II or equal)

✻ **L5978** All lower extremity prostheses, foot, multiaxial ankle/foot

✻ **L5979** All lower extremity prostheses, multiaxial ankle, dynamic response foot, one piece system

✻ **L5980** All lower extremity prostheses, flex foot system

✻ **L5981** All lower extremity prostheses, flexwalk system or equal

✻ **L5982** All exoskeletal lower extremity prostheses, axial rotation unit

✻ **L5984** All endoskeletal lower extremity prostheses, axial rotation unit, with or without adjustability

✻ **L5985** All endoskeletal lower extremity prostheses, dynamic prosthetic pylon

✻ **L5986** All lower extremity prostheses, multiaxial rotation unit ('MCP' or equal)

✻ **L5987** All lower extremity prostheses, shank foot system with vertical loading pylon

✻ **L5988** Addition to lower limb prosthesis, vertical shock reducing pylon feature

✻ **L5990** Addition to lower extremity prosthesis, user adjustable heel height

✻ **L5999** Lower extremity prosthesis, not otherwise specified

Upper Limb (L6000-L6698)

Note: The procedures in L6000-L6599 are considered as base or basic procedures and may be modified by listing procedures from the additions sections. The base procedures include only standard friction wrist and control cable system unless otherwise specified.

Partial Hand

✻ **L6000** Partial hand, thumb remaining

✻ **L6010** Partial hand, little and/or ring finger remaining

✻ **L6020** Partial hand, no finger remaining

✻ **L6026** Transcarpal/metacarpal or partial hand disarticulation prosthesis, external power, self-suspended, inner socket with removable forearm section, electrodes and cables, two batteries, charger, myoelectric control of terminal device, excludes terminal device(s)

Wrist Disarticulation

✻ **L6050** Wrist disarticulation, molded socket, flexible elbow hinges, triceps pad

✻ **L6055** Wrist disarticulation, molded socket with expandable interface, flexible elbow hinges, triceps pad

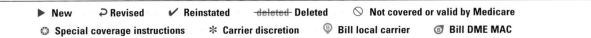

Below Elbow

* ✻ **L6100** Below elbow, molded socket, flexible elbow hinge, triceps pad Ⓑ
* ✻ **L6110** Below elbow, molded socket, (Muenster or Northwestern suspension types) Ⓑ
* ✻ **L6120** Below elbow, molded double wall split socket, step-up hinges, half cuff Ⓑ
* ✻ **L6130** Below elbow, molded double wall split socket, stump activated locking hinge, half cuff Ⓑ

Elbow Disarticulation

* ✻ **L6200** Elbow disarticulation, molded socket, outside locking hinge, forearm Ⓑ
* ✻ **L6205** Elbow disarticulation, molded socket with expandable interface, outside locking hinges, forearm Ⓑ

Above Elbow

* ✻ **L6250** Above elbow, molded double wall socket, internal locking elbow, forearm Ⓑ

Shoulder Disarticulation

* ✻ **L6300** Shoulder disarticulation, molded socket, shoulder bulkhead, humeral section, internal locking elbow, forearm Ⓑ
* ✻ **L6310** Shoulder disarticulation, passive restoration (complete prosthesis) Ⓑ
* ✻ **L6320** Shoulder disarticulation, passive restoration (shoulder cap only) Ⓑ

Interscapular Thoracic

* ✻ **L6350** Interscapular thoracic, molded socket, shoulder bulkhead, humeral section, internal locking elbow, forearm Ⓑ
* ✻ **L6360** Interscapular thoracic, passive restoration (complete prosthesis) Ⓑ
* ✻ **L6370** Interscapular thoracic, passive restoration (shoulder cap only) Ⓑ

Immediate and Early Postsurgical Procedures

* ✻ **L6380** Immediate post surgical or early fitting, application of initial rigid dressing, including fitting alignment and suspension of components, and one cast change, wrist disarticulation or below elbow Ⓑ
* ✻ **L6382** Immediate post surgical or early fitting, application of initial rigid dressing including fitting alignment and suspension of components, and one cast change, elbow disarticulation or above elbow Ⓑ
* ✻ **L6384** Immediate post surgical or early fitting, application of initial rigid dressing including fitting alignment and suspension of components, and one cast change, shoulder disarticulation or interscapular thoracic Ⓑ
* ✻ **L6386** Immediate post surgical or early fitting, each additional cast change and realignment Ⓑ
* ✻ **L6388** Immediate post surgical or early fitting, application of rigid dressing only Ⓑ

Endoskeletal: Below Elbow

* ✻ **L6400** Below elbow, molded socket, endoskeletal system, including soft prosthetic tissue shaping Ⓑ

Endoskeletal: Elbow Disarticulation

* ✻ **L6450** Elbow disarticulation, molded socket, endoskeletal system, including soft prosthetic tissue shaping Ⓑ

Endoskeletal: Above Elbow

* ✻ **L6500** Above elbow, molded socket, endoskeletal system, including soft prosthetic tissue shaping Ⓑ

Endoskeletal: Shoulder Disarticulation

* ✻ **L6550** Shoulder disarticulation, molded socket, endoskeletal system, including soft prosthetic tissue shaping Ⓑ

Endoskeletal: Interscapular Thoracic

* ✻ **L6570** Interscapular thoracic, molded socket, endoskeletal system, including soft prosthetic tissue shaping Ⓑ
* ✻ **L6580** Preparatory, wrist disarticulation or below elbow, single wall plastic socket, friction wrist, flexible elbow hinges, figure of eight harness, humeral cuff, Bowden cable control, USMC or equal pylon, no cover, molded to patient model Ⓑ

* **L6582** Preparatory, wrist disarticulation or below elbow, single wall socket, friction wrist, flexible elbow hinges, figure of eight harness, humeral cuff, Bowden cable control, USMC or equal pylon, no cover, direct formed
* **L6584** Preparatory, elbow disarticulation or above elbow, single wall plastic socket, friction wrist, locking elbow, figure of eight harness, fair lead cable control, USMC or equal pylon, no cover, molded to patient model
* **L6586** Preparatory, elbow disarticulation or above elbow, single wall socket, friction wrist, locking elbow, figure of eight harness, fair lead cable control, USMC or equal pylon, no cover, direct formed
* **L6588** Preparatory, shoulder disarticulation or interscapular thoracic, single wall plastic socket, shoulder joint, locking elbow, friction wrist, chest strap, fair lead cable control, USMC or equal pylon, no cover, molded to patient model
* **L6590** Preparatory, shoulder disarticulation or interscapular thoracic, single wall socket, shoulder joint, locking elbow, friction wrist, chest strap, fair lead cable control, USMC or equal pylon, no cover, direct formed

Additions to Upper Limb

Note: The following procedures/modifications/components may be added to other base procedures. The items in this section should reflect the additional complexity of each modification procedure, in addition to base procedure, at the time of the original order.

* **L6600** Upper extremity additions, polycentric hinge, pair
* **L6605** Upper extremity additions, single pivot hinge, pair
* **L6610** Upper extremity additions, flexible metal hinge, pair
* **L6611** Addition to upper extremity prosthesis, external powered, additional switch, any type
* **L6615** Upper extremity addition, disconnect locking wrist unit
* **L6616** Upper extremity addition, additional disconnect insert for locking wrist unit, each
* **L6620** Upper extremity addition, flexion/extension wrist unit, with or without friction
* **L6621** Upper extremity prosthesis addition, flexion/extension wrist with or without friction, for use with external powered terminal device
* **L6623** Upper extremity addition, spring assisted rotational wrist unit with latch release
* **L6624** Upper extremity addition, flexion/extension and rotation wrist unit
* **L6625** Upper extremity addition, rotation wrist unit with cable lock
* **L6628** Upper extremity addition, quick disconnect hook adapter, Otto Bock or equal
* **L6629** Upper extremity addition, quick disconnect lamination collar with coupling piece, Otto Bock or equal
* **L6630** Upper extremity addition, stainless steel, any wrist
* **L6632** Upper extremity addition, latex suspension sleeve, each
* **L6635** Upper extremity addition, lift assist for elbow
* **L6637** Upper extremity addition, nudge control elbow lock
* **L6638** Upper extremity addition to prosthesis, electric locking feature, only for use with manually powered elbow
* **L6640** Upper extremity additions, shoulder abduction joint, pair
* **L6641** Upper extremity addition, excursion amplifier, pulley type
* **L6642** Upper extremity addition, excursion amplifier, lever type
* **L6645** Upper extremity addition, shoulder flexion-abduction joint, each
* **L6646** Upper extremity addition, shoulder joint, multipositional locking, flexion, adjustable abduction friction control, for use with body powered or external powered system
* **L6647** Upper extremity addition, shoulder lock mechanism, body powered actuator
* **L6648** Upper extremity addition, shoulder lock mechanism, external powered actuator
* **L6650** Upper extremity addition, shoulder universal joint, each
* **L6655** Upper extremity addition, standard control cable, extra

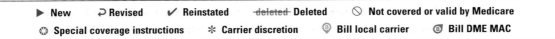

▶ New ↺ Revised ✔ Reinstated ~~deleted~~ Deleted ⊘ Not covered or valid by Medicare
Special coverage instructions * Carrier discretion Bill local carrier Bill DME MAC

✻ **L6660** Upper extremity addition, heavy duty control cable Ⓑ

✻ **L6665** Upper extremity addition, Teflon, or equal, cable lining Ⓑ

✻ **L6670** Upper extremity addition, hook to hand, cable adapter Ⓑ

✻ **L6672** Upper extremity addition, harness, chest or shoulder, saddle type Ⓑ

✻ **L6675** Upper extremity addition, harness, (e.g., figure of eight type), single cable design Ⓑ

✻ **L6676** Upper extremity addition, harness, (e.g., figure of eight type), dual cable design Ⓑ

✻ **L6677** Upper extremity addition, harness, triple control, simultaneous operation of terminal device and elbow Ⓑ

✻ **L6680** Upper extremity addition, test socket, wrist disarticulation or below elbow Ⓑ

✻ **L6682** Upper extremity addition, test socket, elbow disarticulation or above elbow Ⓑ

✻ **L6684** Upper extremity addition, test socket, shoulder disarticulation or interscapular thoracic Ⓑ

✻ **L6686** Upper extremity addition, suction socket Ⓑ

✻ **L6687** Upper extremity addition, frame type socket, below elbow or wrist disarticulation Ⓑ

✻ **L6688** Upper extremity addition, frame type socket, above elbow or elbow disarticulation Ⓑ

✻ **L6689** Upper extremity addition, frame type socket, shoulder disarticulation Ⓑ

✻ **L6690** Upper extremity addition, frame type socket, interscapular-thoracic Ⓑ

✻ **L6691** Upper extremity addition, removable insert, each Ⓑ

✻ **L6692** Upper extremity addition, silicone gel insert or equal, each Ⓑ

✻ **L6693** Upper extremity addition, locking elbow, forearm counterbalance Ⓑ

✻ **L6694** Addition to upper extremity prosthesis, below elbow/above elbow, custom fabricated from existing mold or prefabricated, socket insert, silicone gel, elastomeric or equal, for use with locking mechanism Ⓑ

✻ **L6695** Addition to upper extremity prosthesis, below elbow/above elbow, custom fabricated from existing mold or prefabricated, socket insert, silicone gel, elastomeric or equal, not for use with locking mechanism Ⓑ

✻ **L6696** Addition to upper extremity prosthesis, below elbow/above elbow, custom fabricated socket insert for congenital or atypical traumatic amputee, silicone gel, elastomeric or equal, for use with or without locking mechanism, initial only (for other than initial, use code L6694 or L6695) Ⓑ

✻ **L6697** Addition to upper extremity prosthesis, below elbow/above elbow, custom fabricated socket insert for other than congenital or atypical traumatic amputee, silicone gel, elastomeric or equal, for use with or without locking mechanism, initial only (for other than initial, use code L6694 or L6695) Ⓑ

✻ **L6698** Addition to upper extremity prosthesis, below elbow/above elbow, lock mechanism, excludes socket insert Ⓑ

Terminal Devices (L6703-L9900)

Hooks

✻ **L6703** Terminal device, passive hand/mitt, any material, any size Ⓑ

✻ **L6704** Terminal device, sport/recreational/work attachment, any material, any size Ⓑ

✻ **L6706** Terminal device, hook, mechanical, voluntary opening, any material, any size, lined or unlined Ⓑ

✻ **L6707** Terminal device, hook, mechanical, voluntary closing, any material, any size, lined or unlined Ⓑ

✻ **L6708** Terminal device, hand, mechanical, voluntary opening, any material, any size Ⓑ

✻ **L6709** Terminal device, hand, mechanical, voluntary closing, any material, any size Ⓑ

✻ **L6711** Terminal device, hook, mechanical, voluntary opening, any material, any size, lined or unlined, pediatric Ⓑ

✻ **L6712** Terminal device, hook, mechanical, voluntary closing, any material, any size, lined or unlined, pediatric Ⓑ

✻ **L6713** Terminal device, hand, mechanical, voluntary opening, any material, any size, pediatric Ⓑ

✻ **L6714** Terminal device, hand, mechanical, voluntary closing, any material, any size, pediatric Ⓑ

✻ **L6715** Terminal device, multiple articulating digit, includes motor(s), initial issue or replacement Ⓑ

✻ **L6721** Terminal device, hook or hand, heavy duty, mechanical, voluntary opening, any material, any size, lined or unlined Ⓑ

✻ **L6722** Terminal device, hook or hand, heavy duty, mechanical, voluntary closing, any material, any size, lined or unlined Ⓑ

❂ **L6805** Addition to terminal device, modifier wrist unit Ⓑ

IOM: 100-02, 15, 120; 100-04, 3, 10.4

❂ **L6810** Addition to terminal device, precision pinch device Ⓑ

IOM: 100-02, 15, 120; 100-04, 3, 10.4

Hands

✻ **L6880** Electric hand, switch or myoelectric controlled, independently articulating digits, any grasp pattern or combination of grasp patterns, includes motor(s) Ⓑ

✻ **L6881** Automatic grasp feature, addition to upper limb electric prosthetic terminal device Ⓑ

❂ **L6882** Microprocessor control feature, addition to upper limb prosthetic terminal device Ⓑ

IOM: 100-02, 15, 120; 100-04, 3, 10.4

Replacement Sockets

✻ **L6883** Replacement socket, below elbow/wrist disarticulation, molded to patient model, for use with or without external power Ⓑ

✻ **L6884** Replacement socket, above elbow/elbow disarticulation, molded to patient model, for use with or without external power Ⓑ

✻ **L6885** Replacement socket, shoulder disarticulation/interscapular thoracic, molded to patient model, for use with or without external power Ⓑ

Gloves for Above Hands

✻ **L6890** Addition to upper extremity prosthesis, glove for terminal device, any material, prefabricated, includes fitting and adjustment Ⓑ

✻ **L6895** Addition to upper extremity prosthesis, glove for terminal device, any material, custom fabricated Ⓑ

Hand Restoration

✻ **L6900** Hand restoration (casts, shading and measurements included), partial hand, with glove, thumb or one finger remaining Ⓑ

✻ **L6905** Hand restoration (casts, shading and measurements included), partial hand, with glove, multiple fingers remaining Ⓑ

✻ **L6910** Hand restoration (casts, shading and measurements included), partial hand, with glove, no fingers remaining Ⓑ

✻ **L6915** Hand restoration (shading, and measurements included), replacement glove for above Ⓑ

External Power

Base Devices

✻ **L6920** Wrist disarticulation, external power, self-suspended inner socket, removable forearm shell, Otto Bock or equal switch, cables, two batteries and one charger, switch control of terminal device Ⓑ

✻ **L6925** Wrist disarticulation, external power, self-suspended inner socket, removable forearm shell, Otto Bock or equal electrodes, cables, two batteries and one charger, myoelectronic control of terminal device Ⓑ

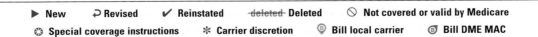

✻ **L6930** Below elbow, external power, self-suspended inner socket, removable forearm shell, Otto Bock or equal switch, cables, two batteries and one charger, switch control of terminal device Ⓑ

✻ **L6935** Below elbow, external power, self-suspended inner socket, removable forearm shell, Otto Bock or equal electrodes, cables, two batteries and one charger, myoelectronic control of terminal device Ⓑ

✻ **L6940** Elbow disarticulation, external power, molded inner socket, removable humeral shell, outside locking hinges, forearm, Otto Bock or equal switch, cables, two batteries and one charger, switch control of terminal device Ⓑ

✻ **L6945** Elbow disarticulation, external power, molded inner socket, removable humeral shell, outside locking hinges, forearm, Otto Bock or equal electrodes, cables, two batteries and one charger, myoelectronic control of terminal device Ⓑ

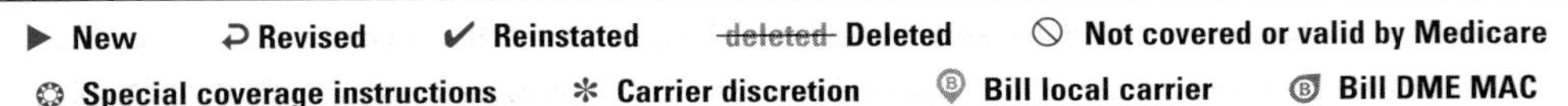

✻ **L6950** Above elbow, external power, molded inner socket, removable humeral shell, internal locking elbow, forearm, Otto Bock or equal switch, cables, two batteries and one charger, switch control of terminal device Ⓑ

✻ **L6955** Above elbow, external power, molded inner socket, removable humeral shell, internal locking elbow, forearm, Otto Bock or equal electrodes, cables, two batteries and one charger, myoelectronic control of terminal device Ⓑ

✻ **L6960** Shoulder disarticulation, external power, molded inner socket, removable shoulder shell, shoulder bulkhead, humeral section, mechanical elbow, forearm, Otto Bock or equal switch, cables, two batteries and one charger, switch control of terminal device Ⓑ

✻ **L6965** Shoulder disarticulation, external power, molded inner socket, removable shoulder shell, shoulder bulkhead, humeral section, mechanical elbow, forearm, Otto Bock or equal electrodes, cables, two batteries and one charger, myoelectronic control of terminal device Ⓑ

✻ **L6970** Interscapular-thoracic, external power, molded inner socket, removable shoulder shell, shoulder bulkhead, humeral section, mechanical elbow, forearm, Otto Bock or equal switch, cables, two batteries and one charger, switch control of terminal device Ⓑ

✻ **L6975** Interscapular-thoracic, external power, molded inner socket, removable shoulder shell, shoulder bulkhead, humeral section, mechanical elbow, forearm, Otto Bock or equal electrodes, cables, two batteries and one charger, myoelectronic control of terminal device Ⓑ

Terminal Devices

✻ **L7007** Electric hand, switch or myoelectric controlled, adult Ⓑ

✻ **L7008** Electric hand, switch or myoelectric controlled, pediatric Ⓑ

✻ **L7009** Electric hook, switch or myoelectric controlled, adult Ⓑ

✻ **L7040** Prehensile actuator, switch controlled Ⓑ

✻ **L7045** Electric hook, switch or myoelectric controlled, pediatric Ⓑ

Elbow

✻ **L7170** Electronic elbow, Hosmer or equal, switch controlled Ⓑ

✻ **L7180** Electronic elbow, microprocessor sequential control of elbow and terminal device Ⓑ

✻ **L7181** Electronic elbow, microprocessor simultaneous control of elbow and terminal device Ⓑ

✻ **L7185** Electronic elbow, adolescent, Variety Village or equal, switch controlled Ⓑ

✻ **L7186** Electronic elbow, child, Variety Village or equal, switch controlled Ⓑ

✻ **L7190** Electronic elbow, adolescent, Variety Village or equal, myoelectronically controlled Ⓑ

✻ **L7191** Electronic elbow, child, Variety Village or equal, myoelectronically controlled Ⓑ

Wrist

✻ **L7259** Electronic wrist rotator, any type Ⓑ

Battery Components

✻ **L7360** Six volt battery, each Ⓑ

✻ **L7362** Battery charger, six volt, each Ⓑ

✻ **L7364** Twelve volt battery, each Ⓑ

✻ **L7366** Battery charger, twelve volt, each Ⓑ

✻ **L7367** Lithium ion battery, rechargeable, replacement Ⓑ

✻ **L7368** Lithium ion battery charger, replacement only Ⓑ

Other/Repair

✻ **L7400** Addition to upper extremity prosthesis, below elbow/wrist disarticulation, ultralight material (titanium, carbon fiber or equal) Ⓑ

✻ **L7401** Addition to upper extremity prosthesis, above elbow disarticulation, ultralight material (titanium, carbon fiber or equal) Ⓑ

✻ **L7402** Addition to upper extremity prosthesis, shoulder disarticulation/interscapular thoracic, ultralight material (titanium, carbon fiber or equal) Ⓑ

✻ **L7403** Addition to upper extremity prosthesis, below elbow/wrist disarticulation, acrylic material Ⓑ

✻ **L7404** Addition to upper extremity prosthesis, above elbow disarticulation, acrylic material Ⓑ

✻ **L7405** Addition to upper extremity prosthesis, shoulder disarticulation/interscapular thoracic, acrylic material Ⓑ

✻ **L7499** Upper extremity prosthesis, not otherwise specified Ⓑ

⚙ **L7510** Repair of prosthetic device, repair or replace minor parts Ⓑ Ⓑ

Bill Local Carrier if repair of implanted prosthetic device. If other, bill DME MAC.

IOM: 100-02, 15, 110.2; 100-02, 15, 120; 100-04, 32, 100

✻ **L7520** Repair prosthetic device, labor component, per 15 minutes Ⓑ Ⓑ

Bill Local Carrier if repair of implanted prosthetic device. If other, bill DME MAC.

⊘ **L7600** Prosthetic donning sleeve, any material, each Ⓑ

Medicare Statute 1862(1)(a)

General

⊘ **L7900** Male vacuum erection system Ⓑ

Medicare Statute 1834a

⊘ **L7902** Tension ring, for vacuum erection device, any type, replacement only, each Ⓑ

Medicare Statute 1834a

Breast Prostheses

⚙ **L8000** Breast prosthesis, mastectomy bra, without integrated breast prosthesis form, any size, any type Ⓑ

IOM: 100-02, 15, 120

⚙ **L8001** Breast prosthesis, mastectomy bra, with integrated breast prosthesis form, unilateral, any size, any type Ⓑ

IOM: 100-02, 15, 120

⚙ **L8002** Breast prosthesis, mastectomy bra, with integrated breast prosthesis form, bilateral, any size, any type Ⓑ

IOM: 100-02, 15, 120

⚙ **L8010** Breast prosthesis, mastectomy sleeve Ⓑ

IOM: 100-02, 15, 120

⚙ **L8015** External breast prosthesis garment, with mastectomy form, post mastectomy Ⓑ

IOM: 100-02, 15, 120

⚙ **L8020** Breast prosthesis, mastectomy form Ⓑ

IOM: 100-02, 15, 120

⚙ **L8030** Breast prosthesis, silicone or equal, without integral adhesive Ⓑ

IOM: 100-02, 15, 120

⚙ **L8031** Breast prosthesis, silicone or equal, with integral adhesive Ⓑ

IOM: 100-02, 15, 120

✻ **L8032** Nipple prosthesis, reusable, any type, each Ⓑ

⚙ **L8035** Custom breast prosthesis, post mastectomy, molded to patient model Ⓑ

IOM: 100-02, 15, 120

✻ **L8039** Breast prosthesis, not otherwise specified Ⓑ

Nasal, Orbital, Auricular Prosthesis

✻ **L8040** Nasal prosthesis, provided by a non-physician Ⓑ

✻ **L8041** Midfacial prosthesis, provided by a non-physician Ⓑ

✻ **L8042** Orbital prosthesis, provided by a non-physician Ⓑ

✻ **L8043** Upper facial prosthesis, provided by a non-physician Ⓑ

✻ **L8044** Hemi-facial prosthesis, provided by a non-physician Ⓑ

✻ **L8045** Auricular prosthesis, provided by a non-physician Ⓑ

✻ **L8046** Partial facial prosthesis, provided by a non-physician Ⓑ

✻ **L8047** Nasal septal prosthesis, provided by a non-physician Ⓑ

✻ **L8048** Unspecified maxillofacial prosthesis, by report, provided by a non-physician Ⓑ

✻ **L8049** Repair or modification of maxillofacial prosthesis, labor component, 15 minute increments, provided by a non-physician Ⓑ

Trusses

⚙ **L8300** Truss, single with standard pad Ⓑ

IOM: 100-02, 15, 120; 100-03, 4, 280.11; 100-03, 4, 280.12; 100-04, 4, 240

⚙ **L8310** Truss, double with standard pads Ⓑ

IOM: 100-02, 15, 120; 100-03, 4, 280.11; 100-03, 4, 280.12; 100-04, 4, 240

⊗ **L8320** Truss, addition to standard pad, water pad Ⓑ

IOM: 100-02, 15, 120; 100-03, 4, 280.11; 100-03, 4, 280.12; 100-04, 4, 240

⊗ **L8330** Truss, addition to standard pad, scrotal pad Ⓑ

IOM: 100-02, 15, 120; 100-03, 4, 280.11; 100-03, 4, 280.12; 100-04, 4, 240

Prosthetic Socks

⊗ **L8400** Prosthetic sheath, below knee, each Ⓑ

IOM: 100-02, 15, 200

⊗ **L8410** Prosthetic sheath, above knee, each Ⓑ

IOM: 100-02, 15, 200

⊗ **L8415** Prosthetic sheath, upper limb, each Ⓑ

IOM: 100-02, 15, 200

* **L8417** Prosthetic sheath/sock, including a gel cushion layer, below knee or above knee, each Ⓑ

⊗ **L8420** Prosthetic sock, multiple ply, below knee, each Ⓑ

IOM: 100-02, 15, 200

⊗ **L8430** Prosthetic sock, multiple ply, above knee, each Ⓑ

IOM: 100-02, 15, 200

⊗ **L8435** Prosthetic sock, multiple ply, upper limb, each Ⓑ

IOM: 100-02, 15, 200

⊗ **L8440** Prosthetic shrinker, below knee, each Ⓑ

IOM: 100-02, 15, 200

⊗ **L8460** Prosthetic shrinker, above knee, each Ⓑ

IOM: 100-02, 15, 200

⊗ **L8465** Prosthetic shrinker, upper limb, each Ⓑ

IOM: 100-02, 15, 200

⊗ **L8470** Prosthetic sock, single ply, fitting, below knee, each Ⓑ

IOM: 100-02, 15, 200

⊗ **L8480** Prosthetic sock, single ply, fitting, above knee, each Ⓑ

IOM: 100-02, 15, 200

⊗ **L8485** Prosthetic sock, single ply, fitting, upper limb, each Ⓑ

IOM: 100-02, 15, 200

* **L8499** Unlisted procedure for miscellaneous prosthetic services Ⓑ Ⓑ

Bill Local Carrier if repair of implanted prosthetic device. If other, bill DME MAC.

Prosthetic Implants (L8500-L9900)

Larynx, Tracheoesophageal

⊗ **L8500** Artificial larynx, any type Ⓑ

IOM: 100-02, 15, 120; 100-03, 1, 50.2; 100-04, 4, 240

⊗ **L8501** Tracheostomy speaking valve Ⓑ

IOM: 100-03, 1, 50.4

* **L8505** Artificial larynx replacement battery/accessory, any type Ⓑ

* **L8507** Tracheo-esophageal voice prosthesis, patient inserted, any type, each Ⓑ

* **L8509** Tracheo-esophageal voice prosthesis, inserted by a licensed health care provider, any type Ⓑ Ⓑ

Bill Local Carrier for dates of service on or after 10/01/2010.

⊗ **L8510** Voice amplifier Ⓑ

IOM: 100-03, 1, 50.2

* **L8511** Insert for indwelling tracheoesophageal prosthesis, with or without valve, replacement only, each Ⓑ Ⓑ

Bill Local Carrier if used with tracheoesophageal voice prostheses inserted by a licensed health care provider. If other, bill DME MAC.

* **L8512** Gelatin capsules or equivalent, for use with tracheoesophageal voice prosthesis, replacement only, per 10 Ⓑ Ⓑ

Bill Local Carrier if used with tracheoesophageal voice prostheses inserted by a licensed health care provider. If other, bill DME MAC.

* **L8513** Cleaning device used with tracheoesophageal voice prosthesis, pipet, brush, or equal, replacement only, each Ⓑ Ⓑ

Bill Local Carrier if used with tracheoesophageal voice prostheses inserted by a licensed health care provider. If other, bill DME MAC.

* **L8514** Tracheoesophageal puncture dilator, replacement only, each Ⓑ Ⓑ

Bill Local Carrier if used with tracheoesophageal voice prostheses inserted by a licensed health care provider. If other, bill DME MAC.

* **L8515** Gelatin capsule, application device for use with tracheoesophageal voice prosthesis, each

Bill Local Carrier if used with tracheoesophageal voice prostheses inserted by a licensed health care provider. If other, bill DME MAC.

Breast

L8600 Implantable breast prosthesis, silicone or equal

IOM: 100-02, 15, 120; 100-3, 2, 140.2

Urinary System

L8603 Injectable bulking agent, collagen implant, urinary tract, 2.5 ml syringe, includes shipping and necessary supplies

Bill on paper, acquisition cost invoice required

IOM: 100-03, 4, 280.1

* **L8604** Injectable bulking agent, dextranomer/ hyaluronic acid copolymer implant, urinary tract, 1 ml, includes shipping and necessary supplies

* **L8605** Injectable bulking agent, dextranomer/ hyaluronic acid copolymer implant, anal canal, 1 ml, includes shipping and necessary supplies

L8606 Injectable bulking agent, synthetic implant, urinary tract, 1 ml syringe, includes shipping and necessary supplies

Bill on paper, acquisition cost invoice required

IOM: 100-03, 4, 280.1

Head (Skull, Facial Bones, and Temporomandibular Joint)

L8607 Injectable bulking agent for vocal cord medialization, 0.1 ml, includes shipping and necessary supplies

IOM: 100-03, 4, 280.1

* **L8609** Artificial cornea

L8610 Ocular implant

IOM: 100-02, 15, 120

L8612 Aqueous shunt

IOM: 100-02, 15, 120

Cross Reference Q0074

L8613 Ossicula implant

IOM: 100-02, 15, 120

L8614 Cochlear device, includes all internal and external components

IOM: 100-02, 15, 120; 100-03, 1, 50.3

L8615 Headset/headpiece for use with cochlear implant device, replacement

IOM: 100-03, 1, 50.3

L8616 Microphone for use with cochlear implant device, replacement

IOM: 100-03, 1, 50.3

L8617 Transmitting coil for use with cochlear implant device, replacement

IOM: 100-03, 1, 50.3

L8618 Transmitter cable for use with cochlear implant device, replacement

IOM: 100-03, 1, 50.3

L8619 Cochlear implant, external speech processor and controller, integrated system, replacement

IOM: 100-03, 1, 50.3

* **L8621** Zinc air battery for use with cochlear implant device and auditory osseointegrated sound processors, replacement, each

* **L8622** Alkaline battery for use with cochlear implant device, any size, replacement, each

* **L8623** Lithium ion battery for use with cochlear implant device speech processor, other than ear level, replacement, each

* **L8624** Lithium ion battery for use with cochlear implant device speech processor, ear level, replacement, each

L8627 Cochlear implant, external speech processor, component, replacement

IOM: 103-03, Part 1, 50.3

L8628 Cochlear implant, external controller component, replacement

IOM: 103-03, Part 1, 50.3

L8629 Transmitting coil and cable, integrated, for use with cochlear implant device, replacement

IOM: 103-03, Part 1, 50.3

Upper Extremity

L8630 Metacarpophalangeal joint implant

IOM: 100-02, 15, 120

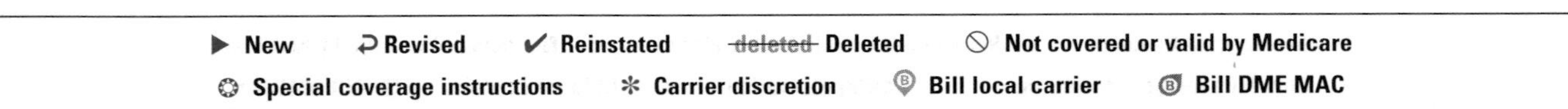

⚙ **L8631** Metacarpal phalangeal joint replacement, two or more pieces, metal (e.g., stainless steel or cobalt chrome), ceramic-like material (e.g., pyrocarbon), for surgical implantation (all sizes, includes entire system) Ⓑ

IOM: 100-02, 15, 120

Lower Extremity (Joint: Knee, Ankle, Toe)

⚙ **L8641** Metatarsal joint implant Ⓑ

IOM: 100-02, 15, 120

⚙ **L8642** Hallux implant Ⓑ

May be billed by ambulatory surgical center or surgeon

IOM: 100-02, 15, 120

Cross Reference Q0073

Miscellaneous Muscular-Skeletal

⚙ **L8658** Interphalangeal joint spacer, silicone or equal, each Ⓑ

IOM: 100-02, 15, 120

⚙ **L8659** Interphalangeal finger joint replacement, 2 or more pieces, metal (e.g., stainless steel or cobalt chrome), ceramic-like material (e.g., pyrocarbon) for surgical implantation, any size Ⓑ

IOM: 100-02, 15, 120

Cardiovascular System

⚙ **L8670** Vascular graft material, synthetic, implant Ⓑ

IOM: 100-02, 15, 120

Neurostimulator

⚙ **L8679** Implantable neurostimulator, pulse generator, any type Ⓑ

IOM: 100-03, 4, 280.4

⦸ **L8680** Implantable neurostimulator electrode, each Ⓑ

Related CPT codes: 43647, 63650, 63655, 64553, 64555, 64560, 64561, 64565, 64573, 64575, 64577, 64580, 64581

⚙ **L8681** Patient programmer (external) for use with implantable programmable neurostimulator pulse generator, replacement only Ⓑ

IOM: 100-03, 4, 280.4

⚙ **L8682** Implantable neurostimulator radiofrequency receiver Ⓑ

IOM: 100-03, 4, 280.4

⚙ **L8683** Radiofrequency transmitter (external) for use with implantable neurostimulator radiofrequency receiver Ⓑ

IOM: 100-03, 4, 280.4

⚙ **L8684** Radiofrequency transmitter (external) for use with implantable sacral root neurostimulator receiver for bowel and bladder management, replacement Ⓑ

IOM: 100-03, 4, 280.4

⦸ **L8685** Implantable neurostimulator pulse generator, single array, rechargeable, includes extension Ⓑ

Related CPT codes: 61885, 64590, 63685

⦸ **L8686** Implantable neurostimulator pulse generator, single array, non-rechargeable, includes extension Ⓑ

Related CPT codes: 61885, 64590, 63685

⦸ **L8687** Implantable neurostimulator pulse generator, dual array, rechargeable, includes extension Ⓑ

Related CPT codes: 64590, 63685, 61886

⦸ **L8688** Implantable neurostimulator pulse generator, dual array, non-rechargeable, includes extension Ⓑ

Related CPT codes: 61885, 64590, 63685

⚙ **L8689** External recharging system for battery (internal) for use with implantable neurostimulator, replacement only Ⓑ

IOM: 100-03, 4, 280.4

✻ **L8690** Auditory osseointegrated device, includes all internal and external components Ⓑ

Related CPT codes: 69714, 69715, 69717, 69718

✻ **L8691** Auditory osseointegrated device, external sound processor, replacement Ⓑ

⦸ **L8692** Auditory osseointegrated device, external sound processor, used without osseointegration, body worn, includes headband or other means of external attachment Ⓑ

Medicare Statute 1862(a)(7)

✻ **L8693** Auditory osseointegrated device abutment, any length, replacement only Ⓑ

▶ New ⤾ Revised ✔ Reinstated ~~deleted~~ Deleted ⦸ Not covered or valid by Medicare
⚙ Special coverage instructions ✻ Carrier discretion Ⓑ Bill local carrier Ⓓ Bill DME MAC

L8695 External recharging system for battery (external) for use with implantable neurostimulator, replacement only

IOM: 100-03, 4, 280.4

L8696 Antenna (external) for use with implantable diaphragmatic/phrenic nerve stimulation device, replacement, each

Miscellaneous Orthotic or Prosthetic Component or Accessory

* **L8699** Prosthetic implant, not otherwise specified

* **L9900** Orthotic and prosthetic supply, accessory, and/or service component of another HCPCS "L" code

Bill Local Carrier if used with implanted prosthetic device. If other, bill DME MAC.

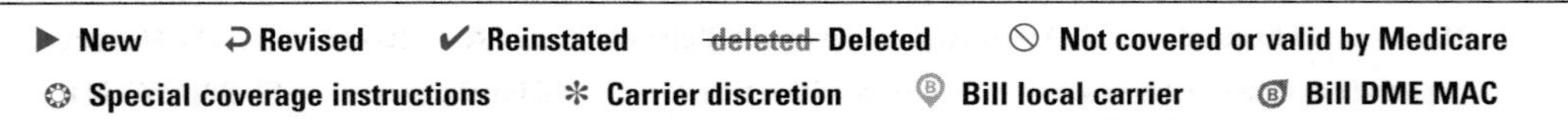

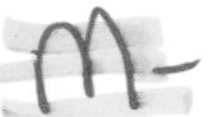
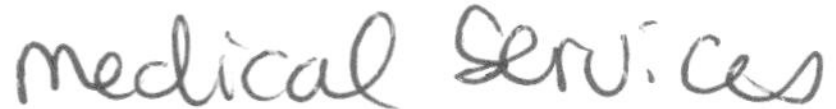

OTHER MEDICAL SERVICES (M0000-M0301)

⃠ **M0075** Cellular therapy Ⓑ

⃠ **M0076** Prolotherapy Ⓑ

Prolotherapy stimulates production of new ligament tissue. Not covered by Medicare.

⃠ **M0100** Intragastric hypothermia using gastric freezing Ⓑ

⃠ **M0300** IV chelation therapy (chemical endarterectomy) Ⓑ

⃠ **M0301** Fabric wrapping of abdominal aneurysm Ⓑ

Treatment for abdominal aneurysms that involves wrapping aneurysms with cellophane or fascia lata. Fabric wrapping of abdominal aneurysms is not a covered Medicare procedure.

▶ New ⤾ Revised ✔ Reinstated ~~deleted~~ Deleted ⃠ Not covered or valid by Medicare
✪ Special coverage instructions ✻ Carrier discretion Ⓑ Bill local carrier Ⓑ Bill DME MAC

LABORATORY SERVICES (P0000-P9999)

Chemistry and Toxicology Tests

P2028 Cephalin floculation, blood

This code appears on a CMS list of codes that represent obsolete and unreliable tests and procedures. Verify before reporting.

IOM: 100-03, 4, 300.1

P2029 Congo red, blood

This code appears on a CMS list of codes that represent obsolete and unreliable tests and procedures. Verify before reporting.

IOM: 100-03, 4, 300.1

P2031 Hair analysis (excluding arsenic)

IOM: 100-03, 4, 300.1

P2033 Thymol turbidity, blood

This code appears on a CMS list of codes that represent obsolete and unreliable tests and procedures. Verify before reporting.

IOM: 100-03, 4, 300.1

P2038 Mucoprotein, blood (seromucoid) (medical necessity procedure)

This code appears on a CMS list of codes that represent obsolete and unreliable tests and procedures. Verify before reporting.

IOM: 100-03, 4, 300.1

Pathology Screening Tests

P3000 Screening Papanicolaou smear, cervical or vaginal, up to three smears, by technician under physician supervision

Co-insurance and deductible waived

Assign for Pap smear ordered for screening purposes only, conventional method, performed by technician

IOM: 100-03, 3, 190.2,

Laboratory Certification: Cytology

P3001 Screening Papanicolaou smear, cervical or vaginal, up to three smears, requiring interpretation by physician

Co-insurance and deductible waived

Report professional component for Pap smears requiring physician interpretation. There are CPT codes assigned for diagnostic Paps, such as, 88141; HCPCS are for screening Paps.

IOM: 100-03, 3, 190.2

Laboratory Certification: Cytology

Microbiology Tests

P7001 Culture, bacterial, urine; quantitative, sensitivity study

Cross Reference CPT

Laboratory Certification: Bacteriology

Miscellaneous Pathology

P9010 Blood (whole), for transfusion, per unit

OPPS recognized blood/blood products

Blood furnished on an outpatient basis, subject to Medicare Part B blood deductible; applicable to first 3 pints of whole blood or equivalent units of packed red cells in calendar year

IOM: 100-01, 3, 20.5; 100-02, 1, 10

P9011 Blood, split unit

OPPS recognized blood/blood products

Reports all splitting activities of any blood component

IOM: 100-01, 3, 20.5; 100-02, 1, 10

P9012 Cryoprecipitate, each unit

OPPS recognized blood/blood products

IOM: 100-01, 3, 20.5; 100-02, 1, 10

P9016 Red blood cells, leukocytes reduced, each unit

OPPS recognized blood/blood products

IOM: 100-01, 3, 20.5; 100-02, 1, 10

P9017 Fresh frozen plasma (single donor), frozen within 8 hours of collection, each unit

OPPS recognized blood/blood products

IOM: 100-01, 3, 20.5; 100-02, 1, 10

P9019 Platelets, each unit

OPPS recognized blood/blood products

IOM: 100-01, 3, 20.5; 100-02, 1, 10

⊛ **P9020** Platelet rich plasma, each unit Ⓑ
OPPS recognized blood/blood products
IOM: 100-01, 3, 20.5; 100-02, 1, 10

⊛ **P9021** Red blood cells, each unit Ⓑ
OPPS recognized blood/blood products
IOM: 100-01, 3, 20.5; 100-02, 1, 10

⊛ **P9022** Red blood cells, washed, each unit Ⓑ
OPPS recognized blood/blood products
IOM: 100-01, 3, 20.5; 100-02, 1, 10

⊛ **P9023** Plasma, pooled multiple donor, solvent/detergent treated, frozen, each unit Ⓑ
OPPS recognized blood/blood products
IOM: 100-01, 3, 20.5; 100-02, 1, 10

⊛ **P9031** Platelets, leukocytes reduced, each unit Ⓑ
OPPS recognized blood/blood products
IOM: 100-01, 3, 20.5; 100-02, 1, 10

⊛ **P9032** Platelets, irradiated, each unit Ⓑ
OPPS recognized blood/blood products
IOM: 100-01, 3, 20.5; 100-02, 1, 10

⊛ **P9033** Platelets, leukocytes reduced, irradiated, each unit Ⓑ
OPPS recognized blood/blood products
IOM: 100-01, 3, 20.5; 100-02, 1, 10

⊛ **P9034** Platelets, pheresis, each unit Ⓑ
OPPS recognized blood/blood products
IOM: 100-01, 3, 20.5; 100-02, 1, 10

⊛ **P9035** Platelets, pheresis, leukocytes reduced, each unit Ⓑ
OPPS recognized blood/blood products
IOM: 100-01, 3, 20.5; 100-02, 1, 10

⊛ **P9036** Platelets, pheresis, irradiated, each unit Ⓑ
OPPS recognized blood/blood products
IOM: 100-01, 3, 20.5; 100-02, 1, 10

⊛ **P9037** Platelets, pheresis, leukocytes reduced, irradiated, each unit Ⓑ
OPPS recognized blood/blood products
IOM: 100-01, 3, 20.5; 100-02, 1, 10

⊛ **P9038** Red blood cells, irradiated, each unit Ⓑ
OPPS recognized blood/blood products
IOM: 100-01, 3, 20.5; 100-02, 1, 10

⊛ **P9039** Red blood cells, deglycerolized, each unit Ⓑ
OPPS recognized blood/blood products
IOM: 100-01, 3, 20.5; 100-02, 1, 10

⊛ **P9040** Red blood cells, leukocytes reduced, irradiated, each unit Ⓑ
OPPS recognized blood/blood products
IOM: 100-01, 3, 20.5; 100-02, 1, 10

* **P9041** Infusion, albumin (human), 5%, 50 ml Ⓑ

⊛ **P9043** Infusion, plasma protein fraction (human), 5%, 50 ml Ⓑ
OPPS recognized blood/blood products
IOM: 100-01, 3, 20.5; 100-02, 1, 10

⊛ **P9044** Plasma, cryoprecipitate reduced, each unit Ⓑ
OPPS recognized blood/blood products
IOM: 100-01, 3, 20.5; 100-02, 1, 10

* **P9045** Infusion, albumin (human), 5%, 250 ml Ⓑ

* **P9046** Infusion, albumin (human), 25%, 20 ml Ⓑ

* **P9047** Infusion, albumin (human), 25%, 50 ml Ⓑ

* **P9048** Infusion, plasma protein fraction (human), 5%, 250 ml Ⓑ
OPPS recognized blood/blood products

* **P9050** Granulocytes, pheresis, each unit Ⓑ
OPPS recognized blood/blood products

⊛ **P9051** Whole blood or red blood cells, leukocytes reduced, CMV-negative, each unit Ⓑ
OPPS recognized blood/blood products
Medicare Statute 1833(t)

⊛ **P9052** Platelets, HLA-matched leukocytes reduced, apheresis/pheresis, each unit Ⓑ
OPPS recognized blood/blood products
Medicare Statute 1833(t)

⊛ **P9053** Platelets, pheresis, leukocytes reduced, CMV-negative, irradiated, each unit Ⓑ
OPPS recognized blood/blood products
Freezing and thawing are reported separately, see Transmittal 1487 (Hospital outpatient)
Medicare Statute 1833(t)

⊛ **P9054** Whole blood or red blood cells, leukocytes reduced, frozen, deglycerol, washed, each unit Ⓑ
OPPS recognized blood/blood products
Medicare Statute 1833(t)

▶ New ⤾ Revised ✔ Reinstated ~~deleted~~ Deleted ⊘ Not covered or valid by Medicare
⊛ Special coverage instructions * Carrier discretion Ⓑ Bill local carrier Ⓓ Bill DME MAC

P9055 Platelets, leukocytes reduced, CMV-negative, apheresis/pheresis, each unit

OPPS recognized blood/blood products

Medicare Statute 1833(t)

P9056 Whole blood, leukocytes reduced, irradiated, each unit

OPPS recognized blood/blood products

Medicare Statute 1833(t)

P9057 Red blood cells, frozen/deglycerolized/washed, leukocytes reduced, irradiated, each unit

OPPS recognized blood/blood products

Medicare Statute 1833(t)

P9058 Red blood cells, leukocytes reduced, CMV-negative, irradiated, each unit

OPPS recognized blood/blood products

Medicare Statute 1833(t)

P9059 Fresh frozen plasma between 8-24 hours of collection, each unit

OPPS recognized blood/blood products

Medicare Statute 1833(t)

P9060 Fresh frozen plasma, donor retested, each unit

OPPS recognized blood/blood products

Medicare Statute 1833(t)

P9070 Plasma, pooled multiple donor, pathogen reduced, frozen, each unit

Medicare Statute 1833T

P9071 Plasma (single donor), pathogen reduced, frozen, each unit

IOM: 100-01, 3, 20.5; 100-02, 1, 10

Medicare Statute 1833T

P9072 Platelets, pheresis, pathogen reduced or rapid bacterial tested, each unit

IOM: 100-01, 3, 20.5; 100-02, 1, 10

Medicare Statute 1833T

P9603 Travel allowance one way in connection with medically necessary laboratory specimen collection drawn from home bound or nursing home bound patient; prorated miles actually traveled

Fee for clinical laboratory travel (P9603) is $0.99 per mile for CY2016

IOM: 100-04, 16, 60

P9604 Travel allowance one way in connection with medically necessary laboratory specimen collection drawn from home bound or nursing home bound patient; prorated trip charge

For CY2016, the fee for clinical laboratory travel is $9.90 per flat rate trip.

IOM: 100-04, 16, 60

P9612 Catheterization for collection of specimen, single patient, all places of service

NCCI edits indicate that when 51701 is comprehensive or is a Column 1 code, P9612 cannot be reported. When the catheter insertion is a component of another procedure, do not report straight catheterization separately.

IOM: 100-04, 16, 60

P9615 Catheterization for collection of specimen(s) (multiple patients)

IOM: 100-04, 16, 60

▶ New ⤾ Revised ✔ Reinstated ~~deleted~~ Deleted ⃠ Not covered or valid by Medicare
Special coverage instructions ✻ Carrier discretion Bill local carrier Bill DME MAC

TEMPORARY CODES ASSIGNED BY CMS (Q0000-Q9999)

Cardiokymography

Q0035 Cardiokymography
Report modifier 26 if professional component only
IOM: 100-03, 1, 20.24

Infusion Therapy

Q0081 Infusion therapy, using other than chemotherapeutic drugs, per visit
IV piggyback only assigned one time per patient encounter per day. Report for hydration or the intravenous administration of antibiotics, anti-emetics, or analgesics. Bill on paper. Requires a report.
IOM: 100-03, 4, 280.14

Chemotherapy Administration

* **Q0083** Chemotherapy administration by other than infusion technique only (e.g., subcutaneous, intramuscular, push), per visit

Q0084 Chemotherapy administration by infusion technique only, per visit
IOM: 100-03, 4, 280.14

* **Q0085** Chemotherapy administration by both infusion technique and other technique(s) (e.g., subcutaneous, intramuscular, push), per visit

Smear Preparation

Q0091 Screening Papanicolaou smear; obtaining, preparing and conveyance of cervical or vaginal smear to laboratory
Medicare does not cover comprehensive preventive medicine services; however, services described by G0101 and Q0091 (only for Medicare patients) are covered. Includes the services necessary to procure and transport the specimen to the laboratory.
IOM: 100-03, 3, 190.2

Portable X-ray Setup

Q0092 Set-up portable x-ray equipment
IOM: 100-04, 13, 90

Miscellaneous Lab Services

* **Q0111** Wet mounts, including preparations of vaginal, cervical or skin specimens
Laboratory Certification: Bacteriology, Mycology, Parasitology

* **Q0112** All potassium hydroxide (KOH) preparations
Laboratory Certification: Mycology

* **Q0113** Pinworm examinations
Laboratory Certification: Parasitology

* **Q0114** Fern test
Laboratory Certification: Routine chemistry

* **Q0115** Post-coital direct, qualitative examinations of vaginal or cervical mucous
Laboratory Certification: Hematology

Drugs

* **Q0138** Injection, ferumoxytol, for treatment of iron deficiency anemia, 1 mg (non-ESRD use)
Feraheme is FDA approved for chronic kidney disease
NDC: Feraheme

* **Q0139** (Revised) Injection, ferumoxytol, for treatment of iron deficiency anemia, 1 mg (for ESRD on dialysis)
NDC: Feraheme

Q0144 (Not covered) Azithromycin dihydrate, oral, capsules/powder, 1 gm
Bill Local Carrier If incident to a physician's service. If other, bill DME MAC.
Other: Zithromax

* **Q0161** Chlorpromazine hydrochloride, 5 mg, oral, FDA approved prescription anti-emetic, for use as a complete therapeutic substitute for an IV anti-emetic at the time of chemotherapy treatment, not to exceed a 48 hour dosage regimen

▶ New ⤺ Revised ✔ Reinstated ~~deleted~~ Deleted ⊘ Not covered or valid by Medicare
Special coverage instructions * Carrier discretion Bill local carrier Bill DME MAC

Q codes - These define drugs, medical equipment, + services that haven't been given permanent code, but need to be billed

⊕ **Q0162** Ondansetron 1 mg, oral, FDA-approved prescription anti-emetic, for use as a complete therapeutic substitute for an iv anti-emetic at the time of chemotherapy treatment, not to exceed a 48 hour dosage regimen Ⓑ

NDC: Zofran

Medicare Statute 4557

⊕ **Q0163** Diphenhydramine hydrochloride, 50 mg, oral, FDA approved prescription anti-emetic, for use as a complete therapeutic substitute for an IV anti-emetic at time of chemotherapy treatment not to exceed a 48 hour dosage regimen Ⓑ

Other: Alercap, Allergy Relief Medicine, Allermax, Alertab, Anti-Hist, Antihistamine, Banophen, Complete Allergy Medication, Complete Allergy medicine, Diphedryl, Diphen, Diphenhist, Diphenyl, Dormin Sleep Aid, Geridryl, Good Sense Antihistamine Allergy Relief, Good Sense Nighttime Sleep Aid, Genahist, Mediphedryl, Night Time Sleep Aid, Nytol Quickcaps, Nytol Quickgels maximum strength, Q-Dryl, Quality Choice Sleep Aid, Quality Choice Rest Simply, Quenalin, Rite Aid Allergy, Serabrina La France, Siladryl Allergy, Silphen, Simply Sleep, Sleep Tabs, Sleepinal, Sominex, Twilite, Valu-Dryl Allergy

Medicare Statute 4557

⊕ **Q0164** Prochlorperazine maleate, 5 mg, oral, FDA approved prescription anti-emetic, for use as a complete therapeutic substitute for an IV anti-emetic at the time of chemotherapy treatment, not to exceed a 48 hour dosage regimen Ⓑ

Other: Compazine

Medicare Statute 4557

⊕ **Q0166** Granisetron hydrochloride, 1 mg, oral, FDA approved prescription anti-emetic, for use as a complete therapeutic substitute for an IV anti-emetic at the time of chemotherapy treatment, not to exceed a 24 hour dosage regimen Ⓑ

Other: Kytril

Medicare Statute 4557

⊕ **Q0167** Dronabinol, 2.5 mg, oral, FDA approved prescription anti-emetic, for use as a complete therapeutic substitute for an IV anti-emetic at the time of chemotherapy treatment, not to exceed a 48 hour dosage regimen Ⓑ

NDC: Marinol

Medicare Statute 4557

⊕ **Q0169** Promethazine hydrochloride, 12.5 mg, oral, FDA approved prescription anti-emetic, for use as a complete therapeutic substitute for an IV anti-emetic at the time of chemotherapy treatment, not to exceed a 48 hour dosage regimen Ⓑ

Other: Phenergan

Medicare Statute 4557

⊕ **Q0173** Trimethobenzamide hydrochloride, 250 mg, oral, FDA approved prescription anti-emetic, for use as a complete therapeutic substitute for an IV anti-emetic at the time of chemotherapy treatment, not to exceed a 48 hour dosage regimen Ⓑ

Other: Ticon, Tigan

Medicare Statute 4557

⊕ **Q0174** Thiethylperazine maleate, 10 mg, oral, FDA approved prescription anti-emetic, for use as a complete therapeutic substitute for an IV anti-emetic at the time of chemotherapy treatment, not to exceed a 48 hour dosage regimen Ⓑ

Other: Torecan

Medicare Statute 4557

⊕ **Q0175** Perphenazine, 4 mg, oral, FDA approved prescription anti-emetic, for use as a complete therapeutic substitute for an IV anti-emetic at the time of chemotherapy treatment, not to exceed a 48 hour dosage regimen Ⓑ

Medicare Statute 4557

⊕ **Q0177** Hydroxyzine pamoate, 25 mg, oral, FDA approved prescription anti-emetic, for use as a complete therapeutic substitute for an IV anti-emetic at the time of chemotherapy treatment, not to exceed a 48 hour dosage regimen Ⓑ

Other: Vistaril

Medicare Statute 4557

⊕ **Q0180** Dolasetron mesylate, 100 mg, oral, FDA approved prescription anti-emetic, for use as a complete therapeutic substitute for an IV anti-emetic at the time of chemotherapy treatment, not to exceed a 24 hour dosage regimen Ⓑ

NDC: Anzemet

Medicare Statute 4557

▶ **New** **Revised** ✔ **Reinstated** ~~deleted~~ **Deleted** ⊘ **Not covered or valid by Medicare**
⊕ **Special coverage instructions** ✻ **Carrier discretion** Ⓑ **Bill local carrier** Ⓑ **Bill DME MAC**

Q0181 Unspecified oral dosage form, FDA approved prescription anti-emetic, for use as a complete therapeutic substitute for a IV anti-emetic at the time of chemotherapy treatment, not to exceed a 48 hour dosage regimen

Medicare Statute 4557

Ventricular Assist Devices

Q0478 Power adapter for use with electric or electric/pneumatic ventricular assist device, vehicle type

CMS has determined the reasonable useful lifetime is one year. Add modifier RA to claims to report when battery is replaced because it was lost, stolen, or irreparably damaged.

Q0479 Power module for use with electric or electric/pneumatic ventricular assist device, replacemment only

CMS has determined the reasonable useful lifetime is one year. Add modifier RA in cases where the battery is being replaced because it was lost, stolen, or irreparably damaged.

Q0480 Driver for use with pneumatic ventricular assist device, replacement only

Q0481 Microprocessor control unit for use with electric ventricular assist device, replacement only

Q0482 Microprocessor control unit for use with electric/pneumatic combination ventricular assist device, replacement only

Q0483 Monitor/display module for use with electric ventricular assist device, replacement only

Q0484 Monitor/display module for use with electric or electric/pneumatic ventricular assist device, replacement only

Q0485 Monitor control cable for use with electric ventricular assist device, replacement only

Q0486 Monitor control cable for use with electric/pneumatic ventricular assist device, replacement only

Q0487 Leads (pneumatic/electrical) for use with any type electric/pneumatic ventricular assist device, replacement only

Q0488 Power pack base for use with electric ventricular assist device, replacement only

Q0489 Power pack base for use with electric/pneumatic ventricular assist device, replacement only

Q0490 Emergency power source for use with electric ventricular assist device, replacement only

Q0491 Emergency power source for use with electric/pneumatic ventricular assist device, replacement only

Q0492 Emergency power supply cable for use with electric ventricular assist device, replacement only

Q0493 Emergency power supply cable for use with electric/pneumatic ventricular assist device, replacement only

Q0494 Emergency hand pump for use with electric or electric/pneumatic ventricular assist device, replacement only

Q0495 Battery/power pack charger for use with electric or electric/pneumatic ventricular assist device, replacement only

Q0496 Battery, other than lithium-ion, for use with electric or electric/pneumatic ventricular assist device, replacement only

Reasonable useful lifetime is 6 months (CR3931).

Q0497 Battery clips for use with electric or electric/pneumatic ventricular assist device, replacement only

Q0498 Holster for use with electric or electric/pneumatic ventricular assist device, replacement only

Q0499 Belt/vest/bag for use to carry external peripheral components of any type ventricular assist device, replacement only

Q0500 Filters for use with electric or electric/pneumatic ventricular assist device, replacement only

Q0501 Shower cover for use with electric or electric/pneumatic ventricular assist device, replacement only

Q0502 Mobility cart for pneumatic ventricular assist device, replacement only

Q0503 Battery for pneumatic ventricular assist device, replacement only, each

Reasonable useful lifetime is 6 months (CR3931).

⊕ **Q0504** Power adapter for pneumatic ventricular assist device, replacement only, vehicle type ⓑ

⊕ **Q0506** Battery, lithium-ion, for use with electric or electric/pneumatic, ventricular assist device, replacement only ⓑ

Reasonable useful lifetime is 12 months. Add RA for replacement if lost, stolen, or irreparable damage.

⊕ **Q0507** Miscellaneous supply or accessory for use with an external ventricular assist device ⓑ

⊕ **Q0508** Miscellaneous supply or accessory for use with an implanted ventricular assist device ⓑ

⊕ **Q0509** Miscellaneous supply or accessory for use with any implanted ventricular assist device for which payment was not made under Medicare Part A ⓑ

Fee, Pharmacy

⊕ **Q0510** Pharmacy supply fee for initial immunosuppressive drug(s), first month following transplant ⓑ

⊕ **Q0511** Pharmacy supply fee for oral anti-cancer, oral anti-emetic or immunosuppressive drug(s); for the first prescription in a 30-day period ⓑ

⊕ **Q0512** Pharmacy supply fee for oral anti-cancer, oral anti-emetic or immunosuppressive drug(s); for a subsequent prescription in a 30-day period ⓑ

⊕ **Q0513** Pharmacy dispensing fee for inhalation drug(s); per 30 days ⓑ

⊕ **Q0514** Pharmacy dispensing fee for inhalation drug(s); per 90 days ⓑ

⊕ **Q0515** Injection, sermorelin acetate, 1 microgram ⓑ

IOM: 100-02, 15, 50

Lens, Intraocular

⊕ **Q1004** New technology intraocular lens category 4 as defined in Federal Register notice ⓑ

⊕ **Q1005** New technology intraocular lens category 5 as defined in Federal Register notice ⓑ

Solutions and Drugs

⊕ **Q2004** Irrigation solution for treatment of bladder calculi, for example renacidin, per 500 ml ⓑ

IOM: 100-02, 15, 50

Medicare Statute 1861S2B

⊕ **Q2009** Injection, fosphenytoin, 50 mg phenytoin equivalent ⓑ

IOM: 100-02, 15, 50

Medicare Statute 1861S2B

⊕ **Q2017** Injection, teniposide, 50 mg ⓑ

IOM: 100-02, 15, 50

Medicare Statute 1861S2B

⊕ **Q2026** Injection, radiesse, 0.1 ml ⓑ

⊕ **Q2028** Injection, sculptra, 0.5 mg ⓑ

⊕ **Q2034** Influenza virus vaccine, split virus, for intramuscular use (Agriflu) Sipuleucel-t, minimum of 50 million autologous CD54+ cells activated with PAP-GM-CSF, including leukapheresis and all other preparatory procedures, per infusion ⓑ

IOM: 100-02, 15, 50

⊕ **Q2035** Influenza virus vaccine, split virus, when administered to individuals 3 years of age and older, for intramuscular use (Afluria) ⓑ

Preventive service; no deductible

IOM: 100-02, 15, 50

⊕ **Q2036** Influenza virus vaccine, split virus, when administered to individuals 3 years of age and older, for intramuscular use (Flulaval) ⓑ

Preventive service; no deductible

IOM: 100-02, 15, 50

⊕ **Q2037** Influenza virus vaccine, split virus, when administered to individuals 3 years of age and older, for intramuscular use (Fluvirin) ⓑ

Preventive service; no deductible

IOM: 100-02, 15, 50

⊕ **Q2038** Influenza virus vaccine, split virus, when administered to individuals 3 years of age or older, for intramuscular use (Fluzone) ⓑ

Preventive service; no deductible

IOM: 100-02, 15, 50

⊕ **Q2039** Influenza virus vaccine, not otherwise specified ⓑ

Preventive service; no deductible

IOM: 100-02, 15, 50

► New Revised ✔ Reinstated ~~deleted~~ Deleted ⊘ Not covered or valid by Medicare
⊕ Special coverage instructions ✻ Carrier discretion ⓑ Bill local carrier ⓑ Bill DME MAC

⊙ **Q2043** Sipuleucel-T, minimum of 50 million autologous CD54+ cells activated with PAP-GM-CSF, including leukapheresis and all other preparatory procedures, per infusion Ⓑ

* **Q2049** Injection, doxorubicin hydrochloride, liposomal, imported lipodox, 10 mg Ⓑ Ⓓ

Bill local carrier if incident to a physician's service or used in an implanted infusion pump. If other, bill DME MAC.

⊙ **Q2050** Injection, doxorubicin hydrochloride, liposomal, not otherwise specified, 10 mg Ⓑ Ⓓ

Bill local carrier if incident to a physician's service or used in an implanted infusion pump. If other, bill DME MAC.

IOM: 100-02, 15, 50

⊙ **Q2052** Services, supplies and accessories used in the home under the Medicare intravenous immune globulin (IVIG) demonstration

Brachytherapy Radioelements

⊙ **Q3001** Radioelements for brachytherapy, any type, each Ⓑ

IOM: 100-04, 12, 70; 100-04, 13, 20

Telehealth

* **Q3014** Telehealth originating site facility fee Ⓑ

Effective January of each year, the fee for telehealth services is increased by the Medicare Economic Index (MEI). The telehealth originating facility site fee (HCPCS code Q3014) for 2011 was 80 percent of the lesser of the actual charge or $24.10.

Drugs

⊙ **Q3027** Injection, interferon beta-1a, 1 mcg for intramuscular use Ⓑ

NDC: Avonex

IOM: 100-02, 15, 50

⊘ **Q3028** Injection, interferon beta-1a, 1 mcg for subcutaneous use Ⓑ

Test, Skin

⊙ **Q3031** Collagen skin test Ⓑ

IOM: 100-03, 4, 280.1

Supplies, Cast

Q4001-Q4051: Payment on a reasonable charge basis is required for splints, casts by regulations contained in 42 CFR 405.501

* **Q4001** Casting supplies, body cast adult, with or without head, plaster Ⓑ

* **Q4002** Cast supplies, body cast adult, with or without head, fiberglass Ⓑ

* **Q4003** Cast supplies, shoulder cast, adult (11 years +), plaster Ⓑ

* **Q4004** Cast supplies, shoulder cast, adult (11 years +), fiberglass Ⓑ

* **Q4005** Cast supplies, long arm cast, adult (11 years +), plaster Ⓑ

* **Q4006** Cast supplies, long arm cast, adult (11 years +), fiberglass Ⓑ

* **Q4007** Cast supplies, long arm cast, pediatric (0-10 years), plaster Ⓑ

* **Q4008** Cast supplies, long arm cast, pediatric (0-10 years), fiberglass Ⓑ

* **Q4009** Cast supplies, short arm cast, adult (11 years +), plaster Ⓑ

* **Q4010** Cast supplies, short arm cast, adult (11 years +), fiberglass Ⓑ

* **Q4011** Cast supplies, short arm cast, pediatric (0-10 years), plaster Ⓑ

* **Q4012** Cast supplies, short arm cast, pediatric (0-10 years), fiberglass Ⓑ

* **Q4013** Cast supplies, gauntlet cast (includes lower forearm and hand), adult (11 years +), plaster Ⓑ

* **Q4014** Cast supplies, gauntlet cast (includes lower forearm and hand), adult (11 years +), fiberglass Ⓑ

* **Q4015** Cast supplies, gauntlet cast (includes lower forearm and hand), pediatric (0-10 years), plaster Ⓑ

* **Q4016** Cast supplies, gauntlet cast (includes lower forearm and hand), pediatric (0-10 years), fiberglass Ⓑ

* **Q4017** Cast supplies, long arm splint, adult (11 years +), plaster Ⓑ

* **Q4018** Cast supplies, long arm splint, adult (11 years +), fiberglass Ⓑ

* **Q4019** Cast supplies, long arm splint, pediatric (0-10 years), plaster Ⓑ
* **Q4020** Cast supplies, long arm splint, pediatric (0-10 years), fiberglass Ⓑ
* **Q4021** Cast supplies, short arm splint, adult (11 years +), plaster Ⓑ
* **Q4022** Cast supplies, short arm splint, adult (11 years +), fiberglass Ⓑ
* **Q4023** Cast supplies, short arm splint, pediatric (0-10 years), plaster Ⓑ
* **Q4024** Cast supplies, short arm splint, pediatric (0-10 years), fiberglass Ⓑ
* **Q4025** Cast supplies, hip spica (one or both legs), adult (11 years +), plaster Ⓑ
* **Q4026** Cast supplies, hip spica (one or both legs), adult (11 years +), fiberglass Ⓑ
* **Q4027** Cast supplies, hip spica (one or both legs), pediatric (0-10 years), plaster Ⓑ
* **Q4028** Cast supplies, hip spica (one or both legs), pediatric (0-10 years), fiberglass Ⓑ
* **Q4029** Cast supplies, long leg cast, adult (11 years +), plaster Ⓑ
* **Q4030** Cast supplies, long leg cast, adult (11 years +), fiberglass Ⓑ
* **Q4031** Cast supplies, long leg cast, pediatric (0-10 years), plaster Ⓑ
* **Q4032** Cast supplies, long leg cast, pediatric (0-10 years), fiberglass Ⓑ
* **Q4033** Cast supplies, long leg cylinder cast, adult (11 years +), plaster Ⓑ
* **Q4034** Cast supplies, long leg cylinder cast, adult (11 years +), fiberglass Ⓑ
* **Q4035** Cast supplies, long leg cylinder cast, pediatric (0-10 years), plaster Ⓑ
* **Q4036** Cast supplies, long leg cylinder cast, pediatric (0-10 years), fiberglass Ⓑ
* **Q4037** Cast supplies, short leg cast, adult (11 years +), plaster Ⓑ
* **Q4038** Cast supplies, short leg cast, adult (11 years +), fiberglass Ⓑ
* **Q4039** Cast supplies, short leg cast, pediatric (0-10 years), plaster Ⓑ
* **Q4040** Cast supplies, short leg cast, pediatric (0-10 years), fiberglass Ⓑ
* **Q4041** Cast supplies, long leg splint, adult (11 years +), plaster Ⓑ
* **Q4042** Cast supplies, long leg splint, adult (11 years +), fiberglass Ⓑ
* **Q4043** Cast supplies, long leg splint, pediatric (0-10 years), plaster Ⓑ
* **Q4044** Cast supplies, long leg splint, pediatric (0-10 years), fiberglass Ⓑ
* **Q4045** Cast supplies, short leg splint, adult (11 years +), plaster Ⓑ
* **Q4046** Cast supplies, short leg splint, adult (11 years +), fiberglass Ⓑ
* **Q4047** Cast supplies, short leg splint, pediatric (0-10 years), plaster Ⓑ
* **Q4048** Cast supplies, short leg splint, pediatric (0-10 years), fiberglass Ⓑ
* **Q4049** Finger splint, static Ⓑ
* **Q4050** Cast supplies, for unlisted types and materials of casts Ⓑ
* **Q4051** Splint supplies, miscellaneous (includes thermoplastics, strapping, fasteners, padding and other supplies) Ⓑ

Drugs

* **Q4074** Iloprost, inhalation solution, FDA-approved final product, non-compounded, administered through DME, unit dose form, up to 20 micrograms Ⓑ Ⓑ

Bill Local Carrier if incident to a physician's service. If other, bill DME MAC.

NDC: Ventavis

⚙ **Q4081** Injection, epoetin alfa, 100 units (for ESRD on dialysis) Ⓑ

NDC: Epogen, Procrit

* **Q4082** Drug or biological, not otherwise classified, Part B drug competitive acquisition program (CAP) Ⓑ

Skin Substitutes

* **Q4100** Skin substitute, not otherwise specified Ⓑ

Other: Surgimend collagen matrix

* **Q4101** Apligraf, per square centimeter Ⓑ
* **Q4102** Oasis Wound Matrix, per square centimeter Ⓑ
* **Q4103** Oasis Burn Matrix, per square centimeter Ⓑ
* **Q4104** Integra Bilayer Matrix Wound Dressing (BMWD), per square centimeter Ⓑ

▶ New   Revised   ✔ Reinstated   ~~deleted~~ Deleted   ⊘ Not covered or valid by Medicare
⚙ Special coverage instructions   * Carrier discretion   Ⓑ Bill local carrier   Ⓑ Bill DME MAC

↩ * **Q4105** Integra Dermal Regeneration Template (DRT) or integra omnigraft dermal regeneration matrix, per square centimeter Ⓑ

* **Q4106** Dermagraft, per square centimeter Ⓑ

* **Q4107** Graftjacket, per square centimeter Ⓑ

  NDC: Graftjacket Maxstrip, Graftjacket Small Ligament Repair Matrix, Graftjacket STD, Handjacket Scaffold Thin, Maxforce Thick, Ulcerjacket Scaffold, Ultra Maxforce

* **Q4108** Integra Matrix, per square centimeter Ⓑ

* **Q4110** Primatrix, per square centimeter Ⓑ

* **Q4111** GammaGraft, per square centimeter Ⓑ

* **Q4112** Cymetra, injectable, 1 cc Ⓑ

* **Q4113** GraftJacket Xpress, injectable, 1 cc Ⓑ

* **Q4114** Integra Flowable Wound Matrix, injectable, 1 cc Ⓑ

* **Q4115** Alloskin, per square centimeter Ⓑ

* **Q4116** Alloderm, per square centimeter Ⓑ

* **Q4117** Hyalomatrix, per square centimeter Ⓑ

  IOM: 100-02, 15, 50

* **Q4118** Matristem micromatrix, 1 mg Ⓑ

~~Q4119 Matristem wound matrix, per square centimeter~~ ✖

~~Q4120 Matristem burn matrix, per square centimeter~~ ✖

* **Q4121** Theraskin, per square centimeter Ⓑ

* **Q4122** Dermacell, per square centimeter Ⓑ

* **Q4123** AlloSkin RT, per square centimeter Ⓑ

* **Q4124** Oasis Ultra Tri-layer Wound Matrix, per square centimeter Ⓑ

* **Q4125** Arthroflex, per square centimeter Ⓑ

* **Q4126** Memoderm, dermaspan, tranzgraft or integuply, per square centimeter Ⓑ

* **Q4127** Talymed, per square centimeter Ⓑ

* **Q4128** FlexHD, Allopatch HD, or Matrix HD, per square centimeter Ⓑ

~~Q4129 Unite Biomatrix, per square centimeter~~ ✖

* **Q4130** Strattice TM, per square centimeter Ⓑ

↩ * **Q4131** Epifix or epicord, per square centimeter Ⓑ

* **Q4132** Grafix core, per square centimeter Ⓑ

* **Q4133** Grafix prime, per square centimeter Ⓑ

* **Q4134** Hmatrix, per square centimeter Ⓑ

* **Q4135** Mediskin, per square centimeter Ⓑ

* **Q4136** Ez-derm, per square centimeter Ⓑ

* **Q4137** Amnioexcel or biodexcel, per square centimeter Ⓑ

* **Q4138** Biodfence dryflex, per square centimeter Ⓑ

* **Q4139** Amniomatrix or biodmatrix, injectable, 1 cc Ⓑ

* **Q4140** Biodfence, per square centimeter Ⓑ

* **Q4141** Alloskin ac, per square centimeter Ⓑ

* **Q4142** XCM biologic tissue matrix, per square centimeter Ⓑ

* **Q4143** Repriza, per square centimeter Ⓑ

* **Q4145** Epifix, injectable, 1 mg Ⓑ

* **Q4146** Tensix, per square centimeter Ⓑ

* **Q4147** Architect, architect PX, or architect FX, extracellular matrix, per square centimeter Ⓑ

* **Q4148** Neox 1k, per square centimeter Ⓑ

* **Q4149** Excellagen, 0.1 cc Ⓑ

* **Q4150** AlloWrap DS or dry, per square centimeter Ⓑ

* **Q4151** Amnioband or guardian, per square centimeter Ⓑ

* **Q4152** DermaPure, per square centimeter Ⓑ

* **Q4153** Dermavest and Plurivest, per square centimeter Ⓑ

* **Q4154** Biovance, per square centimeter Ⓑ

* **Q4155** Neoxflo or clarixflo, 1 mg Ⓑ

* **Q4156** Neox 100, per square centimeter Ⓑ

* **Q4157** Revitalon, per square centimeter Ⓑ

* **Q4158** Marigen, per square centimeter Ⓑ

* **Q4159** Affinity, per square centimeter Ⓑ

* **Q4160** Nushield, per square centimeter Ⓑ

* **Q4161** Bio-ConneKt Wound Matrix, per square centimeter Ⓑ

* **Q4162** Amniopro flow, BioSkin flow, BioRenew flow, WoundEx flow, AmnioGen-A, AmnioGen-C, 0.5 cc Ⓑ

* **Q4163** Amniopro, BioSkin, BioRenew, WoundEx, AmnioGen-45, AmnioGen-200, per square centimeter Ⓑ

* **Q4164** Helicoll, per square centimeter Ⓑ

* **Q4165** Keramatrix, per square centimeter Ⓑ

▶ * **Q4166** Cytal, per square centimeter

▶ * **Q4167** Truskin, per square centimeter

▶ * **Q4168** Amnioband, 1 mg

▶ * **Q4169** Artacent wound, per square centimeter

▶ * **Q4170** Cygnus, per square centimeter

▶ * **Q4171** Interfyl, 1 mg

▶ New ↩ Revised ✔ Reinstated ~~deleted~~ Deleted ⦸ Not covered or valid by Medicare
⊛ Special coverage instructions * Carrier discretion Ⓑ Bill local carrier Ⓓ Bill DME MAC

▶ * **Q4172** PuraPly or PuraPly AM, per square centimeter

▶ * **Q4173** PalinGen or PalinGen XPlus, per square centimeter

▶ * **Q4174** PalinGen or ProMatrX, 0.36 mg per 0.25 cc

▶ * **Q4175** Miroderm, per square centimeter

Hospice Care

Q5001 Hospice or home health care provided in patient's home/residence

Q5002 Hospice or home health care provided in assisted living facility

Q5003 Hospice care provided in nursing long term care facility (LTC) or non-skilled nursing facility (NF)

Q5004 Hospice care provided in skilled nursing facility (SNF)

Q5005 Hospice care provided in inpatient hospital

Q5006 Hospice care provided in inpatient hospice facility

Hospice care provided in an inpatient hospice facility. These are residential facilities, which are places for patients to live while receiving routine home care or continuous home care. These hospice residential facilities are not certified by Medicare or Medicaid for provision of General Inpatient (GIP) or respite care, and regulations at 42 CFR 418.202(e) do not allow provision of GIP or respite care at hospice residential facilities.

Q5007 Hospice care provided in long term care facility

Q5008 Hospice care provided in inpatient psychiatric facility

Q5009 Hospice or home health care provided in place not otherwise specified (NOS)

Q5010 Hospice home care provided in a hospice facility

Miscellaneous

Q5101 Injection, filgrastim (G-CSF), biosimilar, 1 microgram

Bill Local Carrier if incident to a physician's service or used in an implanted infusion pump. If other, bill DME MAC.

NDC: Zarxio

▶ **Q5102** Injection, infliximab, biosimilar, 10 mg

IOM: 100-02, 15, 50

* **Q9950** Injection, sulfur hexafluoride lipid microspheres, per ml

NDC: Lumason

Contrast

Q9951 Low osmolar contrast material, 400 or greater mg/ml iodine concentration, per ml

IOM: 100-04, 12, 70; 100-04, 13, 20; 100-04, 13, 90

Q9953 Injection, iron-based magnetic resonance contrast agent, per ml

IOM: 100-04, 12, 70; 100-04, 13, 20; 100-04, 13, 90

Q9954 Oral magnetic resonance contrast agent, per 100 ml

IOM: 100-04, 12, 70; 100-04, 13, 20; 100-04, 13, 90

* **Q9955** Injection, perflexane lipid microspheres, per ml

* **Q9956** Injection, octafluoropropane microspheres, per ml

NDC: Optison

* **Q9957** Injection, perflutren lipid microspheres, per ml

NDC: Definity

Q9958 High osmolar contrast material, up to 149 mg/ml iodine concentration, per ml

NDC: Conray 30, Cysto-Conray II, Cystografin, Cystografin-Dilute, Reno-Dip

IOM: 100-04, 12, 70; 100-04, 13, 20; 100-04, 13, 90

Q9959 High osmolar contrast material, 150-199 mg/ml iodine concentration, per ml

IOM: 100-04, 12, 70; 100-04, 13, 20; 100-04, 13, 90

Q9960 High osmolar contrast material, 200-249 mg/ml iodine concentration, per ml

NDC: Conray 43

IOM: 100-04, 12, 70; 100-04, 13, 20; 100-04, 13, 90

Q9961 High osmolar contrast material, 250-299 mg/ml iodine concentration, per ml

NDC: Conray, Cholografin Meglumine

IOM: 100-04, 12, 70; 100-04, 13, 20; 100-04, 13, 90

Q9962 High osmolar contrast material, 300-349 mg/ml iodine concentration, per ml

IOM: 100-04, 12, 70; 100-04, 13, 20; 100-04, 13, 90

Q9963 High osmolar contrast material, 350-399 mg/ml iodine concentration, per ml

NDC: Gastrografin, Md-76R, Md Gastroview, Sinografin

IOM: 100-04, 12, 70; 100-04, 13, 20; 100-04, 13, 90

Q9964 High osmolar contrast material, 400 or greater mg/ml iodine concentration, per ml

IOM: 100-04, 12, 70; 100-04, 13, 20; 100-04, 13, 90

Q9965 Low osmolar contrast material, 100-199 mg/ml iodine concentration, per ml

NDC: Omnipaque, Ultravist 150

IOM: 100-04, 12, 70; 100-04, 13, 20; 100-04, 13, 90

Q9966 Low osmolar contrast material, 200-299 mg/ml iodine concentration, per ml

NDC: Isovue, Omnipaque, Optiray, Ultravist 240, Visipaque

IOM: 100-04, 12, 70; 100-04, 13, 20; 100-04, 13, 90

Q9967 Low osmolar contrast material, 300-399 mg/ml iodine concentration, per ml

NDC: Hexabrix 320, Isovue-300, Isovue-370, Omnipaque 300, Omnipaque 350, Optiray, Oxilan, Ultravist 300, Ultravist 370, Vispaque

IOM: 100-04, 12, 70; 100-04, 13, 20; 100-04, 13, 90

* **Q9968** Injection, non-radioactive, non-contrast, visualization adjunct (e.g., Methylene Blue, Isosulfan Blue), 1 mg

Q9969 Tc-99m from non-highly enriched uranium source, full cost recovery add-on, per study dose

~~Q9980 Hyaluronan or derivative, GenVisc 850, for intra-articular injection, 1 mg~~

~~Q9981 Rolapitant, oral, 1 mg~~

Cross Reference J8670

▶ **Q9982** Flutemetamol F18, diagnostic, per study dose, up to 5 millicuries

▶ **Q9983** Florbetaben F18, diagnostic, per study dose, up to 8.1 millicuries

▶ New ↩ Revised ✔ Reinstated ~~deleted~~ Deleted ⊘ Not covered or valid by Medicare
Special coverage instructions * Carrier discretion Bill local carrier Bill DME MAC

DIAGNOSTIC RADIOLOGY SERVICES (R0000-R9999)

Transportation/Setup of Portable Equipment

R0070 Transportation of portable x-ray equipment and personnel to home or nursing home, per trip to facility or location, one patient seen

CMS Transmittal B03-049; specific instructions to contractors on pricing

IOM: 100-04, 13, 90; 100-04, 13, 90.3

R0075 Transportation of portable x-ray equipment and personnel to home or nursing home, per trip to facility or location, more than one patient seen

This code would not apply to the x-ray equipment if stored at the location where the x-ray was performed (e.g., a nursing home).

IOM: 100-04, 13, 90; 100-04, 13, 90.3

R0076 Transportation of portable ECG to facility or location, per patient

EKG procedure code 93000 or 93005 must be submitted on same claim as transportation code. Bundled status on physician fee schedule.

IOM: 100-01, 5, 90.2; 100-02, 15, 80; 100-03, 1, 20.15; 100-04, 13, 90; 100-04, 16, 10; 100-04, 16, 110.4

These codes are for transportation of portable X-ray and/or EKG equipment.

(non-medical)

TEMPORARY NATIONAL CODES ESTABLISHED BY PRIVATE PAYERS (S0000-S9999)

Note: Medicare and other federal payers do not recognize "S" codes; however, S codes may be useful for claims to some private insurers.

- ⃠ **S0012** Butorphanol tartrate, nasal spray, 25 mg
- ⃠ **S0014** Tacrine hydrochloride, 10 mg
- ⃠ **S0017** Injection, aminocaproic acid, 5 grams
- ⃠ **S0020** Injection, bupivacaine hydrochloride, 30 ml
- ⃠ **S0021** Injection, cefoperazone sodium, 1 gram
- ⃠ **S0023** Injection, cimetidine hydrochloride, 300 mg
- ⃠ **S0028** Injection, famotidine, 20 mg
- ⃠ **S0030** Injection, metronidazole, 500 mg
- ⃠ **S0032** Injection, nafcillin sodium, 2 grams
- ⃠ **S0034** Injection, ofloxacin, 400 mg
- ⃠ **S0039** Injection, sulfamethoxazole and trimethoprim, 10 ml
- ⃠ **S0040** Injection, ticarcillin disodium and clavulanate potassium, 3.1 grams
- ⃠ **S0073** Injection, aztreonam, 500 mg

  Other: Cayston
- ⃠ **S0074** Injection, cefotetan disodium, 500 mg
- ⃠ **S0077** Injection, clindamycin phosphate, 300 mg
- ⃠ **S0078** Injection, fosphenytoin sodium, 750 mg
- ⃠ **S0080** Injection, pentamidine isethionate, 300 mg
- ⃠ **S0081** Injection, piperacillin sodium, 500 mg
- ⃠ **S0088** Imatinib, 100 mg
- ⃠ **S0090** Sildenafil citrate, 25 mg
- ⃠ **S0091** Granisetron hydrochloride, 1 mg (for circumstances falling under the Medicare Statute, use Q0166)
- ⃠ **S0092** Injection, hydromorphone hydrochloride, 250 mg (loading dose for infusion pump)
- ⃠ **S0093** Injection, morphine sulfate, 500 mg (loading dose for infusion pump)
- ⃠ **S0104** Zidovudine, oral, 100 mg
- ⃠ **S0106** Bupropion HCl sustained release tablet, 150 mg, per bottle of 60 tablets
- ⃠ **S0108** Mercaptopurine, oral, 50 mg
- ⃠ **S0109** Methadone, oral, 5 mg
- ⃠ **S0117** Tretinoin, topical, 5 grams
- ⃠ **S0119** Ondansetron, oral, 4 mg (for circumstances falling under the medicare statute, use HCPCS Q code)
- ⃠ **S0122** Injection, menotropins, 75 IU
- ⃠ **S0126** Injection, follitropin alfa, 75 IU
- ⃠ **S0128** Injection, follitropin beta, 75 IU
- ⃠ **S0132** Injection, ganirelix acetate, 250 mcg
- ⃠ **S0136** Clozapine, 25 mg
- ⃠ **S0137** Didanosine (DDI), 25 mg
- ⃠ **S0138** Finasteride, 5 mg
- ⃠ **S0139** Minoxidil, 10 mg
- ⃠ **S0140** Saquinavir, 200 mg
- ⃠ **S0142** Colistimethate sodium, inhalation solution administered through DME, concentrated form, per mg
- ⃠ **S0145** Injection, pegylated interferon alfa-2a, 180 mcg per ml
- ⃠ **S0148** Injection, pegylated interferon ALFA-2b, 10 mcg
- ⃠ **S0155** Sterile dilutant for epoprostenol, 50 ml
- ⃠ **S0156** Exemestane, 25 mg
- ⃠ **S0157** Becaplermin gel 0.01%, 0.5 gm
- ⃠ **S0160** Dextroamphetamine sulfate, 5 mg
- ⃠ **S0164** Injection, pantoprazole sodium, 40 mg
- ⃠ **S0166** Injection, olanzapine, 2.5 mg
- ⃠ **S0169** Calcitrol, 0.25 microgram
- ⃠ **S0170** Anastrozole, oral, 1 mg
- ⃠ **S0171** Injection, bumetanide, 0.5 mg
- ⃠ **S0172** Chlorambucil, oral, 2 mg
- ⃠ **S0174** Dolasetron mesylate, oral 50 mg (for circumstances falling under the Medicare Statute, use Q0180)
- ⃠ **S0175** Flutamide, oral, 125 mg
- ⃠ **S0176** Hydroxyurea, oral, 500 mg
- ⃠ **S0177** Levamisole hydrochloride, oral, 50 mg
- ⃠ **S0178** Lomustine, oral, 10 mg
- ⃠ **S0179** Megestrol acetate, oral, 20 mg
- ⃠ **S0182** Procarbazine hydrochloride, oral, 50 mg
- ⃠ **S0183** Prochlorperazine maleate, oral, 5 mg (for circumstances falling under the Medicare Statute, use Q0164)
- ⃠ **S0187** Tamoxifen citrate, oral, 10 mg
- ⃠ **S0189** Testosterone pellet, 75 mg
- ⃠ **S0190** Mifepristone, oral, 200 mg
- ⃠ **S0191** Misoprostol, oral 200 mcg
- ⃠ **S0194** Dialysis/stress vitamin supplement, oral, 100 capsules

USED for Private Payers & Medicaid. NOT MEDICARE

⊘ **S0197** Prenatal vitamins, 30-day supply

⊘ **S0199** Medically induced abortion by oral ingestion of medication including all associated services and supplies (e.g., patient counseling, office visits, confirmation of pregnancy by HCG, ultrasound to confirm duration of pregnancy, ultrasound to confirm completion of abortion) except drugs

⊘ **S0201** Partial hospitalization services, less than 24 hours, per diem

⊘ **S0207** Paramedic intercept, non-hospital-based ALS service (non-voluntary), non-transport

⊘ **S0208** Paramedic intercept, hospital-based ALS service (non-voluntary), non-transport

⊘ **S0209** Wheelchair van, mileage, per mile

⊘ **S0215** Non-emergency transportation; mileage per mile

⊘ **S0220** Medical conference by a physician with interdisciplinary team of health professionals or representatives of community agencies to coordinate activities of patient care (patient is present); approximately 30 minutes

⊘ **S0221** Medical conference by a physician with interdisciplinary team of health professionals or representatives of community agencies to coordinate activities of patient care (patient is present); approximately 60 minutes

⊘ **S0250** Comprehensive geriatric assessment and treatment planning performed by assessment team

⊘ **S0255** Hospice referral visit (advising patient and family of care options) performed by nurse, social worker, or other designated staff

⊘ **S0257** Counseling and discussion regarding advance directives or end of life care planning and decisions, with patient and/or surrogate (list separately in addition to code for appropriate evaluation and management service)

⊘ **S0260** History and physical (outpatient or office) related to surgical procedure (list separately in addition to code for appropriate evaluation and management service)

⊘ **S0265** Genetic counseling, under physician supervision, each 15 minutes

⊘ **S0270** Physician management of patient home care, standard monthly case rate (per 30 days)

⊘ **S0271** Physician management of patient home care, hospice monthly case rate (per 30 days)

⊘ **S0272** Physician management of patient home care, episodic care monthly case rate (per 30 days)

⊘ **S0273** Physician visit at member s home, outside of a capitation arrangement

⊘ **S0274** Nurse practitioner visit at member s home, outside of a capitation arrangement

⊘ **S0280** Medical home program, comprehensive care coordination and planning, initial plan

⊘ **S0281** Medical home program, comprehensive care coordination and planning, maintenance of plan

▶ ⊘ **S0285** Colonoscopy consultation performed prior to a screening colonoscopy procedure

⊘ **S0302** Completed Early Periodic Screening Diagnosis and Treatment (EPSDT) service (list in addition to code for appropriate evaluation and management service)

⊘ **S0310** Hospitalist services (list separately in addition to code for appropriate evaluation and management service)

▶ ⊘ **S0311** Comprehensive management and care coordination for advanced illness, per calendar month

⊘ **S0315** Disease management program; initial assessment and initiation of the program

⊘ **S0316** Disease management program; follow-up/reassessment

⊘ **S0317** Disease management program; per diem

⊘ **S0320** Telephone calls by a registered nurse to a disease management program member for monitoring purposes; per month

⊘ **S0340** Lifestyle modification program for management of coronary artery disease, including all supportive services; first quarter/stage

⊘ **S0341** Lifestyle modification program for management of coronary artery disease, including all supportive services; second or third quarter/stage

⊘ **S0342** Lifestyle modification program for management of coronary artery disease, including all supportive services; fourth quarter/stage

⃠ **S0353** Treatment planning and care coordination management for cancer, initial treatment

⃠ **S0354** Treatment planning and care coordination management for cancer, established patient with a change of regimen

⃠ **S0390** Routine foot care; removal and/or trimming of corns, calluses and/or nails and preventive maintenance in specific medical conditions (e.g., diabetes), per visit

⃠ **S0395** Impression casting of a foot performed by a practitioner other than the manufacturer of the orthotic

⃠ **S0400** Global fee for extracorporeal shock wave lithotripsy treatment of kidney stone(s)

⃠ **S0500** Disposable contact lens, per lens

⃠ **S0504** Single vision prescription lens (safety, athletic, or sunglass), per lens

⃠ **S0506** Bifocal vision prescription lens (safety, athletic, or sunglass), per lens

⃠ **S0508** Trifocal vision prescription lens (safety, athletic, or sunglass), per lens

⃠ **S0510** Non-prescription lens (safety, athletic, or sunglass), per lens

⃠ **S0512** Daily wear specialty contact lens, per lens

⃠ **S0514** Color contact lens, per lens

⃠ **S0515** Scleral lens, liquid bandage device, per lens

⃠ **S0516** Safety eyeglass frames

⃠ **S0518** Sunglasses frames

⃠ **S0580** Polycarbonate lens (list this code in addition to the basic code for the lens)

⃠ **S0581** Nonstandard lens (list this code in addition to the basic code for the lens)

⃠ **S0590** Integral lens service, miscellaneous services reported separately

⃠ **S0592** Comprehensive contact lens evaluation

⃠ **S0595** Dispensing new spectacle lenses for patient supplied frame

⃠ **S0596** Phakic intraocular lens for correction of refractive error

⃠ **S0601** Screening proctoscopy

⃠ **S0610** Annual gynecological examination, new patient

⃠ **S0612** Annual gynecological examination, established patient

⃠ **S0613** Annual gynecological examination; clinical breast examination without pelvic evaluation

⃠ **S0618** Audiometry for hearing aid evaluation to determine the level and degree of hearing loss

⃠ **S0620** Routine ophthalmological examination including refraction; new patient

Many non-Medicare vision plans may require code for routine encounter, no complaints.

⃠ **S0621** Routine ophthalmological examination including refraction; established patient

Many non-Medicare vision plans may require code for routine encounter, no complaints.

⃠ **S0622** Physical exam for college, new or established patient (list separately) in addition to appropriate evaluation and management code

⃠ **S0630** Removal of sutures; by a physician other than the physician who originally closed the wound

⃠ **S0800** Laser in situ keratomileusis (LASIK)

⃠ **S0810** Photorefractive keratectomy (PRK)

⃠ **S0812** Phototherapeutic keratectomy (PTK)

⃠ **S1001** Deluxe item, patient aware (list in addition to code for basic item)

⃠ **S1002** Customized item (list in addition to code for basic item)

⃠ **S1015** IV tubing extension set

⃠ **S1016** Non-PVC (polyvinyl chloride) intravenous administration set, for use with drugs that are not stable in PVC e.g., paclitaxel

⃠ **S1030** Continuous noninvasive glucose monitoring device, purchase (for physician interpretation of data, use CPT code)

⃠ **S1031** Continuous noninvasive glucose monitoring device, rental, including sensor, sensor replacement, and download to monitor (for physician interpretation of data, use CPT code)

⃠ **S1034** Artificial pancreas device system (e.g., low glucose suspend (LGS) feature) including continuous glucose monitor, blood glucose device, insulin pump and computer algorithm that communicates with all of the devices

⃠ **S1035** Sensor; invasive (e.g., subcutaneous), disposable, for use with artificial pancreas device system

⃠ **S1036** Transmitter; external, for use with artificial pancreas device system

⃠ **S1037** Receiver (monitor); external, for use with artificial pancreas device system

⊘ **S1040** Cranial remolding orthosis, pediatric, rigid, with soft interface material, custom fabricated, includes fitting and adjustment(s)

⊘ **S1090** Mometasone furoate sinus implant, 370 micrograms

⊘ **S2053** Transplantation of small intestine and liver allografts

⊘ **S2054** Transplantation of multivisceral organs

⊘ **S2055** Harvesting of donor multivisceral organs, with preparation and maintenance of allografts; from cadaver donor

⊘ **S2060** Lobar lung transplantation

⊘ **S2061** Donor lobectomy (lung) for transplantation, living donor

⊘ **S2065** Simultaneous pancreas kidney transplantation

⊘ **S2066** Breast reconstruction with gluteal artery perforator (GAP) flap, including harvesting of the flap, microvascular transfer, closure of donor site and shaping the flap into a breast, unilateral

⊘ **S2067** Breast reconstruction of a single breast with "stacked" deep inferior epigastric perforator (DIEP) flap(s) and/or gluteal artery perforator (GAP) flap(s), including harvesting of the flap(s), microvascular transfer, closure of donor site(s) and shaping the flap into a breast, unilateral

⊘ **S2068** Breast reconstruction with deep inferior epigastric perforator (DIEP) flap, or superficial inferior epigastric artery (SIEA) flap, including harvesting of the flap, microvascular transfer, closure of donor site and shaping the flap into a breast, unilateral

⊘ **S2070** Cystourethroscopy, with ureteroscopy and/or pyeloscopy; with endoscopic laser treatment of ureteral calculi (includes ureteral catheterization)

⊘ **S2079** Laparoscopic esophagomyotomy (Heller type)

⊘ **S2080** Laser-assisted uvulopalatoplasty (LAUP)

⊘ **S2083** Adjustment of gastric band diameter via subcutaneous port by injection or aspiration of saline

⊘ **S2095** Transcatheter occlusion or embolization for tumor destruction, percutaneous, any method, using yttrium-90 microspheres

⊘ **S2102** Islet cell tissue transplant from pancreas; allogeneic

⊘ **S2103** Adrenal tissue transplant to brain

⊘ **S2107** Adoptive immunotherapy i.e. development of specifi c anti-tumor reactivity (e.g., tumor-infiltrating lymphocyte therapy) per course of treatment

⊘ **S2112** Arthroscopy, knee, surgical for harvesting of cartilage (chondrocyte cells)

⊘ **S2115** Osteotomy, periacetabular, with internal fixation

⊘ **S2117** Arthroereisis, subtalar

⊘ **S2118** Metal-on-metal total hip resurfacing, including acetabular and femoral components

⊘ **S2120** Low density lipoprotein (LDL) apheresis using heparin-induced extracorporeal LDL precipitation

⊘ **S2140** Cord blood harvesting for transplantation, allogeneic

⊘ **S2142** Cord blood-derived stem cell transplantation, allogeneic

⊘ **S2150** Bone marrow or blood-derived stem cells (peripheral or umbilical), allogeneic or autologous, harvesting, transplantation, and related complications; including: pheresis and cell preparation/storage; marrow ablative therapy; drugs, supplies, hospitalization with outpatient follow-up; medical/surgical, diagnostic, emergency, and rehabilitative services; and the number of days of pre- and post-transplant care in the global definition

⊘ **S2152** Solid organ(s), complete or segmental, single organ or combination of organs; deceased or living donor(s), procurement, transplantation, and related complications; including: drugs; supplies; hospitalization with outpatient follow-up; medical/ surgical, diagnostic, emergency, and rehabilitative services, and the number of days of pre- and post-transplant care in the global definition

⊘ **S2202** Echosclerotherapy

⊘ **S2205** Minimally invasive direct coronary artery bypass surgery involving mini-thoracotomy or mini-sternotomy surgery, performed under direct vision; using arterial graft(s), single coronary arterial graft

⊘ **S2206** Minimally invasive direct coronary artery bypass surgery involving mini-thoracotomy or mini-sternotomy surgery, performed under direct vision; using arterial graft(s), two coronary arterial grafts

⊘ **S2207** Minimally invasive direct coronary artery bypass surgery involving mini-thoracotomy or mini-sternotomy surgery, performed under direct vision; using venous graft only, single coronary venous graft

⊘ **S2208** Minimally invasive direct coronary artery bypass surgery involving mini-thoracotomy or mini-sternotomy surgery, performed under direct vision; using single arterial and venous graft(s), single venous graft

⊘ **S2209** Minimally invasive direct coronary artery bypass surgery involving mini-thoracotomy or mini-sternotomy surgery, performed under direct vision; using two arterial grafts and single venous graft

⊘ **S2225** Myringotomy, laser-assisted

⊘ **S2230** Implantation of magnetic component of semi-implantable hearing device on ossicles in middle ear

⊘ **S2235** Implantation of auditory brain stem implant

⊘ **S2260** Induced abortion, 17 to 24 weeks

⊘ **S2265** Induced abortion, 25 to 28 weeks

⊘ **S2266** Induced abortion, 29 to 31 weeks

⊘ **S2267** Induced abortion, 32 weeks or greater

⊘ **S2300** Arthroscopy, shoulder, surgical; with thermally-induced capsulorrhaphy

⊘ **S2325** Hip core decompression

⊘ **S2340** Chemodenervation of abductor muscle(s) of vocal cord

⊘ **S2341** Chemodenervation of adductor muscle(s) of vocal cord

⊘ **S2342** Nasal endoscopy for post-operative debridement following functional endoscopic sinus surgery, nasal and/or sinus cavity(s), unilateral or bilateral

⊘ **S2348** Decompression procedure, percutaneous, of nucleus pulpous of intervertebral disc, using radiofrequency energy, single or multiple levels, lumbar

⊘ **S2350** Diskectomy, anterior, with decompression of spinal cord and/or nerve root(s), including osteophytectomy; lumbar, single interspace

⊘ **S2351** Diskectomy, anterior, with decompression of spinal cord and/or nerve root(s) including osteophytectomy; lumbar, each additional interspace (list separately in addition to code for primary procedure)

⊘ **S2400** Repair, congenital diaphragmatic hernia in the fetus using temporary tracheal occlusion, procedure performed in utero

⊘ **S2401** Repair, urinary tract obstruction in the fetus, procedure performed in utero

⊘ **S2402** Repair, congenital cystic adenomatoid malformation in the fetus, procedure performed in utero

⊘ **S2403** Repair, extralobar pulmonary sequestration in the fetus, procedure performed in utero

⊘ **S2404** Repair, myelomeningocele in the fetus, procedure performed in utero

⊘ **S2405** Repair of sacrococcygeal teratoma in the fetus, procedure performed in utero

⊘ **S2409** Repair, congenital malformation of fetus, procedure performed in utero, not otherwise classified

⊘ **S2411** Fetoscopic laser therapy for treatment of twin-to-twin transfusion syndrome

⊘ **S2900** Surgical techniques requiring use of robotic surgical system (list separately in addition to code for primary procedure)

⊘ **S3000** Diabetic indicator; retinal eye exam, dilated, bilateral

⊘ **S3005** Performance measurement, evaluation of patient self assessment, depression

⊘ **S3600** STAT laboratory request (situations other than S3601)

⊘ **S3601** Emergency STAT laboratory charge for patient who is homebound or residing in a nursing facility

✪ **S3620** Newborn metabolic screening panel, includes test kit, postage and the laboratory tests specified by the state for inclusion in this panel (e.g., galactose; hemoglobin, electrophoresis; hydroxyprogesterone, 17-D; phenylalanine (PKU); and thyroxine, total)

⊘ **S3630** Eosinophil count, blood, direct

⊘ **S3645** HIV-1 antibody testing of oral mucosal transudate

⊘ **S3650** Saliva test, hormone level; during menopause

⊘ **S3652** Saliva test, hormone level; to assess preterm labor risk

▶ New ↩ Revised ✔ Reinstated ~~deleted~~ Deleted ⊘ Not covered or valid by Medicare
✪ Special coverage instructions ✻ Carrier discretion Ⓑ Bill local carrier Ⓓ Bill DME MAC

⊘ **S3655** Antisperm antibodies test (immunobead)

⊘ **S3708** Gastrointestinal fat absorption study

⊘ **S3722** Dose optimization by area under the curve (AUC) analysis, for infusional 5-fluorouracil

⊘ **S3800** Genetic testing for amyotrophic lateral sclerosis (ALS)

⊘ **S3840** DNA analysis for germline mutations of the RET proto-oncogene for susceptibility to multiple endocrine neoplasia type 2

⊘ **S3841** Genetic testing for retinoblastoma

⊘ **S3842** Genetic testing for von Hippel-Lindau disease

⊘ **S3844** DNA analysis of the connexin 26 gene (GJB2) for susceptibility to congenital, profound deafness

⊘ **S3845** Genetic testing for alpha-thalassemia

⊘ **S3846** Genetic testing for hemoglobin E beta-thalassemia

⊘ **S3849** Genetic testing for Niemann-Pick disease

⊘ **S3850** Genetic testing for sickle cell anemia

⊘ **S3852** DNA analysis for APOE epilson 4 allele for susceptibility to Alzheimer s disease

⊘ **S3853** Genetic testing for myotonic muscular dystrophy

✔⊘ **S3854** Gene expression profiling panel for use in the management of breast-cancer treatment

⊘ **S3861** Genetic testing, sodium channel, voltage-gated, type V, alpha subunit (SCN5A) and variants for suspected Brugada syndrome

⊘ **S3865** Comprehensive gene sequence analysis for hypertrophic cardiomyopathy

⊘ **S3866** Genetic analysis for a specific gene mutation for hypertrophic cardiomyopathy (HCM) in an individual with a known HCM mutation in the family

⊘ **S3870** Comparative genomic hybridization (CGH) microarray testing for developmental delay, autism spectrum disorder and/or intellectual disability

⊘ **S3900** Surface electromyography (EMG)

⊘ **S3902** Ballistrocardiogram

⊘ **S3904** Masters two step

Bill on paper. Requires a report.

⊘ **S4005** Interim labor facility global (labor occurring but not resulting in delivery)

⊘ **S4011** In vitro fertilization; including but not limited to identification and incubation of mature oocytes, fertilization with sperm, incubation of embryo(s), and subsequent visualization for determination of development

⊘ **S4013** Complete cycle, gamete intrafallopian transfer (GIFT), case rate

⊘ **S4014** Complete cycle, zygote intrafallopian transfer (ZIFT), case rate

⊘ **S4015** Complete in vitro fertilization cycle, not otherwise specified, case rate

⊘ **S4016** Frozen in vitro fertilization cycle, case rate

⊘ **S4017** Incomplete cycle, treatment cancelled prior to stimulation, case rate

⊘ **S4018** Frozen embryo transfer procedure cancelled before transfer, case rate

⊘ **S4020** In vitro fertilization procedure cancelled before aspiration, case rate

⊘ **S4021** In vitro fertilization procedure cancelled after aspiration, case rate

⊘ **S4022** Assisted oocyte fertilization, case rate

⊘ **S4023** Donor egg cycle, incomplete, case rate

⊘ **S4025** Donor services for in vitro fertilization (sperm or embryo), case rate

⊘ **S4026** Procurement of donor sperm from sperm bank

⊘ **S4027** Storage of previously frozen embryos

⊘ **S4028** Microsurgical epididymal sperm aspiration (MESA)

⊘ **S4030** Sperm procurement and cryopreservation services; initial visit

⊘ **S4031** Sperm procurement and cryopreservation services; subsequent visit

⊘ **S4035** Stimulated intrauterine insemination (IUI), case rate

⊘ **S4037** Cryopreserved embryo transfer, case rate

⊘ **S4040** Monitoring and storage of cryopreserved embryos, per 30 days

⊘ **S4042** Management of ovulation induction (interpretation of diagnostic tests and studies, non-face-to-face medical management of the patient), per cycle

⊘ **S4981** Insertion of levonorgestrel-releasing intrauterine system

⊘ **S4989** Contraceptive intrauterine device (e.g., Progestasert IUD), including implants and supplies

⊘ **S4990** Nicotine patches, legend

⊘ **S4991** Nicotine patches, non-legend

▶ New ⤾ Revised ✔ Reinstated ~~deleted~~ Deleted ⊘ Not covered or valid by Medicare
Special coverage instructions ✻ Carrier discretion Bill local carrier Bill DME MAC

⊘ **S4993** Contraceptive pills for birth control
Only billed by Family Planning Clinics

⊘ **S4995** Smoking cessation gum

⊘ **S5000** Prescription drug, generic

⊘ **S5001** Prescription drug, brand name

⊘ **S5010** 5% dextrose and 0.45% normal saline, 1000 ml

⊘ **S5012** 5% dextrose with potassium chloride, 1000 ml

⊘ **S5013** 5% dextrose/0.45% normal saline with potassium chloride and magnesium sulfate, 1000 ml

⊘ **S5014** 5% dextrose/0.45% normal saline with potassium chloride and magnesium sulfate, 1500 ml

⊘ **S5035** Home infusion therapy, routine service of infusion device (e.g., pump maintenance)

⊘ **S5036** Home infusion therapy, repair of infusion device (e.g., pump repair)

⊘ **S5100** Day care services, adult; per 15 minutes

⊘ **S5101** Day care services, adult; per half day

⊘ **S5102** Day care services, adult; per diem

⊘ **S5105** Day care services, center-based; services not included in program fee, per diem

⊘ **S5108** Home care training to home care client, per 15 minutes

⊘ **S5109** Home care training to home care client, per session

⊘ **S5110** Home care training, family; per 15 minutes

⊘ **S5111** Home care training, family; per session

⊘ **S5115** Home care training, non-family; per 15 minutes

⊘ **S5116** Home care training, non-family; per session

⊘ **S5120** Chore services; per 15 minutes

⊘ **S5121** Chore services; per diem

⊘ **S5125** Attendant care services; per 15 minutes

⊘ **S5126** Attendant care services; per diem

⊘ **S5130** Homemaker service, NOS; per 15 minutes

⊘ **S5131** Homemaker service, NOS; per diem

⊘ **S5135** Companion care, adult (e.g., IADL/ADL); per 15 minutes

⊘ **S5136** Companion care, adult (e.g., IADL/ADL); per diem

⊘ **S5140** Foster care, adult; per diem

⊘ **S5141** Foster care, adult; per month

⊘ **S5145** Foster care, therapeutic, child; per diem

⊘ **S5146** Foster care, therapeutic, child; per month

⊘ **S5150** Unskilled respite care, not hospice; per 15 minutes

⊘ **S5151** Unskilled respite care, not hospice; per diem

⊘ **S5160** Emergency response system; installation and testing

⊘ **S5161** Emergency response system; service fee, per month (excludes installation and testing)

⊘ **S5162** Emergency response system; purchase only

⊘ **S5165** Home modifications; per service

⊘ **S5170** Home delivered meals, including preparation; per meal

⊘ **S5175** Laundry service, external, professional; per order

⊘ **S5180** Home health respiratory therapy, initial evaluation

⊘ **S5181** Home health respiratory therapy, NOS, per diem

⊘ **S5185** Medication reminder service, non-face-to-face; per month

⊘ **S5190** Wellness assessment, performed by non-physician

⊘ **S5199** Personal care item, NOS, each

⊘ **S5497** Home infusion therapy, catheter care/maintenance, not otherwise classified; includes administrative services, professional pharmacy services, care coordination, and all necessary supplies and equipment (drugs and nursing visits coded separately), per diem

⊘ **S5498** Home infusion therapy, catheter care/maintenance, simple (single lumen), includes administrative services, professional pharmacy services, care coordination and all necessary supplies and equipment, (drugs and nursing visits coded separately), per diem

⊘ **S5501** Home infusion therapy, catheter care/maintenance, complex (more than one lumen), includes administrative services, professional pharmacy services, care coordination, and all necessary supplies and equipment (drugs and nursing visits coded separately), per diem

⦸ **S5502** Home infusion therapy, catheter care/maintenance, implanted access device, includes administrative services, professional pharmacy services, care coordination, and all necessary supplies and equipment, (drugs and nursing visits coded separately), per diem (use this code for interim maintenance of vascular access not currently in use)

⦸ **S5517** Home infusion therapy, all supplies necessary for restoration of catheter patency or declotting

⦸ **S5518** Home infusion therapy, all supplies necessary for catheter repair

⦸ **S5520** Home infusion therapy, all supplies (including catheter) necessary for a peripherally inserted central venous catheter (PICC) line insertion

Bill on paper. Requires a report.

⦸ **S5521** Home infusion therapy, all supplies (including catheter) necessary for a midline catheter insertion

⦸ **S5522** Home infusion therapy, insertion of peripherally inserted central venous catheter (PICC), nursing services only (no supplies or catheter included)

⦸ **S5523** Home infusion therapy, insertion of midline central venous catheter, nursing services only (no supplies or catheter included)

⦸ **S5550** Insulin, rapid onset, 5 units

⦸ **S5551** Insulin, most rapid onset (Lispro or Aspart); 5 units

⦸ **S5552** Insulin, intermediate acting (NPH or Lente); 5 units

⦸ **S5553** Insulin, long acting; 5 units

⦸ **S5560** Insulin delivery device, reusable pen; 1.5 ml size

⦸ **S5561** Insulin delivery device, reusable pen; 3 ml size

⦸ **S5565** Insulin cartridge for use in insulin delivery device other than pump; 150 units

⦸ **S5566** Insulin cartridge for use in insulin delivery device other than pump; 300 units

⦸ **S5570** Insulin delivery device, disposable pen (including insulin); 1.5 ml size

⦸ **S5571** Insulin delivery device, disposable pen (including insulin); 3 ml size

⦸ **S8030** Scleral application of tantalum ring(s) for localization of lesions for proton beam therapy

~~S8032~~ ~~Low-dose computer tomography for lung cancer screening~~ ✖

Cross Reference G0297

⦸ **S8035** Magnetic source imaging

⦸ **S8037** Magnetic resonance cholangiopancreatography (MRCP)

⦸ **S8040** Topographic brain mapping

⦸ **S8042** Magnetic resonance imaging (MRI), low-field

⦸ **S8055** Ultrasound guidance for multifetal pregnancy reduction(s), technical component (only to be used when the physician doing the reduction procedure does not perform the ultrasound, guidance is included in the CPT code for multifetal pregnancy reduction - 59866)

⦸ **S8080** Scintimammography (radioimmunoscintigraphy of the breast), unilateral, including supply of radiopharmaceutical

⦸ **S8085** Fluorine-18 fluorodeoxyglucose (F-18 FDG) imaging using dual-head coincidence detection system (non-dedicated PET scan)

⦸ **S8092** Electron beam computed tomography (also known as ultrafast CT, cine CT)

⦸ **S8096** Portable peak flow meter

⦸ **S8097** Asthma kit (including but not limited to portable peak expiratory flow meter, instructional video, brochure, and/or spacer)

⦸ **S8100** Holding chamber or spacer for use with an inhaler or nebulizer; without mask

⦸ **S8101** Holding chamber or spacer for use with an inhaler or nebulizer; with mask

⦸ **S8110** Peak expiratory flow rate (physician services)

⦸ **S8120** Oxygen contents, gaseous, 1 unit equals 1 cubic foot

⦸ **S8121** Oxygen contents, liquid, 1 unit equals 1 pound

⦸ **S8130** Interferential current stimulator, 2 channel

⦸ **S8131** Interferential current stimulator, 4 channel

⦸ **S8185** Flutter device

⦸ **S8186** Swivel adapter

⦸ **S8189** Tracheostomy supply, not otherwise classified

⦸ **S8210** Mucus trap

⦸ **S8265** Haberman feeder for cleft lip/palate

⃠ **S8270** Enuresis alarm, using auditory buzzer and/or vibration device

⃠ **S8301** Infection control supplies, not otherwise specified

⃠ **S8415** Supplies for home delivery of infant

⃠ **S8420** Gradient pressure aid (sleeve and glove combination), custom made

⃠ **S8421** Gradient pressure aid (sleeve and glove combination), ready made

⃠ **S8422** Gradient pressure aid (sleeve), custom made, medium weight

⃠ **S8423** Gradient pressure aid (sleeve), custom made, heavy weight

⃠ **S8424** Gradient pressure aid (sleeve), ready made

⃠ **S8425** Gradient pressure aid (glove), custom made, medium weight

⃠ **S8426** Gradient pressure aid (glove), custom made, heavy weight

⃠ **S8427** Gradient pressure aid (glove), ready made

⃠ **S8428** Gradient pressure aid (gauntlet), ready made

⃠ **S8429** Gradient pressure exterior wrap

⃠ **S8430** Padding for compression bandage, roll

⃠ **S8431** Compression bandage, roll

⃠ **S8450** Splint, prefabricated, digit (specify digit by use of modifier)

⃠ **S8451** Splint, prefabricated, wrist or ankle

⃠ **S8452** Splint, prefabricated, elbow

⃠ **S8460** Camisole, post-mastectomy

⃠ **S8490** Insulin syringes (100 syringes, any size)

⃠ **S8930** Electrical stimulation of auricular acupuncture points; each 15 minutes of personal one-on-one contact with the patient

⃠ **S8940** Equestrian/Hippotherapy, per session

⃠ **S8948** Application of a modality (requiring constant provider attendance) to one or more areas; low-level laser; each 15 minutes

⃠ **S8950** Complex lymphedema therapy, each 15 minutes

⃠ **S8990** Physical or manipulative therapy performed for maintenance rather than restoration

⃠ **S8999** Resuscitation bag (for use by patient on artificial respiration during power failure or other catastrophic event)

⃠ **S9001** Home uterine monitor with or without associated nursing services

⃠ **S9007** Ultrafiltration monitor

⃠ **S9024** Paranasal sinus ultrasound

⃠ **S9025** Omnicardiogram/cardiointegram

⃠ **S9034** Extracorporeal shockwave lithotripsy for gall stones (if performed with ERCP, use 43265)

⃠ **S9055** Procuren or other growth factor preparation to promote wound healing

⃠ **S9056** Coma stimulation per diem

⃠ **S9061** Home administration of aerosolized drug therapy (e.g., pentamidine); administrative services, professional pharmacy services, care coordination, all necessary supplies and equipment (drugs and nursing visits coded separately), per diem

⃠ **S9083** Global fee urgent care centers

⃠ **S9088** Services provided in an urgent care center (list in addition to code for service)

⃠ **S9090** Vertebral axial decompression, per session

⃠ **S9097** Home visit for wound care

⃠ **S9098** Home visit, phototherapy services (e.g., Bili-Lite), including equipment rental, nursing services, blood draw, supplies, and other services, per diem

⃠ **S9110** Telemonitoring of patient in their home, including all necessary equipment; computer system, connections, and software; maintenance; patient education and support; per month

⃠ **S9117** Back school, per visit

⃠ **S9122** Home health aide or certified nurse assistant, providing care in the home; per hour

⃠ **S9123** Nursing care, in the home; by registered nurse, per hour (use for general nursing care only, not to be used when CPT codes 99500-99602 can be used)

⃠ **S9124** Nursing care, in the home; by licensed practical nurse, per hour

⃠ **S9125** Respite care, in the home, per diem

⃠ **S9126** Hospice care, in the home, per diem

⃠ **S9127** Social work visit, in the home, per diem

⃠ **S9128** Speech therapy, in the home, per diem

⃠ **S9129** Occupational therapy, in the home, per diem

⃠ **S9131** Physical therapy; in the home, per diem

⃠ **S9140** Diabetic management program, follow-up visit to non-MD provider

⊘ **S9141** Diabetic management program, follow-up visit to MD provider

⊘ **S9145** Insulin pump initiation, instruction in initial use of pump (pump not included)

⊘ **S9150** Evaluation by ocularist

⊘ **S9152** Speech therapy, re-evaluation

⊘ **S9208** Home management of preterm labor, including administrative services, professional pharmacy services, care coordination, and all necessary supplies or equipment (drugs and nursing visits coded separately), per diem (do not use this code with any home infusion per diem code)

⊘ **S9209** Home management of preterm premature rupture of membranes (PPROM), including administrative services, professional pharmacy services, care coordination, and all necessary supplies or equipment (drugs and nursing visits coded separately), per diem (do not use this code with any home infusion per diem code)

⊘ **S9211** Home management of gestational hypertension, includes administrative services, professional pharmacy services, care coordination, and all necessary supplies and equipment (drugs and nursing visits coded separately); per diem (do not use this code with any home infusion per diem code)

⊘ **S9212** Home management of postpartum hypertension, includes administrative services, professional pharmacy services, care coordination, and all necessary supplies and equipment (drugs and nursing visits coded separately), per diem (do not use this code with any home infusion per diem code)

⊘ **S9213** Home management of preeclampsia, includes administrative services, professional pharmacy services, care coordination, and all necessary supplies and equipment (drugs and nursing services coded separately); per diem (do not use this code with any home infusion per diem code)

⊘ **S9214** Home management of gestational diabetes, includes administrative services, professional pharmacy services, care coordination, and all necessary supplies and equipment (drugs and nursing visits coded separately); per diem (do not use this code with any home infusion per diem code)

⊘ **S9325** Home infusion therapy, pain management infusion; administrative services, professional pharmacy services, care coordination, and all necessary supplies and equipment, (drugs and nursing visits coded separately), per diem (do not use this code with S9326, S9327 or S9328)

⊘ **S9326** Home infusion therapy, continuous (twenty-four hours or more) pain management infusion; administrative services, professional pharmacy services, care coordination, and all necessary supplies and equipment (drugs and nursing visits coded separately), per diem

⊘ **S9327** Home infusion therapy, intermittent (less than twenty-four hours) pain management infusion; administrative services, professional pharmacy services, care coordination, and all necessary supplies and equipment (drugs and nursing visits coded separately), per diem

⊘ **S9328** Home infusion therapy, implanted pump pain management infusion; administrative services, professional pharmacy services, care coordination, and all necessary supplies and equipment (drugs and nursing visits coded separately), per diem

⊘ **S9329** Home infusion therapy, chemotherapy infusion; administrative services, professional pharmacy services, care coordination, and all necessary supplies and equipment (drugs and nursing visits coded separately), per diem (do not use this code with S9330 or S9331)

⊘ **S9330** Home infusion therapy, continuous (twenty-four hours or more) chemotherapy infusion; administrative services, professional pharmacy services, care coordination, and all necessary supplies and equipment (drugs and nursing visits coded separately), per diem

⊘ **S9331** Home infusion therapy, intermittent (less than twenty-four hours) chemotherapy infusion; administrative services, professional pharmacy services, care coordination, and all necessary supplies and equipment (drugs and nursing visits coded separately), per diem

⊘ **S9335** Home therapy, hemodialysis; administrative services, professional pharmacy services, care coordination, and all necessary supplies and equipment (drugs and nursing services coded separately), per diem

▶ New ⤻ Revised ✔ Reinstated ~~deleted~~ Deleted ⊘ Not covered or valid by Medicare
Special coverage instructions ✻ Carrier discretion Bill local carrier Bill DME MAC

⃠ **S9336** Home infusion therapy, continuous anticoagulant infusion therapy (e.g., heparin), administrative services, professional pharmacy services, care coordination, and all necessary supplies and equipment (drugs and nursing visits coded separately), per diem

⃠ **S9338** Home infusion therapy, immunotherapy, administrative services, professional pharmacy services, care coordination, and all necessary supplies and equipment (drug and nursing visits coded separately), per diem

⃠ **S9339** Home therapy; peritoneal dialysis, administrative services, professional pharmacy services, care coordination and all necessary supplies and equipment (drugs and nursing visits coded separately), per diem

⃠ **S9340** Home therapy; enteral nutrition; administrative services, professional pharmacy services, care coordination, and all necessary supplies and equipment (enteral formula and nursing visits coded separately), per diem

⃠ **S9341** Home therapy; enteral nutrition via gravity; administrative services, professional pharmacy services, care coordination, and all necessary supplies and equipment (enteral formula and nursing visits coded separately), per diem

⃠ **S9342** Home therapy; enteral nutrition via pump; administrative services, professional pharmacy services, care coordination, and all necessary supplies and equipment (enteral formula and nursing visits coded separately), per diem

⃠ **S9343** Home therapy; enteral nutrition via bolus; administrative services, professional pharmacy services, care coordination, and all necessary supplies and equipment (enteral formula and nursing visits coded separately), per diem

⃠ **S9345** Home infusion therapy, anti-hemophilic agent infusion therapy (e.g., Factor VIII); administrative services, professional pharmacy services, care coordination, and all necessary supplies and equipment (drugs and nursing visits coded separately), per diem

⃠ **S9346** Home infusion therapy, alpha-1-proteinase inhibitor (e.g., Prolastin); administrative services, professional pharmacy services, care coordination, and all necessary supplies and equipment (drugs and nursing visits coded separately), per diem

⃠ **S9347** Home infusion therapy, uninterrupted, long-term, controlled rate intravenous or subcutaneous infusion therapy (e.g., Epoprostenol); administrative services, professional pharmacy services, care coordination, and all necessary supplies and equipment (drugs and nursing visits coded separately), per diem

⃠ **S9348** Home infusion therapy, sympathomimetic/inotropic agent infusion therapy (e.g., Dobutamine); administrative services, professional pharmacy services, care coordination, all necessary supplies and equipment (drugs and nursing visits coded separately), per diem

⃠ **S9349** Home infusion therapy, tocolytic infusion therapy; administrative services, professional pharmacy services, care coordination, and all necessary supplies and equipment (drugs and nursing visits coded separately), per diem

⃠ **S9351** Home infusion therapy, continuous or intermittent anti-emetic infusion therapy; administrative services, professional pharmacy services, care coordination, and all necessary supplies and equipment (drugs and visits coded separately), per diem

⃠ **S9353** Home infusion therapy, continuous insulin infusion therapy; administrative services, professional pharmacy services, care coordination, and all necessary supplies and equipment (drugs and nursing visits coded separately), per diem

⃠ **S9355** Home infusion therapy, chelation therapy; administrative services, professional pharmacy services, care coordination, and all necessary supplies and equipment (drugs and nursing visits coded separately), per diem

⃠ **S9357** Home infusion therapy, enzyme replacement intravenous therapy; (e.g., Imiglucerase); administrative services, professional pharmacy services, care coordination, and all necessary supplies and equipment (drugs and nursing visits coded separately), per diem

▶ New ↩ Revised ✔ Reinstated ~~deleted~~ Deleted ⃠ Not covered or valid by Medicare
Special coverage instructions ✻ Carrier discretion Bill local carrier Bill DME MAC

⃠ **S9359** Home infusion therapy, anti-tumor necrosis factor intravenous therapy; (e.g., Infliximab); administrative services, professional pharmacy services, care coordination, and all necessary supplies and equipment (drugs and nursing visits coded separately), per diem

⃠ **S9361** Home infusion therapy, diuretic intravenous therapy; administrative services, professional pharmacy services, care coordination, and all necessary supplies and equipment (drugs and nursing visits coded separately), per diem

⃠ **S9363** Home infusion therapy, anti-spasmotic therapy; administrative services, professional pharmacy services, care coordination, and all necessary supplies and equipment (drugs and nursing visits coded separately), per diem

⃠ **S9364** Home infusion therapy, total parenteral nutrition (TPN); administrative services, professional pharmacy services, care coordination, and all necessary supplies and equipment including standard TPN formula (lipids, specialty amino acid formulas, drugs other than in standard formula, and nursing visits coded separately) per diem (do not use with home infusion codes S9365-S9368 using daily volume scales)

⃠ **S9365** Home infusion therapy, total parenteral nutrition (TPN); one liter per day, administrative services, professional pharmacy services, care coordination, and all necessary supplies and equipment including standard TPN formula (lipids, specialty amino acid formulas, drugs other than in standard formula and nursing visits coded separately), per diem

⃠ **S9366** Home infusion therapy, total parenteral nutrition (TPN); more than one liter but no more than two liters per day, administrative services, professional pharmacy services, care coordination, and all necessary supplies and equipment including standard TPN formula; (lipids, specialty amino acid formulas, drugs other than in standard formula and nursing visits coded separately), per diem

⃠ **S9367** Home infusion therapy, total parenteral nutrition (TPN); more than two liters but no more than three liters per day, administrative services, professional pharmacy services, care coordination, and all necessary supplies and equipment including standard TPN formula (lipids, specialty amino acid formulas, drugs other than in standard formula and nursing visits coded separately), per diem

⃠ **S9368** Home infusion therapy, total parenteral nutrition (TPN); more than three liters per day, administrative services, professional pharmacy services, care coordination, and all necessary supplies and equipment (including standard TPN formula; lipids, specialty amino acid formulas, drugs other than in standard formula and nursing visits coded separately), per diem

⃠ **S9370** Home therapy, intermittent anti-emetic injection therapy; administrative services, professional pharmacy services, care coordination, and all necessary supplies and equipment (drugs and nursing visits coded separately), per diem

⃠ **S9372** Home therapy; intermittent anticoagulant injection therapy (e.g., heparin); administrative services, professional pharmacy services, care coordination, and all necessary supplies and equipment (drugs and nursing visits coded separately), per diem (do not use this code for flushing of infusion devices with heparin to maintain patency)

⃠ **S9373** Home infusion therapy, hydration therapy; administrative services, professional pharmacy services, care coordination, and all necessary supplies and equipment (drugs and nursing visits coded separately), per diem (do not use with hydration therapy codes S9374-S9377 using daily volume scales)

⃠ **S9374** Home infusion therapy, hydration therapy; one liter per day, administrative services, professional pharmacy services, care coordination, and all necessary supplies and equipment (drugs and nursing visits coded separately), per diem

⊘ **S9375** Home infusion therapy, hydration therapy; more than one liter but no more than two liters per day, administrative services, professional pharmacy services, care coordination, and all necessary supplies and equipment (drugs and nursing visits coded separately), per diem

⊘ **S9376** Home infusion therapy, hydration therapy; more than two liters but no more than three liters per day, administrative services, professional pharmacy services, care coordination, and all necessary supplies and equipment (drugs and nursing visits coded separately), per diem

⊘ **S9377** Home infusion therapy, hydration therapy; more than three liters per day, administrative services, professional pharmacy services, care coordination, and all necessary supplies (drugs and nursing visits coded separately), per diem

⊘ **S9379** Home infusion therapy, infusion therapy, not otherwise classified; administrative services, professional pharmacy services, care coordination, and all necessary supplies and equipment (drugs and nursing visits coded separately), per diem

⊘ **S9381** Delivery or service to high risk areas requiring escort or extra protection, per visit

⊘ **S9401** Anticoagulation clinic, inclusive of all services except laboratory tests, per session

⊘ **S9430** Pharmacy compounding and dispensing services

⊘ **S9433** Medical food nutritionally complete, administered orally, providing 100% of nutritional intake

⊘ **S9434** Modified solid food supplements for inborn errors of metabolism

⊘ **S9435** Medical foods for inborn errors of metabolism

⊘ **S9436** Childbirth preparation/Lamaze classes, non-physician provider, per session

⊘ **S9437** Childbirth refresher classes, non-physician provider, per session

⊘ **S9438** Cesarean birth classes, non-physician provider, per session

⊘ **S9439** VBAC (vaginal birth after cesarean) classes, non-physician provider, per session

⊘ **S9441** Asthma education, non-physician provider, per session

⊘ **S9442** Birthing classes, non-physician provider, per session

⊘ **S9443** Lactation classes, non-physician provider, per session

⊘ **S9444** Parenting classes, non-physician provider, per session

⊘ **S9445** Patient education, not otherwise classified, non-physician provider, individual, per session

⊘ **S9446** Patient education, not otherwise classified, non-physician provider, group, per session

⊘ **S9447** Infant safety (including CPR) classes, non-physician provider, per session

⊘ **S9449** Weight management classes, non-physician provider, per session

⊘ **S9451** Exercise classes, non-physician provider, per session

⊘ **S9452** Nutrition classes, non-physician provider, per session

⊘ **S9453** Smoking cessation classes, non-physician provider, per session

⊘ **S9454** Stress management classes, non-physician provider, per session

⊘ **S9455** Diabetic management program, group session

⊘ **S9460** Diabetic management program, nurse visit

⊘ **S9465** Diabetic management program, dietitian visit

⊘ **S9470** Nutritional counseling, dietitian visit

⊘ **S9472** Cardiac rehabilitation program, non-physician provider, per diem

⊘ **S9473** Pulmonary rehabilitation program, non-physician provider, per diem

⊘ **S9474** Enterostomal therapy by a registered nurse certified in enterostomal therapy, per diem

⊘ **S9475** Ambulatory setting substance abuse treatment or detoxification services, per diem

⊘ **S9476** Vestibular rehabilitation program, non-physician provider, per diem

⊘ **S9480** Intensive outpatient psychiatric services, per diem

⊘ **S9482** Family stabilization services, per 15 minutes

⊘ **S9484** Crisis intervention mental health services, per hour

⊘ **S9485** Crisis intervention mental health services, per diem

⃠ **S9490** Home infusion therapy, corticosteroid infusion; administrative services, professional pharmacy services, care coordination, and all necessary supplies and equipment (drugs and nursing visits coded separately), per diem

⃠ **S9494** Home infusion therapy, antibiotic, antiviral, or antifungal therapy; administrative services, professional pharmacy services, care coordination, and all necessary supplies and equipment (drugs and nursing visits coded separately) per diem (do not use this code with home infusion codes for hourly dosing schedules S9497-S9504)

⃠ **S9497** Home infusion therapy, antibiotic, antiviral, or antifungal therapy; once every 3 hours; administrative services, professional pharmacy services, care coordination, and all necessary supplies and equipment (drugs and nursing visits coded separately), per diem

⃠ **S9500** Home infusion therapy, antibiotic, antiviral, or antifungal therapy; once every 24 hours; administrative services, professional pharmacy services, care coordination, and all necessary supplies and equipment (drugs and nursing visits coded separately), per diem

⃠ **S9501** Home infusion therapy, antibiotic, antiviral, or antifungal therapy; once every 12 hours; administrative services, professional pharmacy services, care coordination, and all necessary supplies and equipment (drugs and nursing visits coded separately), per diem

⃠ **S9502** Home infusion therapy, antibiotic, antiviral, or antifungal therapy; once every 8 hours, administrative services, professional pharmacy services, care coordination, and all necessary supplies and equipment (drugs and nursing visits coded separately), per diem

⃠ **S9503** Home infusion therapy, antibiotic, antiviral, or antifungal; once every 6 hours; administrative services, professional pharmacy services, care coordination, and all necessary supplies and equipment (drugs and nursing visits coded separately), per diem

⃠ **S9504** Home infusion therapy, antibiotic, antiviral, or antifungal; once every 4 hours; administrative services, professional pharmacy services, care coordination, and all necessary supplies and equipment (drugs and nursing visits coded separately), per diem

⃠ **S9529** Routine venipuncture for collection of specimen(s), single home bound, nursing home, or skilled nursing facility patient

⃠ **S9537** Home therapy; hematopoietic hormone injection therapy (e.g., erythropoietin, G-CSF, GM-CSF); administrative services, professional pharmacy services, care coordination, and all necessary supplies and equipment (drugs and nursing visits coded separately), per diem

⃠ **S9538** Home transfusion of blood product(s); administrative services, professional pharmacy services, care coordination, and all necessary supplies and equipment (blood products, drugs, and nursing visits coded separately), per diem

⃠ **S9542** Home injectable therapy; not otherwise classified, including administrative services, professional pharmacy services, care coordination, and all necessary supplies and equipment (drugs and nursing visits coded separately), per diem

⃠ **S9558** Home injectable therapy; growth hormone, including administrative services, professional pharmacy services, care coordination, and all necessary supplies and equipment (drugs and nursing visits coded separately), per diem

⃠ **S9559** Home injectable therapy; interferon, including administrative services, professional pharmacy services, care coordination, and all necessary supplies and equipment (drugs and nursing visits coded separately), per diem

⃠ **S9560** Home injectable therapy; hormonal therapy (e.g., Leuprolide, Goserelin), including administrative services, professional pharmacy services, care coordination, and all necessary supplies and equipment (drugs and nursing visits coded separately), per diem

⃠ **S9562** Home injectable therapy, palivizumab, including administrative services, professional pharmacy services, care coordination, and all necessary supplies and equipment (drugs and nursing visits coded separately), per diem

⃠ **S9590** Home therapy, irrigation therapy (e.g., sterile irrigation of an organ or anatomical cavity); including administrative services, professional pharmacy services, care coordination, and all necessary supplies and equipment (drugs and nursing visits coded separately), per diem

⃠ **S9810** Home therapy; professional pharmacy services for provision of infusion, specialty drug administration, and/or disease state management, not otherwise classified, per hour (do not use this code with any per diem code)

⃠ **S9900** Services by journal-listed Christian Science Practitioner for the purpose of healing, per diem

⃠ **S9901** Services by a journal-listed Christian Science nurse, per hour

⃠ **S9960** Ambulance service, conventional air service, nonemergency transport, one way (fixed wing)

⃠ **S9961** Ambulance service, conventional air service, nonemergency transport, one way (rotary wing)

⃠ **S9970** Health club membership, annual

⃠ **S9975** Transplant related lodging, meals and transportation, per diem

⃠ **S9976** Lodging, per diem, not otherwise classified

⃠ **S9977** Meals, per diem, not otherwise specified

⃠ **S9981** Medical records copying fee, administrative

⃠ **S9982** Medical records copying fee, per page

⃠ **S9986** Not medically necessary service (patient is aware that service not medically necessary)

⃠ **S9988** Services provided as part of a Phase I clinical trial

⃠ **S9989** Services provided outside of the United States of America (list in addition to code(s) for services(s))

⃠ **S9990** Services provided as part of a Phase II clinical trial

⃠ **S9991** Services provided as part of a Phase III clinical trial

⃠ **S9992** Transportation costs to and from trial location and local transportation costs (e.g., fares for taxicab or bus) for clinical trial participant and one caregiver/companion

⃠ **S9994** Lodging costs (e.g., hotel charges) for clinical trial participant and one caregiver/companion

⃠ **S9996** Meals for clinical trial participant and one caregiver/companion

⃠ **S9999** Sales tax

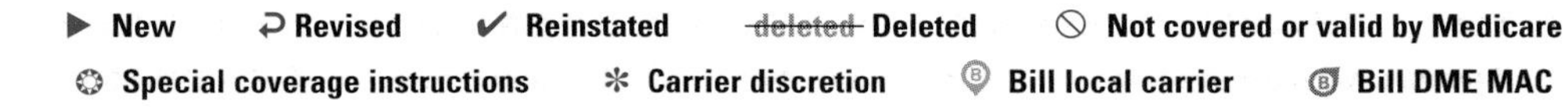

 MEDICAID ONLY

TEMPORARY NATIONAL CODES ESTABLISHED BY MEDICAID (T1000-T9999)

Not Valid For Medicare

⃠ **T1000** Private duty/independent nursing service(s) - licensed, up to 15 minutes

⃠ **T1001** Nursing assessment/evaluation

⃠ **T1002** RN services, up to 15 minutes

⃠ **T1003** LPN/LVN services, up to 15 minutes

⃠ **T1004** Services of a qualified nursing aide, up to 15 minutes

⃠ **T1005** Respite care services, up to 15 minutes

⃠ **T1006** Alcohol and/or substance abuse services, family/couple counseling

⃠ **T1007** Alcohol and/or substance abuse services, treatment plan development and/or modification

⃠ **T1009** Child sitting services for children of the individual receiving alcohol and/or substance abuse services

⃠ **T1010** Meals for individuals receiving alcohol and/or substance abuse services (when meals not included in the program)

⃠ **T1012** Alcohol and/or substance abuse services, skills development

⃠ **T1013** Sign language or oral interpretive services, per 15 minutes

⃠ **T1014** Telehealth transmission, per minute, professional services bill separately

⃠ **T1015** Clinic visit/encounter, all-inclusive

⃠ **T1016** Case Management, each 15 minutes

⃠ **T1017** Targeted Case Management, each 15 minutes

⃠ **T1018** School-based individualized education program (IEP) services, bundled

⃠ **T1019** Personal care services, per 15 minutes, not for an inpatient or resident of a hospital, nursing facility, ICF/MR or IMD, part of the individualized plan of treatment (code may not be used to identify services provided by home health aide or certified nurse assistant)

⃠ **T1020** Personal care services, per diem, not for an inpatient or resident of a hospital, nursing facility, ICF/MR or IMD, part of the individualized plan of treatment (code may not be used to identify services provided by home health aide or certified nurse assistant)

⃠ **T1021** Home health aide or certified nurse assistant, per visit

⃠ **T1022** Contracted home health agency services, all services provided under contract, per day

⃠ **T1023** Screening to determine the appropriateness of consideration of an individual for participation in a specified program, project or treatment protocol, per encounter

⃠ **T1024** Evaluation and treatment by an integrated, specialty team contracted to provide coordinated care to multiple or severely handicapped children, per encounter

⃠ **T1025** Intensive, extended multidisciplinary services provided in a clinic setting to children with complex medical, physical, mental and psychosocial impairments, per diem

⃠ **T1026** Intensive, extended multidisciplinary services provided in a clinic setting to children with complex medical, physical, medical and psychosocial impairments, per hour

⃠ **T1027** Family training and counseling for child development, per 15 minutes

⃠ **T1028** Assessment of home, physical and family environment, to determine suitability to meet patient s medical needs

⃠ **T1029** Comprehensive environmental lead investigation, not including laboratory analysis, per dwelling

⃠ **T1030** Nursing care, in the home, by registered nurse, per diem

⃠ **T1031** Nursing care, in the home, by licensed practical nurse, per diem

▶⃠ **T1040** Medicaid certified community behavioral health clinic services, per diem

▶⃠ **T1041** Medicaid certified community behavioral health clinic services, per month

⃠ **T1502** Administration of oral, intramuscular and/or subcutaneous medication by health care agency/professional, per visit

⃠ **T1503** Administration of medication, other than oral and/or injectable, by a health care agency/professional, per visit

⃠ **T1505** Electronic medication compliance management device, includes all components and accessories, not otherwise classified

▶ New ⤾ Revised ✔ Reinstated ~~deleted~~ Deleted ⃠ Not covered or valid by Medicare
Special coverage instructions * Carrier discretion Bill local carrier Bill DME MAC

⃠ **T1999** Miscellaneous therapeutic items and supplies, retail purchases, not otherwise classified; identify product in "remarks"

⃠ **T2001** Non-emergency transportation; patient attendant/escort

⃠ **T2002** Non-emergency transportation; per diem

⃠ **T2003** Non-emergency transportation; encounter/trip

⃠ **T2004** Non-emergency transport; commercial carrier, multi-pass

⃠ **T2005** Non-emergency transportation: stretcher van

⃠ **T2007** Transportation waiting time, air ambulance and non-emergency vehicle, one-half (1/2) hour increments

⃠ **T2010** Preadmission screening and resident review (PASRR) level I identification screening, per screen

⃠ **T2011** Preadmission screening and resident review (PASRR) level II evaluation, per evaluation

⃠ **T2012** Habilitation, educational, waiver; per diem

⃠ **T2013** Habilitation, educational, waiver; per hour

⃠ **T2014** Habilitation, prevocational, waiver; per diem

⃠ **T2015** Habilitation, prevocational, waiver; per hour

⃠ **T2016** Habilitation, residential, waiver; per diem

⃠ **T2017** Habilitation, residential, waiver; 15 minutes

⃠ **T2018** Habilitation, supported employment, waiver; per diem

⃠ **T2019** Habilitation, supported employment, waiver; per 15 minutes

⃠ **T2020** Day habilitation, waiver; per diem

⃠ **T2021** Day habilitation, waiver; per 15 minutes

⃠ **T2022** Case management, per month

⃠ **T2023** Targeted case management; per month

⃠ **T2024** Service assessment/plan of care development, waiver

⃠ **T2025** Waiver services; not otherwise specified (NOS)

⃠ **T2026** Specialized childcare, waiver; per diem

⃠ **T2027** Specialized childcare, waiver; per 15 minutes

⃠ **T2028** Specialized supply, not otherwise specified, waiver

⃠ **T2029** Specialized medical equipment, not otherwise specified, waiver

⃠ **T2030** Assisted living, waiver; per month

⃠ **T2031** Assisted living; waiver, per diem

⃠ **T2032** Residential care, not otherwise specified (NOS), waiver; per month

⃠ **T2033** Residential care, not otherwise specified (NOS), waiver; per diem

⃠ **T2034** Crisis intervention, waiver; per diem

⃠ **T2035** Utility services to support medical equipment and assistive technology/ devices, waiver

⃠ **T2036** Therapeutic camping, overnight, waiver; each session

⃠ **T2037** Therapeutic camping, day, waiver; each session

⃠ **T2038** Community transition, waiver; per service

⃠ **T2039** Vehicle modifications, waiver; per service

⃠ **T2040** Financial management, self-directed, waiver; per 15 minutes

⃠ **T2041** Supports brokerage, self-directed, waiver; per 15 minutes

⃠ **T2042** Hospice routine home care; per diem

⃠ **T2043** Hospice continuous home care; per hour

⃠ **T2044** Hospice inpatient respite care; per diem

⃠ **T2045** Hospice general inpatient care; per diem

⃠ **T2046** Hospice long term care, room and board only; per diem

⃠ **T2048** Behavioral health; long-term care residential (non-acute care in a residential treatment program where stay is typically longer than 30 days), with room and board, per diem

⃠ **T2049** Non-emergency transportation; stretcher van, mileage; per mile

⃠ **T2101** Human breast milk processing, storage and distribution only

⃠ **T4521** Adult sized disposable incontinence product, brief/diaper, small, each

IOM: 100-03, 4, 280.1

⃠ **T4522** Adult sized disposable incontinence product, brief/diaper, medium, each

IOM: 100-03, 4, 280.1

⊘ **T4523** Adult sized disposable incontinence product, brief/diaper, large, each
IOM: 100-03, 4, 280.1

⊘ **T4524** Adult sized disposable incontinence product, brief/diaper, extra large, each
IOM: 100-03, 4, 280.1

⊘ **T4525** Adult sized disposable incontinence product, protective underwear/pull-on, small size, each
IOM: 100-03, 4, 280.1

⊘ **T4526** Adult sized disposable incontinence product, protective underwear/pull-on, medium size, each
IOM: 100-03, 4, 280.1

⊘ **T4527** Adult sized disposable incontinence product, protective underwear/pull-on, large size, each
IOM: 100-03, 4, 280.1

⊘ **T4528** Adult sized disposable incontinence product, protective underwear/pull-on, extra large size, each
IOM: 100-03, 4, 280.1

⊘ **T4529** Pediatric sized disposable incontinence product, brief/diaper, small/medium size, each
IOM: 100-03, 4, 280.1

⊘ **T4530** Pediatric sized disposable incontinence product, brief/diaper, large size, each
IOM: 100-03, 4, 280.1

⊘ **T4531** Pediatric sized disposable incontinence product, protective underwear/pull-on, small/medium size, each
IOM: 100-03, 4, 280.1

⊘ **T4532** Pediatric sized disposable incontinence product, protective underwear/pull-on, large size, each
IOM: 100-03, 4, 280.1

⊘ **T4533** Youth sized disposable incontinence product, brief/diaper, each
IOM: 100-03, 4, 280.1

⊘ **T4534** Youth sized disposable incontinence product, protective underwear/pull-on, each
IOM: 100-03, 4, 280.1

⊘ **T4535** Disposable liner/shield/guard/pad/ undergarment, for incontinence, each
IOM: 100-03, 4, 280.1

⊘ **T4536** Incontinence product, protective underwear/pull-on, reusable, any size, each
IOM: 100-03, 4, 280.1

⊘ **T4537** Incontinence product, protective underpad, reusable, bed size, each
IOM: 100-03, 4, 280.1

⊘ **T4538** Diaper service, reusable diaper, each diaper
IOM: 100-03, 4, 280.1

⊘ **T4539** Incontinence product, diaper/brief, reusable, any size, each
IOM: 100-03, 4, 280.1

⊘ **T4540** Incontinence product, protective underpad, reusable, chair size, each
IOM: 100-03, 4, 280.1

⊘ **T4541** Incontinence product, disposable underpad, large, each

⊘ **T4542** Incontinence product, disposable underpad, small size, each

⊘ **T4543** Adult sized disposable incontinence product, protective brief/diaper, above extra large, each
IOM: 100-03, 4, 280.1

⊘ **T4544** Adult sized disposable incontinence product, protective underwear/pull-on, above extra large, each
IOM: 100-03, 4, 280.1

⊘ **T5001** Positioning seat for persons with special orthopedic needs, supply, not otherwise specified

⊘ **T5999** Supply, not otherwise specified

VISION SERVICES (V0000-V2999)

Frames

⊕ **V2020** Frames, purchases Ⓑ

Includes cost of frame/replacement and dispensing fee. One unit of service represents one pair of eyeglass frames.

IOM: 100-02, 15, 120

⊘ **V2025** Deluxe frame Ⓑ

Not a benefit. Billing deluxe frames—submit V2020 on one line; V2025 on second line

IOM: 100-04, 1, 30.3.5

Spectacle Lenses

If a CPT procedure code for supply of spectacles or a permanent prosthesis is reported, recode with the specific lens type listed below. For aphakic temporary spectacle correction, CPT.

Single Vision, Glass or Plastic

* * **V2100** Sphere, single vision, plano to plus or minus 4.00, per lens Ⓑ
* * **V2101** Sphere, single vision, plus or minus 4.12 to plus or minus 7.00d, per lens Ⓑ
* * **V2102** Sphere, single vision, plus or minus 7.12 to plus or minus 20.00d, per lens Ⓑ
* * **V2103** Spherocylinder, single vision, plano to plus or minus 4.00d sphere, .12 to 2.00d cylinder, per lens Ⓑ
* * **V2104** Spherocylinder, single vision, plano to plus or minus 4.00d sphere, 2.12 to 4.00d cylinder, per lens Ⓑ
* * **V2105** Spherocylinder, single vision, plano to plus or minus 4.00d sphere, 4.25 to 6.00d cylinder, per lens Ⓑ
* * **V2106** Spherocylinder, single vision, plano to plus or minus 4.00d sphere, over 6.00d cylinder, per lens Ⓑ
* * **V2107** Spherocylinder, single vision, plus or minus 4.25 to plus or minus 7.00 sphere, .12 to 2.00d cylinder, per lens Ⓑ
* * **V2108** Spherocylinder, single vision, plus or minus 4.25d to plus or minus 7.00d sphere, 2.12 to 4.00d cylinder, per lens Ⓑ
* * **V2109** Spherocylinder, single vision, plus or minus 4.25 to plus or minus 7.00d sphere, 4.25 to 6.00d cylinder, per lens Ⓑ
* * **V2110** Sperocylinder, single vision, plus or minus 4.25 to 7.00d sphere, over 6.00d cylinder, per lens Ⓑ
* * **V2111** Spherocylinder, single vision, plus or minus 7.25 to plus or minus 12.00d sphere, .25 to 2.25d cylinder, per lens Ⓑ
* * **V2112** Spherocylinder, single vision, plus or minus 7.25 to plus or minus 12.00d sphere, 2.25d to 4.00d cylinder, per lens Ⓑ
* * **V2113** Spherocylinder, single vision, plus or minus 7.25 to plus or minus 12.00d sphere, 4.25 to 6.00d cylinder, per lens Ⓑ
* * **V2114** Spherocylinder, single vision, sphere over plus or minus 12.00d, per lens Ⓑ
* * **V2115** Lenticular, (myodisc), per lens, single vision Ⓑ
* * **V2118** Aniseikonic lens, single vision Ⓑ

⊕ **V2121** Lenticular lens, per lens, single Ⓑ

IOM: 100-02, 15, 120; 100-04, 3, 10.4

* **V2199** Not otherwise classified, single vision lens Ⓑ

Bill on paper. Requires report of type of single vision lens and optical lab invoice.

Bifocal, Glass or Plastic

* * **V2200** Sphere, bifocal, plano to plus or minus 4.00d, per lens Ⓑ
* * **V2201** Sphere, bifocal, plus or minus 4.12 to plus or minus 7.00d, per lens Ⓑ
* * **V2202** Sphere, bifocal, plus or minus 7.12 to plus or minus 20.00d, per lens Ⓑ
* * **V2203** Spherocylinder, bifocal, plano to plus or minus 4.00d sphere, .12 to 2.00d cylinder, per lens Ⓑ
* * **V2204** Spherocylinder, bifocal, plano to plus or minus 4.00d sphere, 2.12 to 4.00d cylinder, per lens Ⓑ
* * **V2205** Spherocylinder, bifocal, plano to plus or minus 4.00d sphere, 4.25 to 6.00d cylinder, per lens Ⓑ
* * **V2206** Spherocylinder, bifocal, plano to plus or minus 4.00d sphere, over 6.00d cylinder, per lens Ⓑ
* * **V2207** Spherocylinder, bifocal, plus or minus 4.25 to plus or minus 7.00d sphere, .12 to 2.00d cylinder, per lens Ⓑ

* **V2208** Spherocylinder, bifocal, plus or minus 4.25 to plus or minus 7.00d sphere, 2.12 to 4.00d cylinder, per lens Ⓑ

* **V2209** Spherocylinder, bifocal, plus or minus 4.25 to plus or minus 7.00d sphere, 4.25 to 6.00d cylinder, per lens Ⓑ

* **V2210** Spherocylinder, bifocal, plus or minus 4.25 to plus or minus 7.00d sphere, over 6.00d cylinder, per lens Ⓑ

* **V2211** Spherocylinder, bifocal, plus or minus 7.25 to plus or minus 12.00d sphere, .25 to 2.25d cylinder, per lens Ⓑ

* **V2212** Spherocylinder, bifocal, plus or minus 7.25 to plus or minus 12.00d sphere, 2.25 to 4.00d cylinder, per lens Ⓑ

* **V2213** Spherocylinder, bifocal, plus or minus 7.25 to plus or minus 12.00d sphere, 4.25 to 6.00d cylinder, per lens Ⓑ

* **V2214** Spherocylinder, bifocal, sphere over plus or minus 12.00d, per lens Ⓑ

* **V2215** Lenticular (myodisc), per lens, bifocal Ⓑ

* **V2218** Aniseikonic, per lens, bifocal Ⓑ

* **V2219** Bifocal seg width over 28 mm Ⓑ

* **V2220** Bifocal add over 3.25d Ⓑ

⚙ **V2221** Lenticular lens, per lens, bifocal Ⓑ

IOM: 100-02, 15, 120; 100-04, 3, 10.4

* **V2299** Specialty bifocal (by report) Ⓑ

Bill on paper. Requires report of type of specialty bifocal lens and optical lab invoice.

Trifocal, Glass or Plastic

* **V2300** Sphere, trifocal, plano to plus or minus 4.00d, per lens Ⓑ

* **V2301** Sphere, trifocal, plus or minus 4.12 to plus or minus 7.00d per lens Ⓑ

* **V2302** Sphere, trifocal, plus or minus 7.12 to plus or minus 20.00, per lens Ⓑ

* **V2303** Spherocylinder, trifocal, plano to plus or minus 4.00d sphere, .12 to 2.00d cylinder, per lens Ⓑ

* **V2304** Spherocylinder, trifocal, plano to plus or minus 4.00d sphere, 2.25-4.00d cylinder, per lens Ⓑ

* **V2305** Spherocylinder, trifocal, plano to plus or minus 4.00d sphere, 4.25 to 6.00 cylinder, per lens Ⓑ

* **V2306** Spherocylinder, trifocal, plano to plus or minus 4.00d sphere, over 6.00d cylinder, per lens Ⓑ

* **V2307** Spherocylinder, trifocal, plus or minus 4.25 to plus or minus 7.00d sphere, .12 to 2.00d cylinder, per lens Ⓑ

* **V2308** Spherocylinder, trifocal, plus or minus 4.25 to plus or minus 7.00d sphere, 2.12 to 4.00d cylinder, per lens Ⓑ

* **V2309** Spherocylinder, trifocal, plus or minus 4.25 to plus or minus 7.00d sphere, 4.25 to 6.00d cylinder, per lens Ⓑ

* **V2310** Spherocylinder, trifocal, plus or minus 4.25 to plus or minus 7.00d sphere, over 6.00d cylinder, per lens Ⓑ

* **V2311** Spherocylinder, trifocal, plus or minus 7.25 to plus or minus 12.00d sphere, .25 to 2.25d cylinder, per lens Ⓑ

* **V2312** Spherocylinder, trifocal, plus or minus 7.25 to plus or minus 12.00d sphere, 2.25 to 4.00d cylinder, per lens Ⓑ

* **V2313** Spherocylinder, trifocal, plus or minus 7.25 to plus or minus 12.00d sphere, 4.25 to 6.00d cylinder, per lens Ⓑ

* **V2314** Spherocylinder, trifocal, sphere over plus or minus 12.00d, per lens Ⓑ

* **V2315** Lenticular, (myodisc), per lens, trifocal Ⓑ

* **V2318** Aniseikonic lens, trifocal Ⓑ

* **V2319** Trifocal seg width over 28 mm Ⓑ

* **V2320** Trifocal add over 3.25d Ⓑ

⚙ **V2321** Lenticular lens, per lens, trifocal Ⓑ

IOM: 100-02, 15, 120; 100-04, 3, 10.4

* **V2399** Specialty trifocal (by report) Ⓑ

Bill on paper. Requires report of type of trifocal lens and optical lab invoice.

Variable Asphericity

* **V2410** Variable asphericity lens, single vision, full field, glass or plastic, per lens Ⓑ

* **V2430** Variable asphericity lens, bifocal, full field, glass or plastic, per lens Ⓑ

* **V2499** Variable sphericity lens, other type Ⓑ

Bill on paper. Requires report of other ptical lab invoice.

▶ New   Revised   ✔ Reinstated   ~~deleted~~ Deleted   ⦸ Not covered or valid by Medicare
⚙ Special coverage instructions   * Carrier discretion   Ⓑ Bill local carrier   Ⓑ Bill DME MAC

Contact Lenses

If a CPT procedure code for supply of contact lens is reported, recode with specific lens type listed below (per lens).

✻ **V2500** Contact lens, PMMA, spherical, per lens
Requires prior authorization for patients under age 21.

✻ **V2501** Contact lens, PMMA, toric or prism ballast, per lens
Requires prior authorization for clients under age 21.

✻ **V2502** Contact lens, PMMA, bifocal, per lens
Requires prior authorization for clients under age 21. Bill on paper. Requires optical lab invoice.

✻ **V2503** Contact lens PMMA, color vision deficiency, per lens
Requires prior authorization for clients under age 21. Bill on paper. Requires optical lab invoice.

✻ **V2510** Contact lens, gas permeable, spherical, per lens
Requires prior authorization for clients under age 21.

✻ **V2511** Contact lens, gas permeable, toric, prism ballast, per lens
Requires prior authorization for clients under age 21.

✻ **V2512** Contact lens, gas permeable, bifocal, per lens
Requires prior authorization for clients under age 21.

✻ **V2513** Contact lens, gas permeable, extended wear, per lens
Requires prior authorization for clients under age 21.

V2520 Contact lens, hydrophilic, spherical, per lens
Bill Local Carrier if incident to a physician's service. If other, bill DME MAC.
Requires prior authorization for clients under age 21.
IOM: 100-03, 1, 80.1; 100-03, 1, 80.4

V2521 Contact lens, hydrophilic, toric, or prism ballast, per lens
Bill Local Carrier if incident to a physician's service. If other, bill DME MAC.
Requires prior authorization for clients under age 21.
IOM: 100-03, 1, 80.1; 100-03, 1, 80.4

V2522 Contact lens, hydrophilic, bifocal, per lens
Bill Local Carrier if incident to a physician's service. If other, bill DME MAC.
Requires prior authorization for clients under age 21.
IOM: 100-03, 1, 80.1; 100-03, 1, 80.4

V2523 Contact lens, hydrophilic, extended wear, per lens
Bill Local Carrier if incident to a physician's service. If other, bill DME MAC.
Requires prior authorization for clients under age 21.
IOM: 100-03, 1, 80.1; 100-03, 1, 80.4

✻ **V2530** Contact lens, scleral, gas impermeable, per lens (for contact lens modification, see 92325)
Requires prior authorization for clients under age 21.

V2531 Contact lens, scleral, gas permeable, per lens (for contact lens modification, see 92325)
Requires prior authorization for clients under age 21. Bill on paper. Requires optical lab invoice.
IOM: 100-03, 1, 80.5

✻ **V2599** Contact lens, other type
Bill Local Carrier if incident to a physician's service. If other, bill DME MAC.
Requires prior authorization for clients under age 21. Bill on paper. Requires report of other type of contact lens and optical invoice.

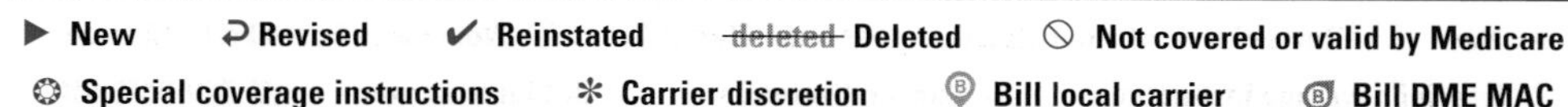

Low Vision Aids

If a CPT procedure code for supply of low vision aid is reported, recode with specific systems listed below.

✻ **V2600** Hand held low vision aids and other nonspectacle mounted aids
Requires prior authorization.

✻ **V2610** Single lens spectacle mounted low vision aids
Requires prior authorization.

✻ **V2615** Telescopic and other compound lens system, including distance vision telescopic, near vision telescopes and compound microscopic lens system
Requires prior authorization. Bill on paper. Requires optical lab invoice.

Prosthetic Eye

V2623 Prosthetic eye, plastic, custom
DME regional carrier. Requires prior authorization. Bill on paper. Requires optical lab invoice.

✻ **V2624** Polishing/resurfacing of ocular prosthesis
Requires prior authorization. Bill on paper. Requires optical lab invoice.

✻ **V2625** Enlargement of ocular prosthesis
Requires prior authorization. Bill on paper. Requires optical lab invoice.

✻ **V2626** Reduction of ocular prosthesis
Requires prior authorization. Bill on paper. Requires optical lab invoice.

V2627 Scleral cover shell
DME regional carrier
Requires prior authorization. Bill on paper. Requires optical lab invoice.
IOM: 100-03, 4, 280.2

✻ **V2628** Fabrication and fitting of ocular conformer
Requires prior authorization. Bill on paper. Requires optical lab invoice.

✻ **V2629** Prosthetic eye, other type
Requires prior authorization. Bill on paper. Requires optical lab invoice.

Intraocular Lenses

V2630 Anterior chamber intraocular lens
IOM: 100-02, 15, 120

V2631 Iris supported intraocular lens
IOM: 100-02, 15, 120

V2632 Posterior chamber intraocular lens
IOM: 100-02, 15, 120

Miscellaneous Vision Services

✻ **V2700** Balance lens, per lens

⊘ **V2702** Deluxe lens feature
IOM: 100-02, 15, 120; 100-04, 3, 10.4

✻ **V2710** Slab off prism, glass or plastic, per lens

✻ **V2715** Prism, per lens

✻ **V2718** Press-on lens, Fresnel prism, per lens

✻ **V2730** Special base curve, glass or plastic, per lens

V2744 Tint, photochromatic, per lens
Requires prior authorization.
IOM: 100-02, 15, 120; 100-04, 3, 10.4

V2745 Addition to lens, tint, any color, solid, gradient or equal, excludes photochroatic, any lens material, per lens
Includes photochromatic lenses (V2744) used as sunglasses, which are prescribed in addition to regular prosthetic lenses for aphakic patient will be denied as not medically necessary.
IOM: 100-02, 15, 120; 100-04, 3, 10.4

V2750 Anti-reflective coating, per lens
Requires prior authorization.
IOM: 100-02, 15, 120; 100-04, 3, 10.4

V2755 U-V lens, per lens
IOM: 100-02, 15, 120; 100-04, 3, 10.4

✻ **V2756** Eye glass case

✻ **V2760** Scratch resistant coating, per lens

V2761 Mirror coating, any type, solid, gradient or equal, any lens material, per lens
IOM: 100-02, 15, 120; 100-04, 3, 10.4

V2762 Polarization, any lens material, per lens
IOM: 100-02, 15, 120; 100-04, 3, 10.4

▶ New Revised ✔ Reinstated ~~deleted~~ Deleted ⊘ Not covered or valid by Medicare
Special coverage instructions ✻ Carrier discretion Bill local carrier Bill DME MAC

✻ **V2770** Occluder lens, per lens Ⓑ
Requires prior authorization.

✻ **V2780** Oversize lens, per lens Ⓑ
Requires prior authorization.

✻ **V2781** Progressive lens, per lens Ⓑ
Requires prior authorization.

✪ **V2782** Lens, index 1.54 to 1.65 plastic or 1.60 to 1.79 glass, excludes polycarbonate, per lens Ⓑ
Do not bill in addition to V2784
IOM: 100-02, 15, 120; 100-04, 3, 10.4

✪ **V2783** Lens, index greater than or equal to 1.66 plastic or greater than or equal to 1.80 glass, excludes polycarbonate, per lens Ⓑ
Do not bill in addition to V2784
IOM: 100-02, 15, 120; 100-04, 3, 10.4

✪ **V2784** Lens, polycarbonate or equal, any index, per lens Ⓑ
Covered only for patients with functional vision in one eye—in this situation, an impact-resistant material is covered for both lenses if eyeglasses are covered. Claims with V2784 that do not meet this coverage criterion will be denied as not medically necessary.
IOM: 100-02, 15, 120; 100-04, 3, 10.4

✻ **V2785** Processing, preserving and transporting corneal tissue Ⓑ
For ASC, bill on paper. Must attach eye bank invoice to claim.
For Hospitals, bill charges for corneal tissue to receive cost based reimbursement.

✪ **V2786** Specialty occupational multifocal lens, per lens Ⓑ
IOM: 100-02, 15, 120; 100-04, 3, 10.4

⃠ **V2787** Astigmatism correcting function of intraocular lens Ⓑ
Medicare Statute 1862(a)(7)

⃠ **V2788** Presbyopia correcting function of intraocular lens Ⓑ
Medicare Statute 1862a7

✻ **V2790** Amniotic membrane for surgical reconstruction, per procedure Ⓑ

✻ **V2797** Vision supply, accessory and/or service component of another HCPCS vision code Ⓑ

✻ **V2799** Vision item or service, miscellaneous Ⓑ
Bill on paper. Requires report of miscellaneous service and optical lab invoice.

HEARING SERVICES (V5000-V5999)

Note: These codes are for non-physician services.

⃠ **V5008** Hearing screening Ⓑ
IOM: 100-02, 16, 90

⃠ **V5010** Assessment for hearing aid Ⓑ
Medicare Statute 1862a7

⃠ **V5011** Fitting/orientation/checking of hearing aid Ⓑ
Medicare Statute 1862a7

⃠ **V5014** Repair/modification of a hearing aid Ⓑ
Medicare Statute 1862a7

⃠ **V5020** Conformity evaluation Ⓑ
Medicare Statute 1862a7

⃠ **V5030** Hearing aid, monaural, body worn, air conduction Ⓑ
Medicare Statute 1862a7

⃠ **V5040** Hearing aid, monaural, body worn, bone conduction Ⓑ
Medicare Statute 1862a7

⃠ **V5050** Hearing aid, monaural, in the ear Ⓑ
Medicare Statute 1862a7

⃠ **V5060** Hearing aid, monaural, behind the ear Ⓑ
Medicare Statute 1862a7

⃠ **V5070** Glasses, air conduction Ⓑ
Medicare Statute 1862a7

⃠ **V5080** Glasses, bone conduction Ⓑ
Medicare Statute 1862a7

⃠ **V5090** Dispensing fee, unspecified hearing aid Ⓑ
Medicare Statute 1862a7

⃠ **V5095** Semi-implantable middle ear hearing prosthesis Ⓑ
Medicare Statute 1862a7

⃠ **V5100** Hearing aid, bilateral, body worn Ⓑ
Medicare Statute 1862a7

⃠ **V5110** Dispensing fee, bilateral Ⓑ
Medicare Statute 1862a7

⃠ **V5120** Binaural, body Ⓑ
Medicare Statute 1862a7

⃠ **V5130** Binaural, in the ear Ⓑ
Medicare Statute 1862a7

⊘ **V5140** Binaural, behind the ear Ⓑ
Medicare Statute 1862a7

⊘ **V5150** Binaural, glasses Ⓑ
Medicare Statute 1862a7

⊘ **V5160** Dispensing fee, binaural Ⓑ
Medicare Statute 1862a7

⊘ **V5170** Hearing aid, CROS, in the ear Ⓑ
Medicare Statute 1862a7

⊘ **V5180** Hearing aid, CROS, behind the ear Ⓑ
Medicare Statute 1862a7

⊘ **V5190** Hearing aid, CROS, glasses Ⓑ
Medicare Statute 1862a7

⊘ **V5200** Dispensing fee, CROS Ⓑ
Medicare Statute 1862a7

⊘ **V5210** Hearing aid, BICROS, in the ear Ⓑ
Medicare Statute 1862a7

⊘ **V5220** Hearing aid, BICROS, behind the ear Ⓑ
Medicare Statute 1862a7

⊘ **V5230** Hearing aid, BICROS, glasses Ⓑ
Medicare Statute 1862a7

⊘ **V5240** Dispensing fee, BICROS Ⓑ
Medicare Statute 1862a7

⊘ **V5241** Dispensing fee, monaural hearing aid, any type Ⓑ
Medicare Statute 1862a7

⊘ **V5242** Hearing aid, analog, monaural, CIC (completely in the ear canal) Ⓑ
Medicare Statute 1862a7

⊘ **V5243** Hearing aid, analog, monaural, ITC (in the canal) Ⓑ
Medicare Statute 1862a9

⊘ **V5244** Hearing aid, digitally programmable analog, monaural, CIC Ⓑ
Medicare Statute 1862a7

⊘ **V5245** Hearing aid, digitally programmable, analog, monaural, ITC Ⓑ
Medicare Statute 1862a7

⊘ **V5246** Hearing aid, digitally programmable analog, monaural, ITE (in the ear) Ⓑ
Medicare Statute 1862a7

⊘ **V5247** Hearing aid, digitally programmable analog, monaural, BTE (behind the ear) Ⓑ
Medicare Statute 1862a7

⊘ **V5248** Hearing aid, analog, binaural, CIC Ⓑ
Medicare Statute 1862a7

⊘ **V5249** Hearing aid, analog, binaural, ITC Ⓑ
Medicare Statute 1862a7

⊘ **V5250** Hearing aid, digitally programmable analog, binaural, CIC Ⓑ
Medicare Statute 1862a7

⊘ **V5251** Hearing aid, digitally programmable analog, binaural, ITC Ⓑ
Medicare Statute 1862a7

⊘ **V5252** Hearing aid, digitally programmable, binaural, ITE Ⓑ
Medicare Statute 1862a7

⊘ **V5253** Hearing aid, digitally programmable, binaural, BTE Ⓑ
Medicare Statute 1862a7

⊘ **V5254** Hearing aid, digital, monaural, CIC Ⓑ
Medicare Statute 1862a7

⊘ **V5255** Hearing aid, digital, monaural, ITC Ⓑ
Medicare Statute 1862a7

⊘ **V5256** Hearing aid, digital, monaural, ITE Ⓑ
Medicare Statute 1862a7

⊘ **V5257** Hearing aid, digital, monaural, BTE Ⓑ
Medicare Statute 1862a7

⊘ **V5258** Hearing aid, digital, binaural, CIC Ⓑ
Medicare Statute 1862a7

⊘ **V5259** Hearing aid, digital, binaural, ITC Ⓑ
Medicare Statute 1862a7

⊘ **V5260** Hearing aid, digital, binaural, ITE Ⓑ
Medicare Statute 1862a7

⊘ **V5261** Hearing aid, digital, binaural, BTE Ⓑ
Medicare Statute 1862a7

⊘ **V5262** Hearing aid, disposable, any type, monaural Ⓑ
Medicare Statute 1862a7

⊘ **V5263** Hearing aid, disposable, any type, binaural Ⓑ
Medicare Statute 1862a7

⊘ **V5264** Ear mold/insert, not disposable, any type Ⓑ
Medicare Statute 1862a7

⊘ **V5265** Ear mold/insert, disposable, any type Ⓑ
Medicare Statute 1862a7

⊘ **V5266** Battery for use in hearing device Ⓑ
Medicare Statute 1862a7

⊘ **V5267** Hearing aid or assistive listening device/supplies/accessories, not otherwise specified Ⓑ
Medicare Statute 1862a7

⃠ **V5268** Assistive listening device, telephone amplifier, any type Ⓑ
Medicare Statute 1862a7

⃠ **V5269** Assistive listening device, alerting, any type Ⓑ
Medicare Statute 1862a7

⃠ **V5270** Assistive listening device, television amplifier, any type Ⓑ
Medicare Statute 1862a7

⃠ **V5271** Assistive listening device, television caption decoder Ⓑ
Medicare Statute 1862a7

⃠ **V5272** Assistive listening device, TDD Ⓑ
Medicare Statute 1862a7

⃠ **V5273** Assistive listening device, for use with cochlear implant Ⓑ
Medicare Statute 1862a7

⃠ **V5274** Assistive listening device, not otherwise specified Ⓑ
Medicare Statute 1862a7

⃠ **V5275** Ear impression, each Ⓑ
Medicare Statute 1862a7

⃠ **V5281** Assistive listening device, personal FM/DM system, monaural, (1 receiver, transmitter, microphone), any type Ⓑ
Medicare Statute 1862a7

⃠ **V5282** Assistive listening device, personal FM/DM system, binaural, (2 receivers, transmitter, microphone), any type Ⓑ
Medicare Statute 1862a7

⃠ **V5283** Assistive listening device, personal FM/DM neck, loop induction receiver Ⓑ
Medicare Statute 1862a7

⃠ **V5284** Assistive listening device, personal FM/DM, ear level receiver Ⓑ
Medicare Statute 1862a7

⃠ **V5285** Assistive listening device, personal FM/DM, direct audio input receiver Ⓑ
Medicare Statute 1862a7

⃠ **V5286** Assistive listening device, personal blue tooth FM/DM receiver Ⓑ
Medicare Statute 1862a7

⃠ **V5287** Assistive listening device, personal FM/DM receiver, not otherwise specified Ⓑ
Medicare Statute 1862a7

⃠ **V5288** Assistive listening device, personal FM/DM transmitter assistive listening device Ⓑ
Medicare Statute 1862a7

⃠ **V5289** Assistive listening device, personal FM/DM adapter/boot coupling device for receiver, any type Ⓑ
Medicare Statute 1862a7

⃠ **V5290** Assistive listening device, transmitter microphone, any type Ⓑ
Medicare Statute 1862a7

⃠ **V5298** Hearing aid, not otherwise classified Ⓑ
Medicare Statute 1862a7

✪ **V5299** Hearing service, miscellaneous Ⓑ
IOM: 100-02, 16, 90

Repair/Modification

⃠ **V5336** Repair/modification of augmentative communicative system or device (excludes adaptive hearing aid) Ⓓ
Medicare Statute 1862a7

Speech, Language, and Pathology Screening

These codes are for non-physician services.

⃠ **V5362** Speech screening Ⓑ
Medicare Statute 1862a7

⃠ **V5363** Language screening Ⓑ
Medicare Statute 1862a7

⃠ **V5364** Dysphagia screening Ⓑ
Medicare Statute 1862a7

▶ New ⤾ Revised ✔ Reinstated ~~deleted~~ Deleted ⃠ Not covered or valid by Medicare
✪ Special coverage instructions ✻ Carrier discretion Ⓑ Bill local carrier Ⓓ Bill DME MAC

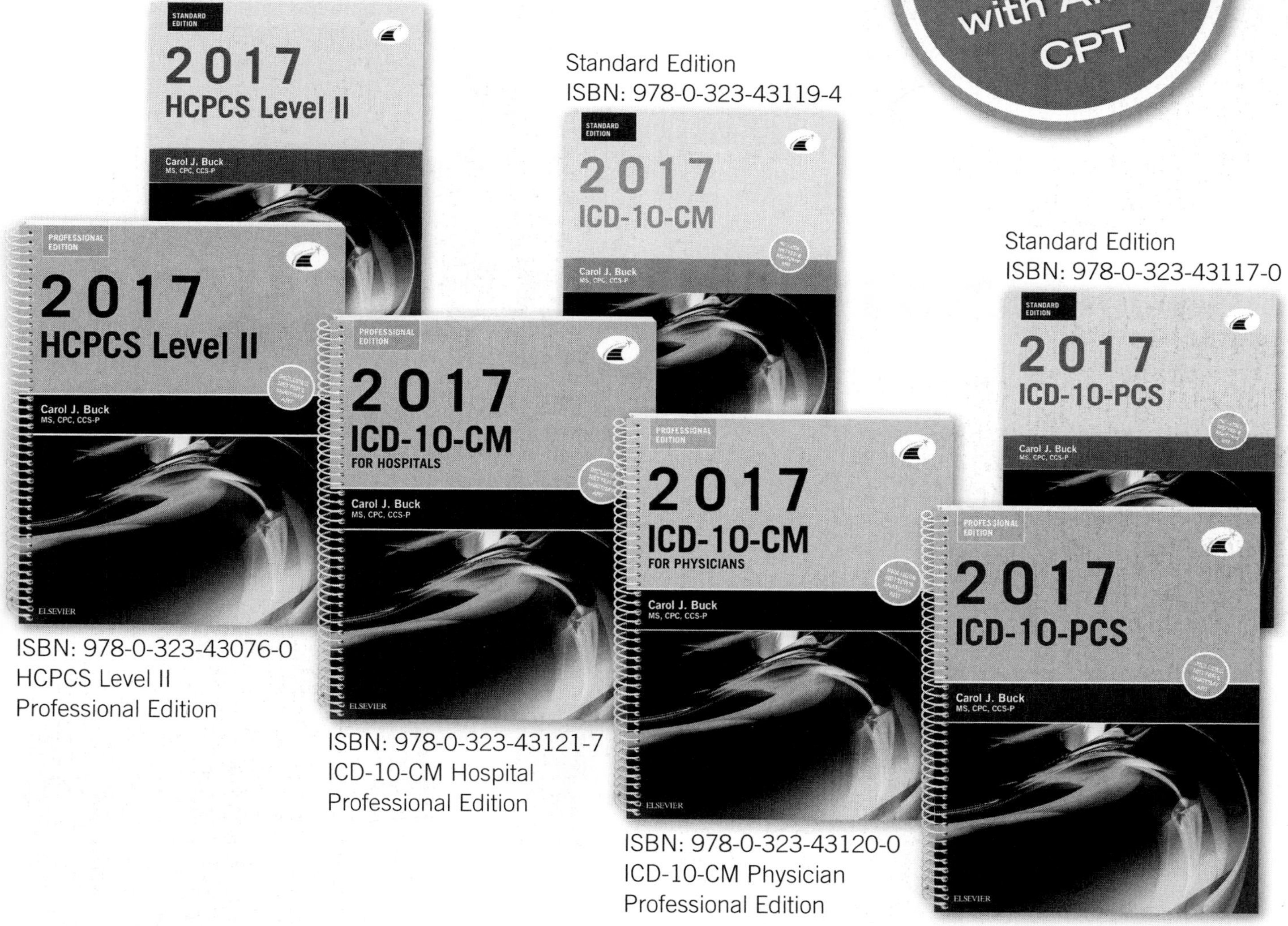

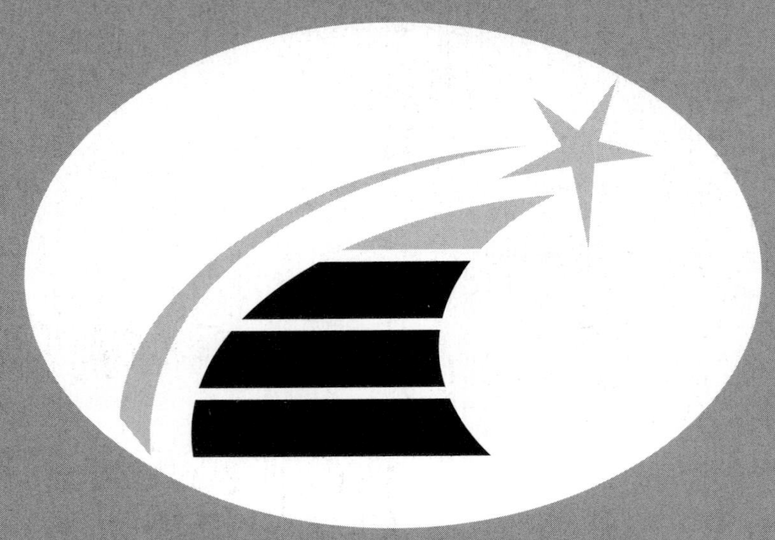

Step 4: Professional Resources

"Nothing is particularly hard if you divide it into small jobs."

— Henry Ford

We want to applaud you for taking this step in your career.

Medical coding is a fine profession that has the ability to intrigue and captivate you for a lifetime. Practice your craft carefully, with due diligence, patience for the process, and always the highest ethical standards.

— Carol J. Buck, MS, CPC, CCS-P

— Jackie L. Grass, CPC

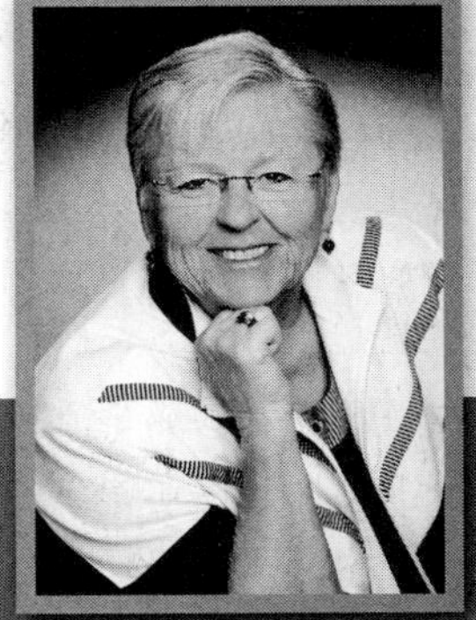

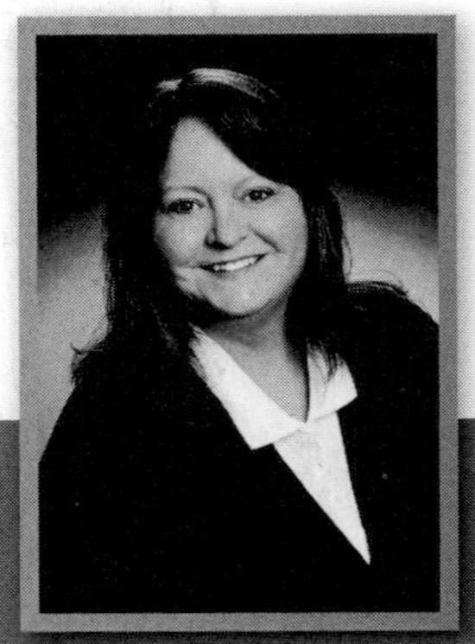

Track your progress!

See the checklist in the back of this book to learn more about your steps toward coding success!

TRAVEL THE WORLD ATLAS

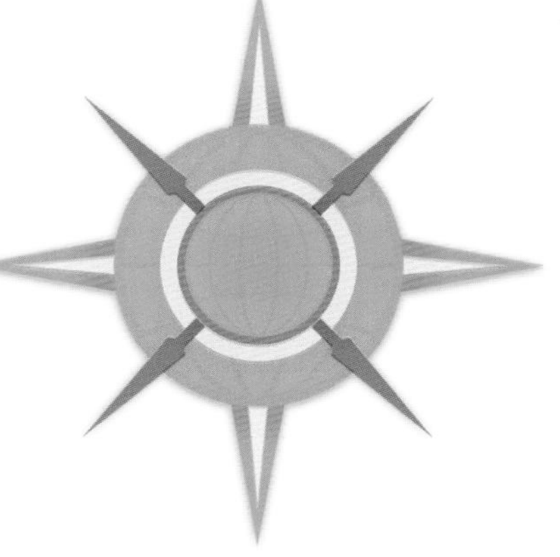

WRITTEN BY
Shirley Willis

ILLUSTRATED BY
Nick Hewetson

CREATED AND DESIGNED BY
David Salariya

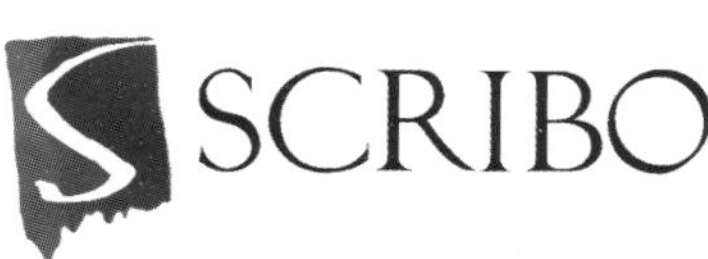

SCRIBO

Contents

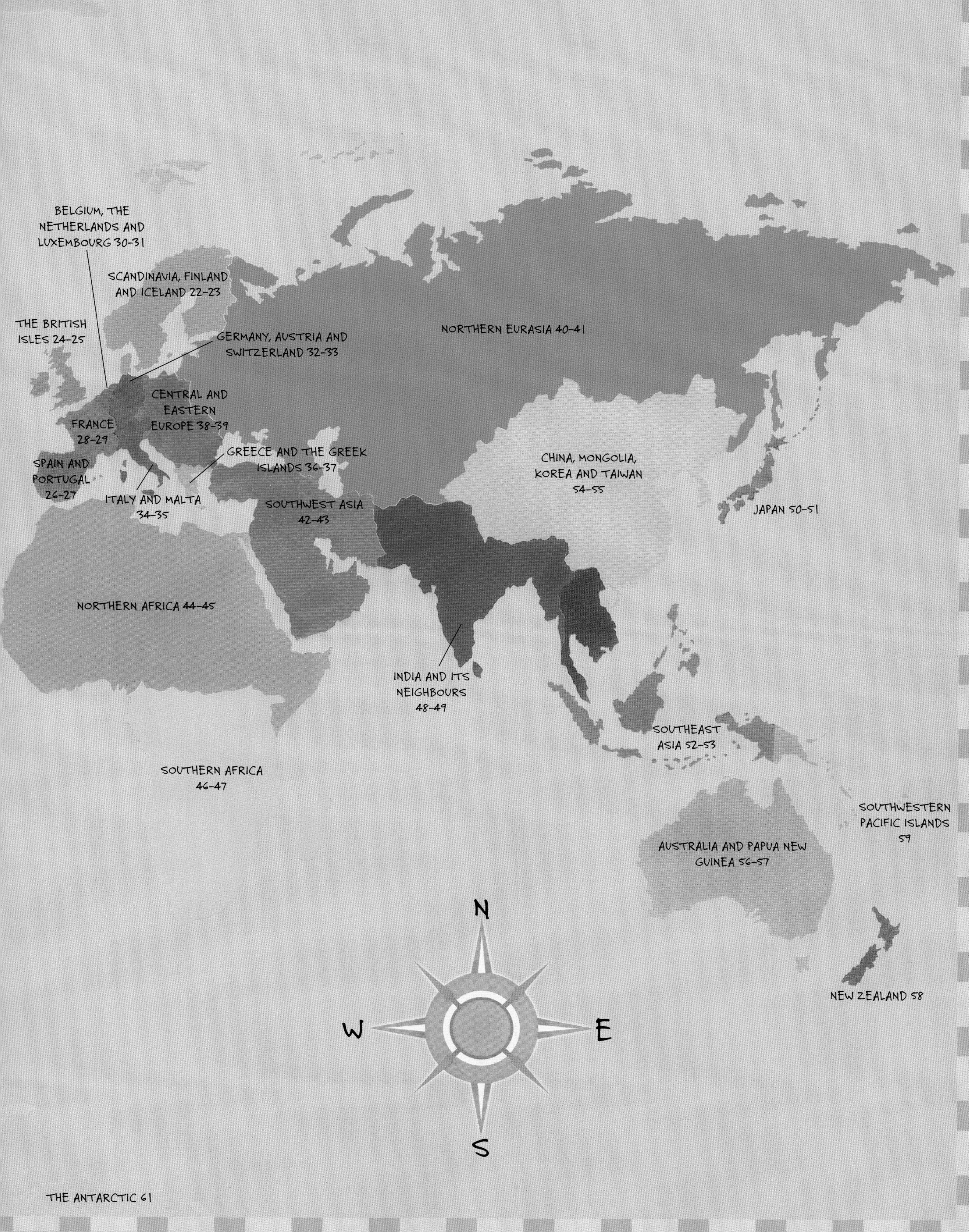
BELGIUM, THE NETHERLANDS AND LUXEMBOURG 30–31
SCANDINAVIA, FINLAND AND ICELAND 22–23
THE BRITISH ISLES 24–25
GERMANY, AUSTRIA AND SWITZERLAND 32–33
NORTHERN EURASIA 40–41
CENTRAL AND EASTERN EUROPE 38–39
FRANCE 28–29
GREECE AND THE GREEK ISLANDS 36–37
SPAIN AND PORTUGAL 26–27
ITALY AND MALTA 34–35
SOUTHWEST ASIA 42–43
CHINA, MONGOLIA, KOREA AND TAIWAN 54–55
JAPAN 50–51
NORTHERN AFRICA 44–45
INDIA AND ITS NEIGHBOURS 48–49
SOUTHEAST ASIA 52–53
SOUTHERN AFRICA 46–47
SOUTHWESTERN PACIFIC ISLANDS 59
AUSTRALIA AND PAPUA NEW GUINEA 56–57
N
W
E
S
NEW ZEALAND 58
THE ANTARCTIC 61

The Earth in space

The Earth is a ball of rock that orbits the Sun. It depends on the Sun's energy for warmth and light.

The Earth is one of eight planets that orbit (circle) the Sun. Together they form the Solar System.
Each planet orbits the Sun in an elliptical (oval) path. The length of a planet's orbit depends on its distance from the Sun. Mercury is closest and takes 88 days to orbit the Sun, but Neptune takes almost 165 years because it is so far away from the Sun. The Earth's orbit takes about 365 days. Beyond Neptune are 'dwarf' planets such as Pluto.

Uranus

Saturn

Neptune

The Earth is always moving. As it orbits the Sun, the planet spins on its axis, making one complete turn every 24 hours. While one side of its surface is lit by the Sun, the other side is in darkness. This is why we have day-time and night-time.

The Earth's axis is an imaginary line running through its center.

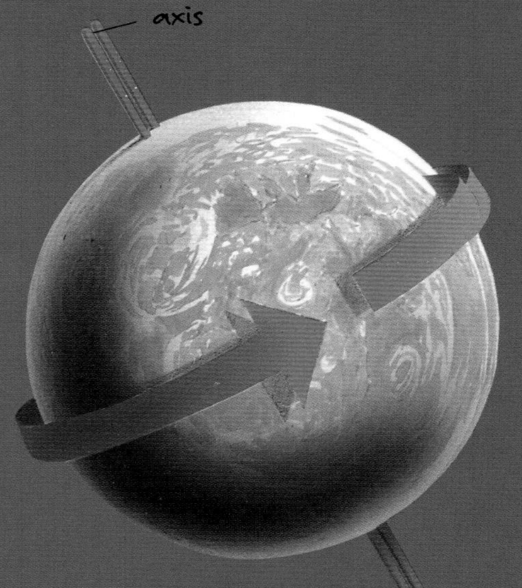

The Earth seen from space

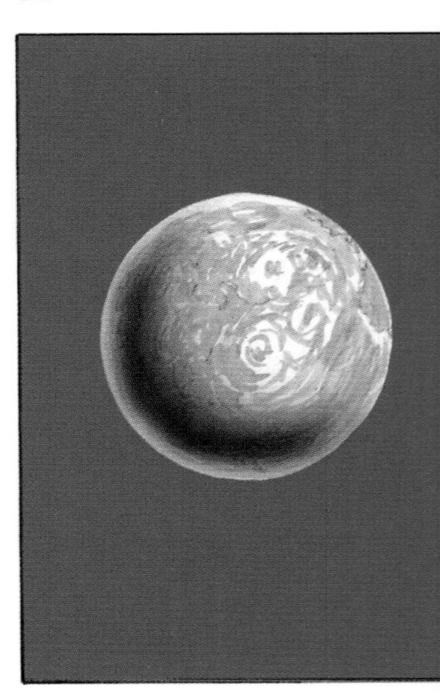

The Earth is 93 million miles (148,800,000 km) from the Sun, making it neither too hot nor too cold to live on. It is the only planet in the Solar System where life is known to exist.

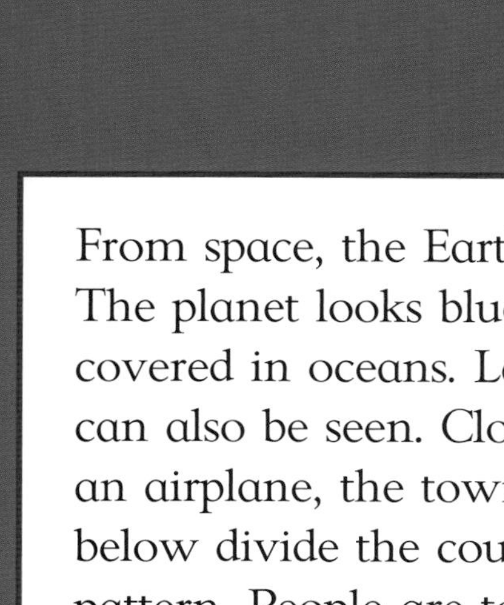

Sun

Jupiter

From space, the Earth is seen as a huge round ball. The planet looks blue because much of its surface is covered in oceans. Large landmasses, called continents, can also be seen. Closer up, the Earth looks flat. From an airplane, the towns, roads, rivers, and railway tracks below divide the countryside into a huge patchwork pattern. People are too small to be seen from this distance. If you look down from a skyscraper, people below can be seen but look as small as ants. Cars on the streets look like children's toys.

The Earth seen from an airplane

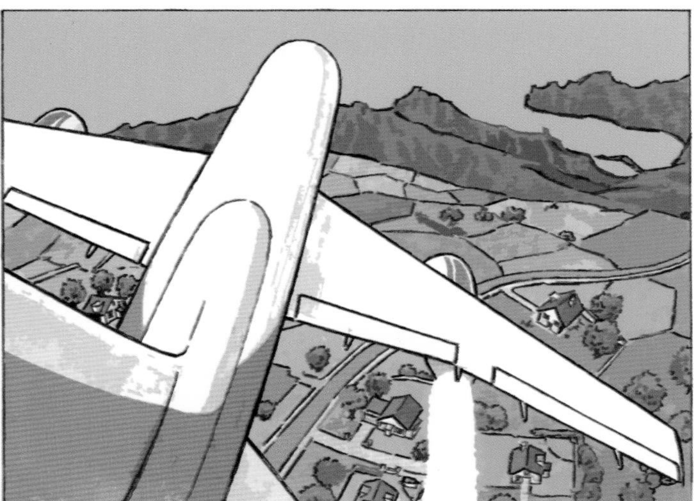

The Earth seen from a tall building

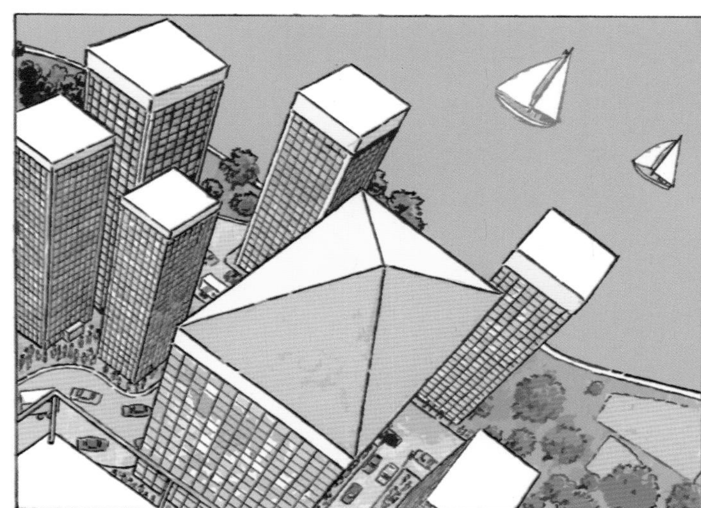

How the world becomes a flat map

A globe is a round map of the world. Mapmakers make a flat map of the world for an atlas.

Our planet is made up of four layers (below). We live on the surface of the Earth which is called the crust. Every continent and ocean lies on the Earth's crust. Beneath the crust is a layer of rock called the mantle. Parts of the mantle are hot and molten (liquid) and can break through the crust to form a volcano. The core of the planet has two parts: the outer core is hot, molten metal and the inner core is solid metal.

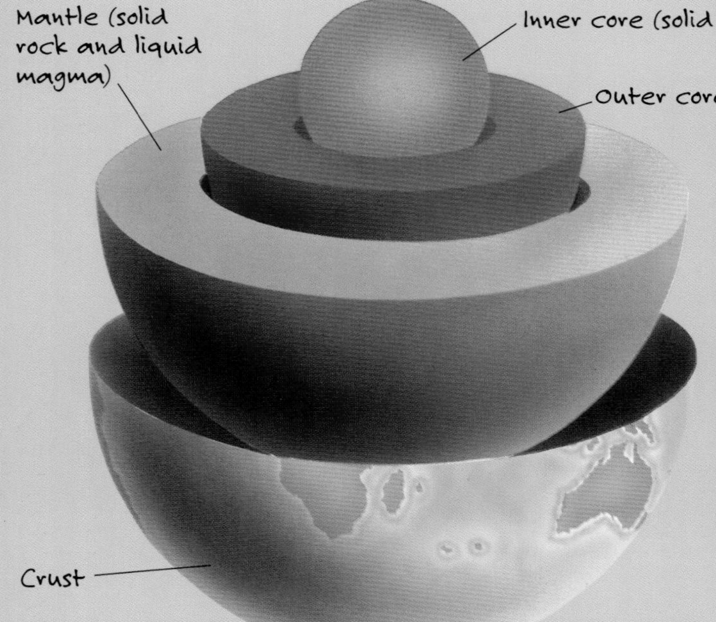

Map-makers divide the world's surface into segments. These are laid side by side like the skin of an orange, but this leaves gaps in the map (above). Parts of the world have to be 'stretched' so that the map joins up. This process is called map projection. On the flat maps in an atlas, the countries are shaped slightly differently than they are on a globe.

Map-makers use a grid of imaginary lines across the globe to help plot the exact positions of places. Lines of longitude are drawn from north to south and lines of latitude from east to west.

The equator is an imaginary line dividing the world in half. It is positioned at latitude o (zero degrees). The northern hemisphere is above the equator and the southern hemisphere is below.

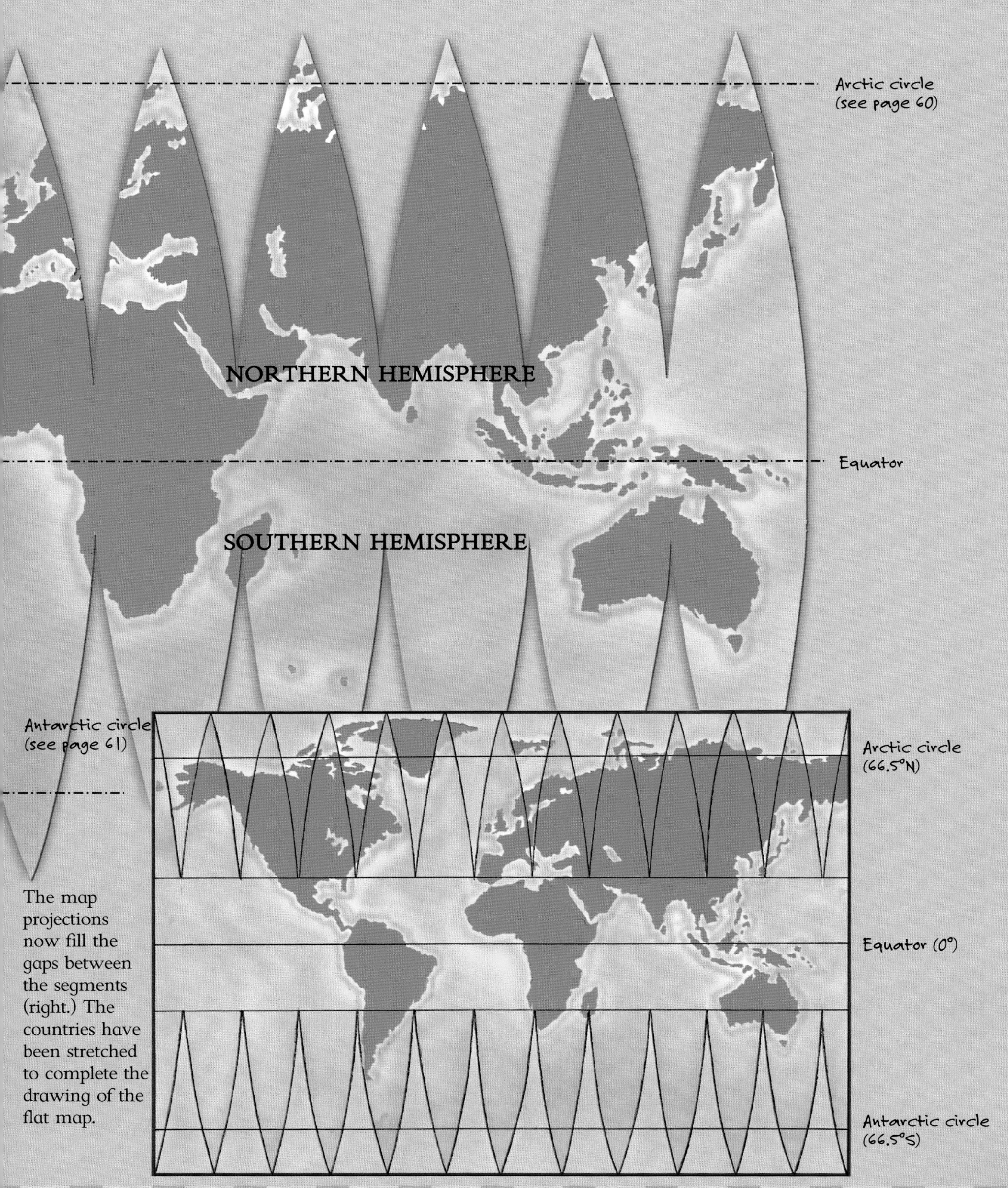

The map projections now fill the gaps between the segments (right.) The countries have been stretched to complete the drawing of the flat map.

How the pages work in this atlas

This is the kind of map you will find in this atlas. Each page shows a map of different countries of the world. The notes on this page explain the type of information given on each map.

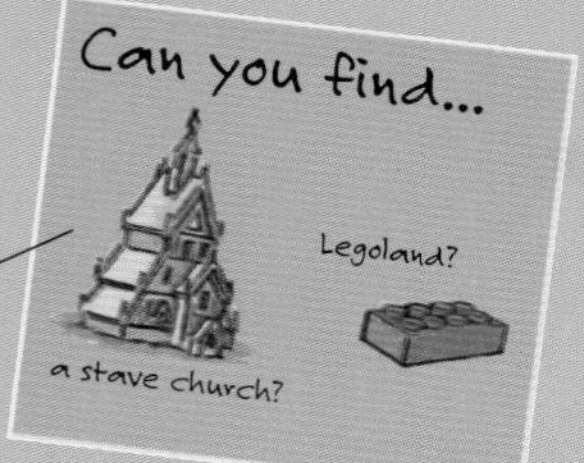
Scandinavia, Fi
and Iceland
Norway, Sweden and Denmark are known as Scandinavia. These countries are rich in natural resources: timber, fish, oil and natural gas. They have warm summers but bitterly cold winters.
Can you find...
Legoland?
a stave church?

"Can you find..." Look at the map to find the buildings or places of interest shown in the box.

A large label in capital letters shows a country's name.

A thick dotted line shows the border between countries. A thin dotted line shows state borders within a country.

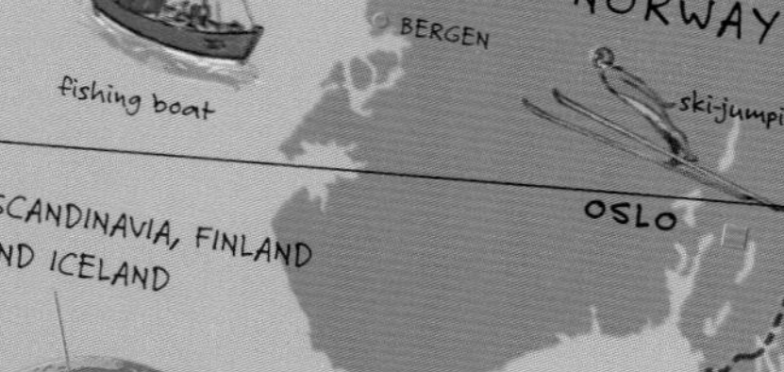
oil rig
stave church
skiing
NORWAY
BERGEN
fishing boat
ski-jumping
OSLO
Drottningholm Palace
Norway spruce
SCANDINAVIA, FINLAND AND ICELAND

The globe shows where each country is in the world.

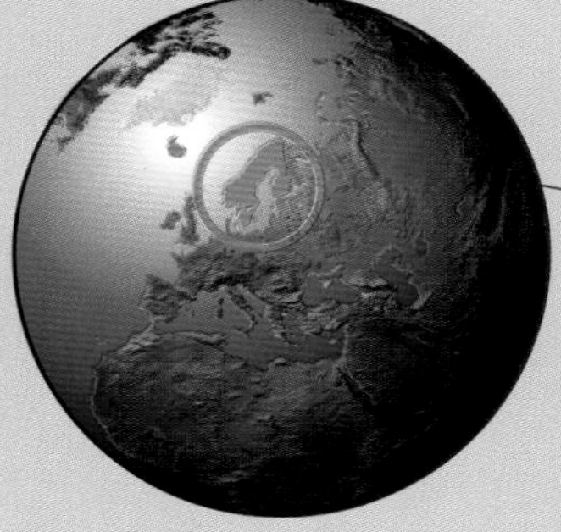

A small label like this shows the name of a lake or river.

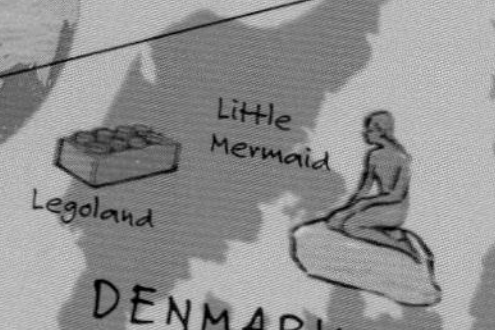
Little Mermaid
Legoland
GOTHENBURG

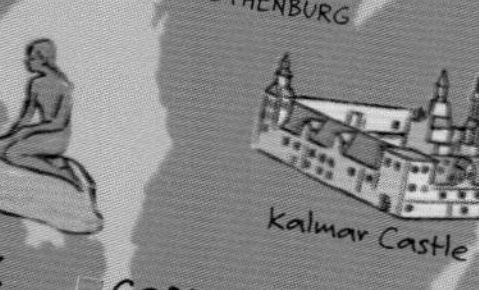

A curved label like this shows the name of a sea or ocean.

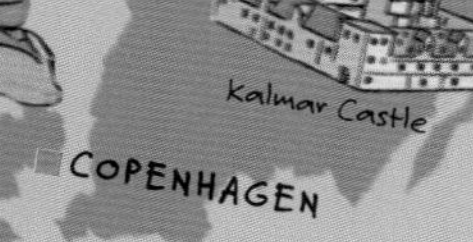

Fact boxes give extra information about each country or continent.

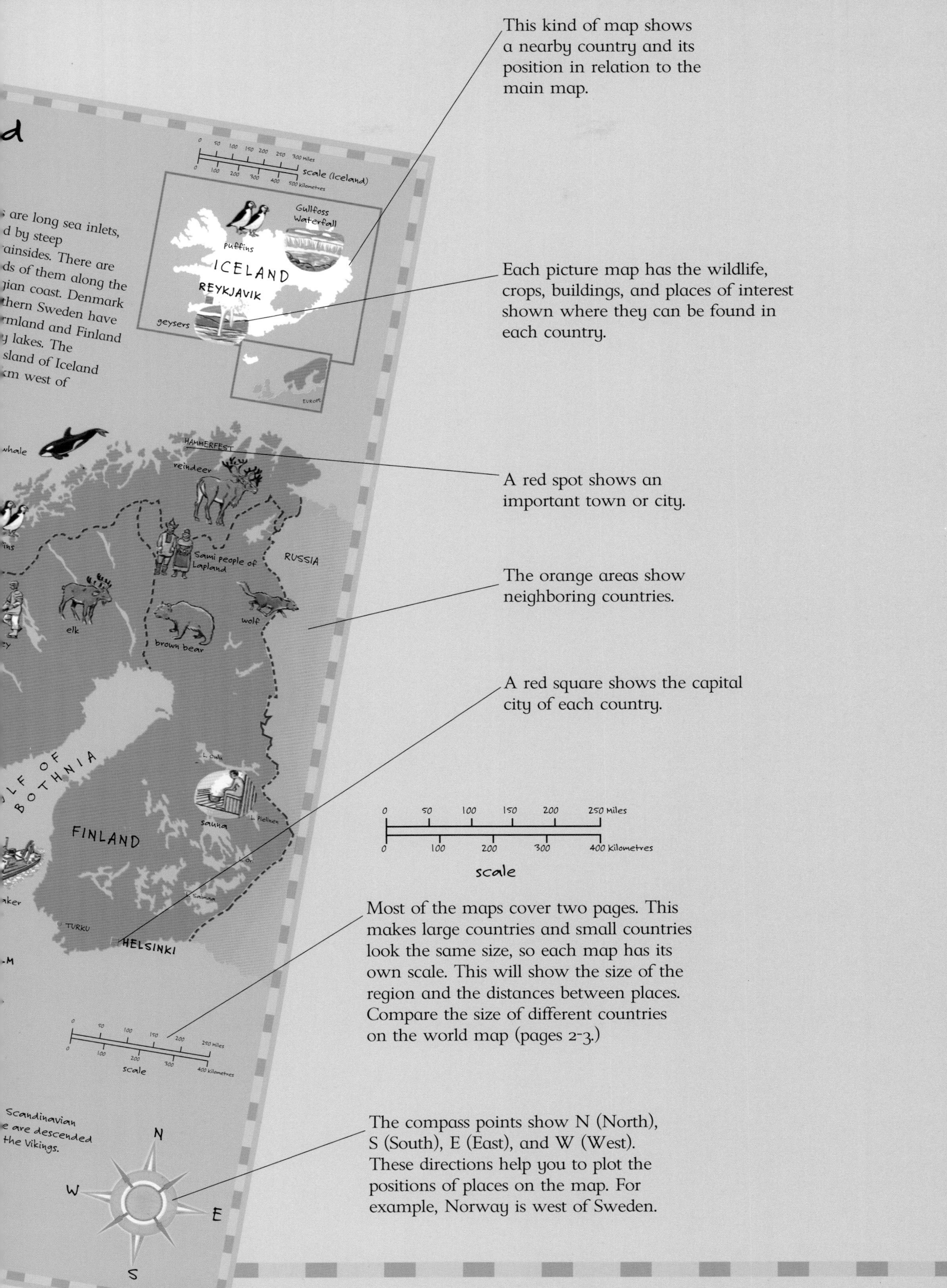

This kind of map shows a nearby country and its position in relation to the main map.
Each picture map has the wildlife, crops, buildings, and places of interest shown where they can be found in each country.
A red spot shows an important town or city.
The orange areas show neighboring countries.
A red square shows the capital city of each country.
Most of the maps cover two pages. This makes large countries and small countries look the same size, so each map has its own scale. This will show the size of the region and the distances between places. Compare the size of different countries on the world map (pages 2-3.)
The compass points show N (North), S (South), E (East), and W (West). These directions help you to plot the positions of places on the map. For example, Norway is west of Sweden.
scale (Iceland)
puffins
Gullfoss Waterfall
ICELAND
REYKJAVIK
geysers
HAMMERFEST
reindeer
Sami people of Lapland
RUSSIA
elk
brown bear
wolf
L. Oulu
sauna
FINLAND
TURKU
HELSINKI
0 50 100 150 200 250 Miles
0 100 200 300 400 Kilometres
scale
N
W
E
S

Canada and Greenland

Canada is the second biggest country in the world but it does not have a large population. Few people live in northern Canada as the climate there is too cold.

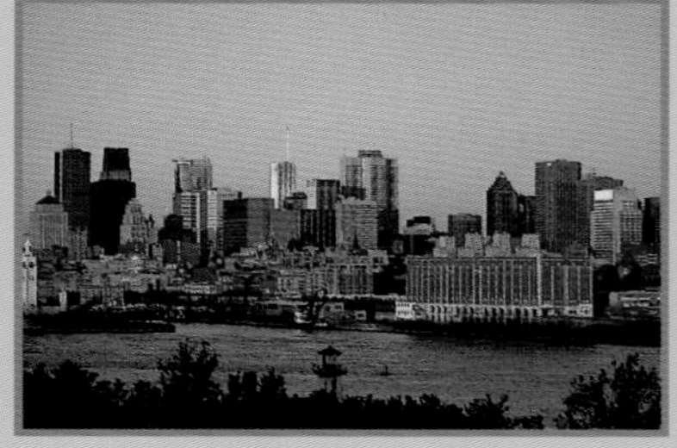

Canada has two official languages: English and French. Montreal (above) in Quebec is the largest French-speaking city in the world after Paris.

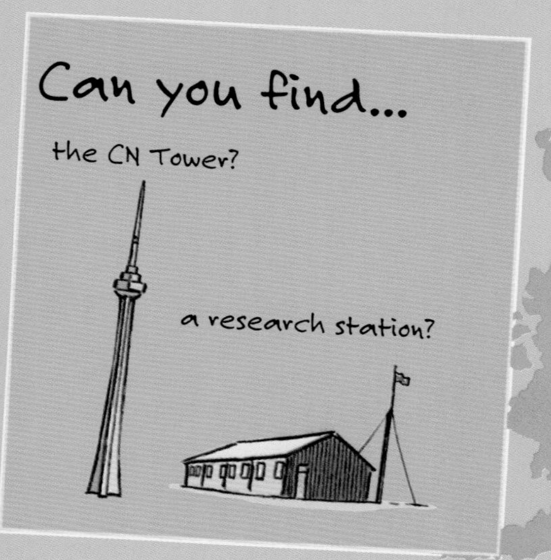

Can you find...
the CN Tower?
a research station?

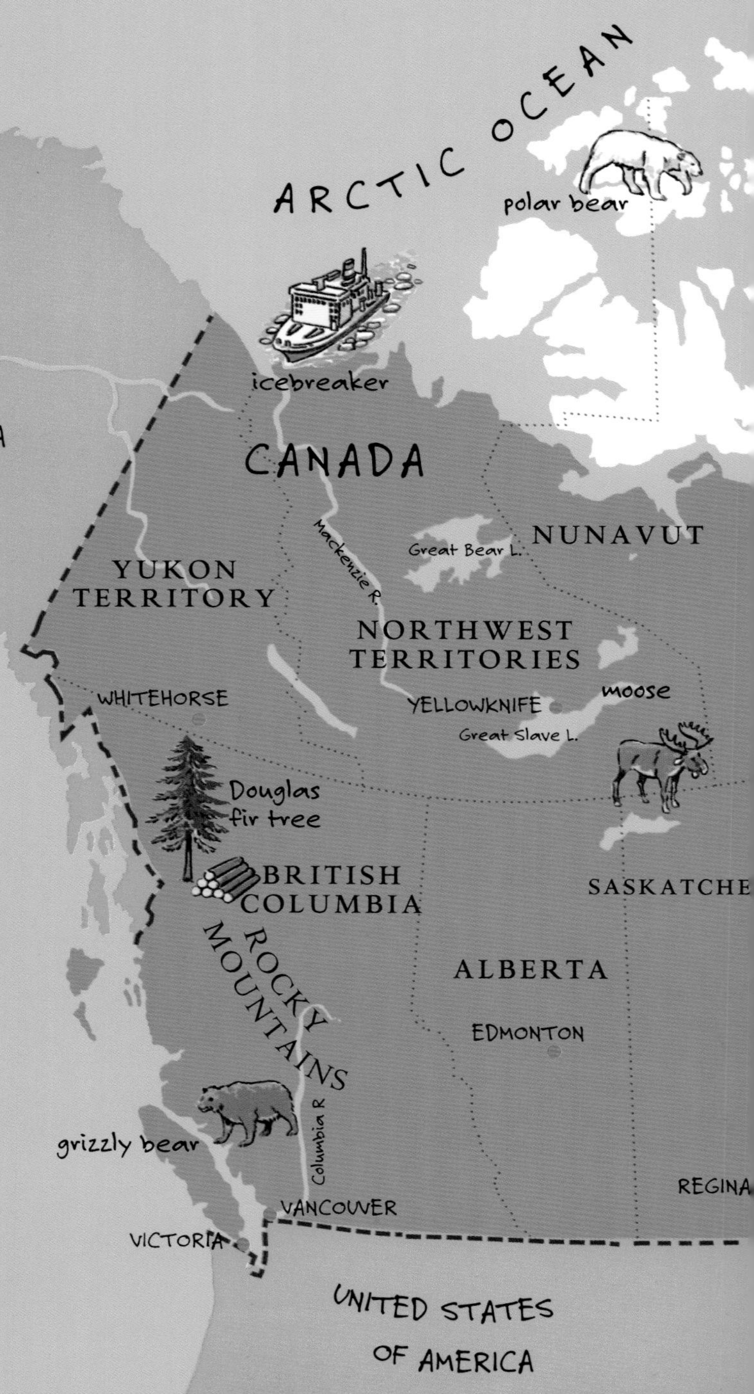

There are high, rocky mountain ranges in the west and rich, flat farmlands called "prairies" in the central area of Canada. Most Canadians live in the big cities in the east where the climate is less cold.

Greenland is the largest island in the world. It belongs to Denmark but has its own government. The Inuit people who live in northern Canada and Greenland still hunt seals and polar bears.

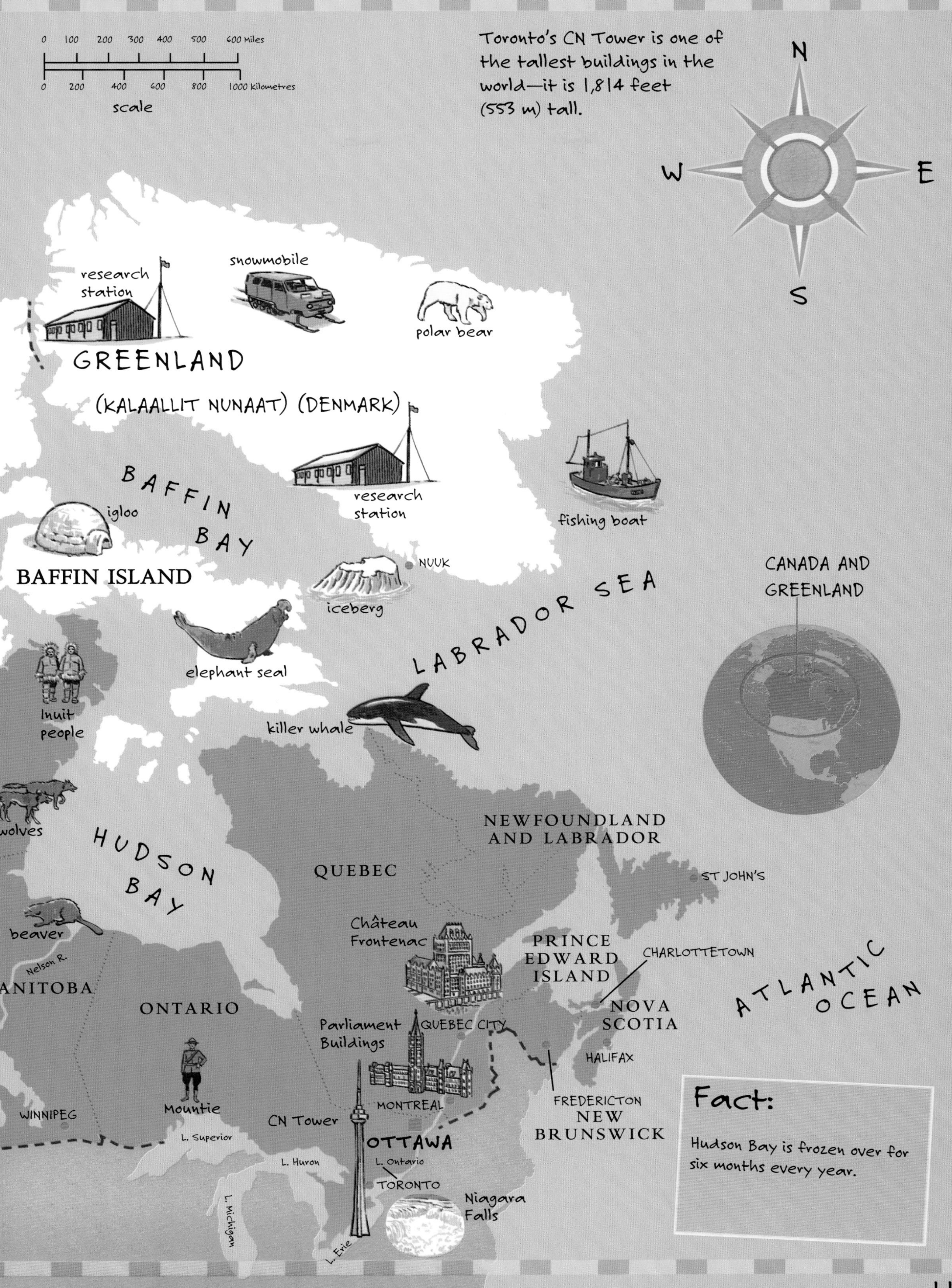

0 100 200 300 400 500 600 Miles
0 200 400 600 800 1000 Kilometres
scale
Toronto's CN Tower is one of the tallest buildings in the world—it is 1,814 feet (553 m) tall.
N
W
E
S
research station
snowmobile
polar bear
GREENLAND
(KALAALLIT NUNAAT) (DENMARK)
research station
fishing boat
BAFFIN BAY
igloo
BAFFIN ISLAND
NUUK
iceberg
LABRADOR SEA
CANADA AND GREENLAND
elephant seal
Inuit people
killer whale
wolves
HUDSON BAY
NEWFOUNDLAND AND LABRADOR
QUEBEC
ST JOHN'S
beaver
Château Frontenac
PRINCE EDWARD ISLAND
CHARLOTTETOWN
ATLANTIC OCEAN
Nelson R.
MANITOBA
ONTARIO
NOVA SCOTIA
Parliament Buildings
QUEBEC CITY
HALIFAX
FREDERICTON
NEW BRUNSWICK
Mountie
MONTREAL
WINNIPEG
CN Tower
L. Superior
OTTAWA
L. Huron
L. Ontario
TORONTO
L. Michigan
Niagara Falls
L. Erie
Fact:
Hudson Bay is frozen over for six months every year.

USA: The West and Midwest

The United States of America (USA) is one of the wealthiest countries in the world. It is made up of fifty states. The western states include Alaska in the far north and Hawaii, 2,485 miles (4,000 km) out in the Pacific Ocean.

The rugged landscape of the western states is dominated by the Rocky Mountains. California is the largest state in the region. More people live there than in any other American state.

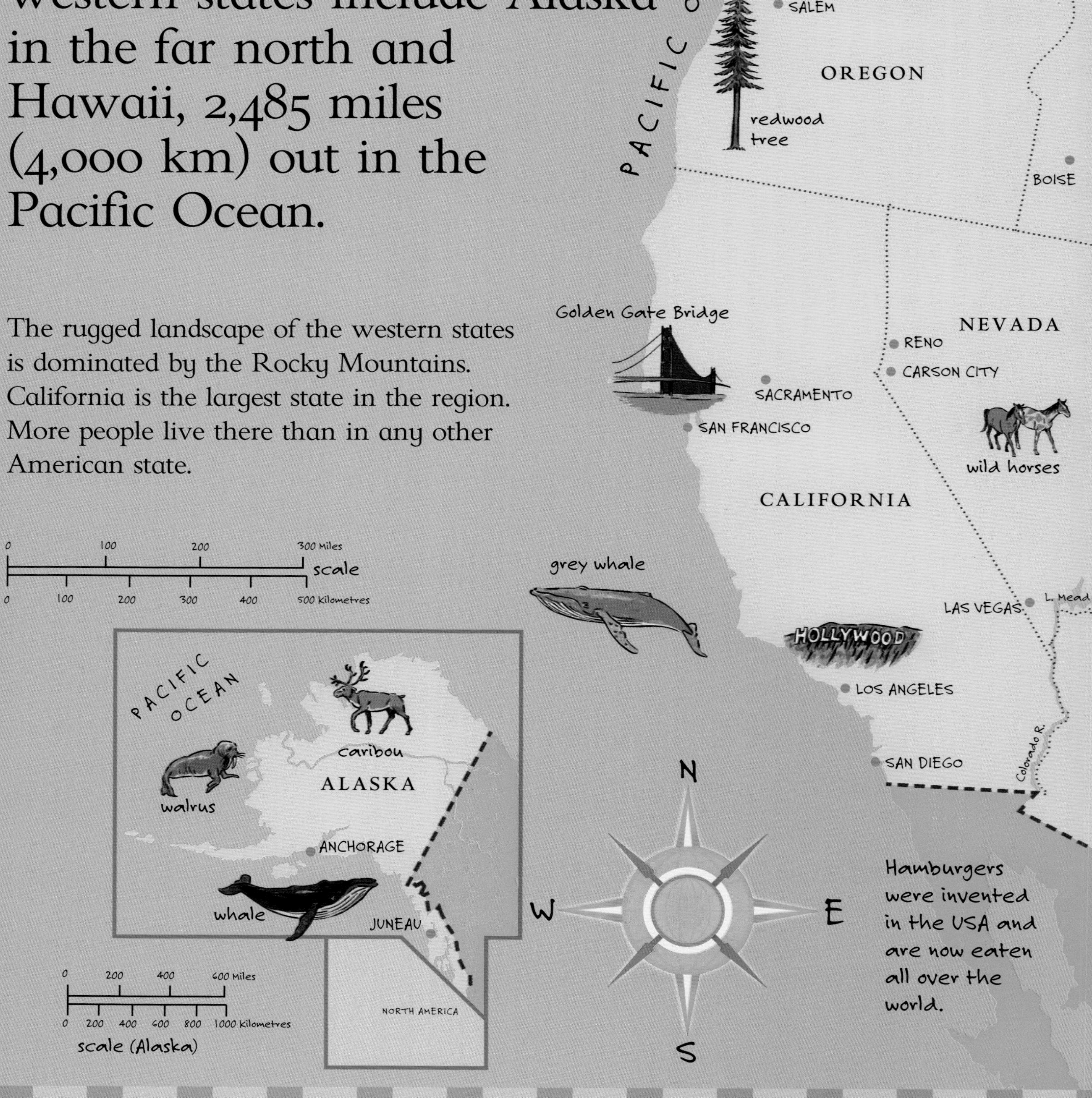

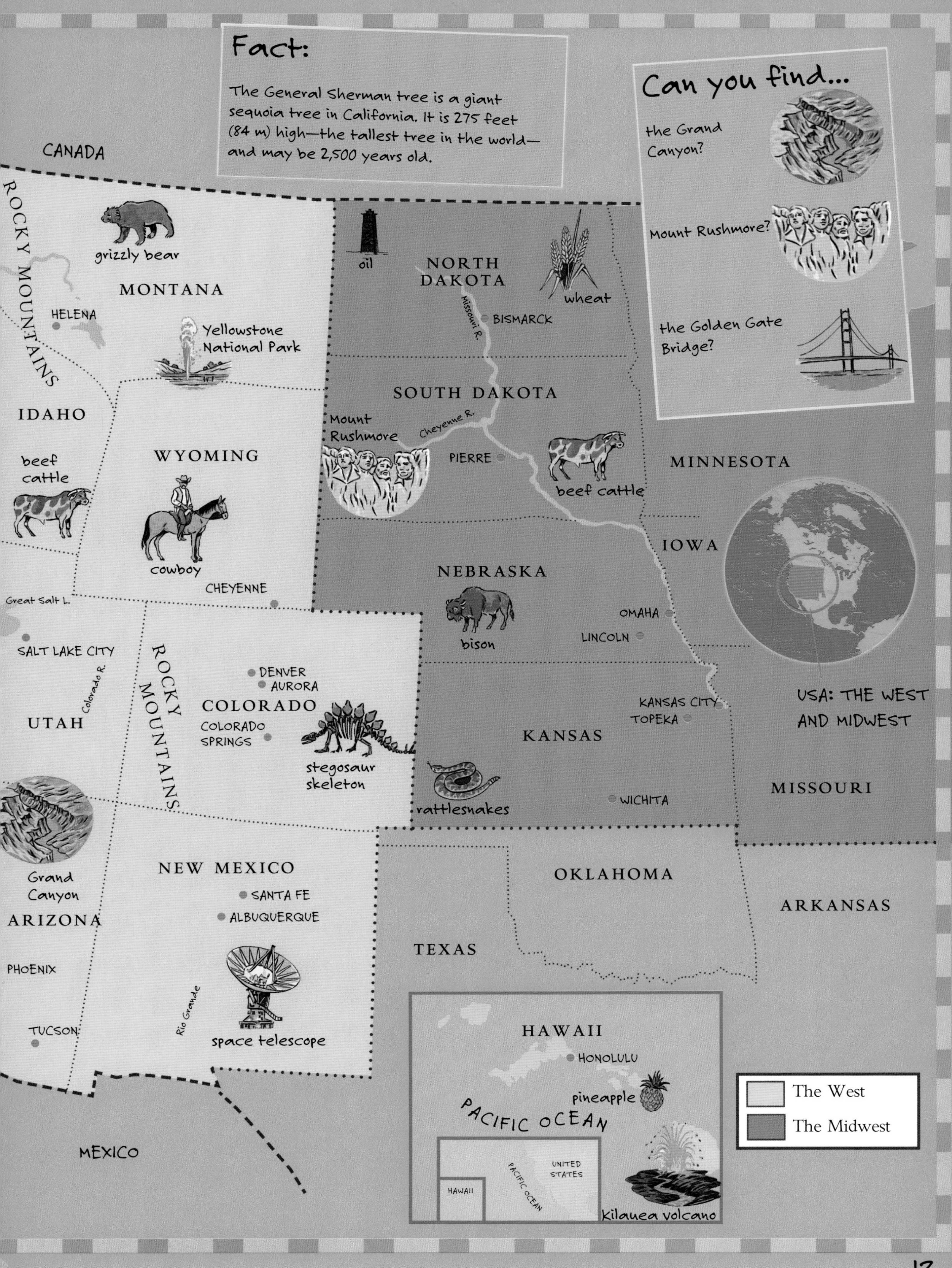
Fact:
The General Sherman tree is a giant sequoia tree in California. It is 275 feet (84 m) high—the tallest tree in the world—and may be 2,500 years old.
Can you find...
the Grand Canyon?
Mount Rushmore?
the Golden Gate Bridge?
CANADA
ROCKY MOUNTAINS
grizzly bear
MONTANA
HELENA
Yellowstone National Park
oil
NORTH DAKOTA
Missouri R.
BISMARCK
wheat
SOUTH DAKOTA
Mount Rushmore
Cheyenne R.
PIERRE
beef cattle
MINNESOTA
IDAHO
beef cattle
WYOMING
cowboy
CHEYENNE
IOWA
NEBRASKA
bison
OMAHA
LINCOLN
Great Salt L.
SALT LAKE CITY
Colorado R.
UTAH
ROCKY MOUNTAINS
DENVER
AURORA
COLORADO
COLORADO SPRINGS
stegosaur skeleton
KANSAS CITY
TOPEKA
KANSAS
rattlesnakes
WICHITA
USA: THE WEST AND MIDWEST
MISSOURI
Grand Canyon
ARIZONA
PHOENIX
TUCSON
NEW MEXICO
SANTA FE
ALBUQUERQUE
Rio Grande
space telescope
OKLAHOMA
ARKANSAS
TEXAS
HAWAII
HONOLULU
pineapple
PACIFIC OCEAN
UNITED STATES
PACIFIC OCEAN
HAWAII
Kilauea volcano
The West
The Midwest
MEXICO

USA: The Midwest and Northeast

The United States is the world's most industrialized country. The area around the Great Lakes supplies most of the USA's iron and steel. Detroit was famous as the center of the American car industry.

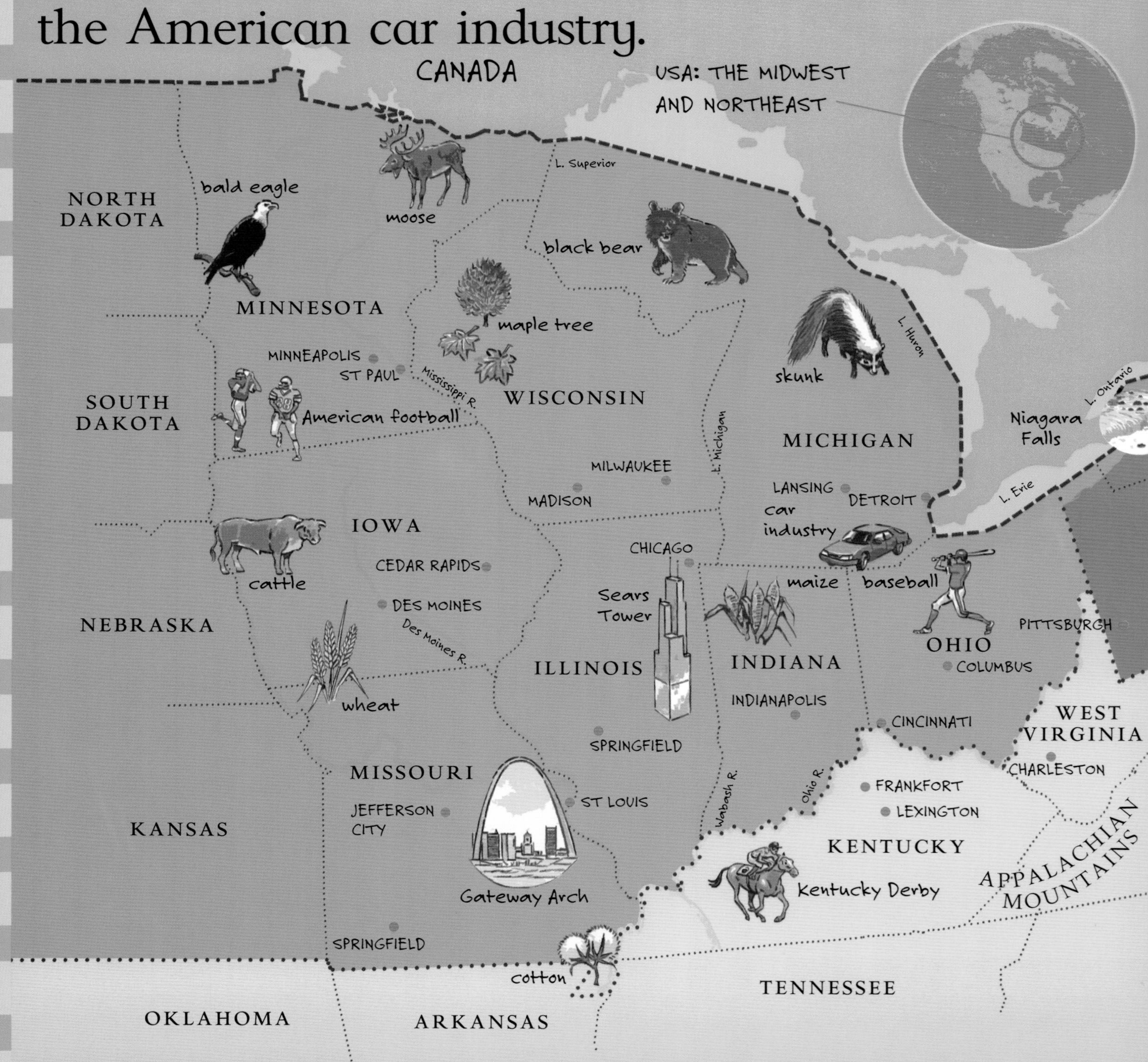

The flat, fertile plains south of the Great Lakes produce so much wheat and maize that the area is known as the "breadbasket of the world." Over the Appalachian Mountains lie the great cities of the Atlantic coast. New York City is the largest city in the USA, with a population of 8.5 million.

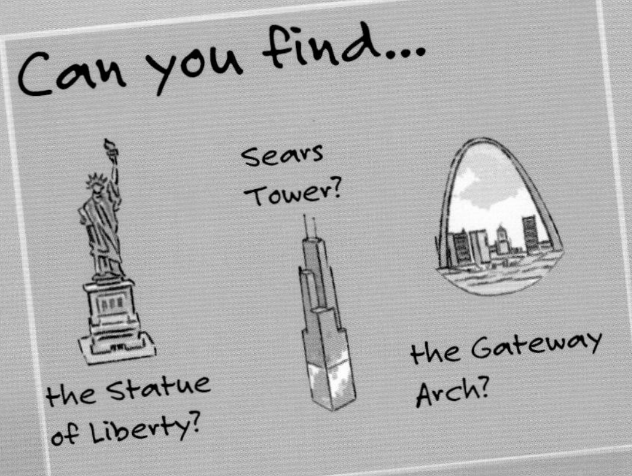

Fact:

The White House in Washington, D.C. (District of Columbia) has been the home of United States presidents for nearly 200 years.

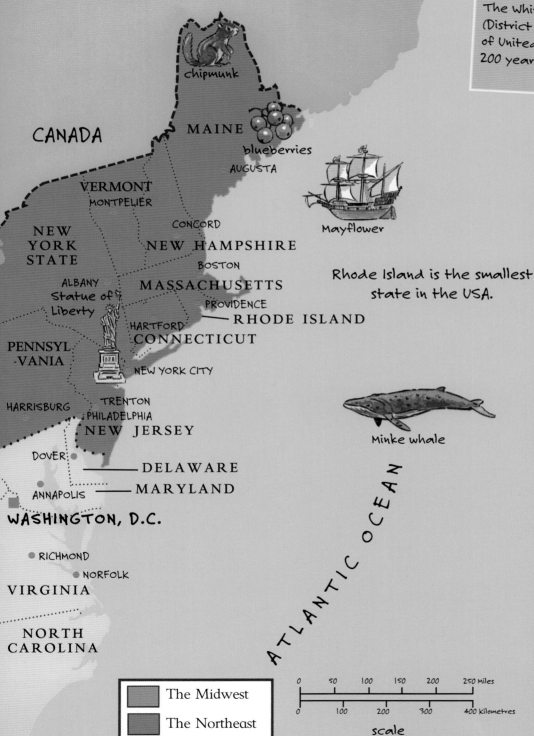

CANADA
chipmunk
MAINE
blueberries
AUGUSTA
VERMONT
MONTPELIER
Mayflower
CONCORD
NEW YORK STATE
NEW HAMPSHIRE
BOSTON
Rhode Island is the smallest state in the USA.
ALBANY
MASSACHUSETTS
Statue of Liberty
PROVIDENCE
RHODE ISLAND
HARTFORD
CONNECTICUT
PENNSYLVANIA
NEW YORK CITY
HARRISBURG
TRENTON
PHILADELPHIA
NEW JERSEY
Minke whale
DOVER
DELAWARE
ANNAPOLIS
MARYLAND
WASHINGTON, D.C.
ATLANTIC OCEAN
RICHMOND
NORFOLK
VIRGINIA
NORTH CAROLINA

The Midwest
The Northeast

0 50 100 150 200 250 Miles
0 100 200 300 400 Kilometres
scale

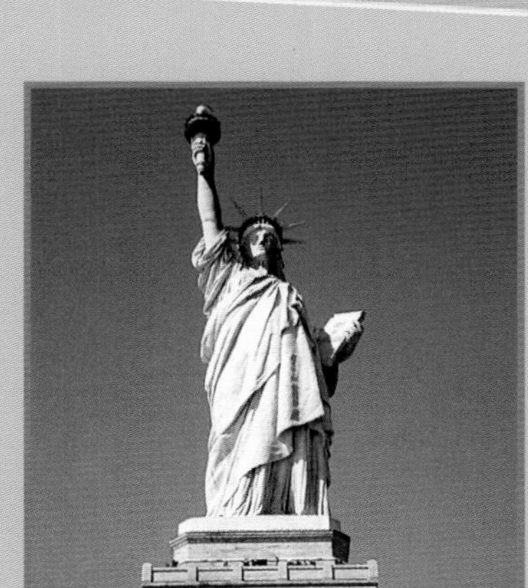

The Statue of Liberty was built by Gustave Eiffel in Paris, France. It was shipped to America in pieces and put together there. A staircase inside its hollow structure allows visitors to climb up to Liberty's crown.

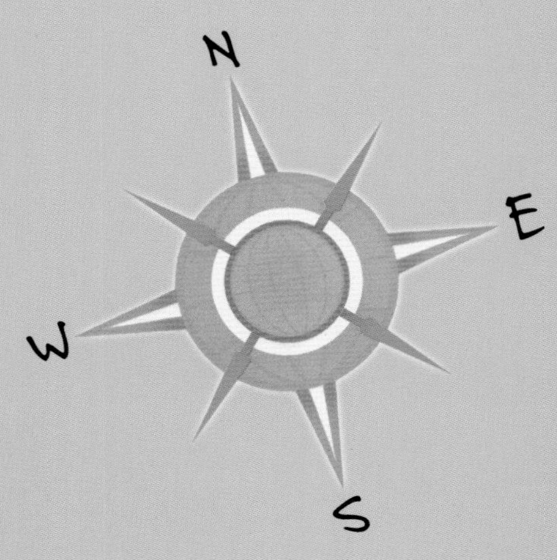

USA: The South

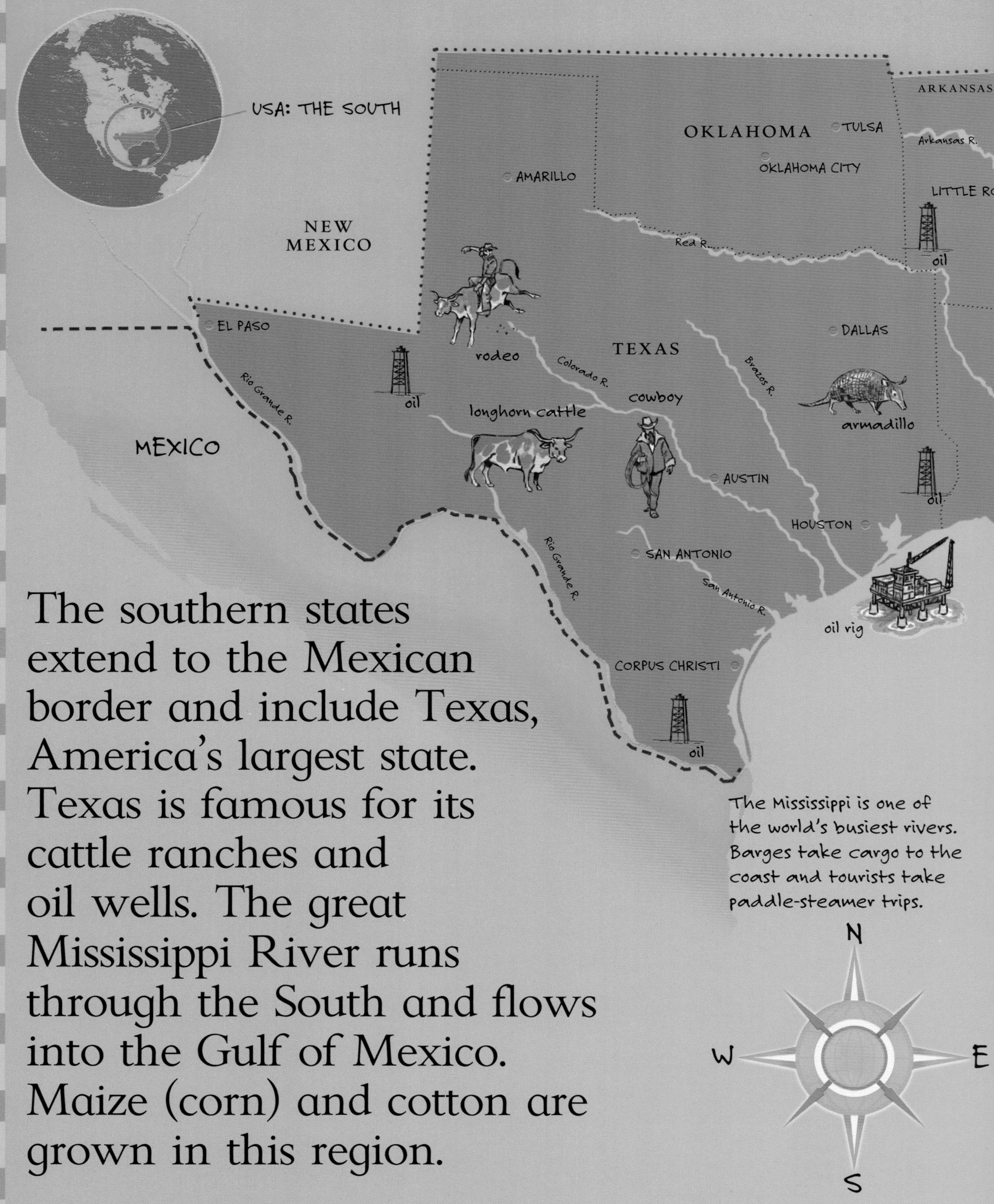

The southern states extend to the Mexican border and include Texas, America's largest state. Texas is famous for its cattle ranches and oil wells. The great Mississippi River runs through the South and flows into the Gulf of Mexico. Maize (corn) and cotton are grown in this region.

The Mississippi is one of the world's busiest rivers. Barges take cargo to the coast and tourists take paddle-steamer trips.

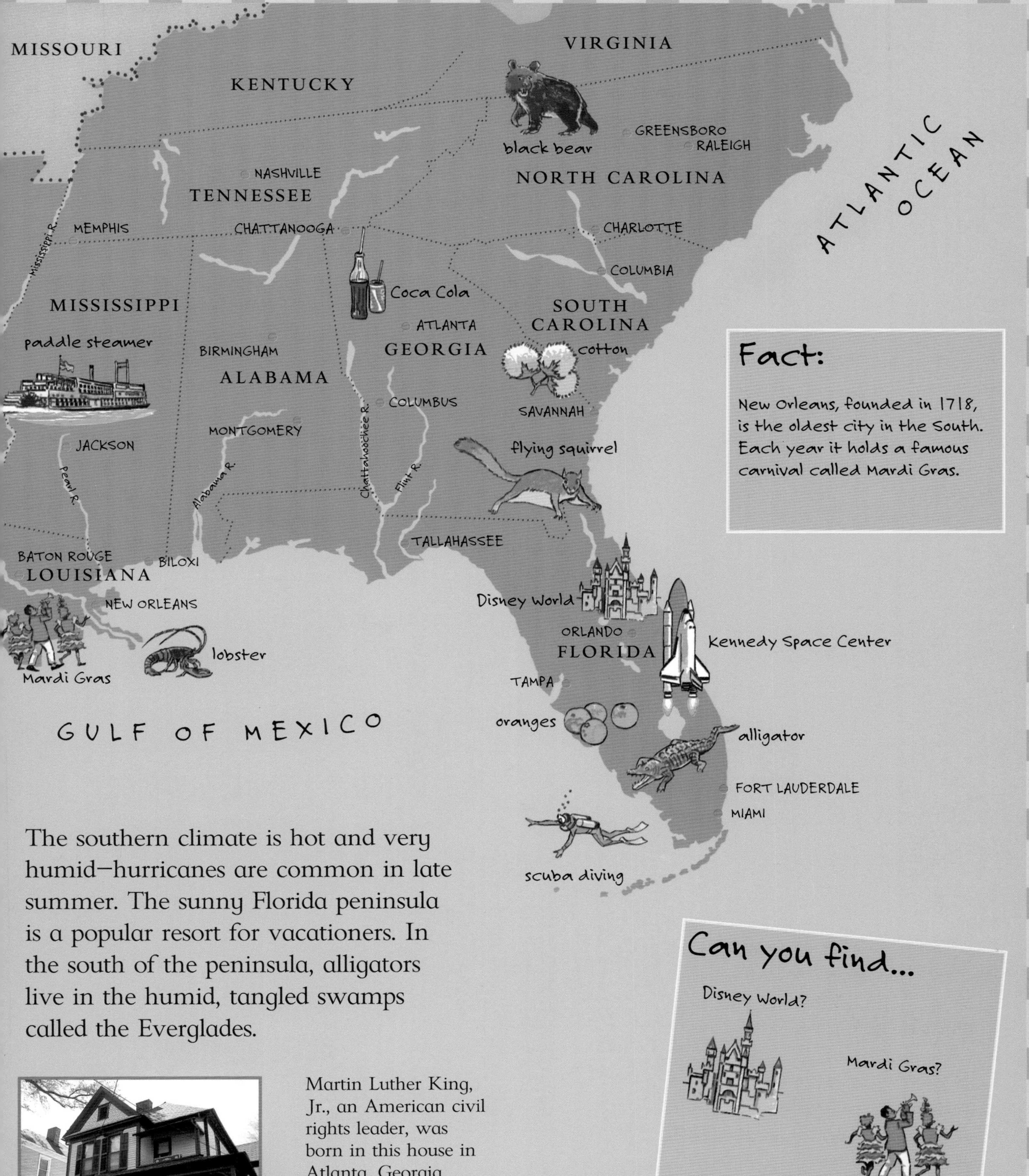

Fact:

New Orleans, founded in 1718, is the oldest city in the South. Each year it holds a famous carnival called Mardi Gras.

The southern climate is hot and very humid—hurricanes are common in late summer. The sunny Florida peninsula is a popular resort for vacationers. In the south of the peninsula, alligators live in the humid, tangled swamps called the Everglades.

Can you find...

Disney World?

Mardi Gras?

Martin Luther King, Jr., an American civil rights leader, was born in this house in Atlanta, Georgia.

0 50 100 150 200 250 300 Miles

0 100 200 300 400 500 Kilometres

scale

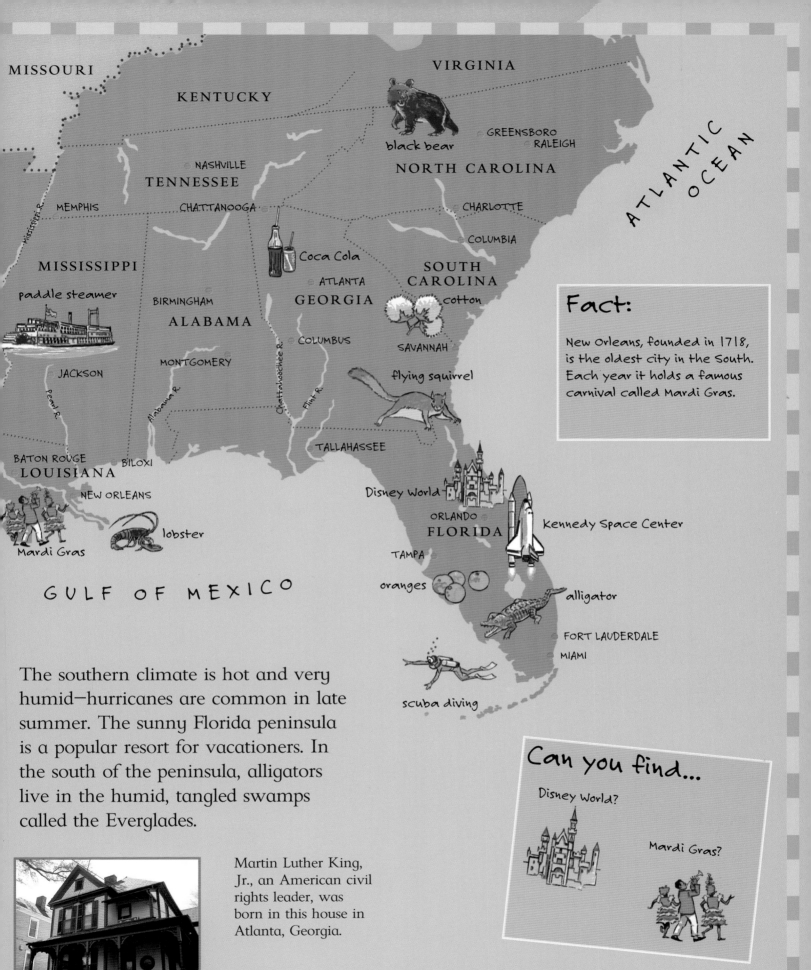

Mexico, Central America, and the Caribbean

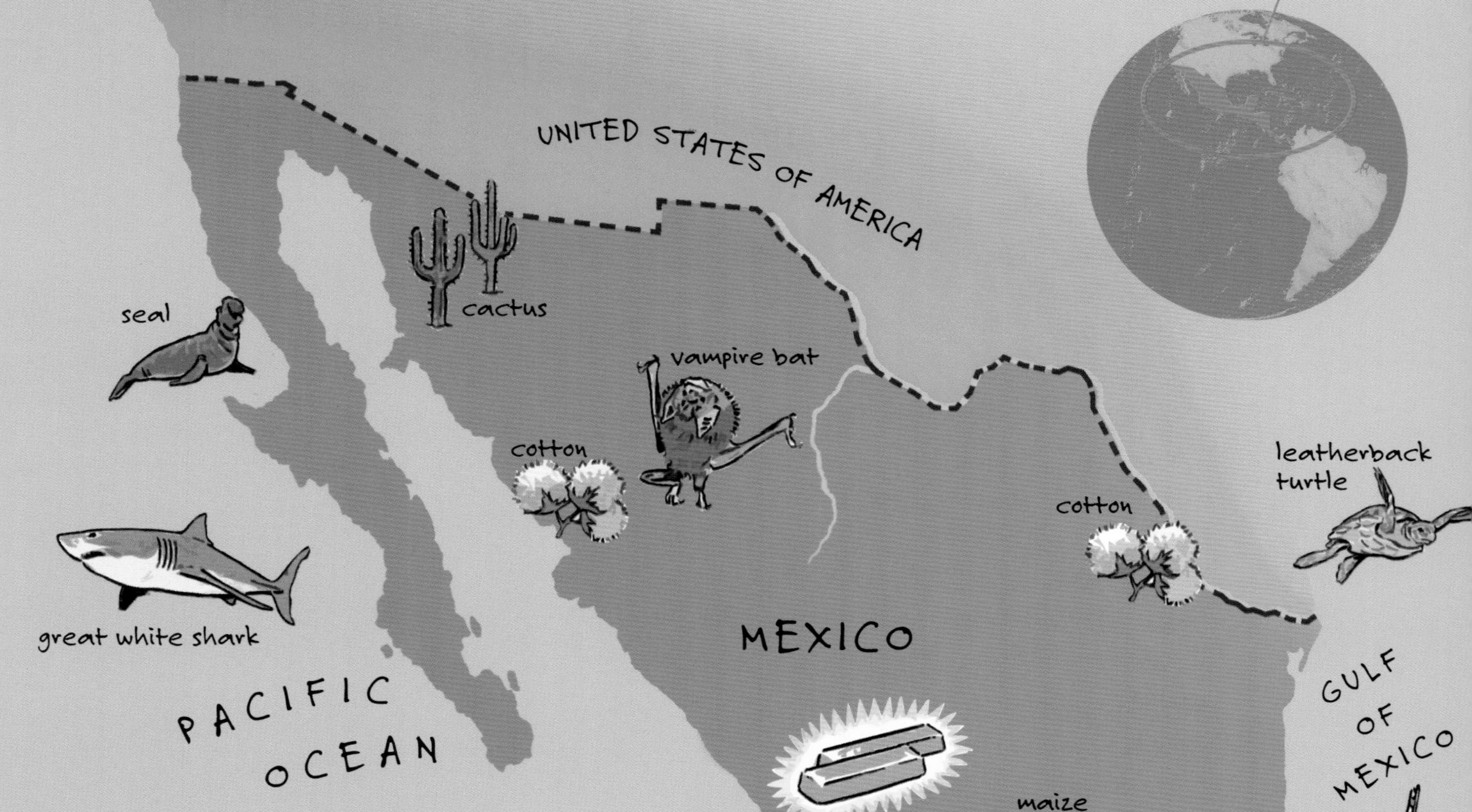

Mexico and Central America link the continents of North and South America. The land is mountainous and much of it is covered by tropical rainforests. The Panama Canal, in the south of the region, provides a link for ships between the Atlantic and Pacific Oceans.

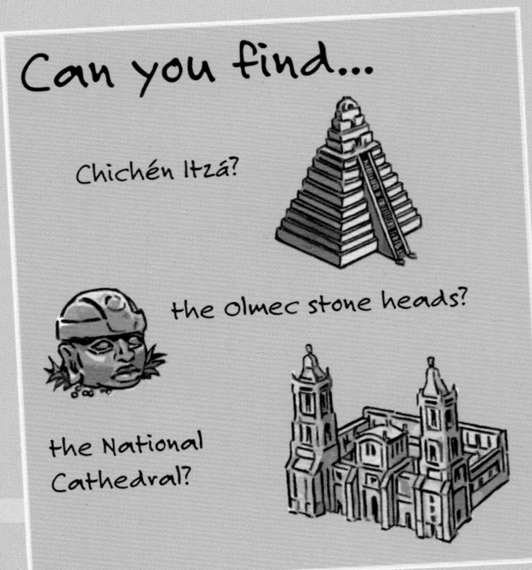

Can you find...
Chichén Itzá?
the Olmec stone heads?
the National Cathedral?

Mexico is this region's largest country. It is rich in silver and oil. Bananas and coffee grow in Central America and the Caribbean. The warm seas and climate of the Caribbean's volcanic islands attract many tourists. This region is a hurricane zone. Fierce tropical storms around the Gulf of Mexico create enormous waves that can cause a lot of damage.

Fact:

Mexico City is slowly sinking each year because it is built on the bed of an ancient lake.

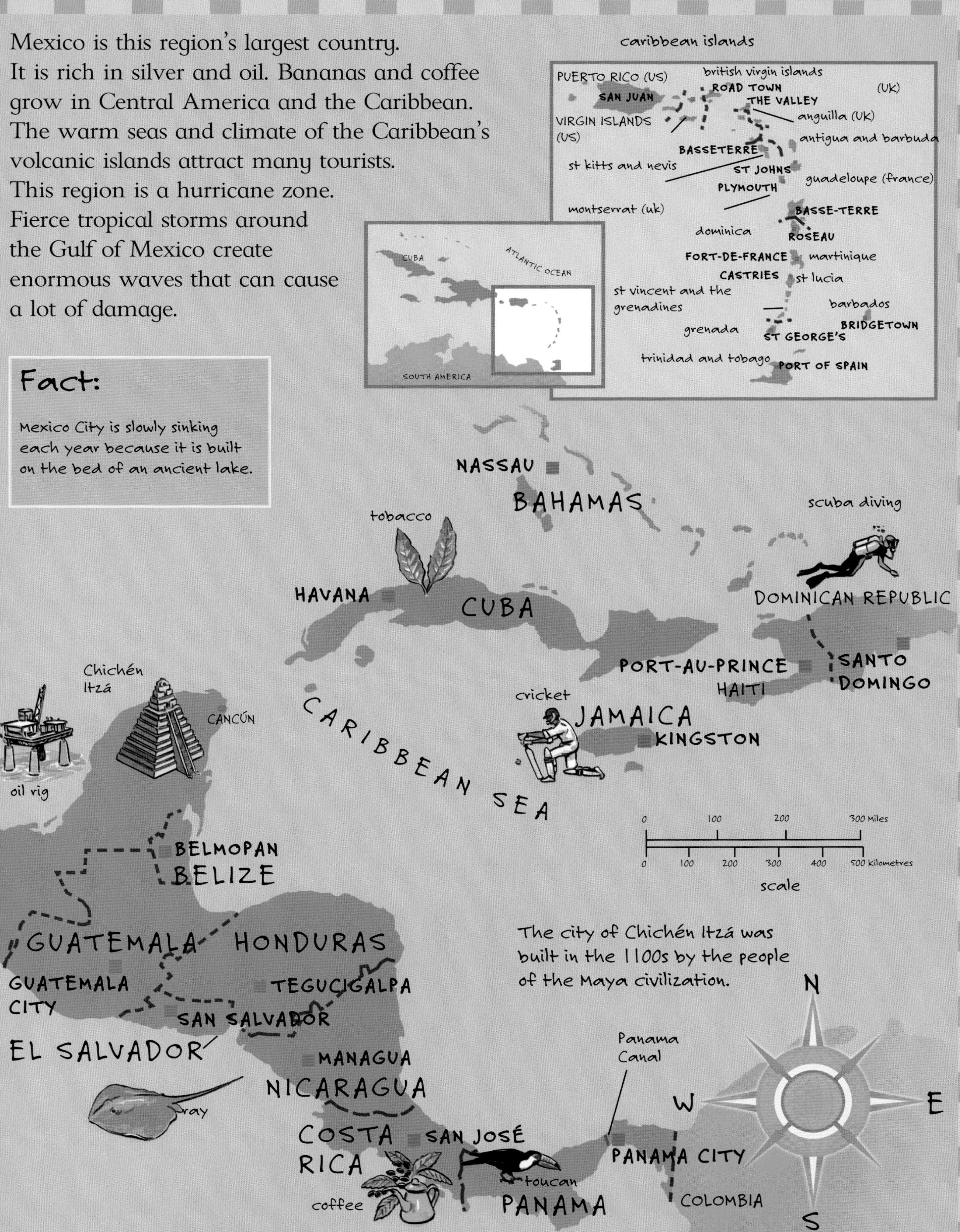

The city of Chichén Itzá was built in the 1100s by the people of the Maya civilization.

South America

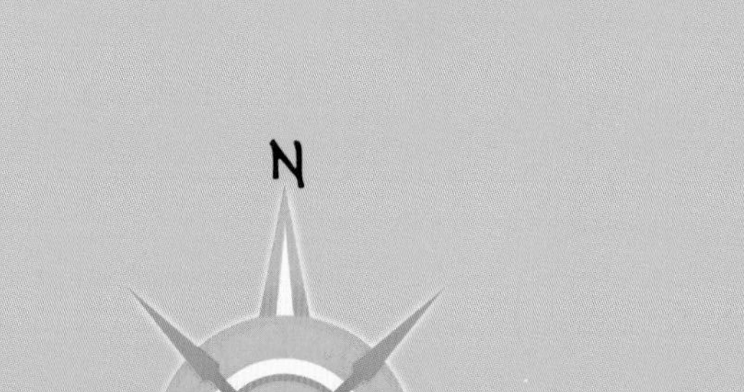

Tomatoes were first discovered growing in South America.

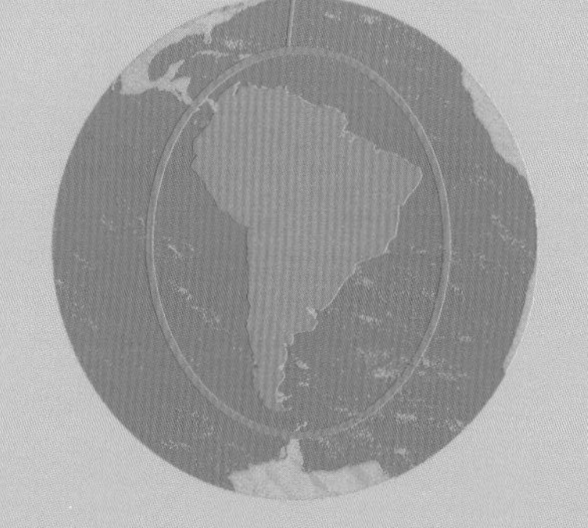

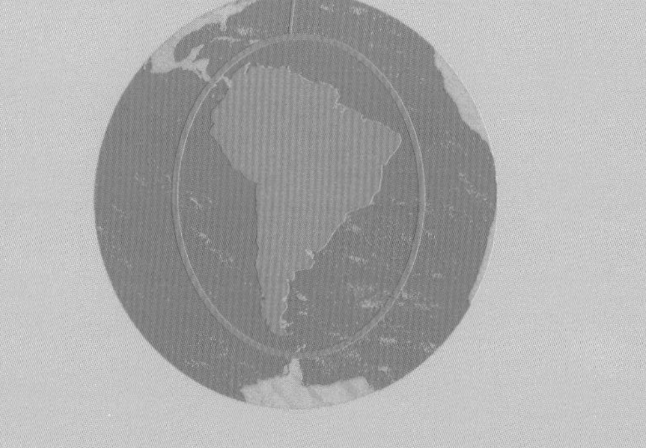

Machu Picchu was a holy city, built by the Inca civilization in the 15th century. The ancient mountain-top settlement in the Peruvian Andes was rediscovered in 1911.

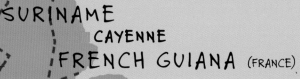

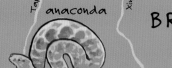

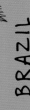

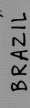

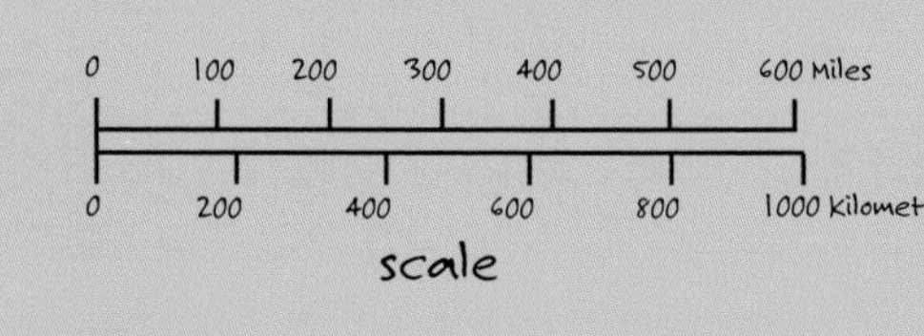

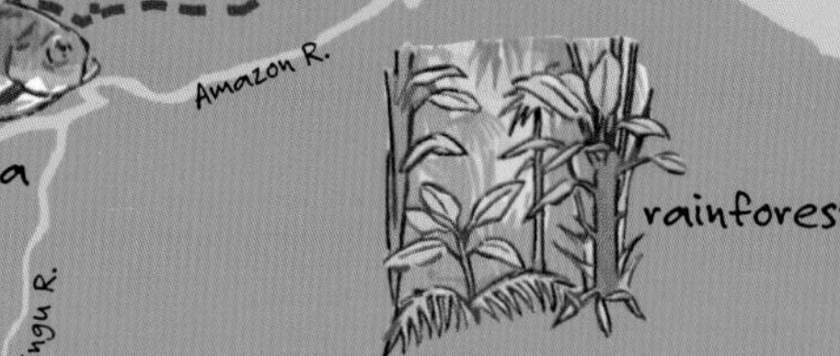

The Andes mountains run the length of the huge continent of South America. In the north, the Amazon River runs through vast tropical rainforests full of wildlife. In the south, millions of cattle and sheep are reared on fertile grasslands called Pampas.

South America is rich in oil, silver, copper, coal, and iron ore. The continent's largest country, Brazil, is also the richest and most industrialized and is the world's leading coffee producer. Spanish is spoken throughout South America except in Brazil, where the language is Portuguese.

Fact:

Angel Falls in Venezuela is the highest waterfall in the world at over 2,600 feet (800 m) high.

Can you find...

Angel Falls?

the Statue of Christ?

Machu Picchu?

Scandinavia, Finland, and Iceland

Norway, Sweden, and Denmark are known as Scandinavia. These countries are rich in natural resources: timber, fish, oil, and natural gas. They have warm summers, but bitterly cold winters.

Fjords are long sea inlets, banked by steep mountainsides. There are hundreds of them along the Norwegian coast. Denmark and southern Sweden have fertile farmland, and Finland has many lakes. The volcanic island of Iceland lies 620 miles (1,000 km) west of Norway.

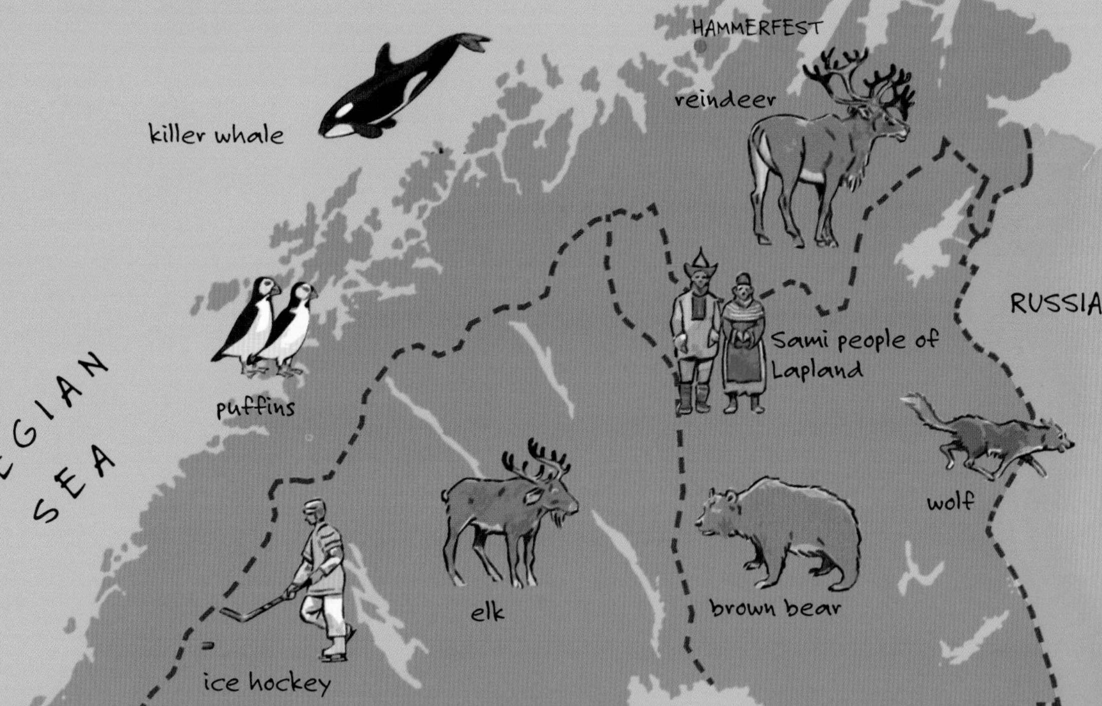

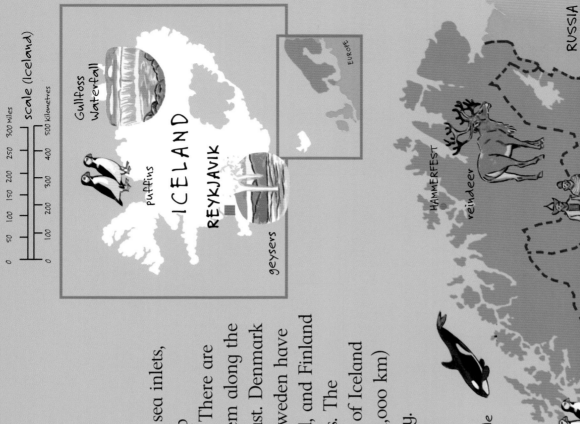

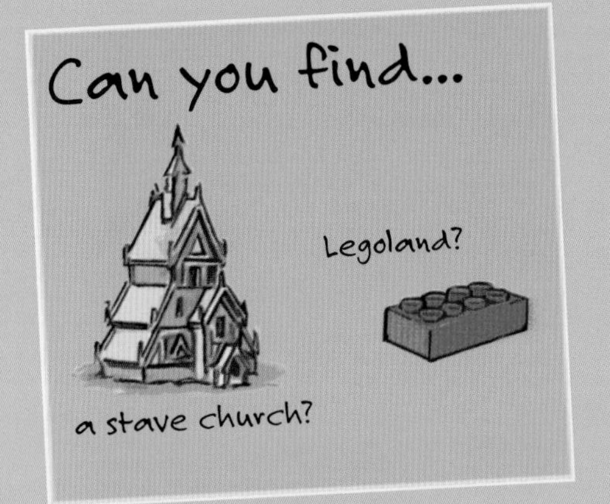

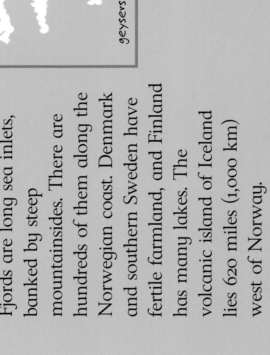

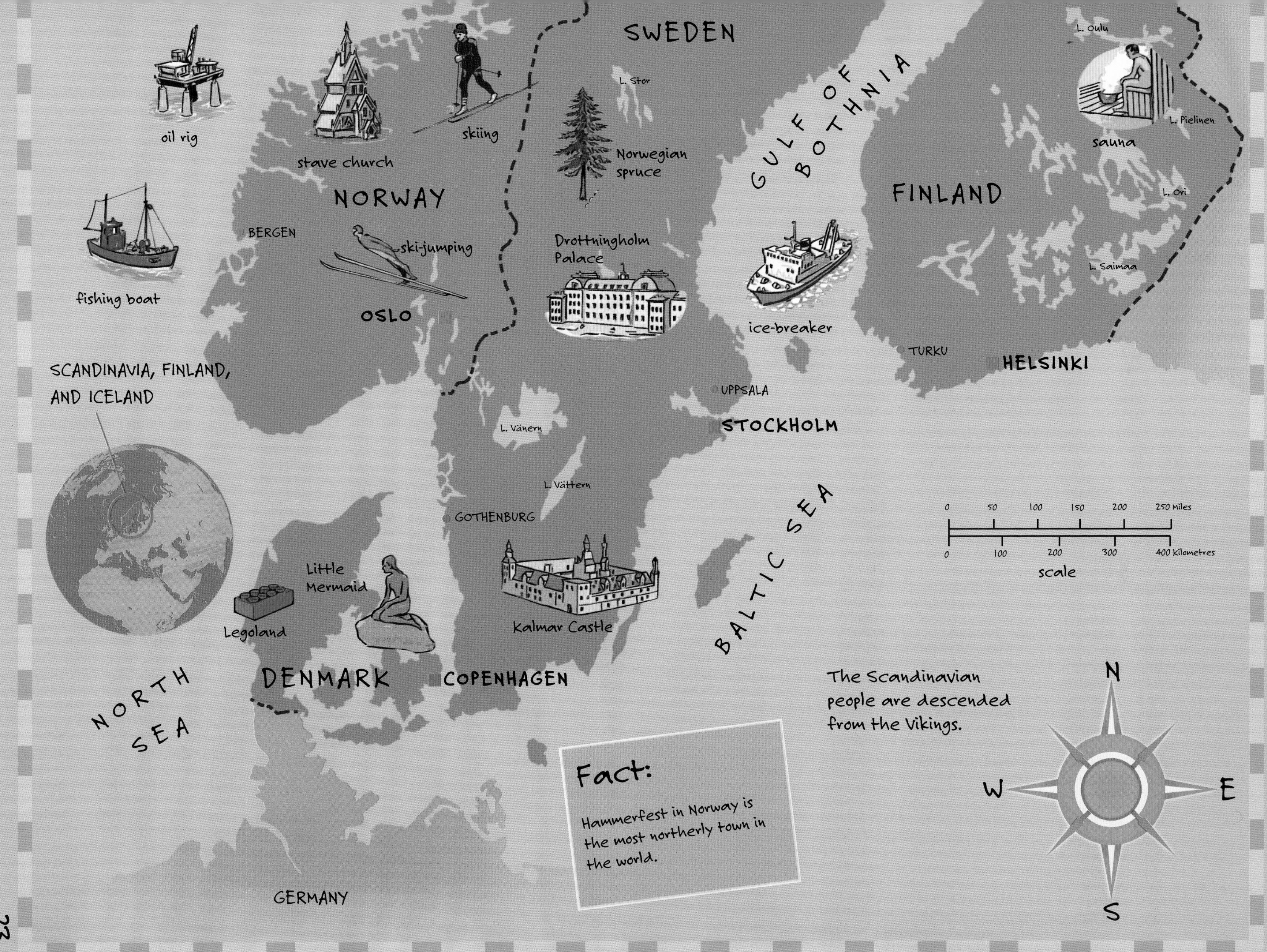

The Scandinavian people are descended from the Vikings.

Fact:

Hammerfest in Norway is the most northerly town in the world.

The British Isles

The United Kingdom (UK) and Ireland are known as the British Isles. Much of the land is farmed, but there are many large cities. London, the biggest city and the capital of the UK, is a major financial and cultural center. The Channel Tunnel links the UK with mainland Europe.

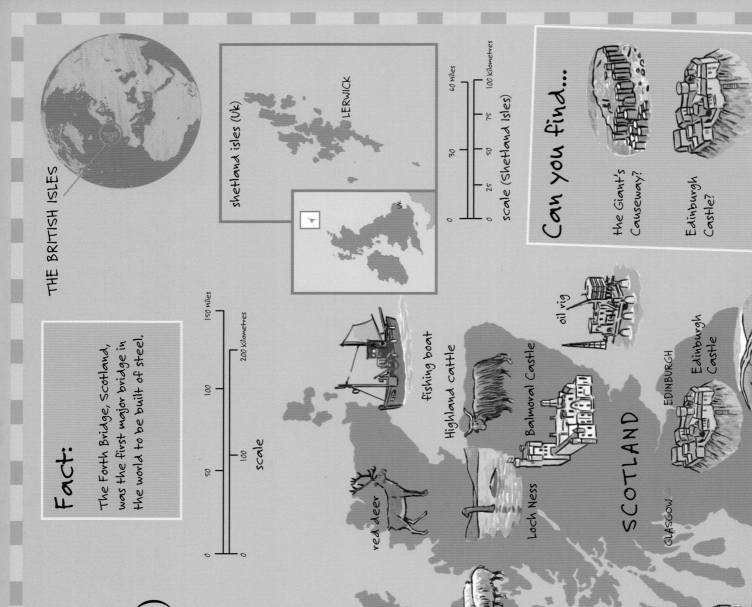

Fact:

The Forth Bridge, Scotland, was the first major bridge in the world to be built of steel.

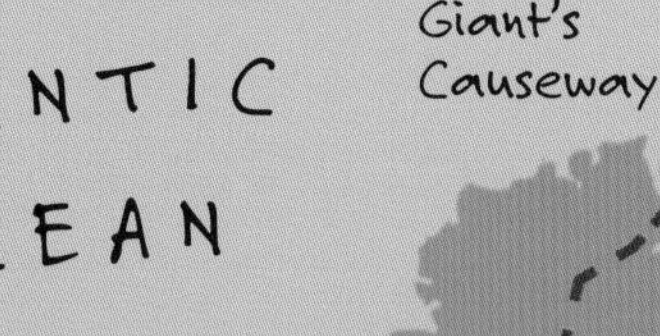

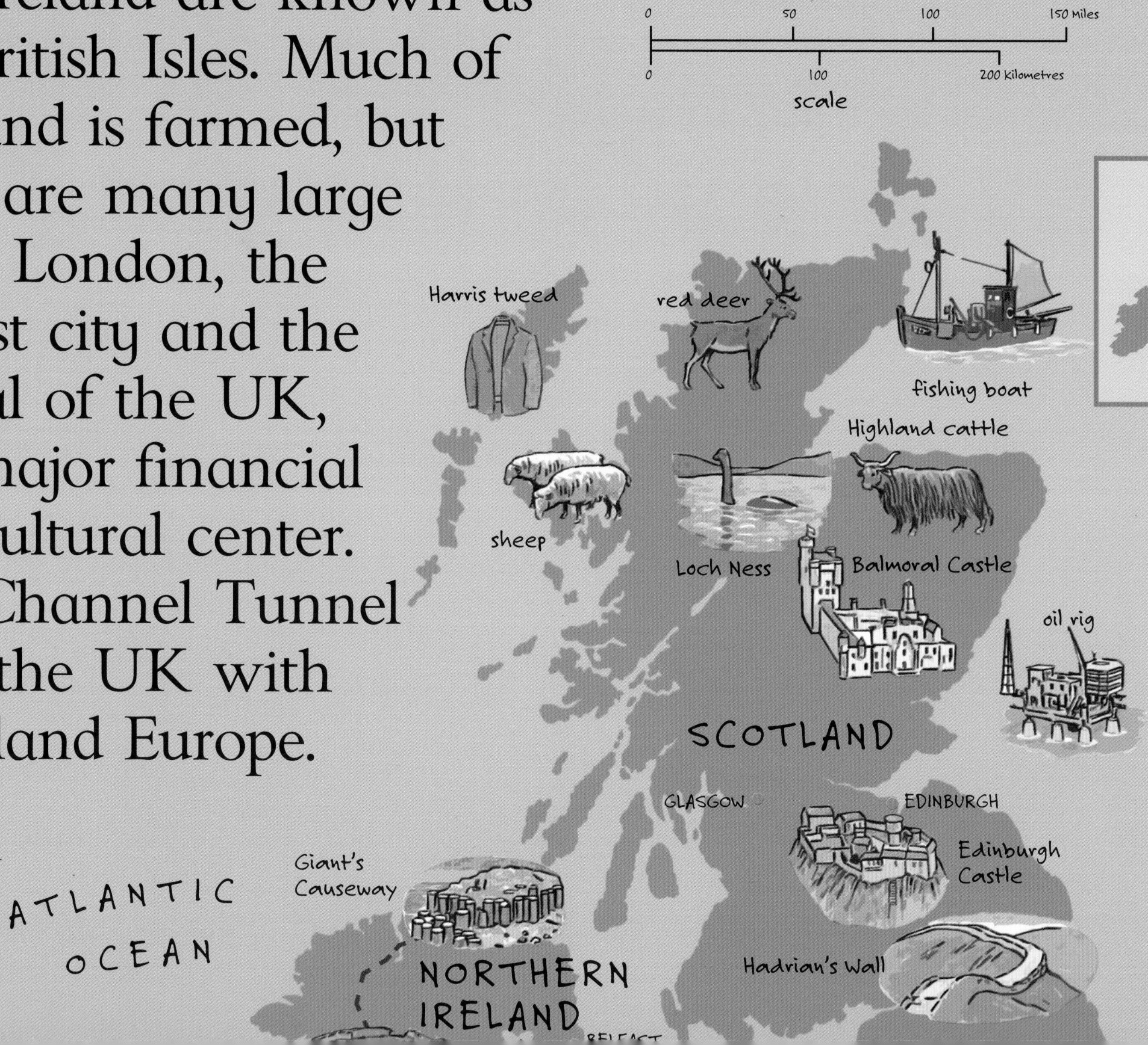

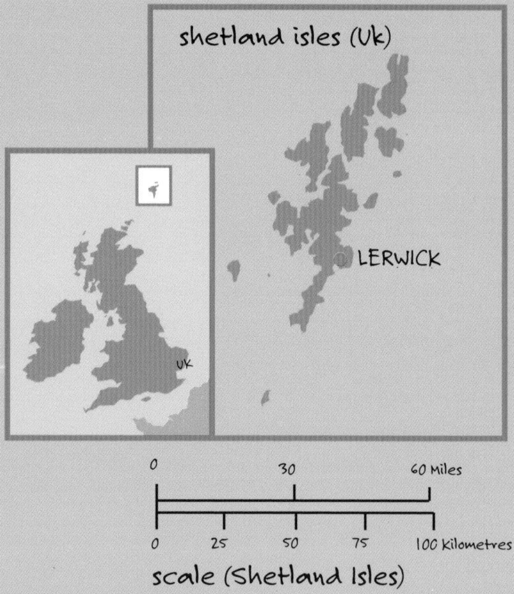

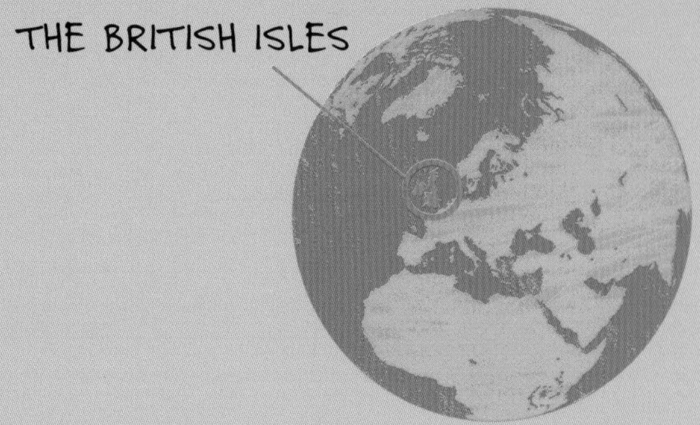

Can you find...

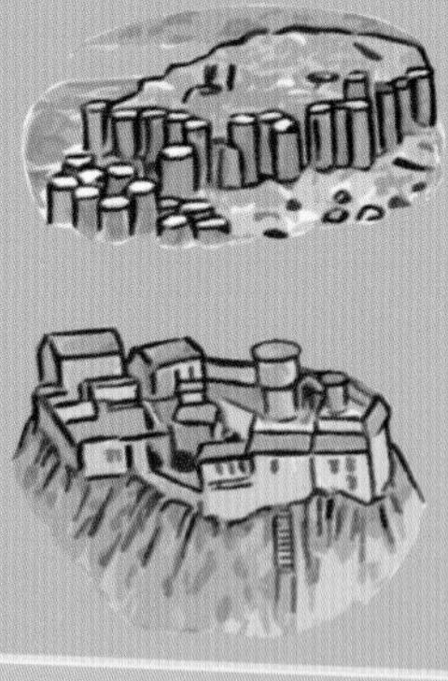

the Giant's Causeway?

Edinburgh Castle?

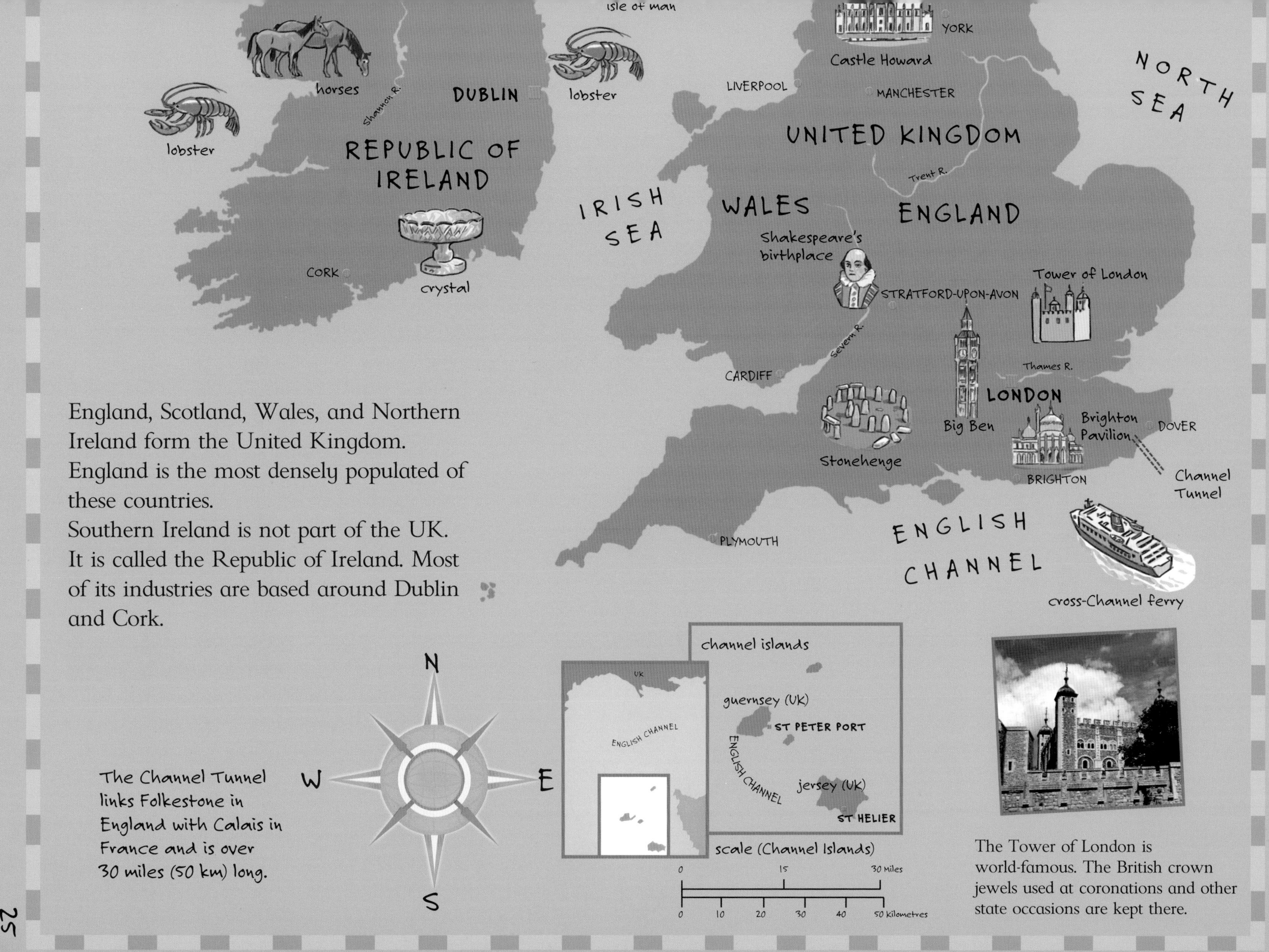

England, Scotland, Wales, and Northern Ireland form the United Kingdom. England is the most densely populated of these countries. Southern Ireland is not part of the UK. It is called the Republic of Ireland. Most of its industries are based around Dublin and Cork.

The Channel Tunnel links Folkestone in England with Calais in France and is over 30 miles (50 km) long.

The Tower of London is world-famous. The British crown jewels used at coronations and other state occasions are kept there.

Spain and Portugal

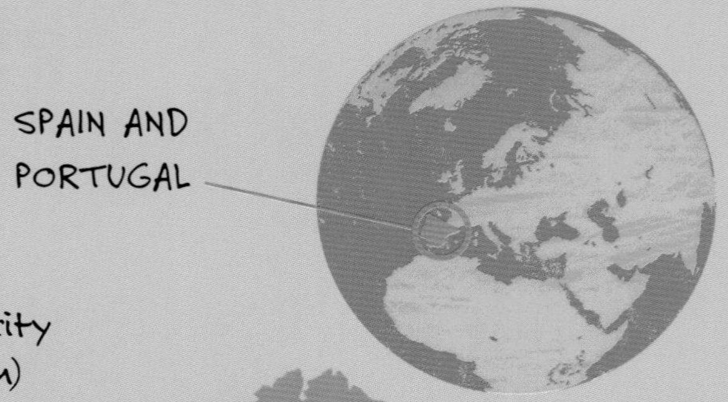

SPAIN AND
PORTUGAL

Madrid is the highest capital city in Europe at 2,099 feet (640 m) above sea level.

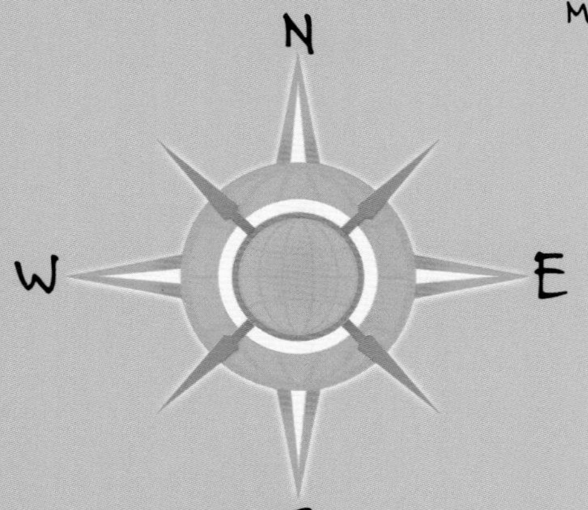

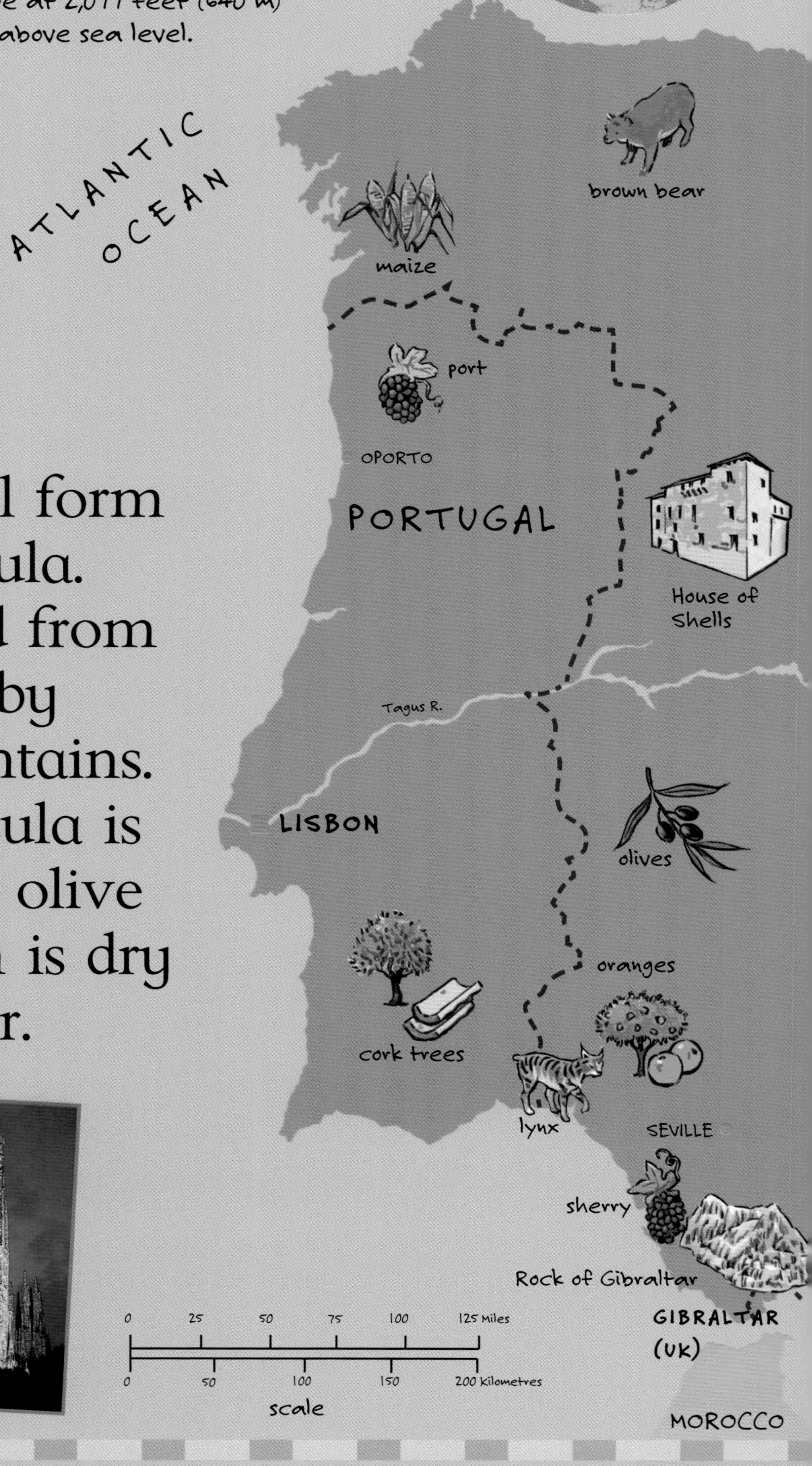

Spain and Portugal form the Iberian Peninsula. They are separated from the rest of Europe by the Pyrenees mountains. Most of the peninsula is dry grassland with olive groves. This region is dry and hot in summer.

brown bear

maize

port

OPORTO

PORTUGAL

House of Shells

Tagus R.

LISBON

olives

oranges

cork trees

lynx

SEVILLE

sherry

Rock of Gibraltar

GIBRALTAR (UK)

MOROCCO

Antoní Gaudi began work on Barcelona's famous church, the Sagrada Familia, in 1883. The building work still continues today because the church has not yet been completed.

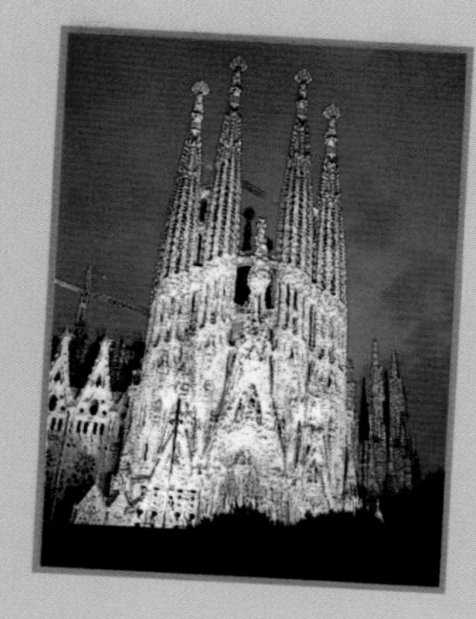

0 25 50 75 100 125 Miles

0 50 100 150 200 kilometres

scale

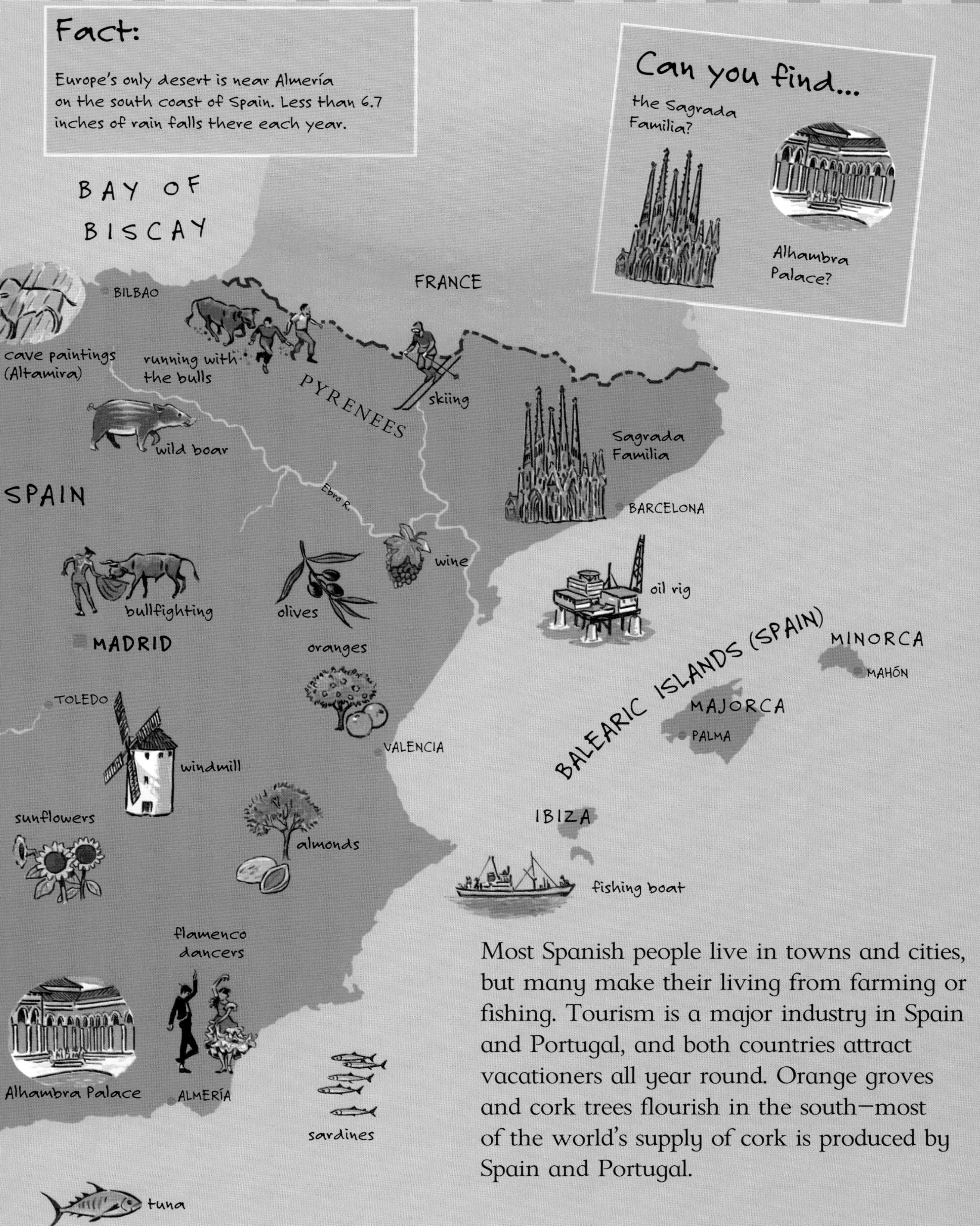

Most Spanish people live in towns and cities, but many make their living from farming or fishing. Tourism is a major industry in Spain and Portugal, and both countries attract vacationers all year round. Orange groves and cork trees flourish in the south—most of the world's supply of cork is produced by Spain and Portugal.

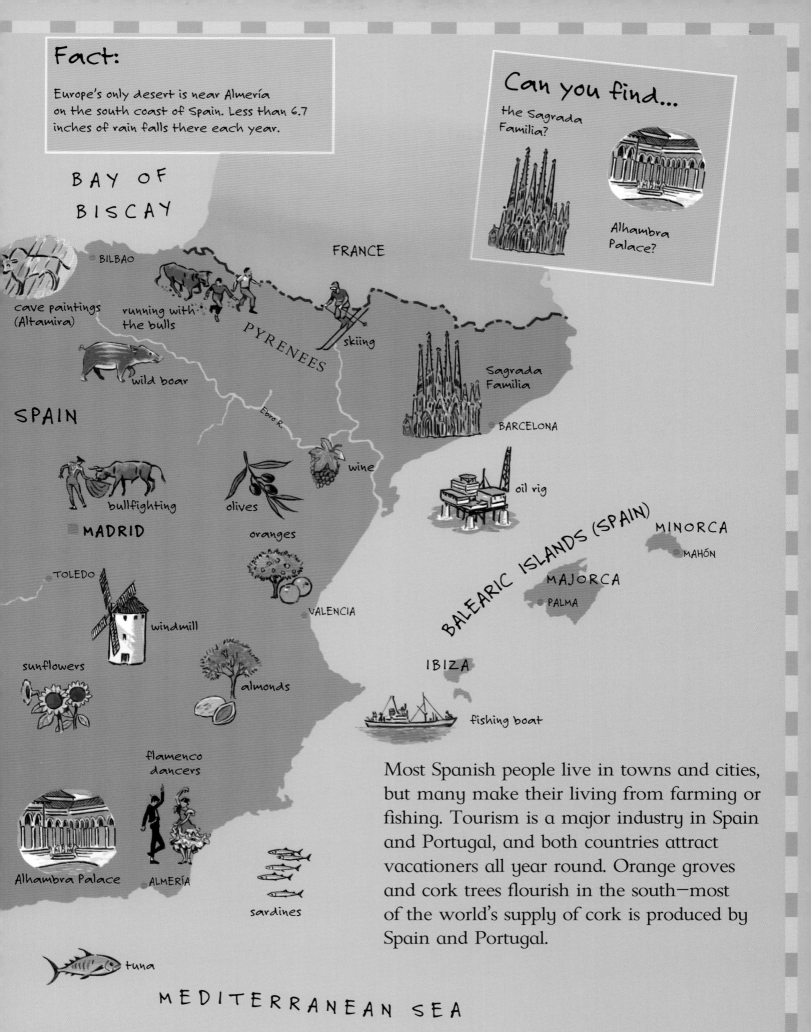

France

France is one of Europe's largest farming and industrial countries. Its mild climate becomes hotter and drier towards its southern borders with Italy and Spain. France is famous for its fine food and wines.

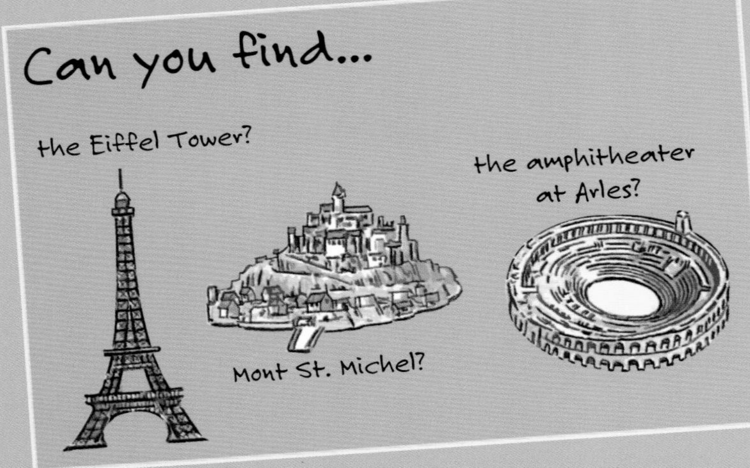

Can you find...
the Eiffel Tower?

the amphitheater at Arles?

Much of France is farmland but most people now live in towns and cities.

The area around Paris, the capital city, is densely populated. Paris is famous for its great fashion houses, its smart restaurants, and as a center for the arts.

Andorra and Monaco are small, independent countries. Many wealthy people choose to live in Monaco because of its tax laws.

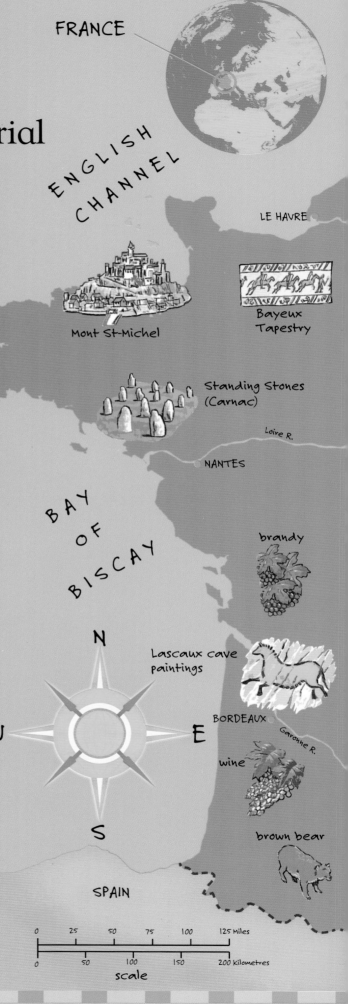

FRANCE

ENGLISH CHANNEL

LE HAVRE

Mont St-Michel

Bayeux Tapestry

Standing Stones (Carnac)

Loire R.

NANTES

BAY OF BISCAY

brandy

N

W

E

S

Lascaux cave paintings

BORDEAUX

Garonne R.

wine

brown bear

SPAIN

0 25 50 75 100 125 Miles

0 50 100 150 200 Kilometres

scale

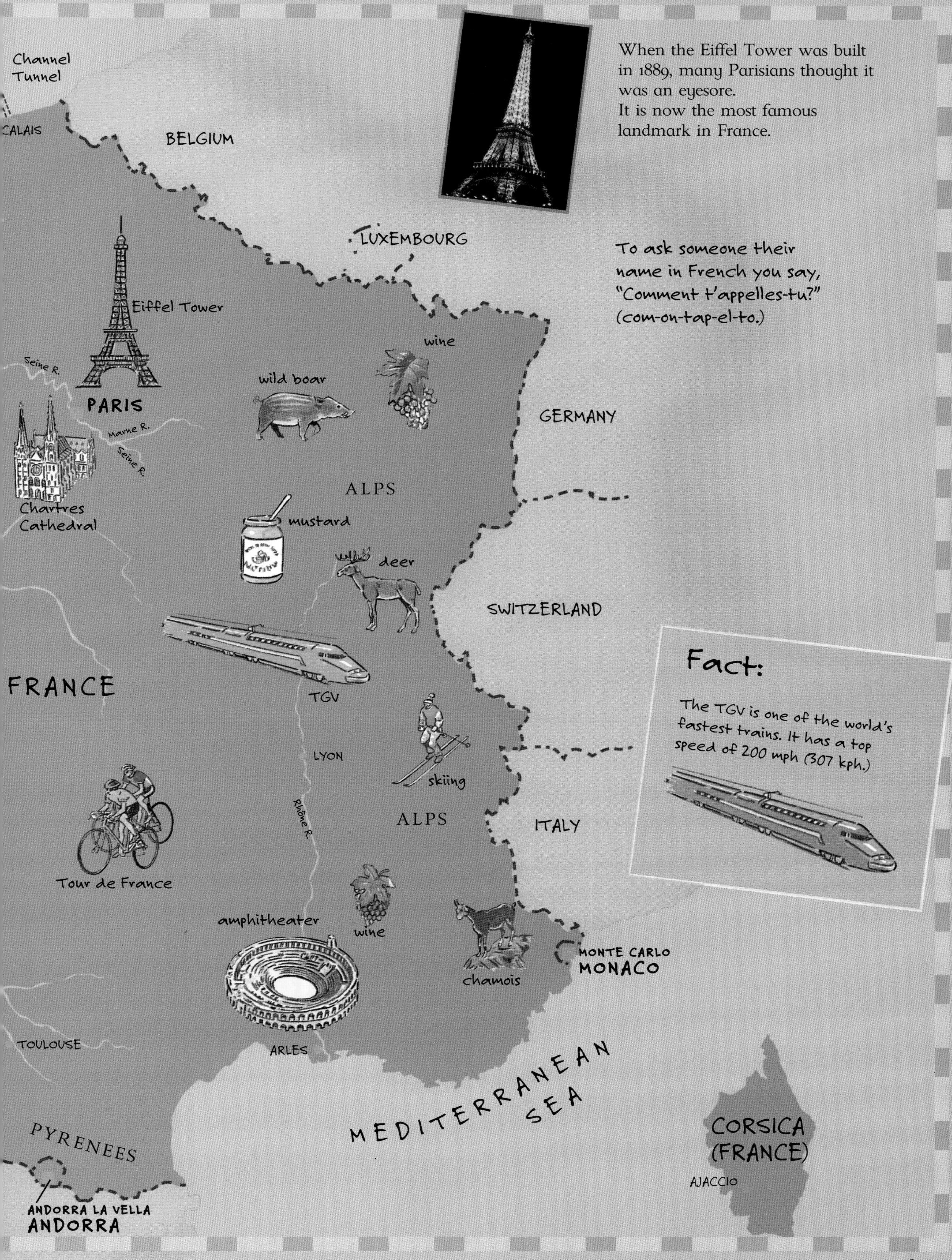
Channel Tunnel
CALAIS
BELGIUM
When the Eiffel Tower was built in 1889, many Parisians thought it was an eyesore.
It is now the most famous landmark in France.
LUXEMBOURG
To ask someone their name in French you say, "Comment t'appelles-tu?" (com-on-tap-el-to.)
Eiffel Tower
wine
Seine R.
wild boar
PARIS
GERMANY
Marne R.
Seine R.
ALPS
Chartres Cathedral
mustard
deer
SWITZERLAND
FRANCE
TGV
Fact:
The TGV is one of the world's fastest trains. It has a top speed of 200 mph (307 kph.)
LYON
skiing
Rhône R.
ALPS
ITALY
Tour de France
amphitheater
wine
chamois
MONTE CARLO
MONACO
TOULOUSE
ARLES
MEDITERRANEAN SEA
CORSICA (FRANCE)
AJACCIO
PYRENEES
ANDORRA LA VELLA
ANDORRA

Belgium, the Netherlands, and Luxembourg

This part of Europe is called “the Low Countries.” Most of the land in these countries is flat. Large areas of land have been reclaimed from the sea by draining it and building long dykes (walls) to protect the land from flooding.

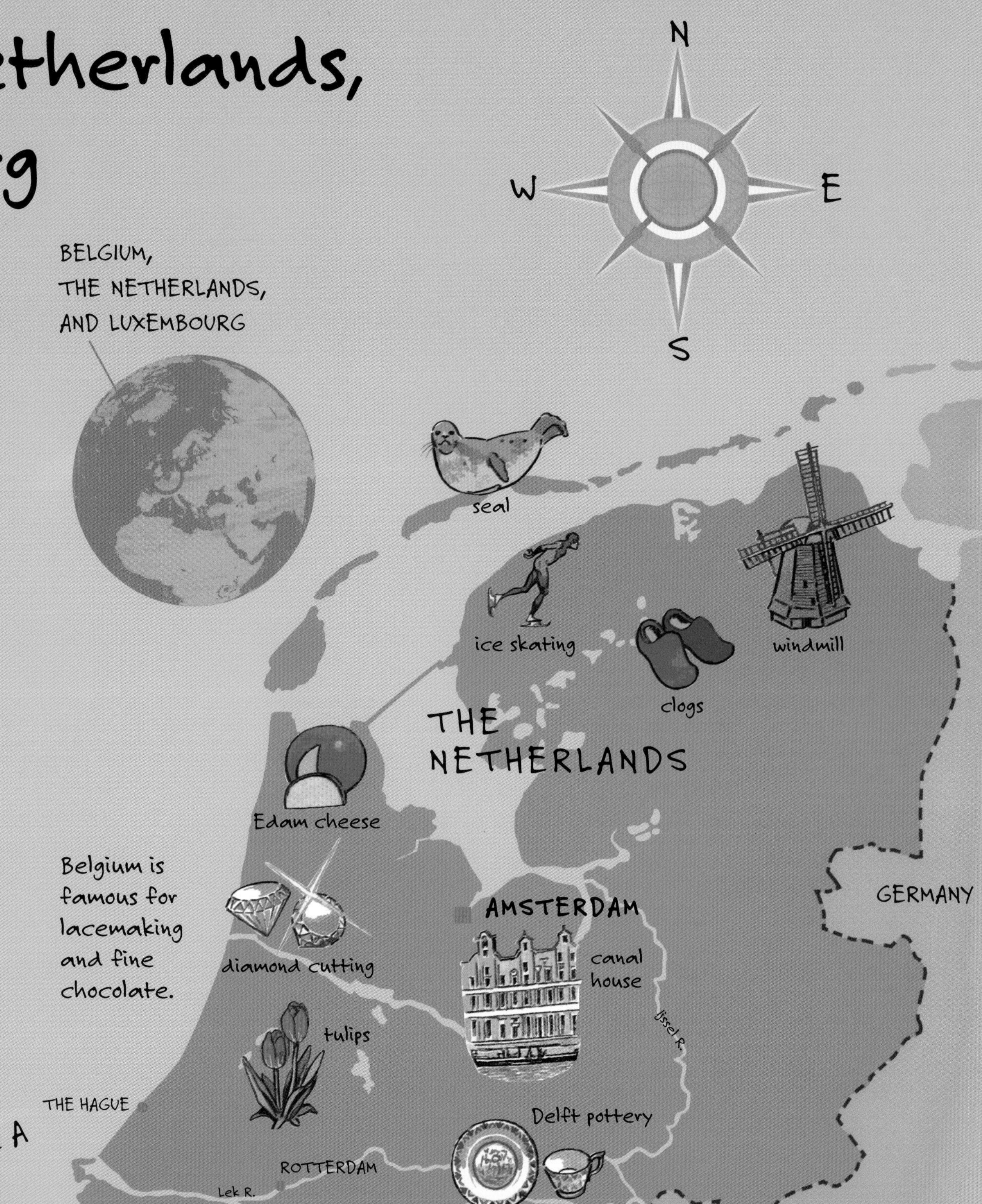

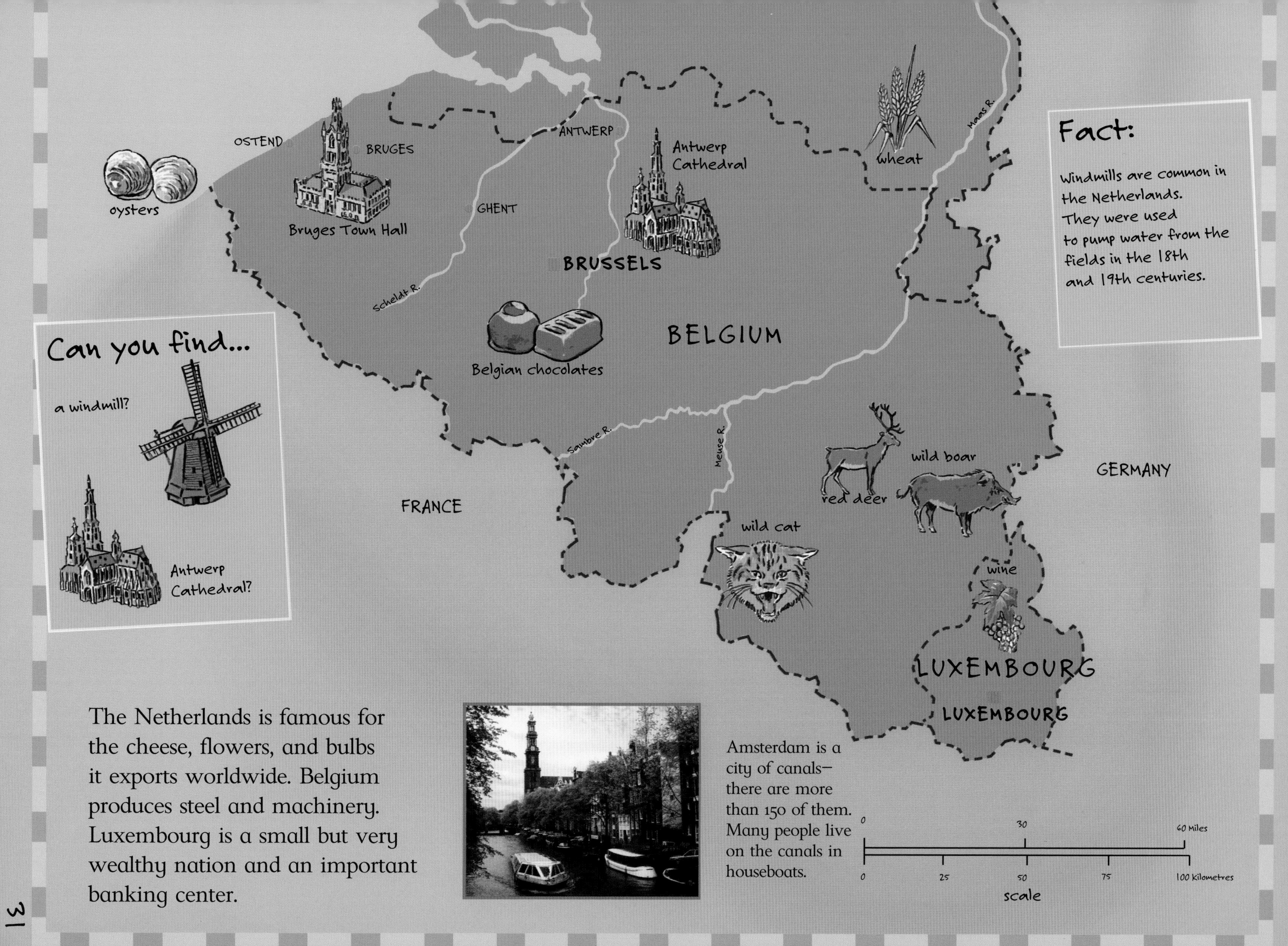

Fact:

Windmills are common in the Netherlands. They were used to pump water from the fields in the 18th and 19th centuries.

Can you find...

a windmill?

Antwerp Cathedral?

The Netherlands is famous for the cheese, flowers, and bulbs it exports worldwide. Belgium produces steel and machinery. Luxembourg is a small but very wealthy nation and an important banking center.

Amsterdam is a city of canals—there are more than 150 of them. Many people live on the canals in houseboats.

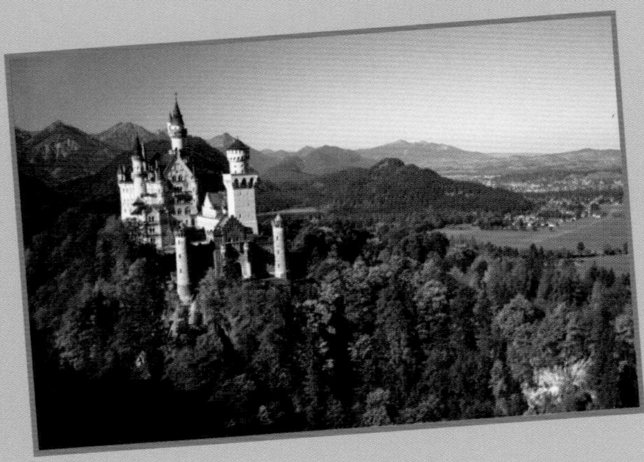

Neuschwanstein Castle was built by King Ludwig of Bavaria. Walt Disney based his fairy-tale castle on this fantastic building.

NORTH SEA

GERMANY, AUSTRIA, AND SWITZERLAND

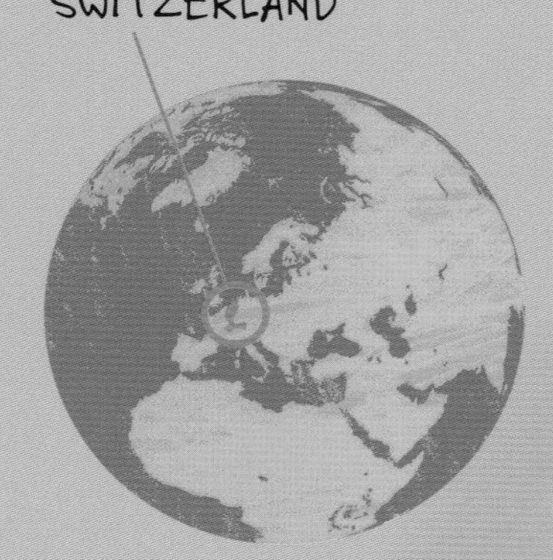

NETHERLANDS

Weser R.

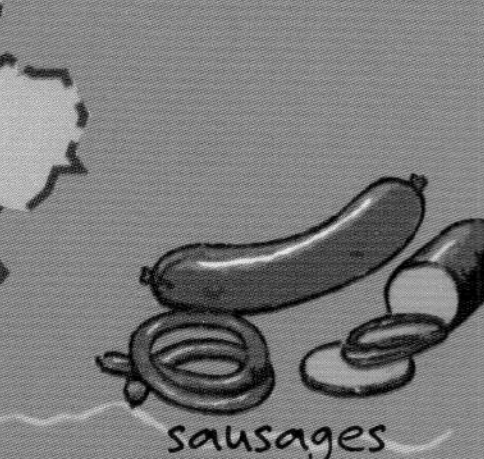

Rhine R.

Cologne Cathedral

DÜSSELDORF

COLOGNE

BONN

Beethoven's birthplace

BELGIUM

LUXEMBOURG

Germany, Austria, and Switzerland

Germany is a wealthy industrial nation. It produces cars, electrical goods, wines, and beers. It has a large population and many large cities. There are forests, long rivers, and lots of fine castles. Germany's large rivers are important for transporting goods around the country.

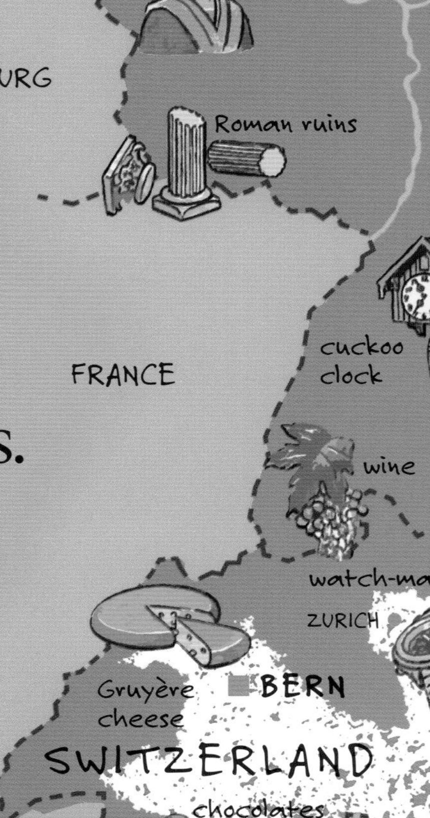

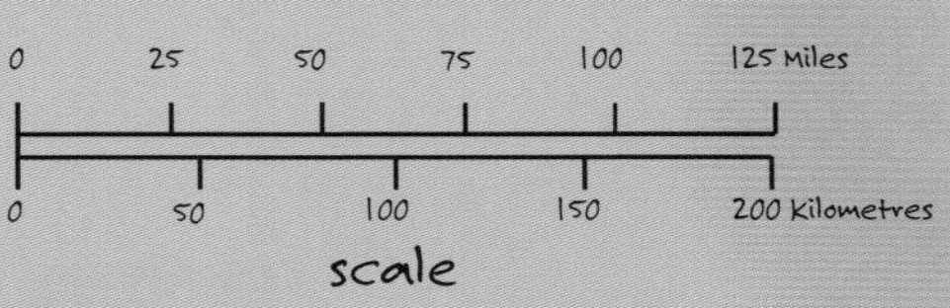

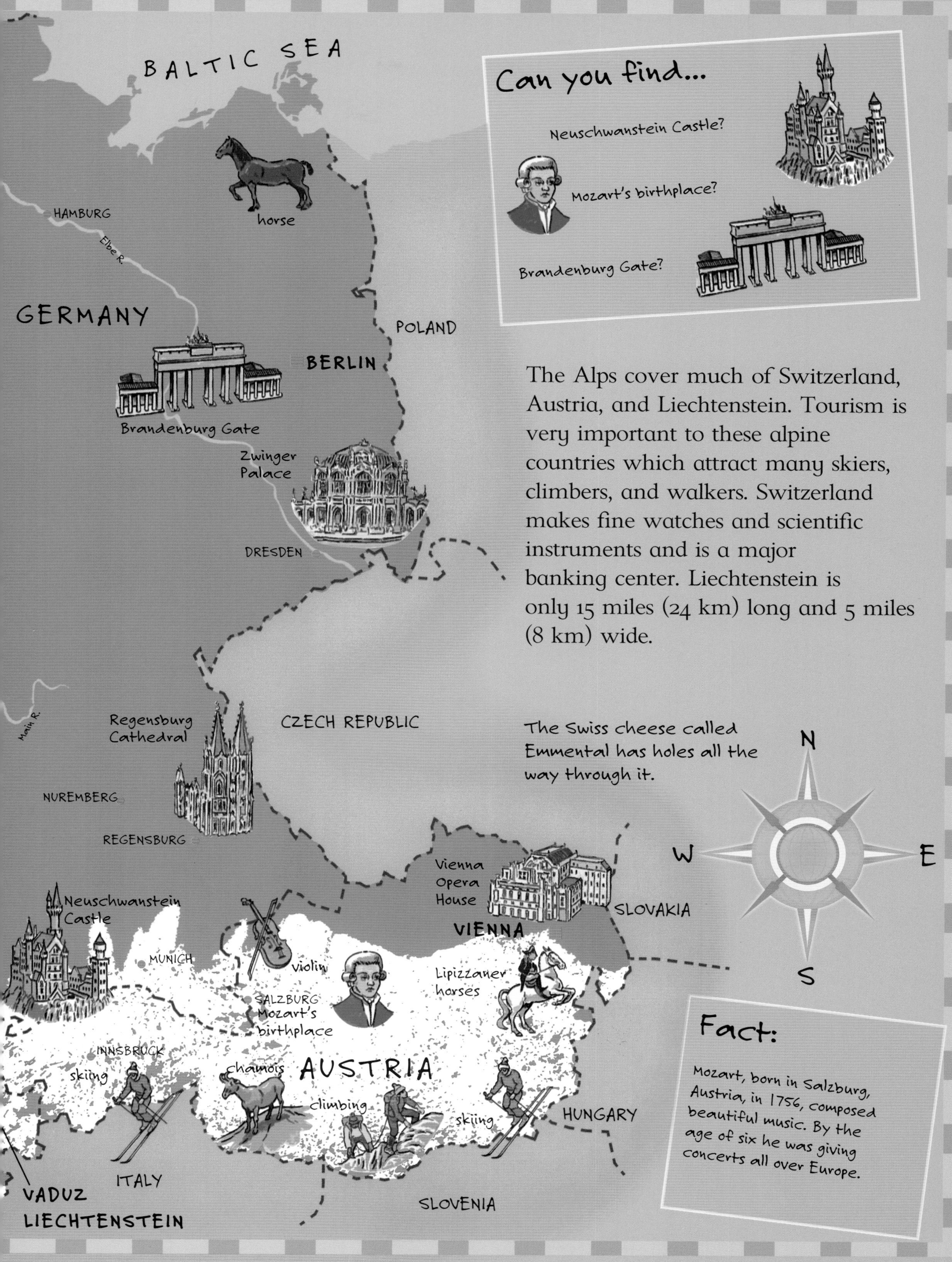
BALTIC SEA
Can you find...
Neuschwanstein Castle?
Mozart's birthplace?
Brandenburg Gate?
horse
HAMBURG
Elbe R.
GERMANY
POLAND
BERLIN
Brandenburg Gate
Zwinger Palace
DRESDEN
The Alps cover much of Switzerland, Austria, and Liechtenstein. Tourism is very important to these alpine countries which attract many skiers, climbers, and walkers. Switzerland makes fine watches and scientific instruments and is a major banking center. Liechtenstein is only 15 miles (24 km) long and 5 miles (8 km) wide.
Main R.
Regensburg Cathedral
CZECH REPUBLIC
The Swiss cheese called Emmental has holes all the way through it.
N
W
E
S
NUREMBERG
REGENSBURG
Vienna Opera House
Neuschwanstein Castle
SLOVAKIA
VIENNA
MUNICH
violin
Lipizzaner horses
SALZBURG
Mozart's birthplace
Fact:
Mozart, born in Salzburg, Austria, in 1756, composed beautiful music. By the age of six he was giving concerts all over Europe.
INNSBRUCK
skiing
chamois
AUSTRIA
climbing
skiing
HUNGARY
ITALY
VADUZ
LIECHTENSTEIN
SLOVENIA

Italy and Malta

Italy is famous for its art, food, fashion, and cars. Most of its population, industry, and farmland are concentrated along the River Po in the north.

Fact:

Pizza is a traditional food that was invented in Italy. It is now eaten worldwide.

scale: 0 25 50 75 100 125 Miles; 0 50 100 150 200 Kilometres

AUSTRIA

SWITZERLAND

SLOVENIA

CROATIA

FRANCE

ALPS

ALPS

Milan Cathedral

MILAN

TURIN

violin

L. Garda

St. Mark's Square

VENICE

gondolier

Po R.

Parmesan cheese

Parma ham

pasta

wine

olives

The city of Venice is built on islands in a shallow lagoon.

Leaning Tower of Pisa

PISA

FLORENCE

Florence Cathedral

SAN MARINO

SAN MARINO

Tiber R.

ITALY

LIGURIAN SEA

CORSICA (FRANCE)

Colosseum

Vatican

ROME

VATICAN CITY

ADRIATIC SEA

Can you find...

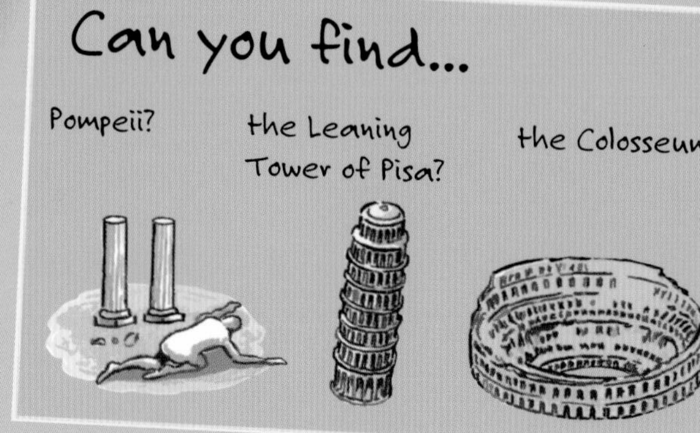

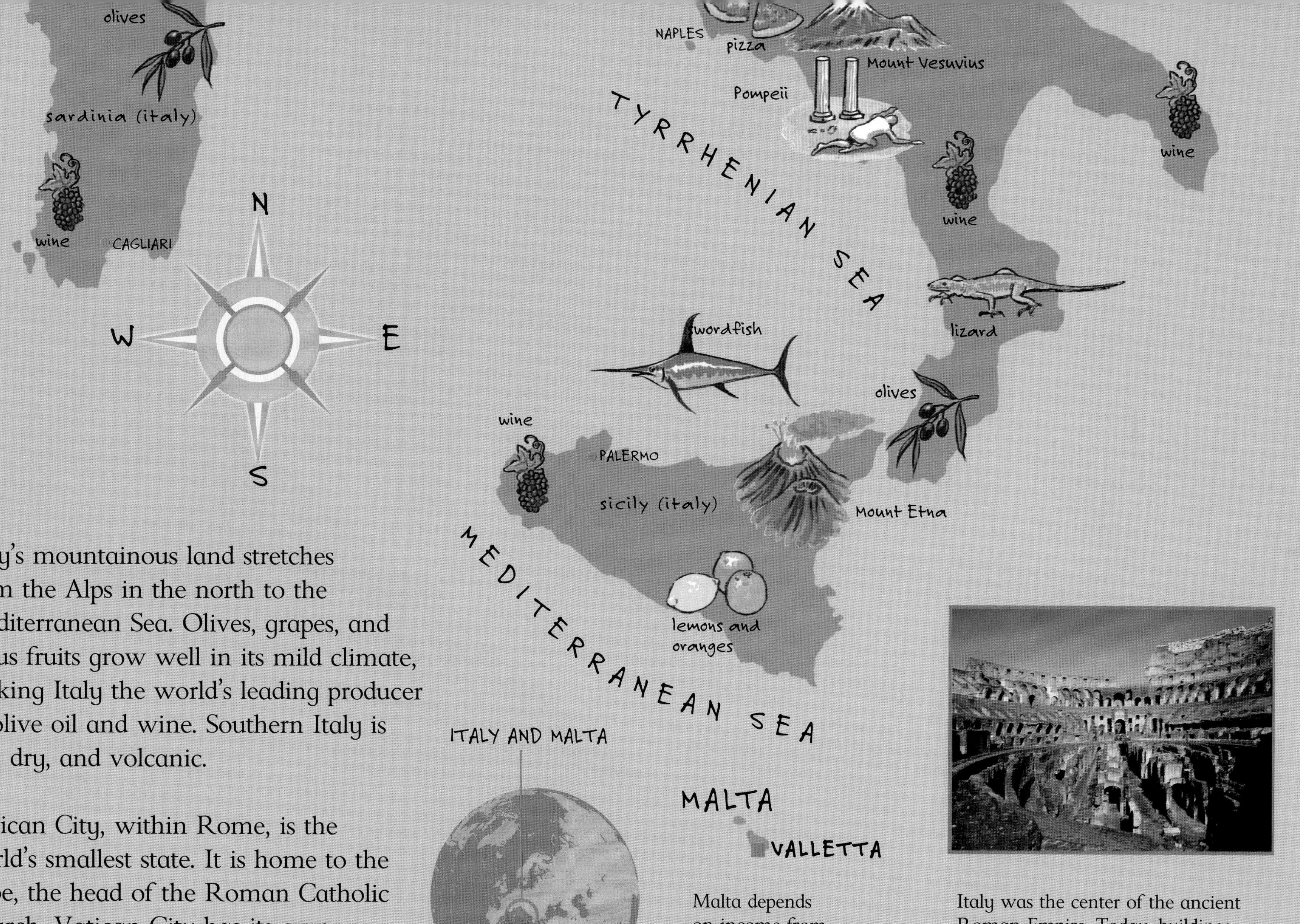

Italy's mountainous land stretches from the Alps in the north to the Mediterranean Sea. Olives, grapes, and citrus fruits grow well in its mild climate, making Italy the world's leading producer of olive oil and wine. Southern Italy is hot, dry, and volcanic.

Vatican City, within Rome, is the world's smallest state. It is home to the Pope, the head of the Roman Catholic Church. Vatican City has its own government, newspaper, coins, stamps, and radio station.

Malta depends on income from tourism and its shipping ports.

Italy was the center of the ancient Roman Empire. Today, buildings such as the Roman Colosseum attract thousands of tourists.

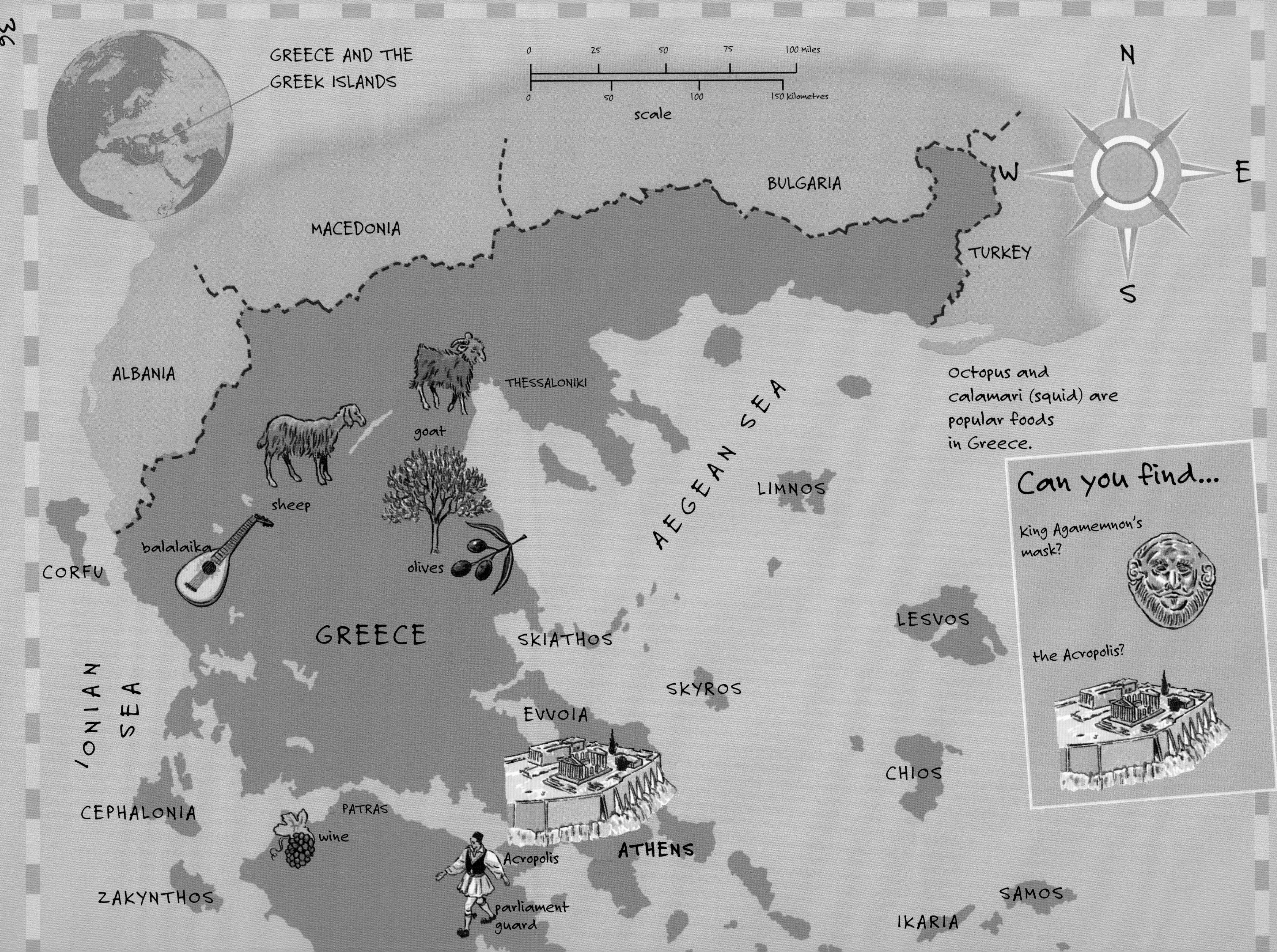
GREECE AND THE
GREEK ISLANDS
0
25
50
75
100 Miles
0
50
100
150 Kilometres
scale
N
E
S
W
MACEDONIA
BULGARIA
TURKEY
ALBANIA
THESSALONIKI
goat
sheep
olives
balalaika
CORFU
AEGEAN SEA
LIMNOS
Octopus and
calamari (squid) are
popular foods
in Greece.
Can you find...
King Agamemnon's
mask?
the Acropolis?
GREECE
SKIATHOS
LESVOS
IONIAN SEA
SKYROS
EVVOIA
CHIOS
CEPHALONIA
PATRAS
wine
Acropolis
ATHENS
ZAKYNTHOS
parliament
guard
SAMOS
IKARIA

Fact:

Ancient Greece was the birthplace of democracy.

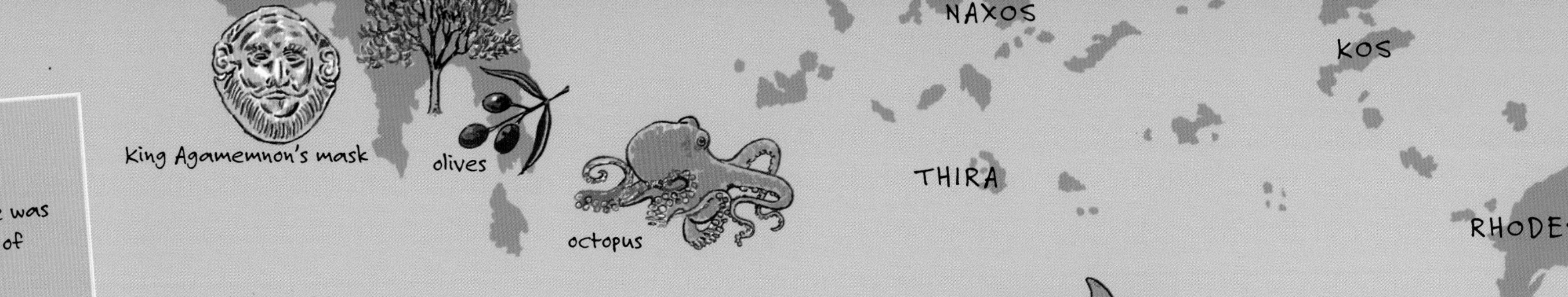

Greece and the Greek Islands

Greece is in southern Europe. It is a dry, mountainous country with many islands. The capital city, Athens, is home to more than one third of Greece's population. Farming and tourism are the major industries.

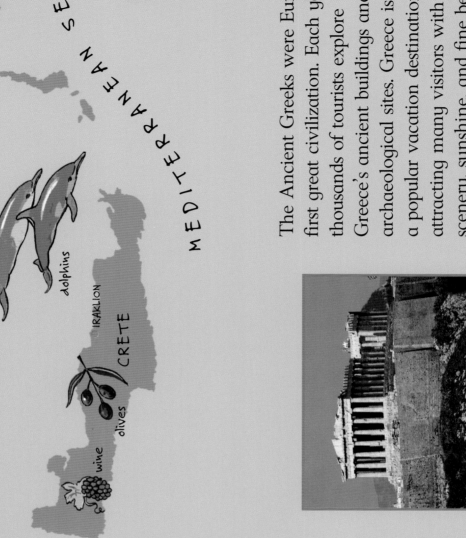

The Parthenon is an ancient Greek temple. It stands on the Acropolis—a rocky hill that towers over the city of Athens.

The Ancient Greeks were Europe's first great civilization. Each year, thousands of tourists explore Greece's ancient buildings and archaeological sites. Greece is a popular vacation destination, attracting many visitors with its scenery, sunshine, and fine beaches. Its hot climate is ideal for growing olives, grapes, and citrus fruits.

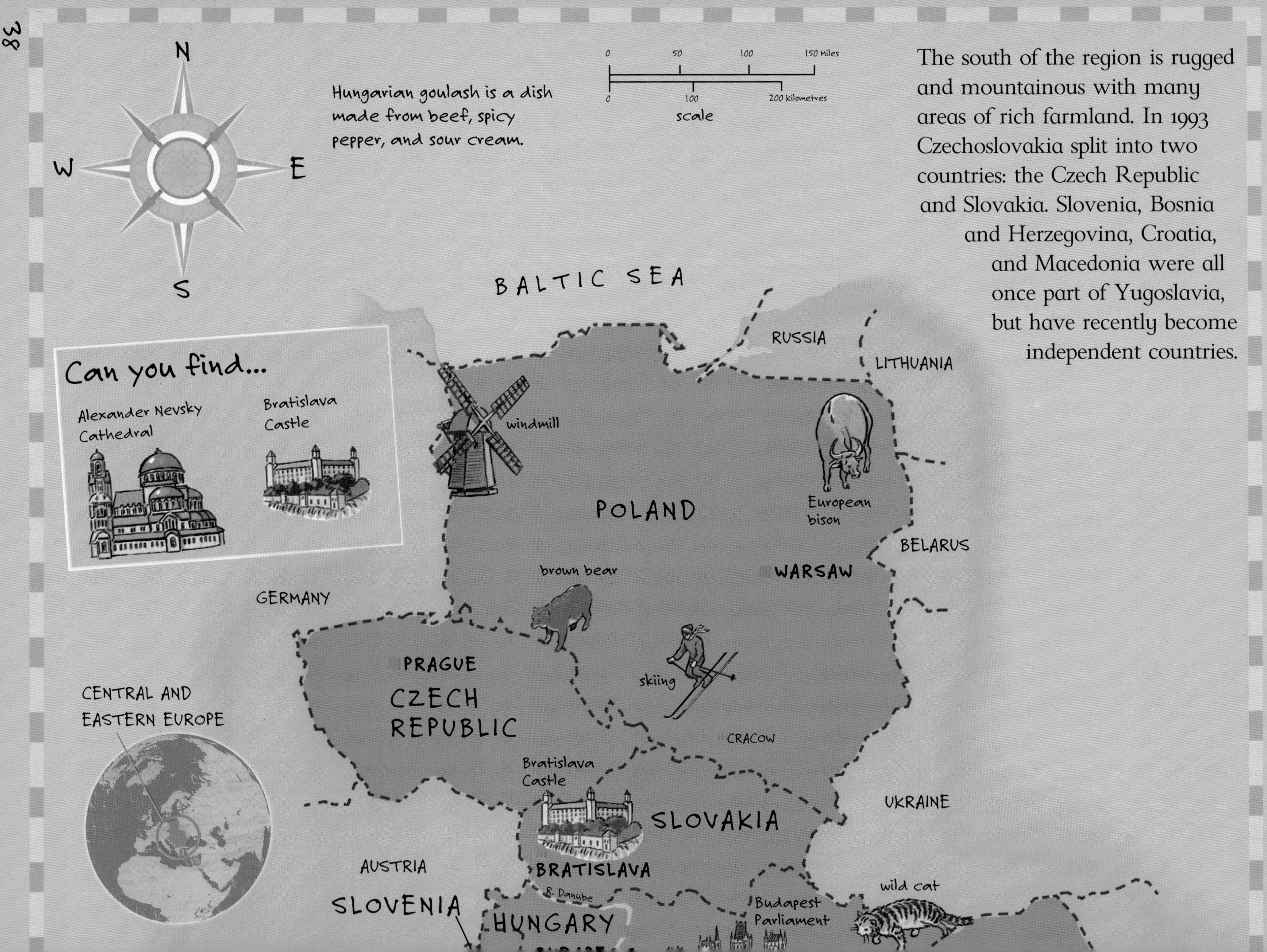
The south of the region is rugged and mountainous with many areas of rich farmland. In 1993 Czechoslovakia split into two countries: the Czech Republic and Slovakia. Slovenia, Bosnia and Herzegovina, Croatia, and Macedonia were all once part of Yugoslavia, but have recently become independent countries.
Hungarian goulash is a dish made from beef, spicy pepper, and sour cream.
N
E
S
W
0
50
100
150 Miles
0
100
200 Kilometres
scale
BALTIC SEA
Can you find...
Alexander Nevsky Cathedral
Bratislava Castle
windmill
RUSSIA
LITHUANIA
POLAND
European bison
BELARUS
GERMANY
brown bear
WARSAW
PRAGUE
CZECH REPUBLIC
skiing
CRACOW
CENTRAL AND EASTERN EUROPE
Bratislava Castle
SLOVAKIA
UKRAINE
AUSTRIA
BRATISLAVA
R. Danube
SLOVENIA
HUNGARY
Budapest Parliament
wild cat

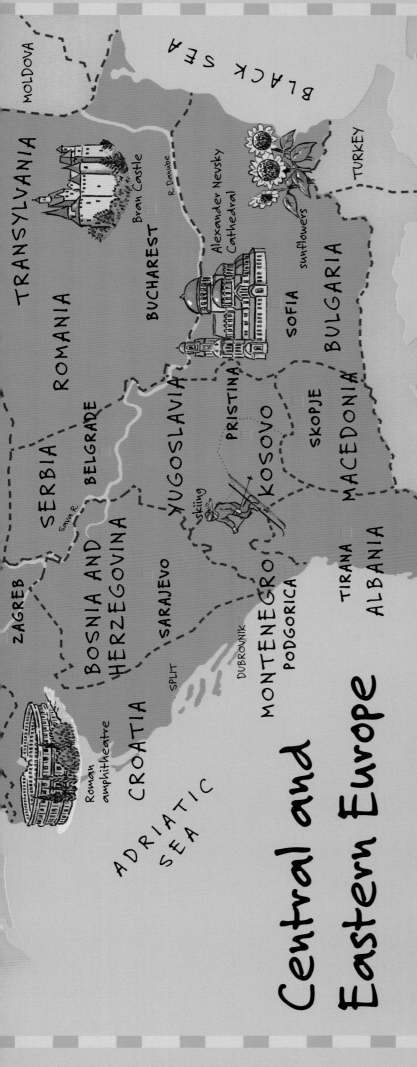

Central and Eastern Europe

Parts of this region suffered bitter fighting during the 1990s. Borders were redrawn and new countries have been created. Poland, the largest and most populated country in the region, has major iron, steel, and shipbuilding industries.

Facts:

- Heavy industry has caused serious pollution problems in Poland, Hungary, and the Czech Republic.
- Budapest, the capital city of Hungary, was once two towns separated by the River Danube. One town was called Buda and the other Pest.

Northern Eurasia

This vast region stretches across Asia and Europe. Until 1991 it was one single country, the Soviet Union. Today, it is made up of 15 independent nations including Russia, the largest country in the world.

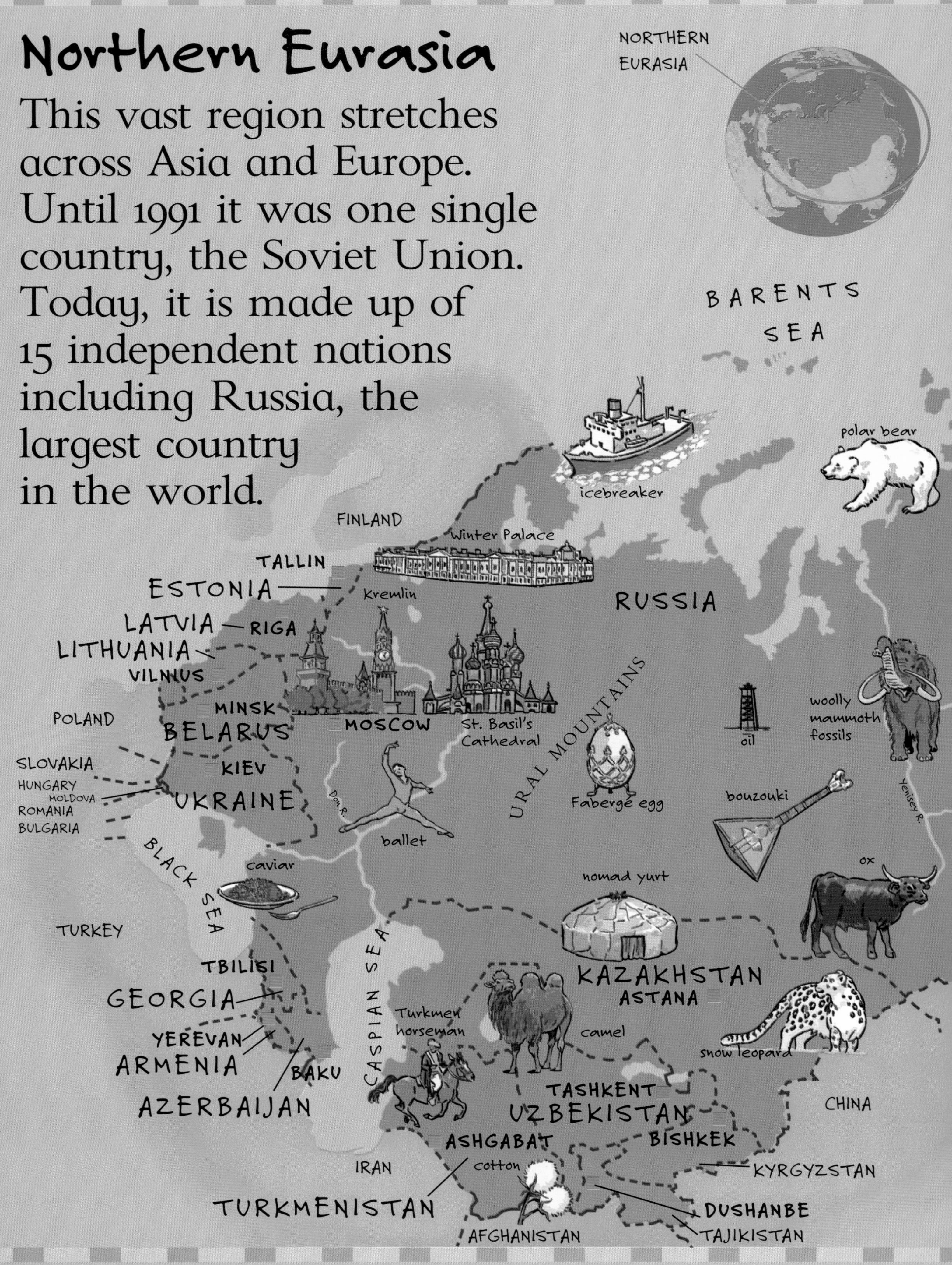

Can you find...

St Basil's Cathedral?

the Trans-Siberian Railway?

Vast forests and grasslands separate the Arctic land in the north from the deserts which cover most of Kazakhstan, Uzbekistan, and Turkmenistan in the south. Most of Russia's population, industry, and fertile land are west of the Ural Mountains. To the east, Siberia is rich in oil and coal but few people live there as the climate is bitterly cold.

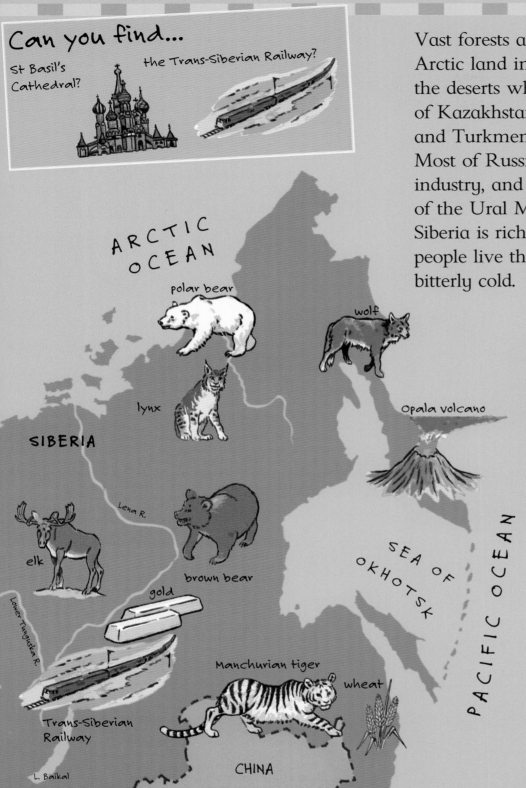

ARCTIC OCEAN

polar bear

wolf

lynx

Opala volcano

SIBERIA

Lena R.

elk

brown bear

gold

Lower Tunguska R.

SEA OF OKHOTSK

PACIFIC OCEAN

Manchurian tiger

wheat

Trans-Siberian Railway

L. Baikal

CHINA

VLADIVOSTOK

MONGOLIA

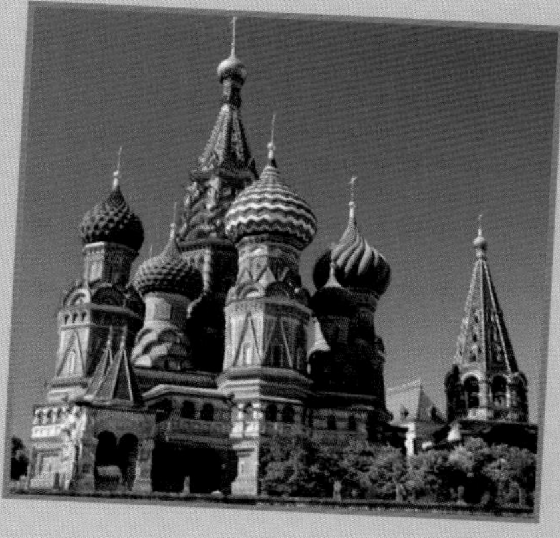

St. Basil's Cathedral was built in 1555 by Ivan the Terrible. It stands next to Red Square in the center of Moscow.

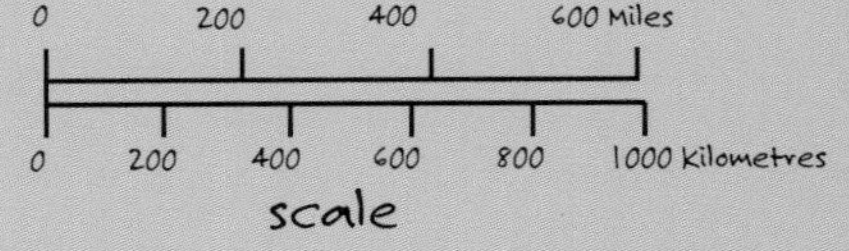

scale

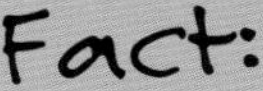

Fact:

Siberia is a vast wilderness. It is one of the world's coldest places. A temperature as low as -95.8°F (-71°C) has been recorded there.

It takes eight days to travel the length of the Trans-Siberian Railway line from Moscow to Vladivostok 5,777 miles (9,297 km.)

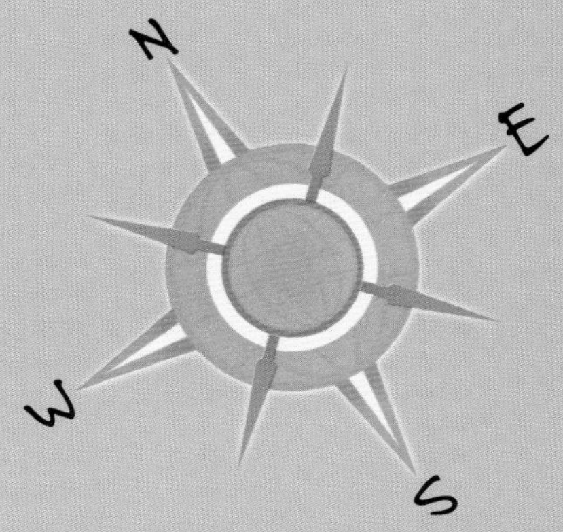

Can you find...

the Royal Tomb at Petra?

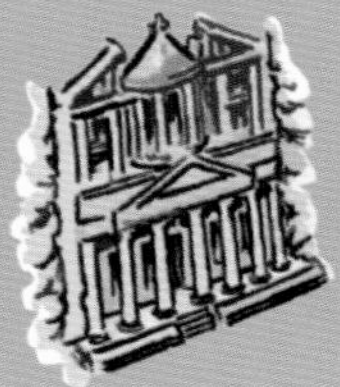

the Suleymaniye Mosque?

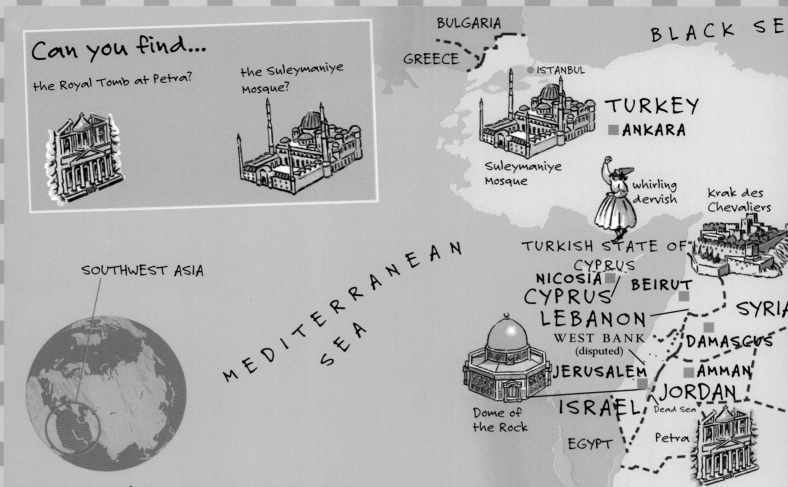

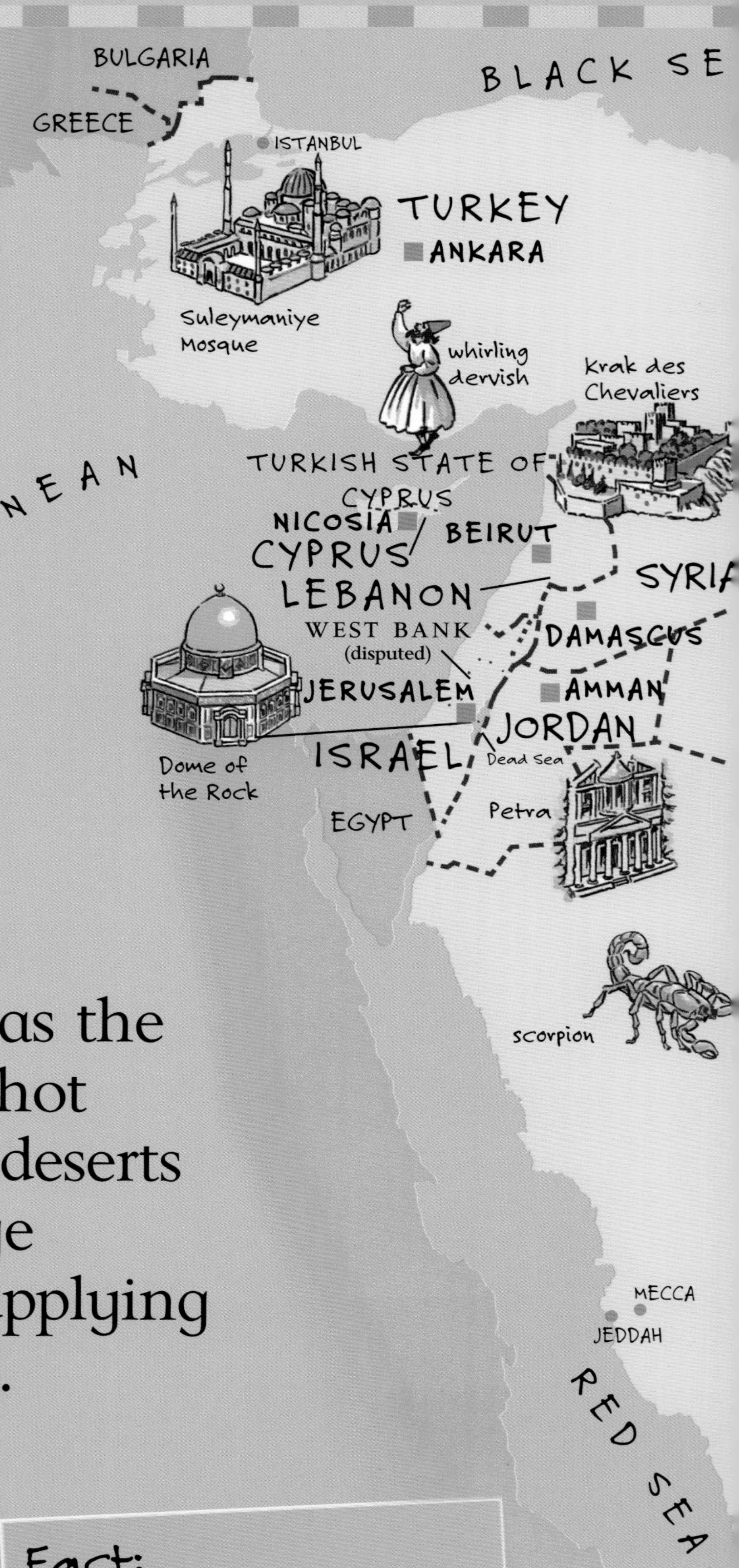

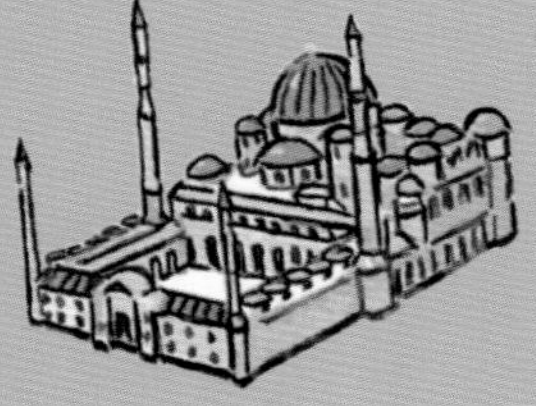

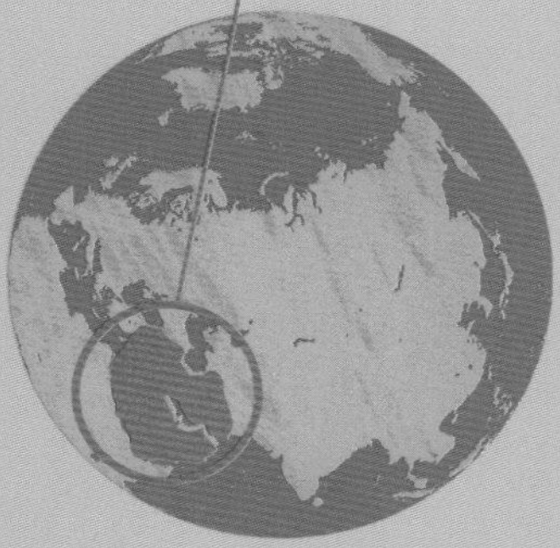

BULGARIA
GREECE
BLACK SEA
ISTANBUL
TURKEY
ANKARA
Suleymaniye Mosque
whirling dervish
Krak des Chevaliers
TURKISH STATE OF CYPRUS
NICOSIA
CYPRUS
BEIRUT
SYRIA
LEBANON
WEST BANK (disputed)
DAMASCUS
JERUSALEM
AMMAN
JORDAN
Dome of the Rock
ISRAEL
Dead Sea
EGYPT
Petra
MEDITERRANEAN SEA
SOUTHWEST ASIA

scorpion

MECCA
JEDDAH
RED SEA

Southwest Asia

This area, also known as the Middle East, is mainly hot and dry with vast arid deserts to the south. It is a huge oil-producing region, supplying much of the world's oil.

The Middle East has long been troubled by wars between neighbouring countries. The discovery of large amounts of oil and natural gas around the Persian Gulf has brought great wealth to the region.

Fact:

The Dead Sea lies on the border of Israel and Jordan. Its water is so salty that people can float in it without swimming—it is impossible to sink.

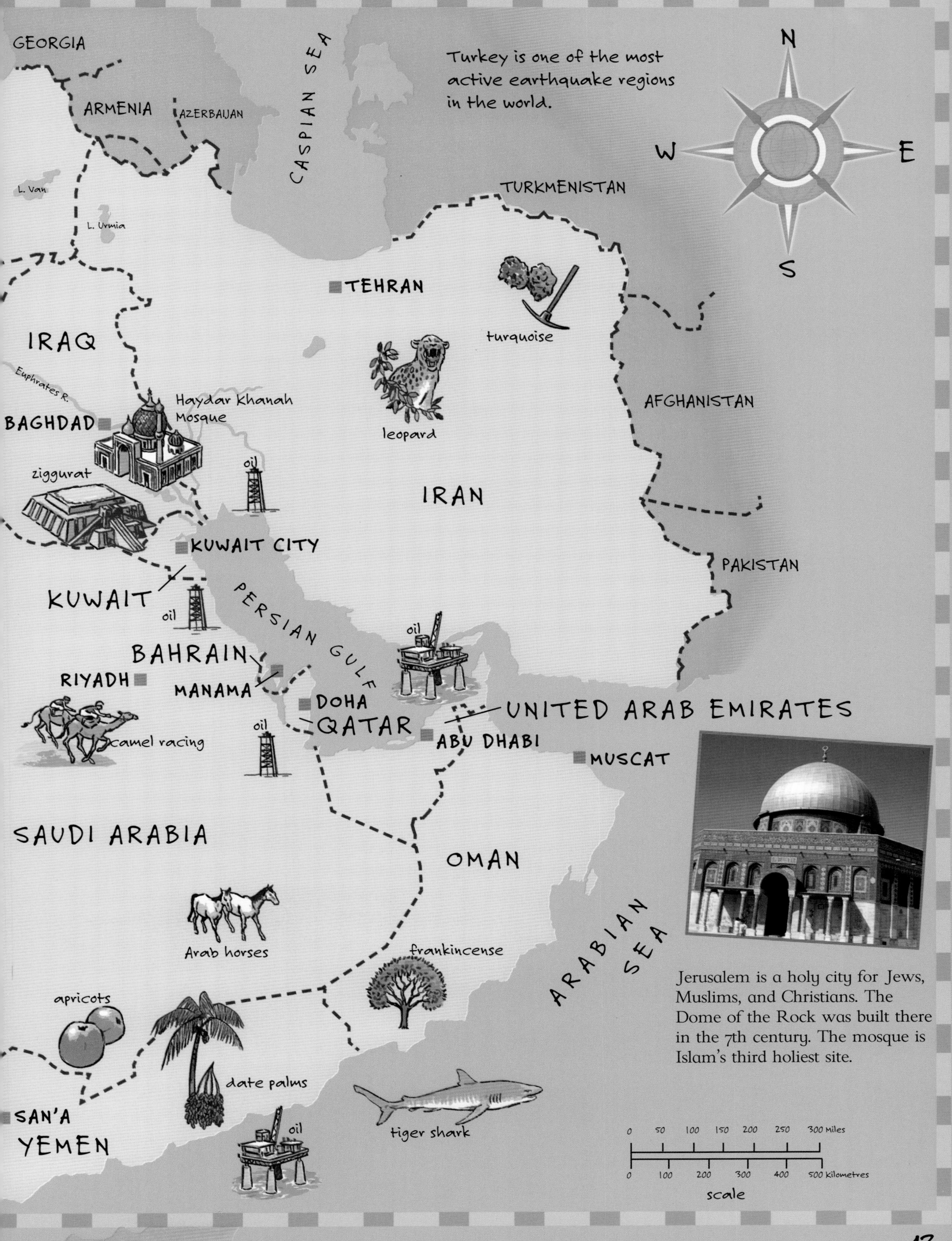

Jerusalem is a holy city for Jews, Muslims, and Christians. The Dome of the Rock was built there in the 7th century. The mosque is Islam's third holiest site.

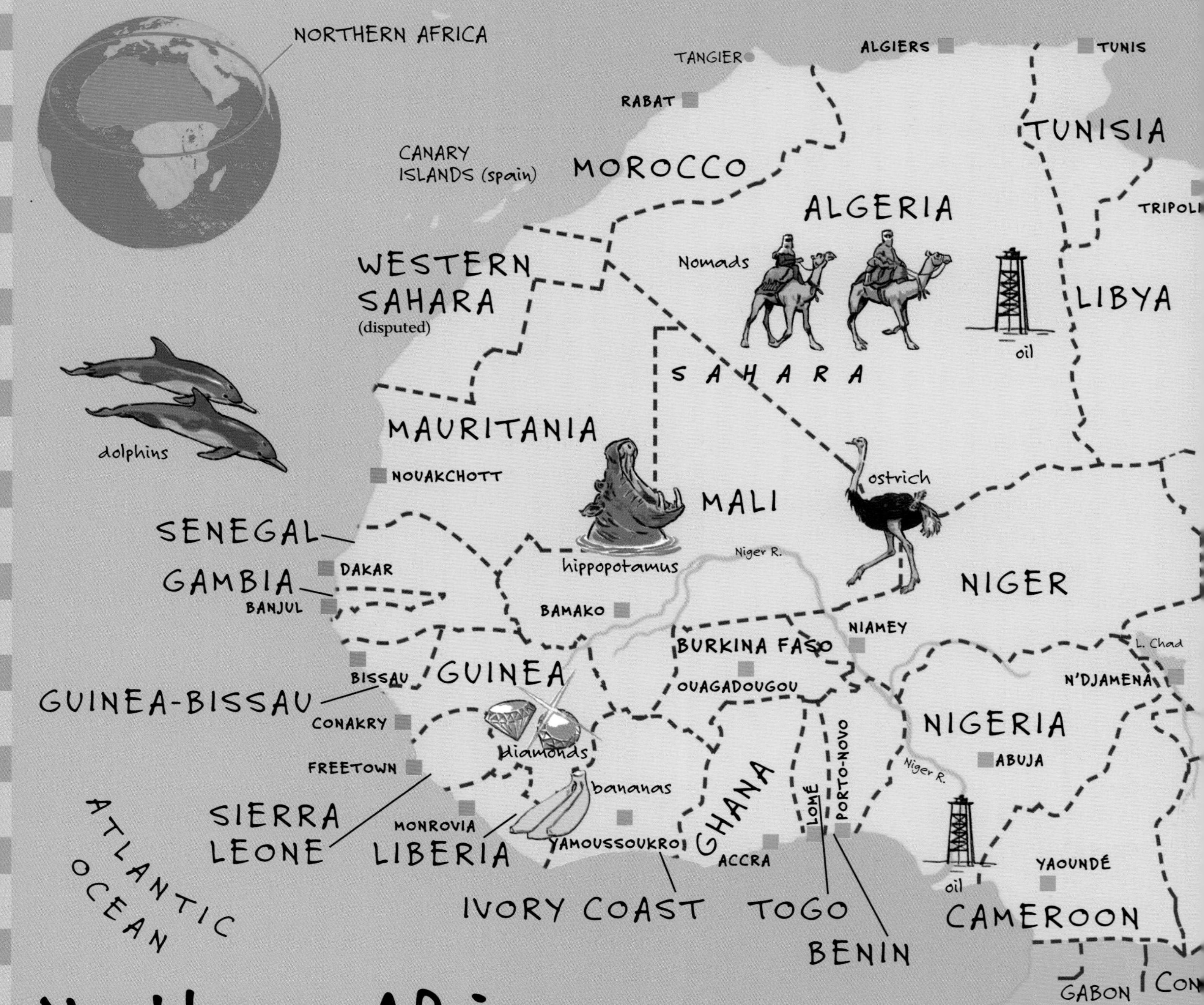

Northern Africa

Much of the huge continent of Africa is hot and dry. The land along the Mediterranean coast and the Nile Valley is rich and fertile. The vast Sahara Desert covers more than half of north Africa.

Facts:

- The Sahara Desert is the largest desert in the world, covering about 5.6 million square miles (9 million sq. km.)
- Nigeria's oil industry makes it one of the richest countries in Africa.

The Nile Valley in Egypt is the most densely populated region. Lagos in Nigeria is Africa's largest city.

The Nile is the longest river in the world, stretching 4,132 miles (6,650 km.) Huge crocodiles live in it.

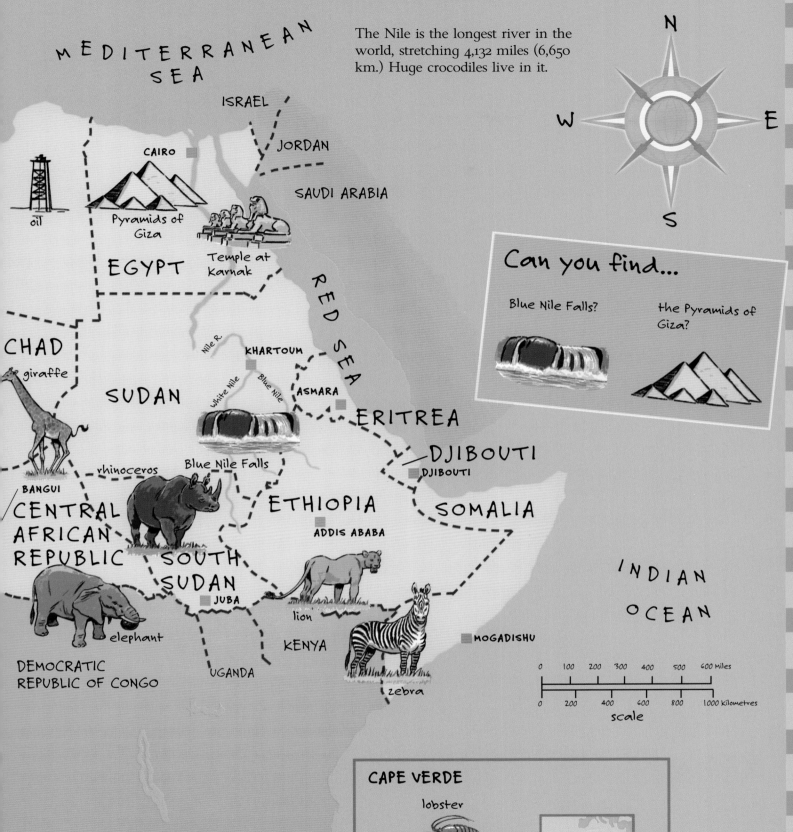

MEDITERRANEAN SEA

N
W
E
S

ISRAEL
JORDAN
CAIRO
oil
Pyramids of Giza
SAUDI ARABIA
Temple at Karnak
EGYPT
RED SEA

Can you find...

Blue Nile Falls?

the Pyramids of Giza?

CHAD
giraffe
Nile R.
KHARTOUM
SUDAN
White Nile
Blue Nile
ASMARA
ERITREA
DJIBOUTI
DJIBOUTI
Blue Nile Falls
rhinoceros
BANGUI
CENTRAL AFRICAN REPUBLIC
ETHIOPIA
SOMALIA
ADDIS ABABA
SOUTH SUDAN
JUBA
INDIAN OCEAN
lion
elephant
KENYA
MOGADISHU
DEMOCRATIC REPUBLIC OF CONGO
UGANDA
zebra

0 100 200 300 400 500 600 Miles
0 200 400 600 800 1000 Kilometres
scale

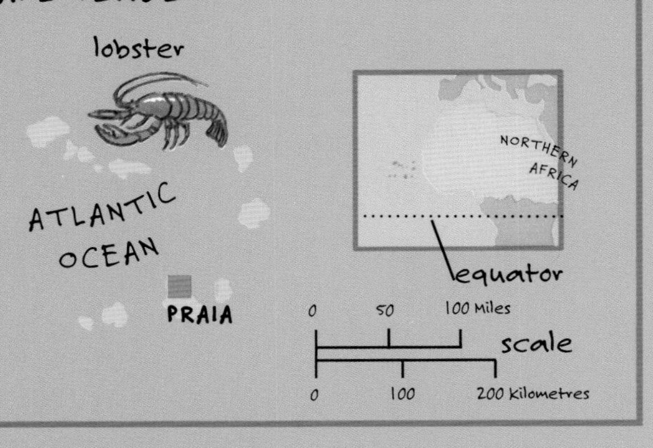

Africa was home to the civilization of ancient Egypt. Tourists visit Egypt's many ancient sites, such as the Great Pyramid, which was built around 2500 BC.

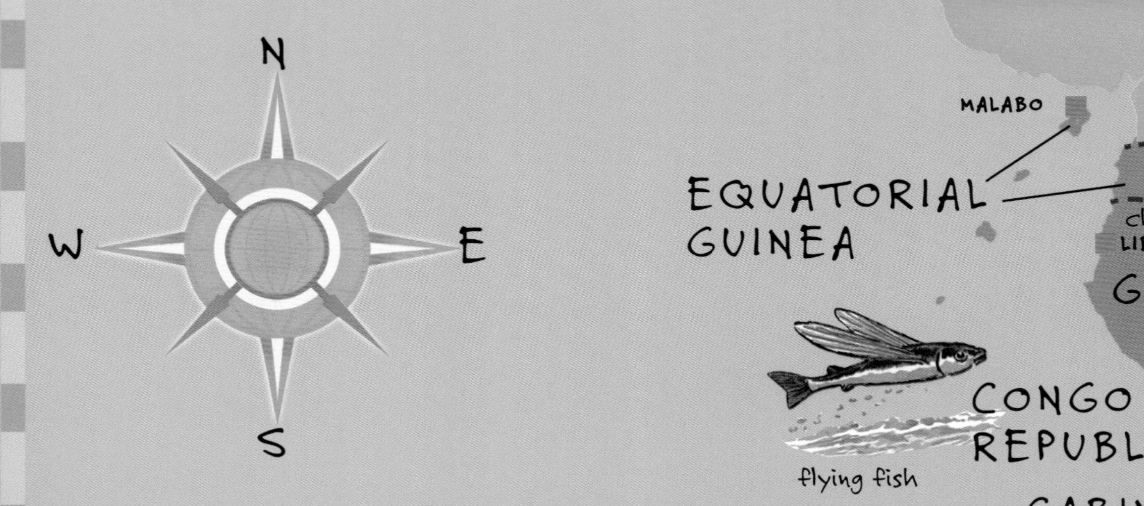

Southern Africa

The mighty Congo River runs through dense, tropical rainforests in Central Africa. Crocodiles, chimpanzees, and gorillas live in these hot, steamy forests. Grasslands and deserts make up much of Southern Africa, but there is rich farmland in the far south.

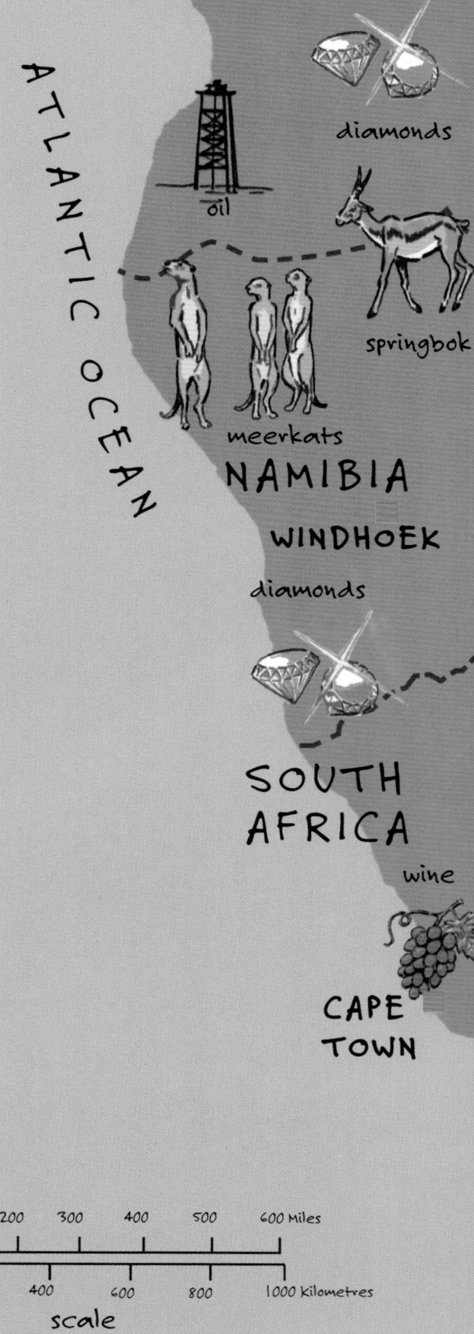

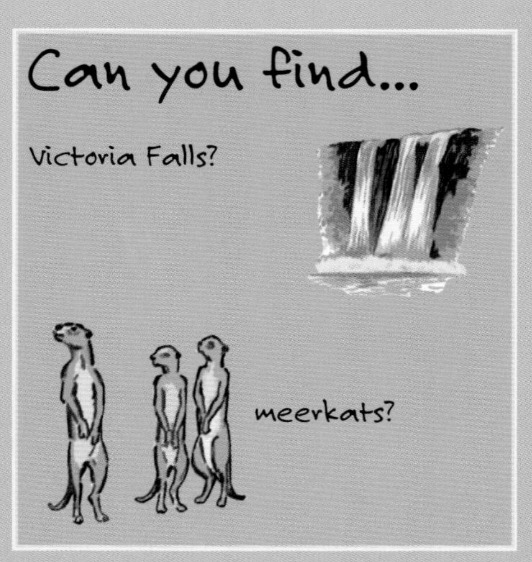

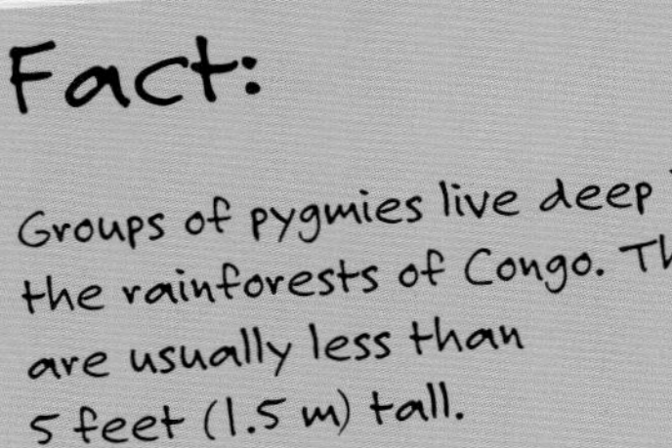

Fact:

Groups of pygmies live deep in the rainforests of Congo. They are usually less than 5 feet (1.5 m) tall.

scale: 0 100 200 300 400 500 600 Miles / 0 200 400 600 800 1000 Kilometres

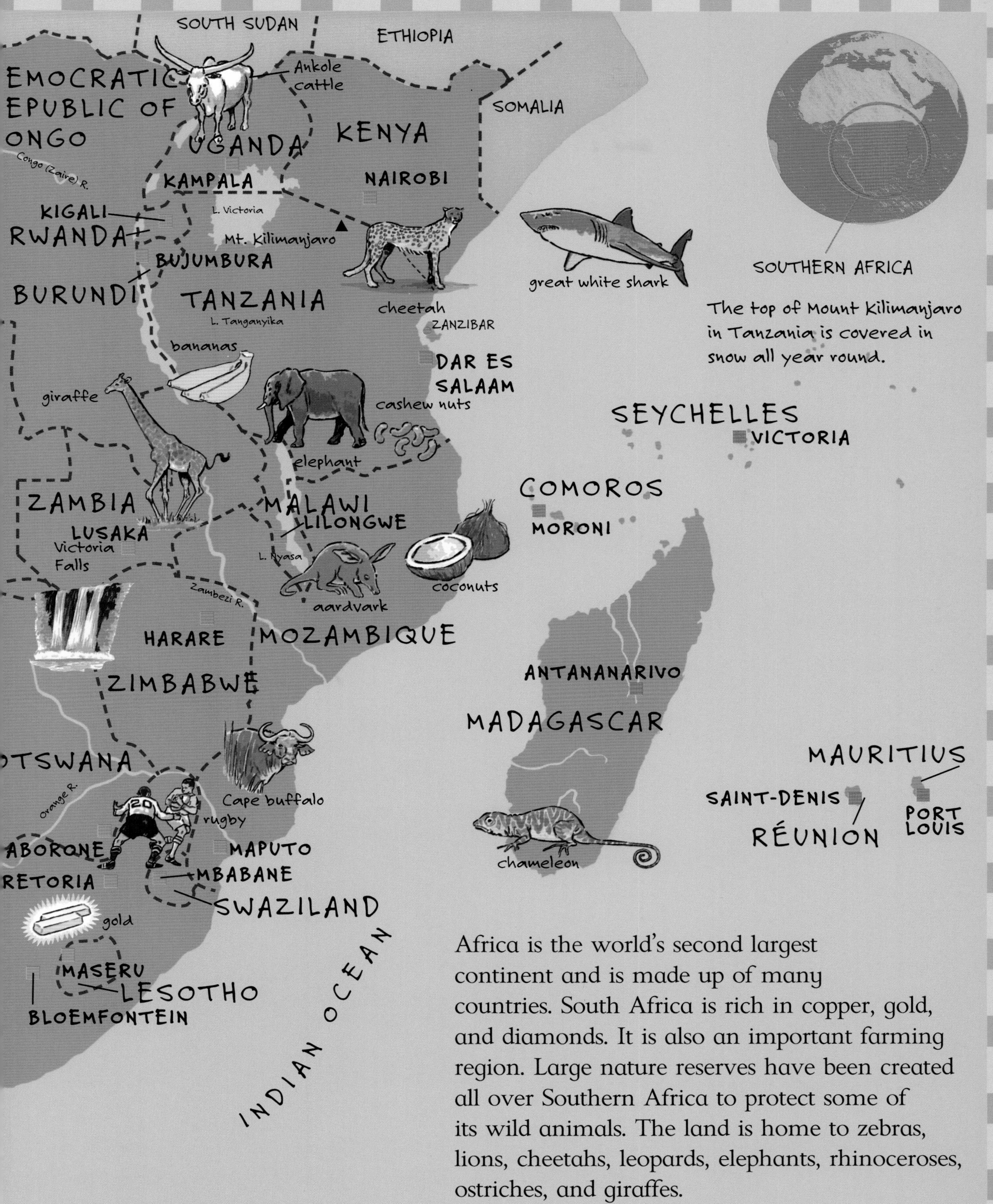

Africa is the world's second largest continent and is made up of many countries. South Africa is rich in copper, gold, and diamonds. It is also an important farming region. Large nature reserves have been created all over Southern Africa to protect some of its wild animals. The land is home to zebras, lions, cheetahs, leopards, elephants, rhinoceroses, ostriches, and giraffes.

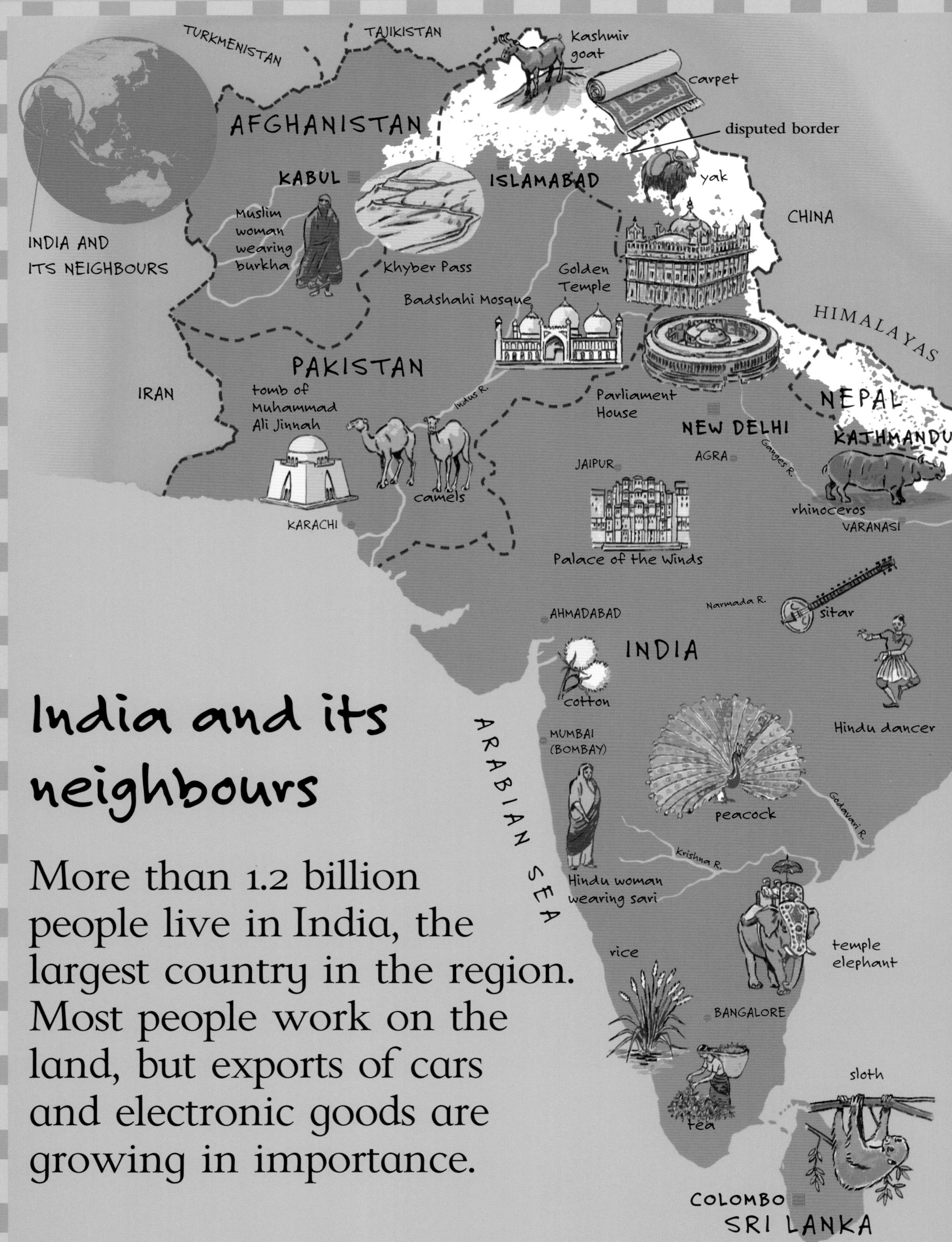

India and its neighbours

More than 1.2 billion people live in India, the largest country in the region. Most people work on the land, but exports of cars and electronic goods are growing in importance.

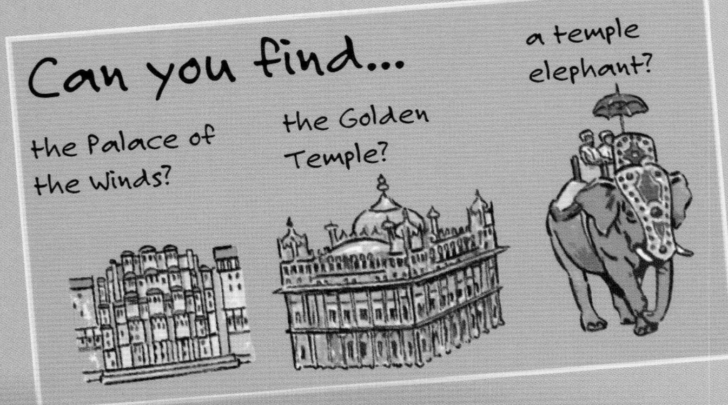
Can you find...
the Palace of the Winds?
the Golden Temple?
a temple elephant?

Vast mountain ranges separate this region from Central Asia. The climate is hot and dry, so many people live on the coast or on the fertile plains along the Ganges and Indus rivers. India, Bangladesh, and Sri Lanka are some of the world's main tea-growing nations. Most industries are concentrated in the large crowded cities of India and Pakistan.

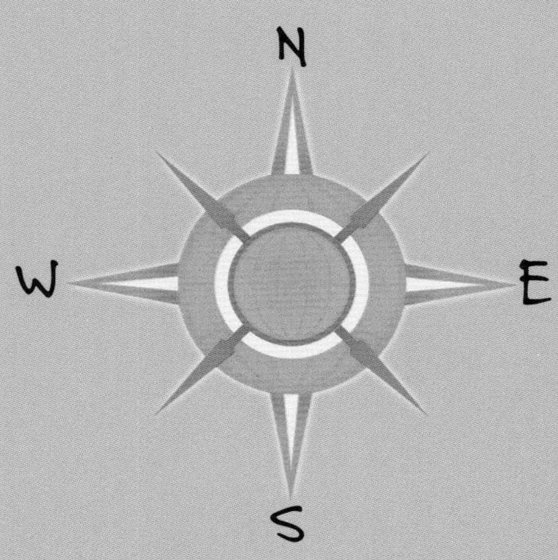

BHUTAN
Mount Everest
THIMPHU
Brahmaputra R.
tea
tea
INDIA
BANGLADESH
Ganges R.
DHAKA
KOLKATTA (CALCUTTA)
CHINA
logging elephant
MYANMAR (BURMA)
LAOS
THAILAND
Irrawaddy R.
Buddhist monk
YANGON (RANGOON)
BAY OF BENGAL
INDIAN OCEAN
rubber trees
ANDAMAN AND NICOBAR ISLANDS

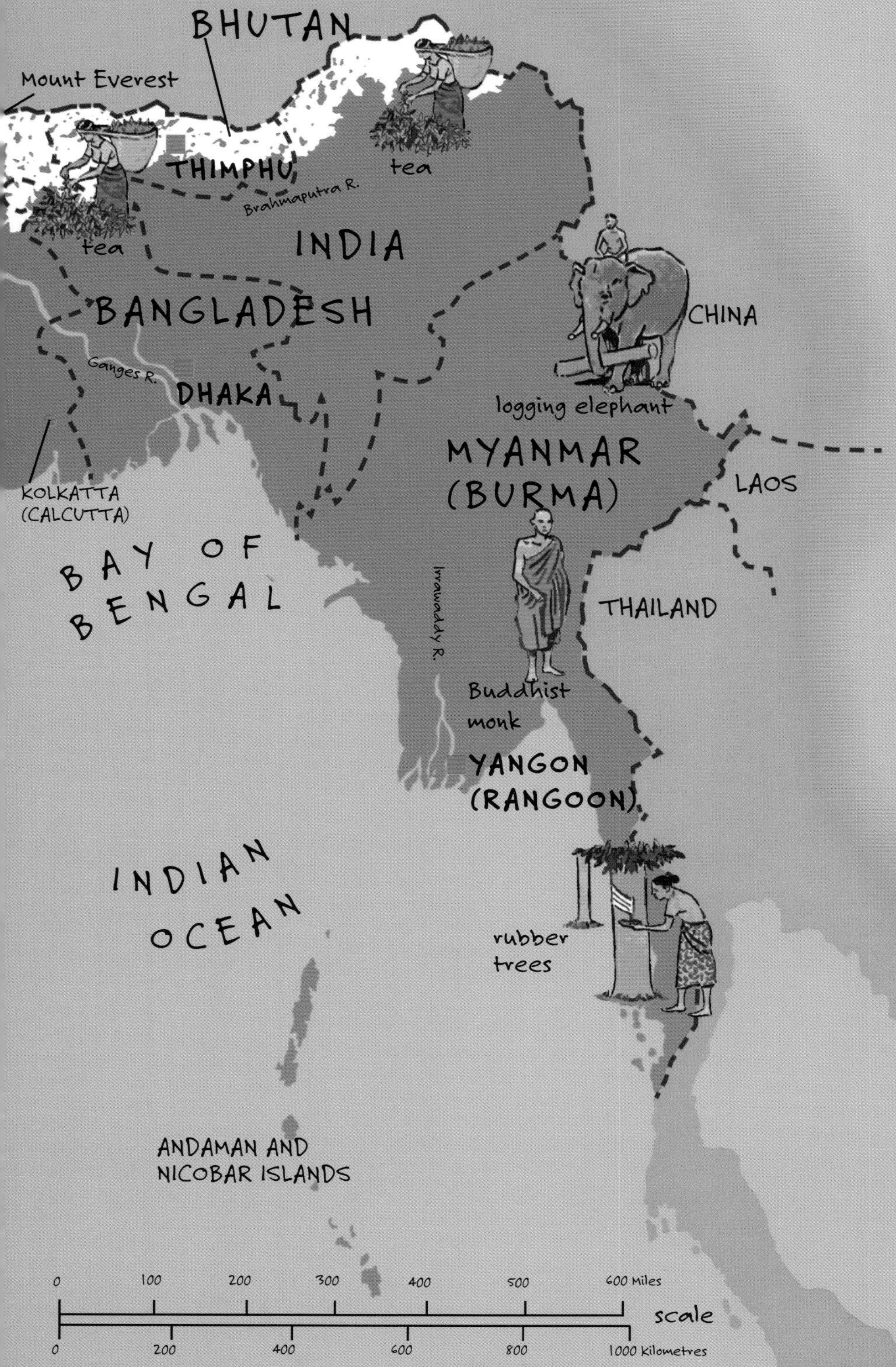

Mount Everest, in the Himalayas, is the tallest mountain above sea level. It is 29,028 feet (8,848 m) tall.

Fact:

Indian cobras are poisonous snakes. They can grow up to 18 feet (5.5 m) long.

scale
0 100 200 300 400 500 600 Miles
0 200 400 600 800 1000 Kilometres

Fact:

Sushi is a dish made of balls of cold rice served with vegetables and raw fish.

About 38 million people live in and around Tokyo, Japan's capital city.

Japan

Japan is made up of four large islands and thousands of smaller ones. It lies off the east coast of China. Japan's cities are built along its flat coastland because mountains and forests cover much of the country inland.

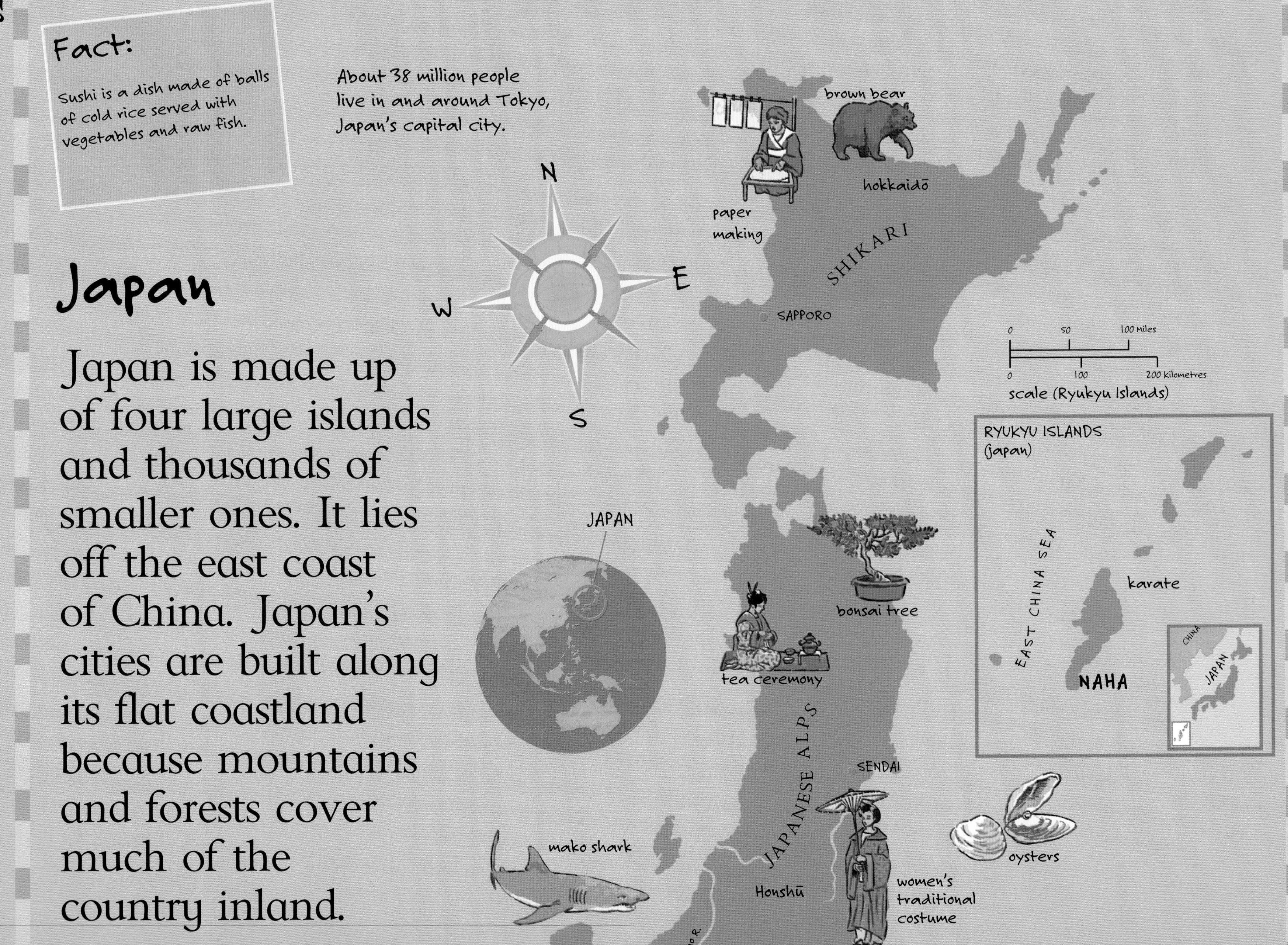

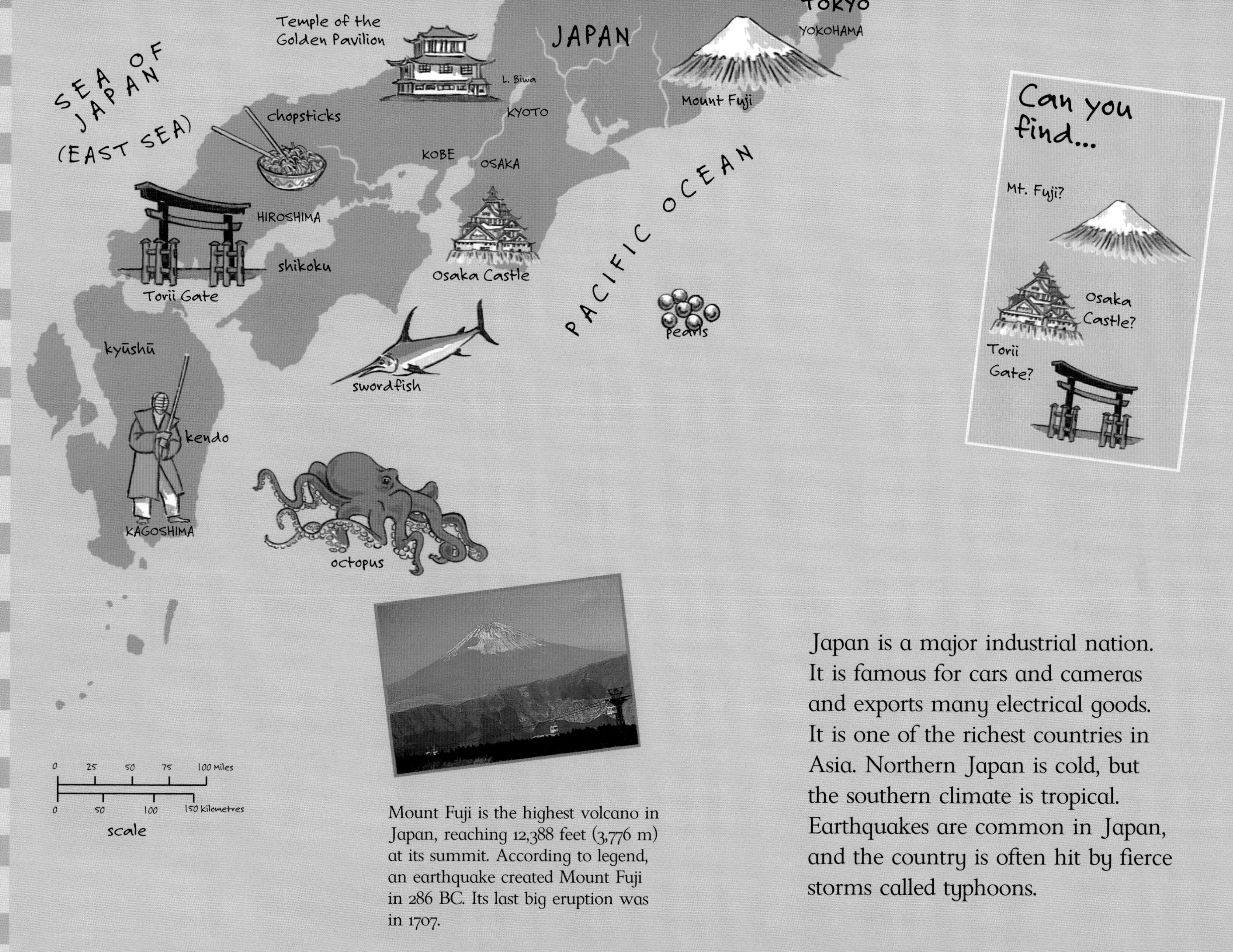

Mount Fuji is the highest volcano in Japan, reaching 12,388 feet (3,776 m) at its summit. According to legend, an earthquake created Mount Fuji in 286 BC. Its last big eruption was in 1707.

Japan is a major industrial nation. It is famous for cars and cameras and exports many electrical goods. It is one of the richest countries in Asia. Northern Japan is cold, but the southern climate is tropical. Earthquakes are common in Japan, and the country is often hit by fierce storms called typhoons.

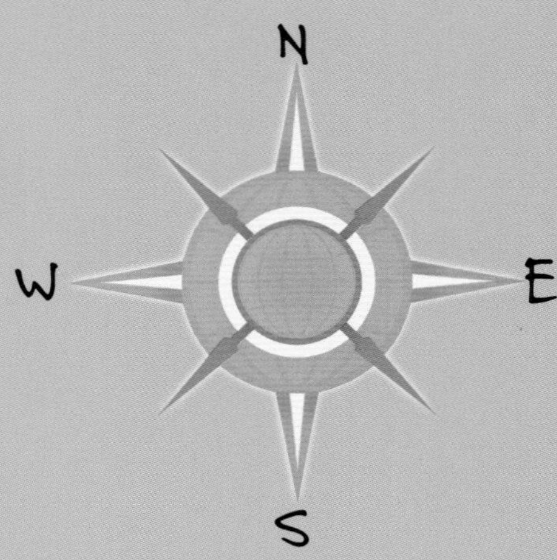

Southeast Asia

Southeast Asia is made up of two small areas of mainland and almost 20,000 islands. The climate is hot and humid. Tropical rainforests cover much of this mountainous region and provide the world with most of its hardwoods.

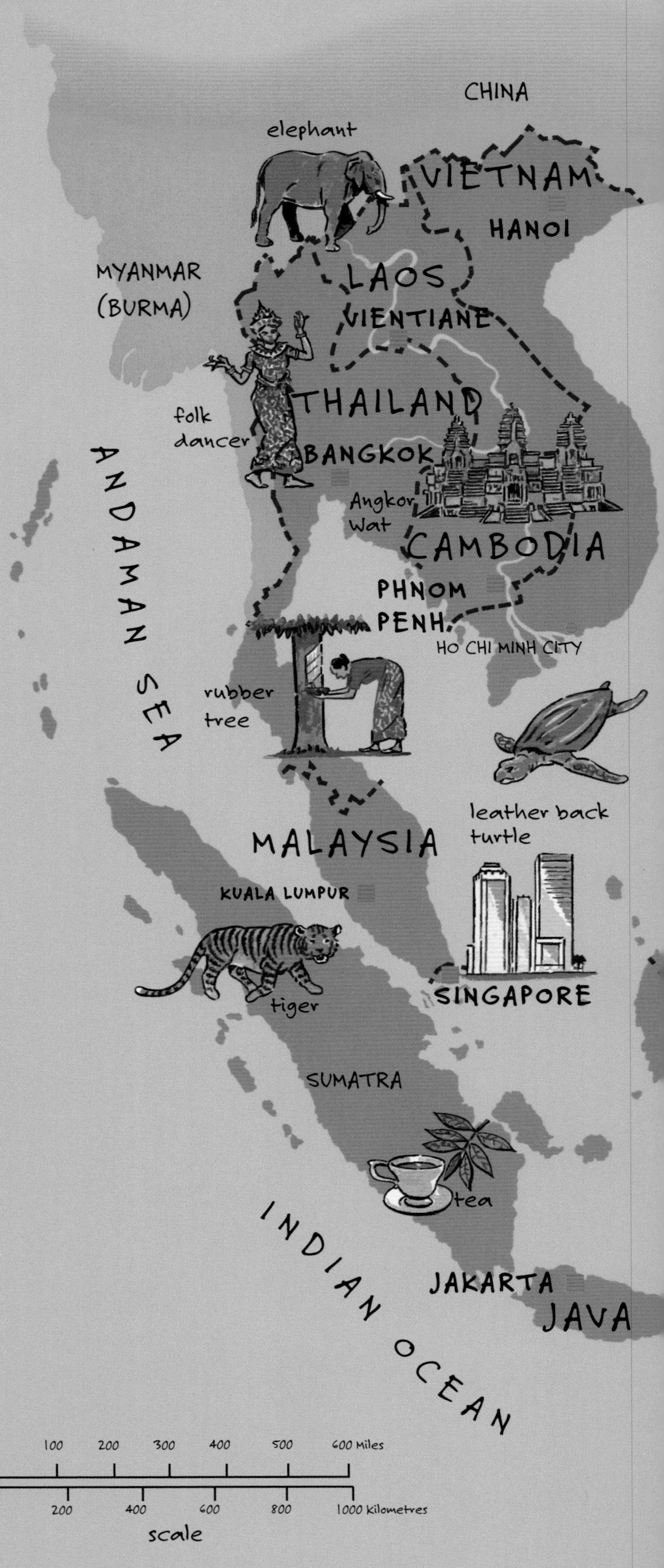

CHINA
elephant
VIETNAM
HANOI
MYANMAR (BURMA)
LAOS
VIENTIANE
THAILAND
folk dancer
BANGKOK
Angkor Wat
CAMBODIA
ANDAMAN SEA
PHNOM PENH
HO CHI MINH CITY
rubber tree
leather back turtle
MALAYSIA
KUALA LUMPUR
tiger
SINGAPORE
SUMATRA
tea
INDIAN OCEAN
JAKARTA
JAVA

0 100 200 300 400 500 600 Miles
0 200 400 600 800 1000 Kilometres
scale

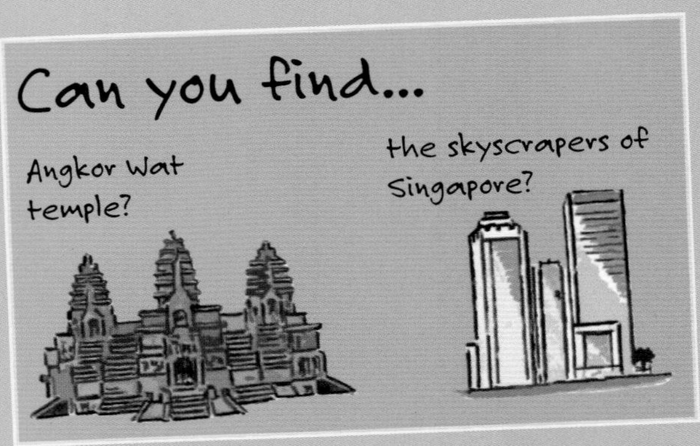
Can you find...
Angkor Wat temple?
the skyscrapers of Singapore?

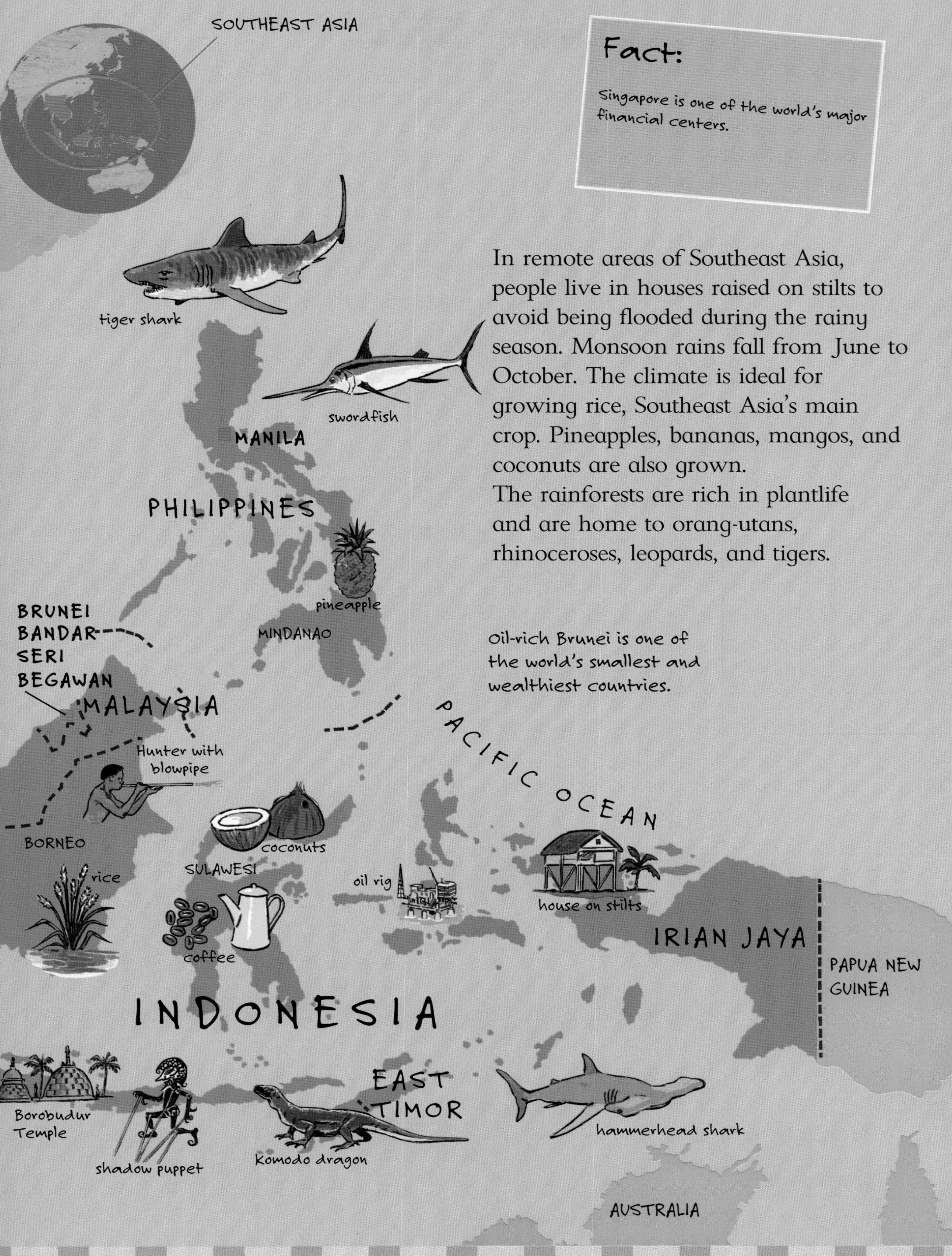

In remote areas of Southeast Asia, people live in houses raised on stilts to avoid being flooded during the rainy season. Monsoon rains fall from June to October. The climate is ideal for growing rice, Southeast Asia's main crop. Pineapples, bananas, mangos, and coconuts are also grown.
The rainforests are rich in plantlife and are home to orang-utans, rhinoceroses, leopards, and tigers.

China, Mongolia, Korea, and Taiwan

CHINA, MONGOLIA, KOREA, AND TAIWAN

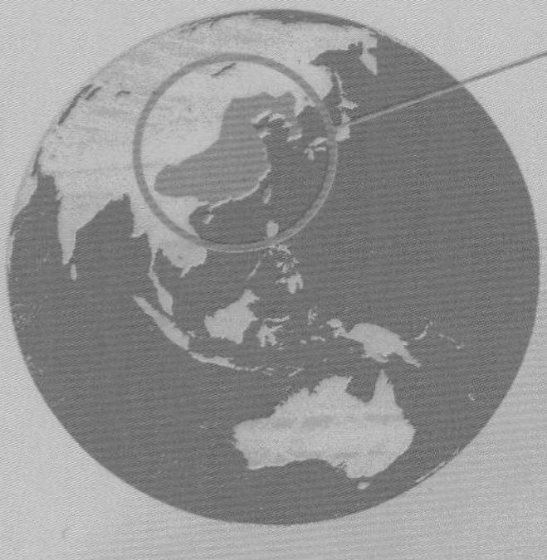

More people live in China than in any other country. Most of the population farm the fertile land in the east, growing rice, wheat, maize, and tea. China is also an industrial nation and has many large cities.

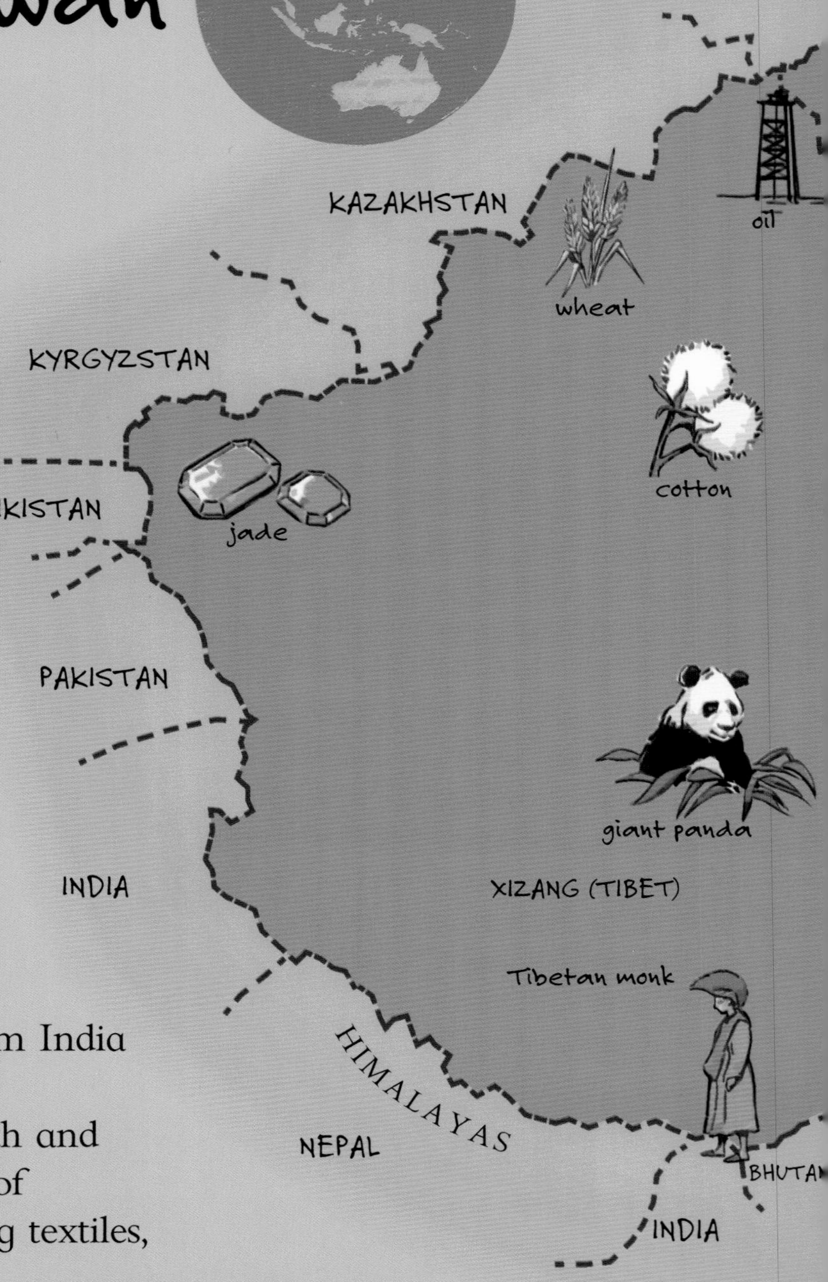

KAZAKHSTAN
oil
wheat
KYRGYZSTAN
cotton
TAJIKISTAN
jade
PAKISTAN
giant panda
INDIA
XIZANG (TIBET)
Tibetan monk
HIMALAYAS
NEPAL
BHUTAN
INDIA

High mountain ranges separate China from India and there are vast deserts to the north. The Korean peninsula is divided into North and South Korea. South Korea and the island of Taiwan have successful industries including textiles, cars, and electrical goods.

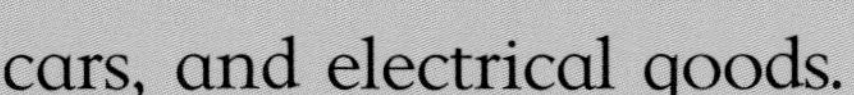

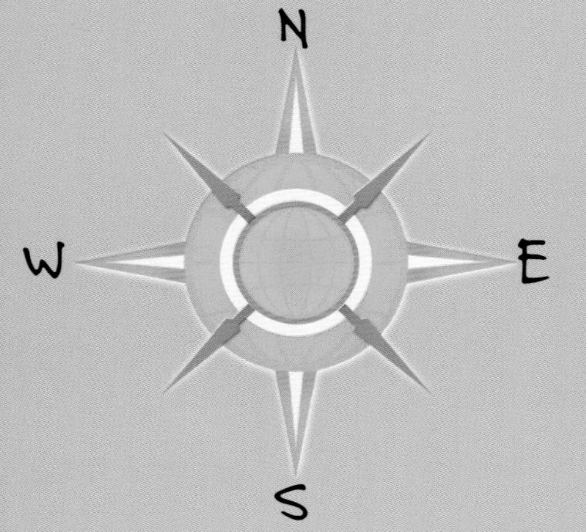

The Great Wall of China is 2,145 miles (3,460 km) long. But it's not true that you can see it from the Moon.

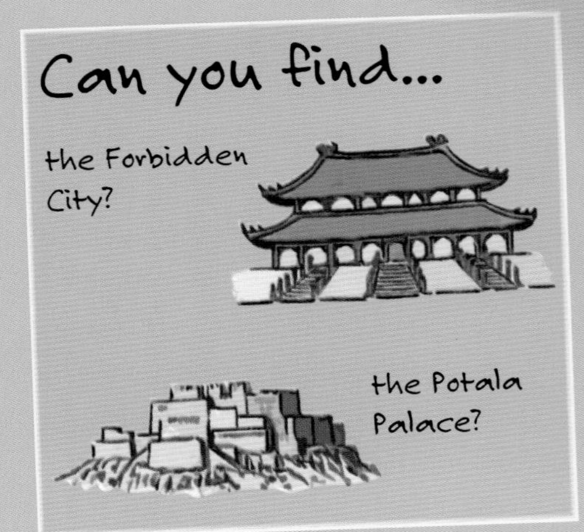

Can you find...
the Forbidden City?
the Potala Palace?

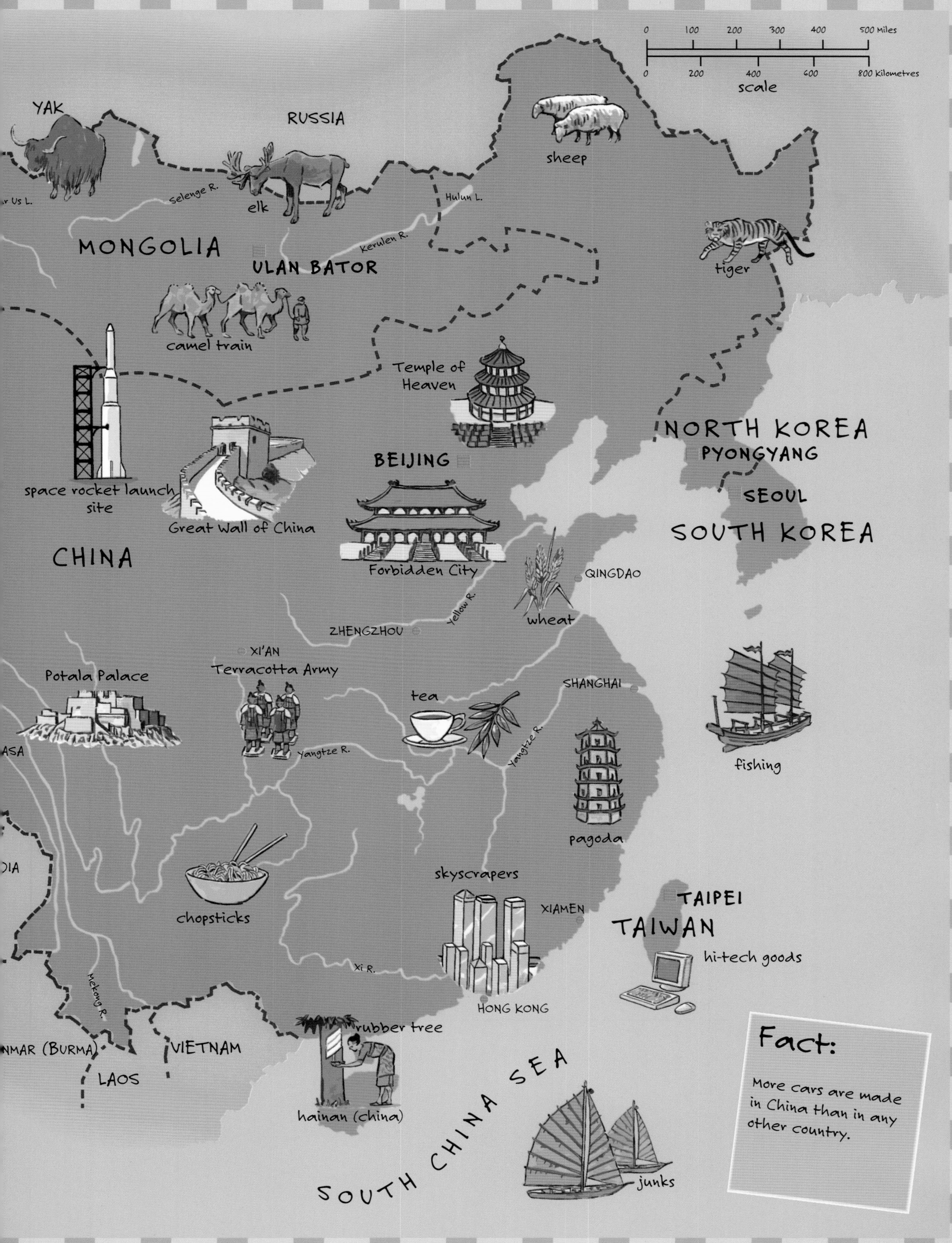
0 100 200 300 400 500 Miles
0 200 400 600 800 Kilometres
scale
YAK
RUSSIA
sheep
Selenge R.
elk
Hulun L.
MONGOLIA
ULAN BATOR
Kerulen R.
tiger
camel train
Temple of Heaven
NORTH KOREA
PYONGYANG
BEIJING
space rocket launch site
SEOUL
SOUTH KOREA
Great Wall of China
CHINA
Forbidden City
QINGDAO
Yellow R.
wheat
ZHENGZHOU
XI'AN
Terracotta Army
Potala Palace
SHANGHAI
tea
Yangtze R.
Yangtze R.
fishing
pagoda
chopsticks
skyscrapers
TAIPEI
XIAMEN
TAIWAN
hi-tech goods
Xi R.
Mekong R.
HONG KONG
rubber tree
VIETNAM
LAOS
hainan (china)
SOUTH CHINA SEA
junks
Fact:
More cars are made in China than in any other country.

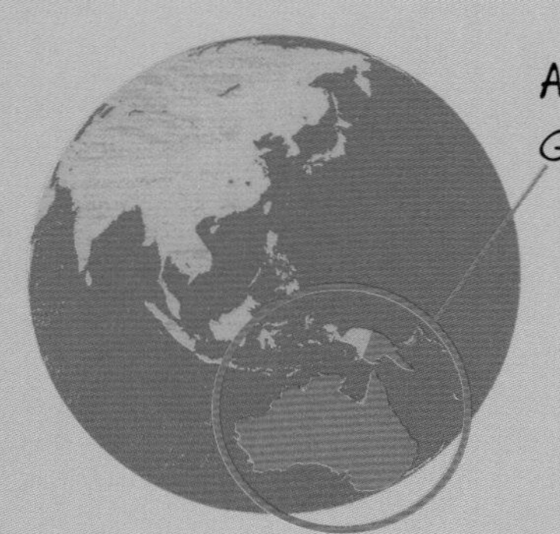
AUSTRALIA AND PAPUA NEW GUINEA

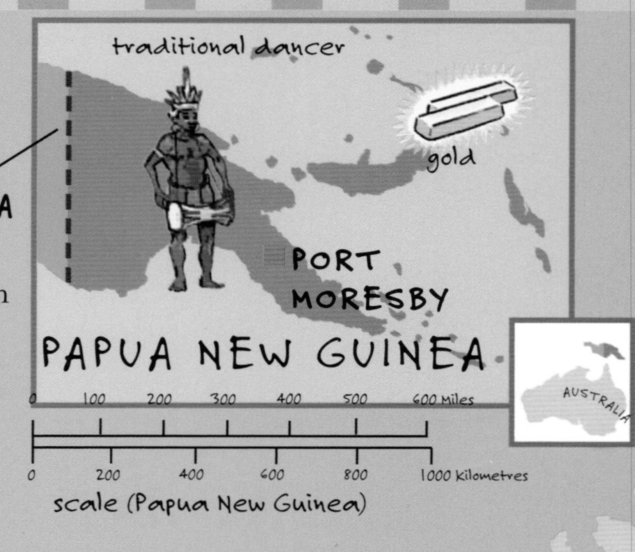

Papua New Guinea has over 700 languages—more than any other country.

Australia and Papua New Guinea

Australia is the world's smallest continent. It is a wealthy country with a small population. It is hot and dry inland, so most people live in large coastal cities. Much of Australia's wealth comes from farming, mining, and tourism.

Central Australia is called the 'outback.' It is mainly deserts and grasslands.
Few people live there, but vast numbers of sheep and cattle graze on stations (large farms.) Australia produces more wool than any other country. It also has large deposits of opals, diamonds, gold, and silver.

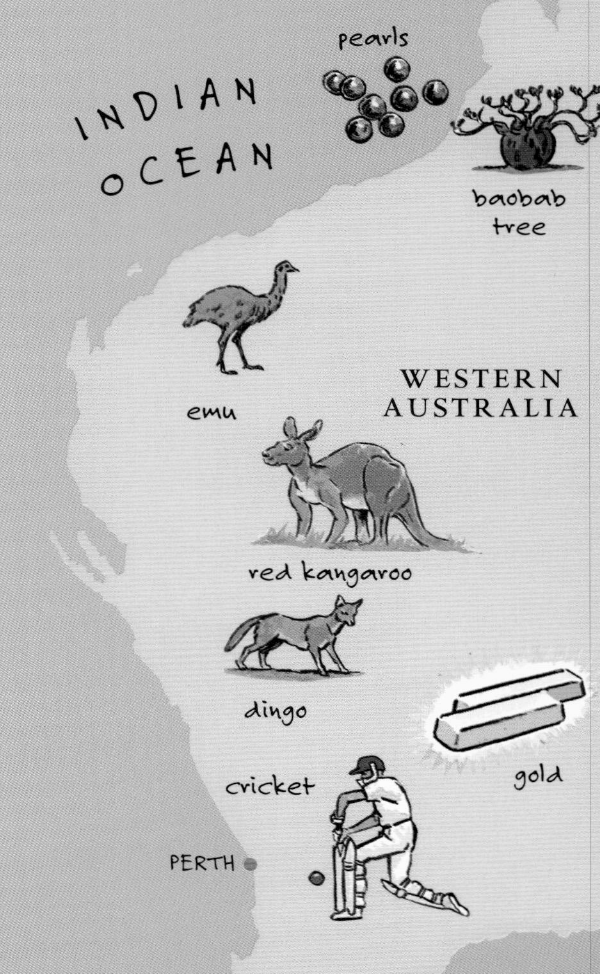

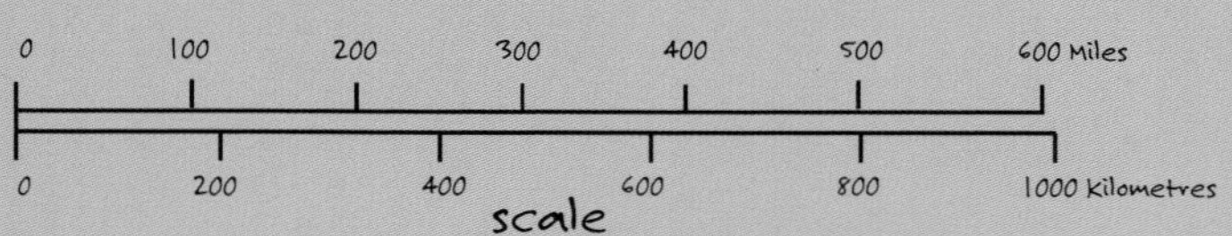

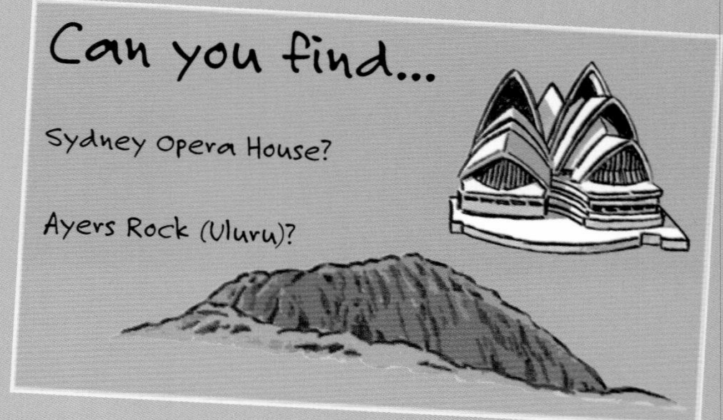
Can you find...
Sydney Opera House?
Ayers Rock (Uluru)?

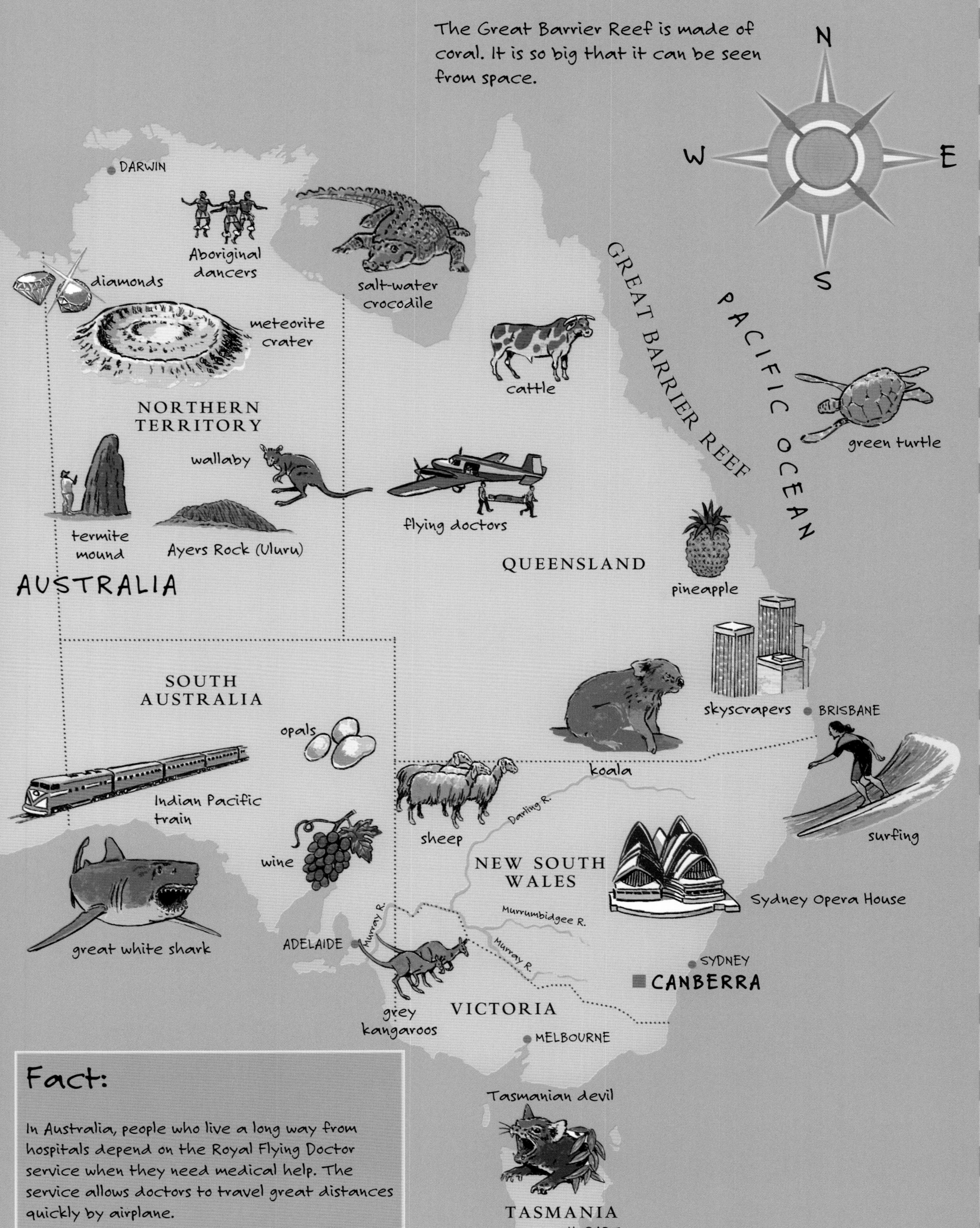

Fact:

In Australia, people who live a long way from hospitals depend on the Royal Flying Doctor service when they need medical help. The service allows doctors to travel great distances quickly by airplane.

New Zealand

New Zealand is divided into two islands. Most people live on the volcanic North Island. It has large cattle and sheep ranches and exports lamb and dairy products.

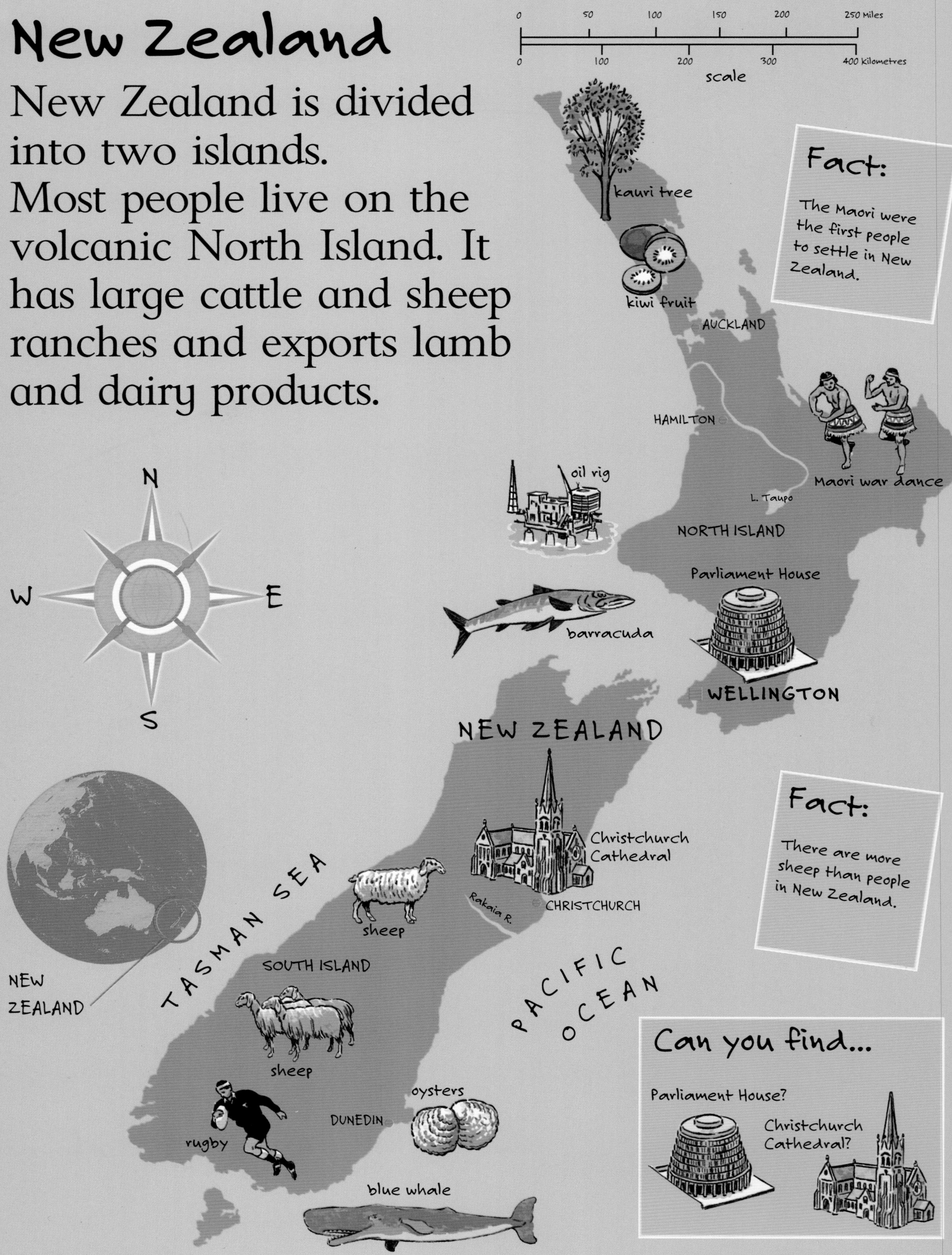

Southwestern Pacific Islands

Thousands of small tropical islands are scattered across the Pacific Ocean east of Australia. Most islanders live in small villages. They fish and grow tropical fruit, including bananas and coconuts.

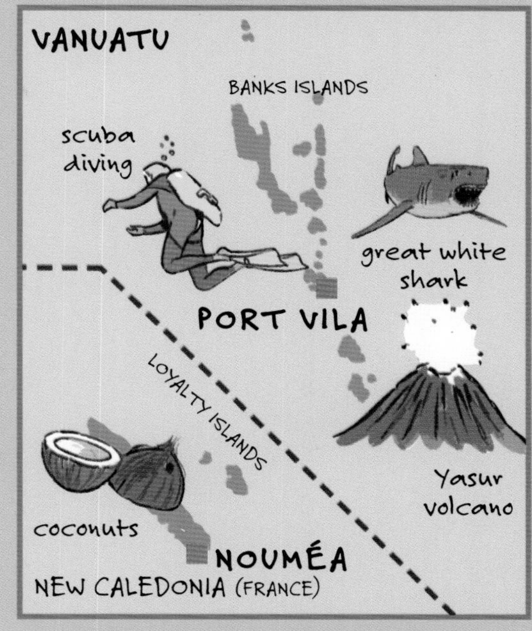

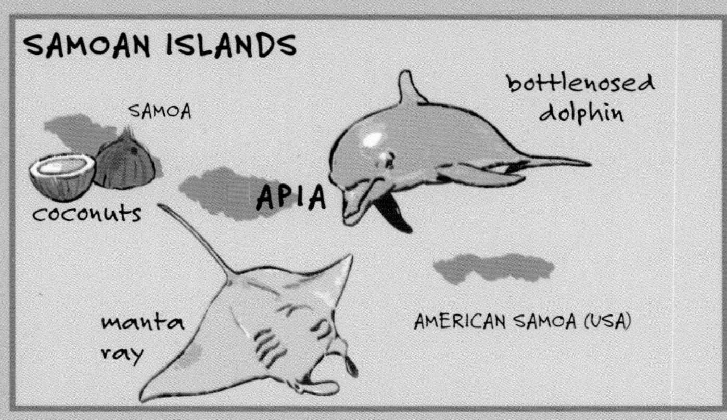

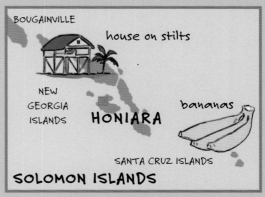

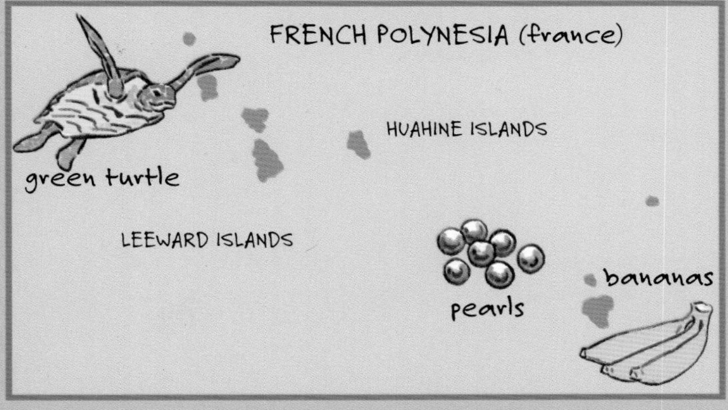

Fact:

The people of Bougainville in the Solomon Islands have discovered how to use coconut oil as a fuel for cars.

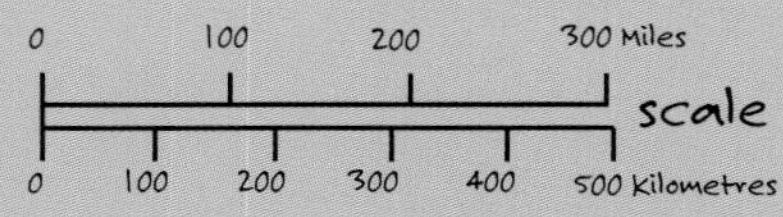

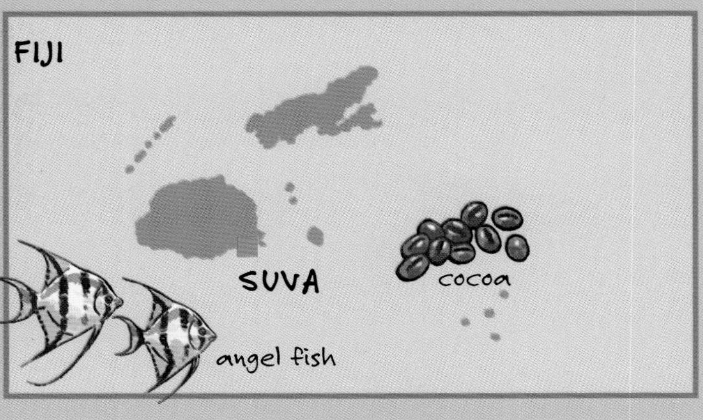

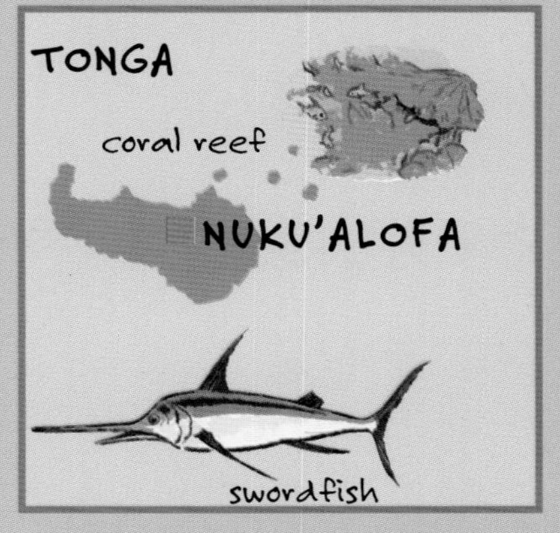

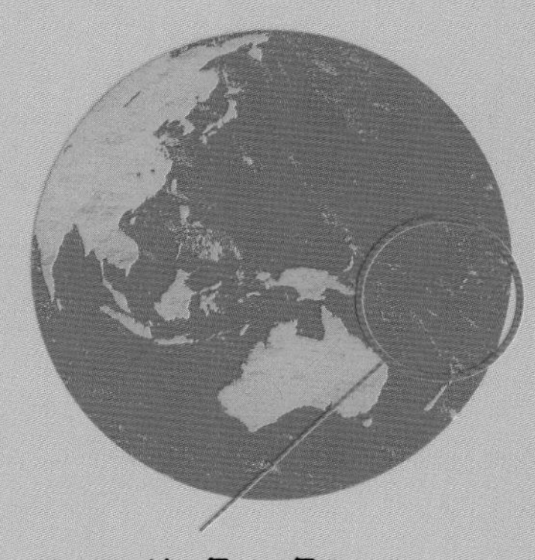

SOUTHWESTERN PACIFIC ISLANDS

The Arctic

The Arctic Ocean is covered in thick ice at the North Pole. The Inuit and Sami are the only people who live in this harsh environment, but many animals and plants survive there.

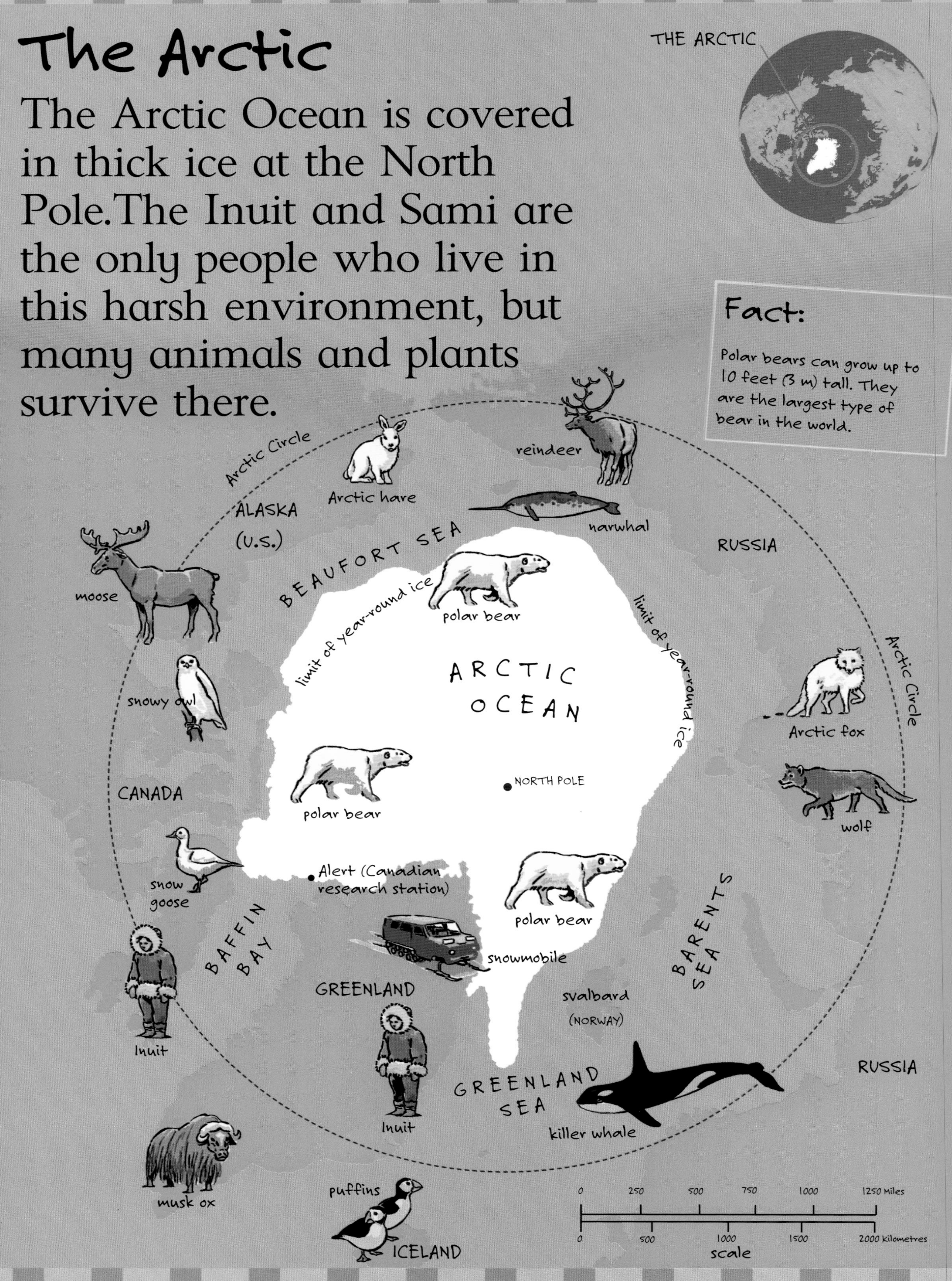

The Antarctic

The South Pole in the Antarctic is the coldest place on Earth. No country owns this frozen continent, but many have set up scientific research stations there.

Facts:

- The world's coldest temperature, -128.6°F (-89.2°C) was recorded at Vostok research station in July 1983.
- The sun does not appear at the Poles during the winter.

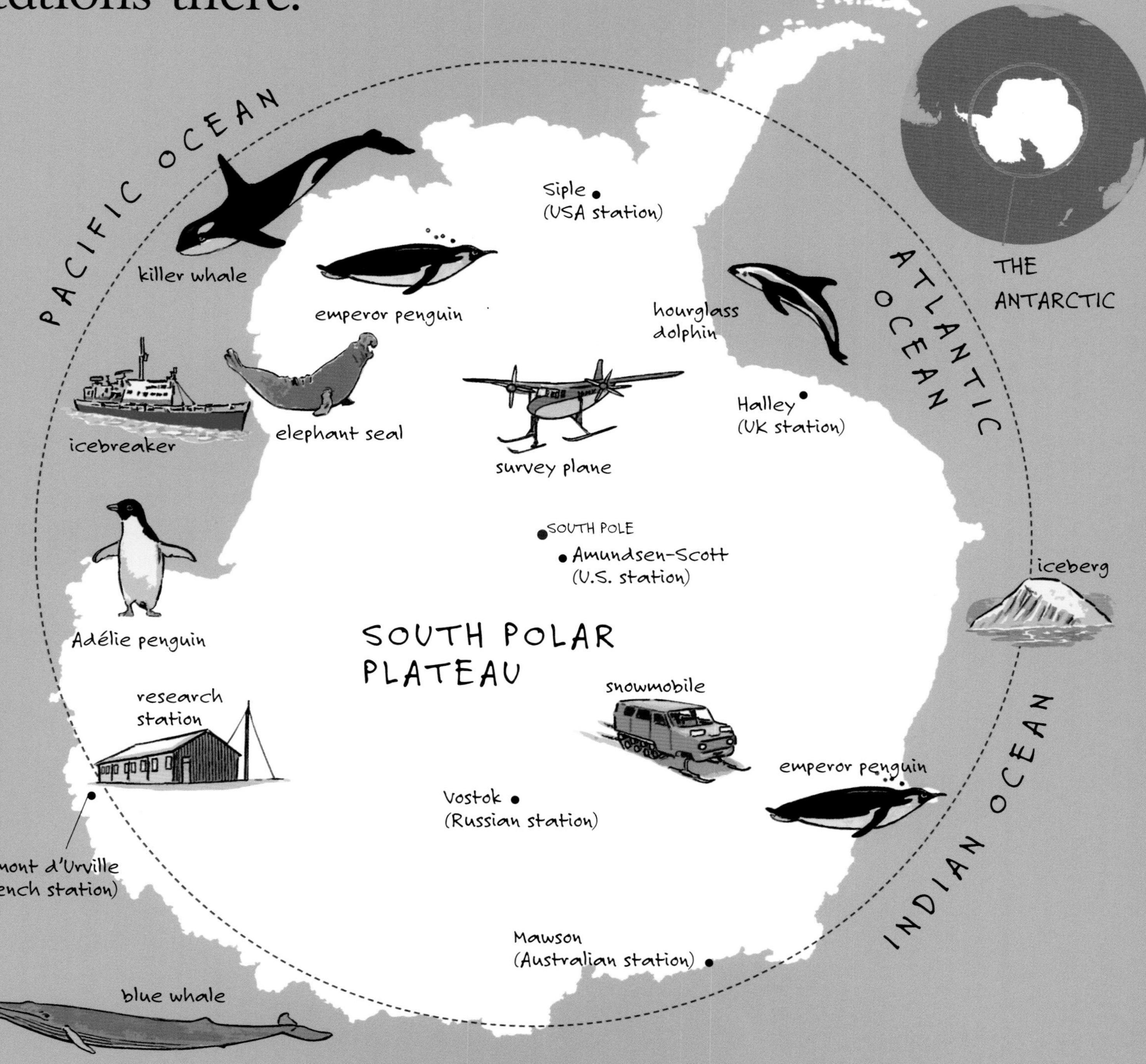

Glossary

climate The average weather of a region.

continent One of the large masses of land on the Earth's surface.

desert An area that has very little or no rainfall.

equator The imaginary line around the center of the Earth. The areas around the equator are the parts of the planet closest to the Sun.

export Something that is sent from one country to be sold in another.

fertile (of soil) Able to grow plenty of crops.

humid Warm and damp.

hurricane A storm with very strong winds.

independence A country ruled by another country gains independence when it begins ruling itself.

latitude Imaginary lines that run horizontally around the Earth.

longitude Imaginary lines that run vertically around the Earth.

magma Molten rock beneath the Earth's crust.

map projection The process of forming a flat atlas map by "stretching" a globe.

monsoon A strong South-Asian wind that usually also brings heavy rain.

northern hemisphere The northern half of the Earth above the equator.

peninsula A narrow area of land that sticks out far into the sea.

permanent Likely to last a very long time.

population The people who live in a place or country.

southern hemisphere The southern half of the Earth below the equator.

summit The highest point of a mountain.

tropical Having a very warm and humid climate, as found in the areas around the equator.

volcanic Formed by a volcano.

Index

Editors: Karen Barker Smith, Stephanie Cole

Picture Research: Nicola Roe

Consultant: Penny Clarke

Photographic credits
Digital Stock/Corbis Corporation: 20, 25, 32, 35, 37, 41
John Foxx Images: 29, 31, 43, 45
Pictor International: 10, 17, 26, 51
Salariya Book Company: 15

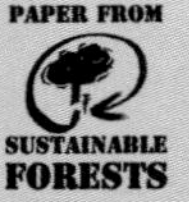

Published in Great Britain in MMXVI by
Book House, an imprint of
The Salariya Book Company Ltd
25 Marlborough Place, Brighton BN1 1UB
www.salariya.com
www.book-house.co.uk

ISBN: 978-1-910706-85-5

SALARIYA

1 3 5 7 9 8 6 4 2

A CIP catalogue record for this book is available from the British Library.

Printed and bound in Malaysia.